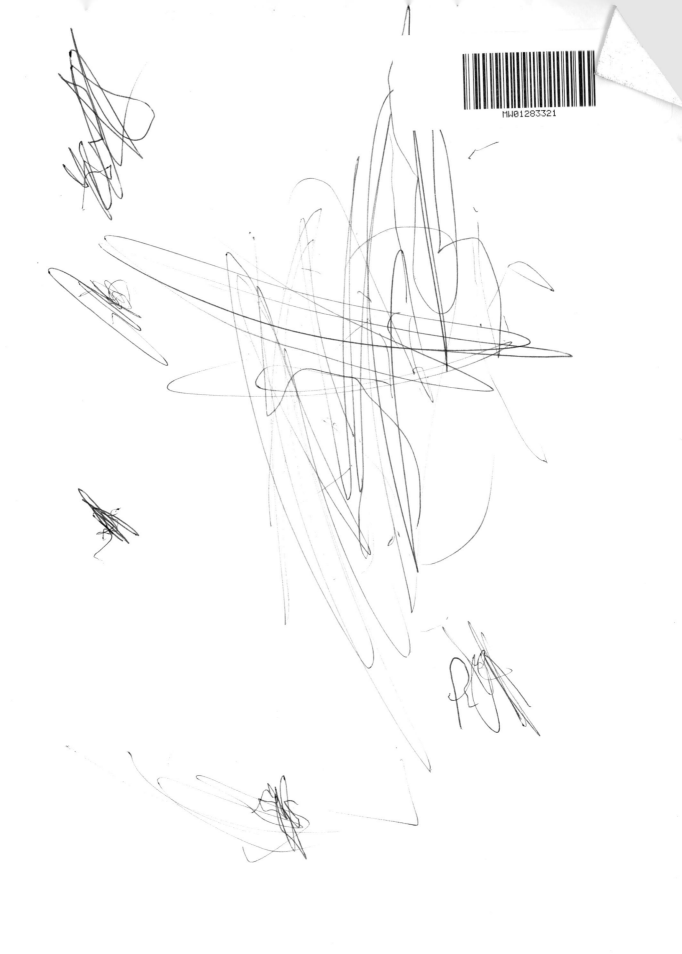

MW01283321

MILADY

STANDARD

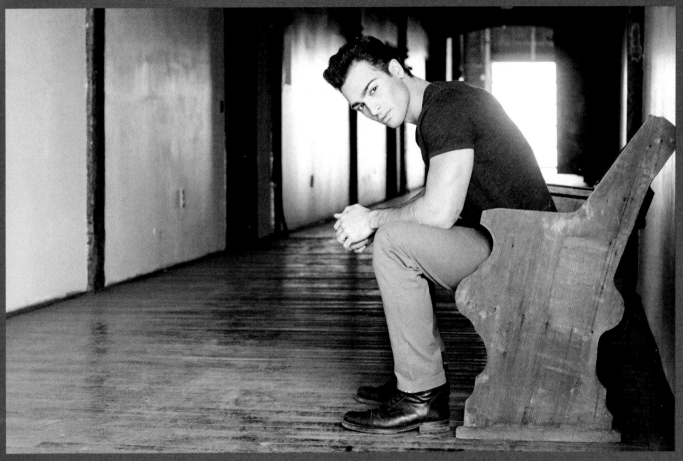

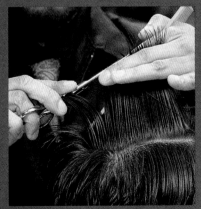
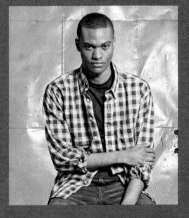
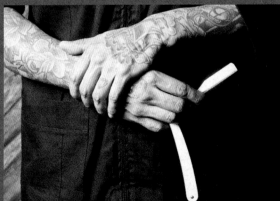

Barbering

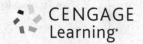
CENGAGE
Learning®

Milady Standard Barbering, Sixth Edition
Main Author: Maura Scali-Sheahan
Contributing Authors: Leslie Roste,
  Linnea Linquest, Amy Burness,
  Dennis "Denny Moe" Mitchell

Executive Director, Milady: Sandra Bruce

Product Director: Corina Santoro

Associate Content Developer: Sarah Prediletto

Product Assistants: Harry Garrott
  Michelle Whitehead

Senior Director of Sales and Marketing:
  Gerard McAvey

Marketing Manager: Elizabeth Bushey

Community Manager: Matthew McGuire

Senior Production Director: Wendy Troeger

Production Director: Andrew Crouth

Senior Content Project Manager:
  Nina Tucciarelli

Senior Art Director: Benj Gleeksman

Cover images:

  Hair by: Fern Andong and Jes Sutton

  Makeup by: Amy Elizabeth

  Photography: Joseph and Yuki Paradiso

Library of Congress Control Number: 2016934303

ISBN: 978-1-305-10055-8

Milady
20 Channel Center Street
Boston, MA 02210
USA

Cengage Learning is a leading provider of customized learning solutions with employees residing in nearly 40 different countries and sales in more than 125 countries around the world. Find your local representative at **www.cengage.com**.

Cengage Learning products are represented in Canada by Nelson Education, Ltd.

For your lifelong learning solutions, visit **milady.cengage.com**

Purchase any of our products at your local college store or at our preferred online store **www.cengagebrain.com**

Visit our corporate website at **cengage.com**.

Printed in the United States of America
Print Number: 03   Print Year: 2018

BRIEF CONTENTS

CONTENTS

PART *3*

THE PRACTICE
OF BARBERING | 272

PART *4*

ADVANCED BARBERING SERVICES | 526

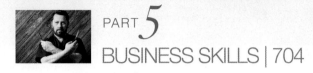

Milady Standard Barbering

Congratulations! You have chosen a career filled with unlimited potential, one that can propel you in many directions as you become a confident and successful professional. As a barber, you will play an important role in your client's lives and in your community. You will be relied on to provide professional services and expertise that enable your clients to look and feel their absolute best.

Milady Standard Barbering, 6th Edition, has been created using student and industry feedback to provide you with the information you need to pass your state licensure exam. This edition includes the classic techniques paired with the most contemporary looks to ensure your success in school and beyond to employment. This text not only teaches you the technical skills needed for success but also provides comprehensive education on the soft skills you need to cultivate to become a successful professional.

This edition has brought together some of the best and brightest minds in the barbering industry to provide you with the very best in education. We here at Milady wish you an enjoyable and successful journey as you embark on this chapter of your life.

The Industry Standard

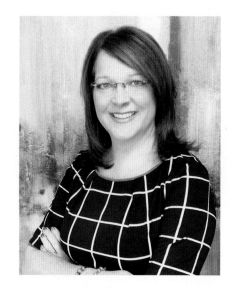

Since 1927, Milady has been committed to quality education for beauty professionals. Over the years, tens of millions of licensed professionals have begun their careers studying from Milady's industry-leading textbooks.

We at Milady are dedicated to providing the most comprehensive learning solutions in the widest variety of formats to serve you, today's student. The newest edition of *Milady Standard Barbering* is available to in multiple formats including the traditional print version, an eBook version, and Mindtap, which provides an interactive learning experience complete with activities, learning tools, and brand new video content.

Milady would like to thank the educators and professionals who participated in surveys and reviews to best determine the changes that needed to be made for this edition. We would also like to thank our students, past and present, for being vocal about your needs and giving Milady the opportunity to provide you with the very best in barbering education.

Thank you for trusting Milady to provide you with the valuable information you need to build the foundation of your career. Our content, combined with your passion, creativity, and devotion to your craft and your customers will set you on the path to a lifetime of success. Congratulations for taking the first step toward your future as a Barber!

Sandra Bruce
Executive Director, Milady

New to This Edition

Design

For this edition, the Milady Team worked to dramatically modernize and transform the look and feel of *Milady Standard Barbering* from the cover to the interior design. Using feedback from students, we created a new sleek and clean design. By using fewer background colors, we have provided more white space for you to take your own notes on the pages themselves!

Photography and Art

Milady conducted a photoshoot and worked with a wide network of barbers and models to capture over 400 new, four-color photographs that appear throughout the book. All of the new procedure photographs were taken using models, not mannequins.

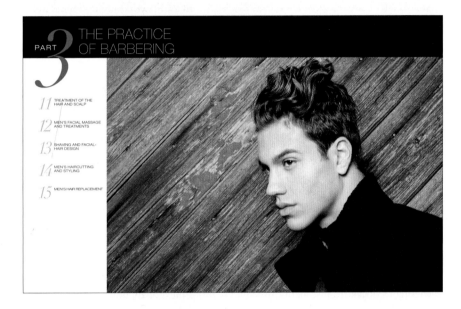

Learning Objectives

At the beginning of each chapter is a list of learning objectives that tell you what important information you will be expected to know after studying the chapter. Throughout the chapter, learning objectives also originate below the main topic, where the objectives will be met in subsequent paragraphs. This is done for ease of reference and to reinforce the main competencies that are critical to learn in each chapter to prepare for licensure. This duplication is an indication to the reader that the objective can be accurately measured by reading, understanding, and practicing to achieve all of the outcomes for the lesson.

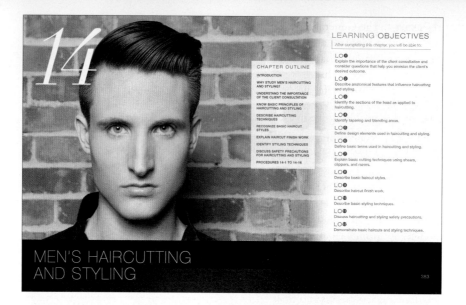

Combination of Key Terms and Glossary List

A complete list of key terms now appears as part of the glossary located at the end of each chapter. In addition to the key terms, you will find the page number references for where the key terms are defined and discussed in the chapter material. The combined key term and chapter glossary is a way to learn important terms that are used in the barbering industry and in preparation for licensure. This list is a one-stop resource to create flashcards or study for quizzes on a particular chapter.

All key terms are re-included in the *Glossary*, as well as in the *Index* at the end of the text.

New Organization of Chapters

In this edition of *Milady Standard Barbering*, Milady wanted to hear what you had to say. Using feedback from students, instructors, and professionals around the country, we made drastic changes to the order of the chapters and the content within them. We worked to provide you, the students, with the most relevant content in a digestible format to make your path to licensure a bit more enjoyable.

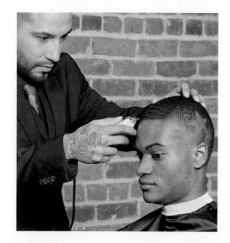

In Part 1: Orientation to Barbering, The history of Barbering now appears first as the foundation of your education, because you must know where you came from to really grasp where you are going. The other change we made was creating the Chapter 2, Life Skills, from the previously names Study Skills chapter. While this chapter includes the important information on studying you will need for your education, it also includes the skills you will need to be successful in your life and career.

Orientation to Barbering consists of three chapters that cover the field of barbering and the personal skills you will need to become successful. Chapter 1, The History of Barbering, outlines the enthralling history of the barbering profession and the opportunities of its future. In Chapter 2, Life Skills, the ability to set goals and maintain a healthy attitude is highlighted, along with the psychology of success. Chapter 3, Professional Image, stresses the importance of inward beauty and health, as well as the importance of maintaining an outward appearance that remains true to you and your environment as a professional.

In Part 2: In the General Sciences we combined two chapters, Microbiology and Infection Control and Safe Work Practices, from previous editions into one comprehensive Chapter 4, Infection Control: Principles and Practices. This combined chapter includes the most valuable in infection control to keep yourself and your clients safe. While the order of the chapters in the rest of Part 2 remains the same, the content in each chapter was revised to be relevant to today's student.

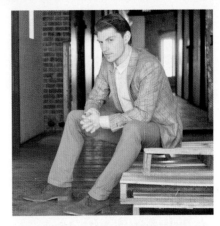

General Sciences includes vital information you need to know to keep yourself and your clients safe and healthy. Chapter 4, Infection Control: Principles and Practices, offers the most current infection control practices and information on preventing the spread of viruses and bacteria, such as hepatitis, HIV, and MRSA. Chapter 5, Implements, Tools, and Equipment, covers the basics for every tool you will need during your barbering career. The other chapters in this section: Chapter 6, General Anatomy and Physiology; Chapter 7, Basics of Chemistry; Chapter 8, Basics of Electricity; Chapter 9, The Skin—Structure, Disorders, and Diseases; and Chapter 10, Properties and Disorders of the Hair and Scalp—provide essential information that will affect how you interact with your clients and how you use service products and tools.

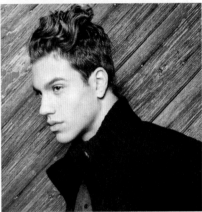

In Part 3: The Practice of Barbering, we made significant changes to the art and procedures. Each procedure in the Men's Haircutting chapter was reviewed and revised with both in-person and digital reviewers to ensure the steps are clear and accurate. A photo shoot was held to capture new photos for the chapters and many of the procedures in this section.

The order of the chapters in Part 3 may have remained the same, but each chapter was examined closely and revised to have the relevant content for today's student. The chapters in this section—Chapter 11, Treatment of the Hair and Scalp; Chapter 12, Men's Facial Massage and Treatments; Chapter 13, Shaving and Facial-Hair Design; Chapter 14, Men's Haircutting and Styling; and Chapter 15, Men's Hair Replacement—cover the technical skills needed to treat the basic needs of your clients.

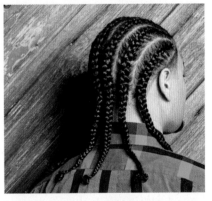

In Part 4: Advanced Barbering Services, Milady listened to the reviewers and decided to make a significant change. The Nails and Manicuring chapter was removed from this section and placed in the Appendix of this edition. Since many states do not require Nails and Manicuring for their State Board Examinations, the content is now still accessible for the states that need it, but does not interrupt the flow of the book for states that do not require the subject.

The content that has remained in this section—Chapter 16, Women's Haircutting and Styling; Chapter 17, Chemical Texture Services; and Chapter 18, Haircoloring and Lightening—provides you with theory and practical step-by-step procedures you will need to master to perform these advanced services for your clients.

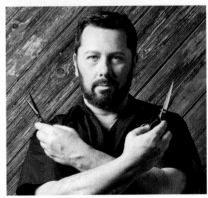

In Part 5: Business Skills, we updated the business content to reflect the current and projected markets and environment of the Barbering Industry. The updated content in Chapter 19, Preparing for Licensure and Employment; Chapter 20, Working behind the Chair; and Chapter 21, The Business of Barbering is the gateway to your future. From preparing you for licensure to working behind the chair and running your own shop, this section is designed to help you successfully launch into a vibrant career.

Additional Features of This Edition

FOCUS ON

Being a Good Teammate

While each individual may be concerned with getting ahead and being successful, a good teammate knows that no one can be successful alone. You will be truly successful if you entire shop is successful!

Throughout the text, short paragraphs in the outer column draw attention to various skills and concepts that will help you reach your goal. The *Focus On* pieces target sharpening technical and personal skills, ticket upgrading, client consultation, and building your client base. These topics are key to your success as a student and as a professional.

DID YOU KNOW?

Histology, also known as *microscopic anatomy*, is the study of tiny structures found in living tissues.

This feature provides interesting information that will enhance your understanding of the material in the text and call attention to a special point.

ACTIVITY

Research the Web for local and state procedures for licensing electrical, light, and laser therapy devised.

The *Activity* boxes describe hands-on classroom exercises that will help you understand the concepts explained in the text.

HERE'S A TIP

Barbering professionals are not allowed to treat or recommend treatments for infections, diseases, or abnormal conditions. Clients with such problems should be referred to their physicians.

These helpful tips draw attention to situations that might arise and provide quick ways of doing things. Look for these tips throughout the text.

CAUTION

Read labels carefully! Manufacturers take great care to develop safe and highly effective products. However, when used improperly, many otherwise safe products can be dangerous. If you do not follow proper guidelines and instructions, any professional product can be dangerous. As with all products, disinfectants must be used exactly as the label instructs.

Some information is so critical for your safety and the safety of your clients that is deserves special attention. Be sure to direct your attention to the information in the *Caution* boxes.

STATE REGULATORY ALERT!

Always be certain that you are in compliance with your state's regulations for licensing and use of electric current devices.

This feature alerts you to check the laws in your region for procedures and practices that are regulated differently from state to state. It is important, while you are studying, to contact state boards and provincial regulatory agencies to learn what is allowed and not allowed. Your instructor will provide you with contact information.

WEB RESOURCES

For more information on electricity and energy, visit the U.S. Energy Information Administration's website at loc.gov and enter the search words electricity or energy.

The *Web Resources* provide you with Web addresses where you can find more information on a topic and references to additional site for more information.

Why Study This?

Milady knows, understands, and appreciates how excited you are to jump right into the newest and most excited haircutting, shaving, and haircoloring chapters. We also recognize that you can sometimes feel restless spending time learning the basics of barbering, such as history, the sciences, and business. To help you understand why you need to learn each chapter's material, and to help you see the role it will play in your future barbering career, we have added a *Why Study* section to the beginning of each chapter. This section tells you why the material is important and how you will use it in your professional career.

Procedures

At the beginning of each procedure you will be provided with a list of all needed implements and materials, as well as any preparation that must be completed before starting the procedure. At the introduction of many procedures we have added images showing the final, styled result of the cut you are about to perform.

In previous editions, the procedures interrupted the flow of the chapter material, making it necessary for you to flip through many pages in order to continue your studying. To avoid this interruption, in this edition we have placed all procedures in a special *Procedure* section at the end of each chapter.

For those students who wish to review a procedure at the time it is mentioned, Milady has added Procedure icons with page numbers to direct you to the proper procedure. Many procedures have undergone significant changes and updates for this edition, specifically in Chapters 4, 5, 11, 12, 13, 14, 16, 17, and 18.

Review Questions

Each chapter ends with questions designed to test your understanding of the chapter's information. Your instructor may ask you to write the answer to these questions as an assignment or to answer them during class time. If you have trouble answering a chapter review question, go back to the chapter to review the material and then try again! The answers to these review questions are located in your Instructor's *Course Management Guide*.

Meet the Team

Main Author
Maura Scali-Sheahan

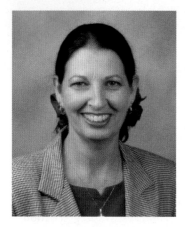

MAURA SCALI-SHEAHAN, ED.D.

Master Barber, Author, Educator, and Consultant

In addition to earning a master barber license in the 1970s, Maura has a doctorate in education and a master's degree in workforce education training and development. She has served the barbering profession in a variety of capacities, from instructor and program director to state board member and author. In 2008, she was inducted into the NABBA Barbering Hall of Fame *for her many years of service to the Barber profession.*

Maura is also an adjunct instructor for Southern Illinois University's Workforce Education and Development program. In this capacity, she provides instruction in courses that range from occupational analysis and curriculum development to instructional methods and materials.

Dr. Scali-Sheahan is dedicated to promoting the longevity of the barbering profession through enhanced barbering education. To this end, she provides professional development and enrichment venues for barbering programs, instructors, and students to help prepare the next generation of educators and barbers for the profession.

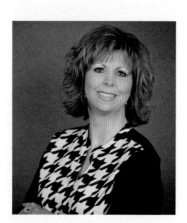

Contributing Authors

Amy Burness

Chapter 15 Men's Hair Replacement

As a second-generation hair stylist and educator, Amy has been building and expanding her knowledge in the hair care industry for over 25 years. Early in her career, Amy learned the art of hair replacement, helping men and women restore their confidence. As an educator for one of the world's most recognized fine and thinning hair care company, she is exceptionally passionate about training stylists about fine and thinning hair, the art of styling, and the integrity of exceptional service. She is honored to have had this opportunity to share her passion and knowledge of the second fastest growing market in our industry.

Linnea Lindquist

Chapter 16 Women's Haircutting and Styling

Chapter 17 Chemical Texture Services

Chapter 18 Haircoloring and Lightening

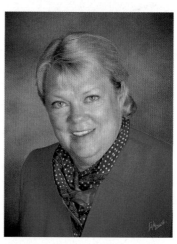

Linnea Lindquist has been in the cosmetology industry for over 30 years. After receiving her bachelor's degree in education and history from Augustana College (IL), she decided to follow her passion and enrolled in cosmetology school. She was eventually able to combine her educational knowledge with her cosmetology skills and become a cosmetology instructor. She has taught at both private and public educational institutions including Horst Institute (now Aveda Institute), Cosmetology Training Center (MN), and Minneapolis Community & Technical College. Throughout her career, Linnea has written multiple cosmetology curricula, for both hour- and credit-based programs, and has developed and managed extensive cosmetology, barber, and esthetician testing programs. In her work as an instructional designer, she has developed training materials for classroom facilitation, self-guided study, and online training. Training materials she has developed include facilitator guides, participant guides, visual presentations, reference materials, classroom activities, and evaluations. Linnea is the author of a variety of cosmetology-related educational books, including *Milady's Preparing for the State Exam, Milady's Standard Theory Workbook,* and *Milady's Nail Technology Workbook.* She received her master's degree from the University of Minnesota in vocational education with a focus on instructional design and testing and measurement.

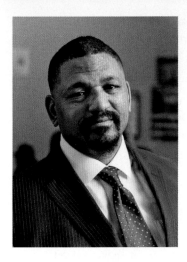

Dennis "Denny Moe" Mitchell

Chapter 14 Men's Haircutting and Styling (Procedures 14-9: Pompadour Fade, 14-10: Fade Haircut with Star Design)

Celebrity barber Dennis "Denny Moe" Mitchell is owner of Denny Moe's Superstar Barbershop in Harlem. He began his career at the age of 15 and he is now a master barber with over 35 years of experience and a client roster including the likes of entertainers such as Eddie Murphy, P. Diddy, Jason Williams, Jerry Stackhouse, and many more. While being proud of these accomplishments, Denny Moe considers all of his clients to be superstars and ensures that each person receives a high-caliber haircut with every visit to his barbershop. Whether it is his legendary sculpted afro or a classic fade, his clients receive nothing but the best.

Since opening its doors in 2006, Denny Moe's Superstar Barbershop has consistently given back by hosting a number of events that aim to uplift and empower the community. Through initiatives including an annual Back to School Drive, Christmas Toy Drive, and College Scholarship Drive, Denny Moe strives to create a positive impact in his community. His largest effort Cutting for a Cure, a health fair that provides free medical screenings, live entertainment, and more has received national recognition and further proves that his barbershop not only makes dollars but also makes a difference. Among his leadership roles, Denny Moe is also a member of the community advisory board for an NIH-funded study to improve organ donor registration among black men with the NYU School of Medicine.

Leslie Roste

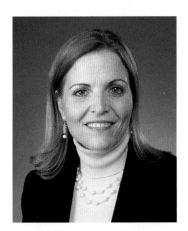

Chapter 4 Infection Control: Principles and Practices
Chapter 6 General Anatomy and Physiology
Chapter 9 The Skin—Structure, Disorders, and Diseases
Chapter 10 Properties and Disorders of the Hair and Scalp

Leslie Roste, RN, BSN, graduated from the University of Kansas, where she studied nursing and microbiology. She worked in various nursing positions including obstetrical nursing and infection control in the Kansas City area prior to beginning work in the cosmetology industry. Her main focus in the industry has been on health and safety in the professional beauty environment and general education about the sciences involved. She has written many articles for publications such as the *Modern Salon* and the *NAILS Magazine* and has spoken to audiences large and small on infection control in the work environment, minimum health and safety standards, and safety-based licensure. She is very involved with the industry at all levels, from students to legislators, in making sure that professional beauty industry services are performed safely.

Leslie currently serves on the NACAS National Career Programs Standardization Committee, the Professional Beauty Coalition for Legislative Education & Reform, and the NIC Education Committee. She also spends a large portion of her time working with individual states and revising rules and/or legislation surrounding infection control in the professional beauty industry. She recently wrote and launched a free Web-based infection control certification and has already certified over 9,000 professionals and students. Her certification is being widely used in the schools.

Acknowledgments

Milady recognizes, with gratitude and respect, the many professionals who have offered their time to contribute to this edition of *Milady Standard Barbering*. We wish to extend an enormous thank you to the following people who have played an invaluable role in the creation of this edition.

- Milady would like to send a huge thank you to our on-camera professionals who performed the procedures for our photoshoot.
  - Fern Andong
  - Lilly Benitez
  - John Gould
  - Courtney Harris
  - Dekar Lawson
  - Daiwan Perry
  - Jes Sutton
  - Christie Valentie

- Thank you, to the amazing duo Joseph and Yuki Paradiso for their creativity, vision, and dedication in bringing this product and its photos to life.

- Amy Elizabeth, makeup artist, for your incredible work at the shoot. Not only was the makeup amazing, but you saved the day more than once with your beauty first aid kit! You were always willing to jump on set and go the extra mile to ensure everything was clean, crisp, and smooth for the shoot.

- Harry Garrott, Product Assistant, for working to revise and align the content for this edition. Your dedication and wiliness to jump onto any task for this project has truly made a huge difference in the finished product.

- Michelle Whitehead, Product Assistant, for your work at the photoshoot and beyond. Your creativity and artistic eye resulted in stunning and unique backgrounds for our finished looks and amazing art from your art research. Thank you, for offering to help with every aspect of this project from the planning phone calls, to the post-shoot work. In addition, your attention to detail while assisting with the development of this edition.

- Alyssa Hardy, Social Media Manager and Fashion Stylist at the shoot, for your hours of work gathering outfits for our models. You went above and beyond to ensure that the finished looks were modern and on trend, while remaining sleek and classic.

- Jessica Mahoney, Senior Content Developer, for lending your knowledge, experience, and time to this edition.

Subject Matter Expert Reviewers of *Milady Standard Barbering*, 6e

Jes Sutton, Barber, Cosmetologist at Barbetorium, Rochester, NY.

Thomas S. Torres, Barber and Educator, Continental School of Beauty, Rochester, NY.

Reviewers of *Milady Standard Barbering*, 6e

Sam Barcelona, Executive Director of the Arizona State Board of Barbers, Past President of NABBA, Member of the Board of Directors: Barbers International, Captain of PBA, Phoenix, AZ.

Johnathan Cifredo, barber, educator, Owner of Cifredo'z Barber Salon, Reading, PA.

Kimberly Cutter-Williams, M.Ed., Savannah Technical College, Savannah, GA.

Derek Davis, District of Columbia examiner, and President, District of Columbia Career and Technical Education, Washington, DC.

Christopher Diaz, Owner, Master Barber, NYS Examiner, The Long Island Barber Institute, Inc. and Star Studded Cutz, Inc. Hempstead, NY.

JoAnn DiPrete, Sales and Education Manager of Ultronics, Copley, OH.

Debbie Eckstone-Weidner, Owner, Supervisor, Director at DeRielle Cosmetology Academy and Revelations A Day Spa, Mechanicsburg, PA.

Christopher D. Felder, Owner, Director of The Long Island Barber Institute, Inc., Hempstead, NY.

Lauren Geller-Henderson, Campus Director, Evergreen Beauty College, Everett, WA.

Laureen Gillis, RLCI, RLC, Consultant Trainer, Grand Rapids, MI.

Thamer Hite, Owner, Operator of The Barber School, Midvale, UT.

Lynell Hite, Owner, Operator of The Barber School, Midvale, UT.

Larry Little, President, Owner of AR College of Barbering and Hair Design, Inc., Little Rock, AR.

Walter J Lupu, School Director, Barber Instructor at Barber Styling College of Lansing, Lansing, MI.

Johnnie T. Major, Director of Hair Services, SC Department of Mental Health Master Barber/Barber Instructor, B.S. Business Administration University, SC.

Sophia Markus, Instructor at the Avalon School of Cosmetology, Worthington, MN.

Jeffery L. Olson, Barber Instructor at Bates Technical College, Tacoma, WA.

Renee Patton, Barbershop Owner/Instructor, The Barber Shop of Boiling Springs, 1st Vice President of National Association for Barber Boards of America (NABBA), Vice Chair, South Carolina Board of Barber Examiners, Innman, SC.

Ernestine Pledger-Peete, Master Instructor of Barbering & Cosmetology, Tennessee College of Applied Technology at Memphis, Memphis, TN.

Lloyd Dale Sheffield, Barber/Stylist at Alberti's, Parrish, FL.

Donna Simmons, Master Educator, Tulsa Tech, Clinsville, OK.

Jon C. Stone, Barber Member, Minnesota Board of Barber Examiners, Detroit Lakes, MN.

Theodore W. Taylor, Barber Instructor, Flint Institute of Barbering Inc., Flint, MI.

Milady's Infection Control Advisory Panel Reviewers

Barbara Accello, RN, Innovations in Health Care, Denton, TX.

Mike Kennamer, Director of Workforce Development at Northeast Alabama Community College, Rainsville, AL and President/CEO Kennamer Media Group, Inc., Henagar, AL.

Janet McCormick, Co-Founder, Nailcare Academy, LLC, Frostproof, FL.

Leslie Roste, RN, National Director of Education and Market Development, King Research/Barbicide, WI.

Dr. Robert Spaulding, Podiatrist DPM, Medinail Learning Center, Signal Mountain, TN.

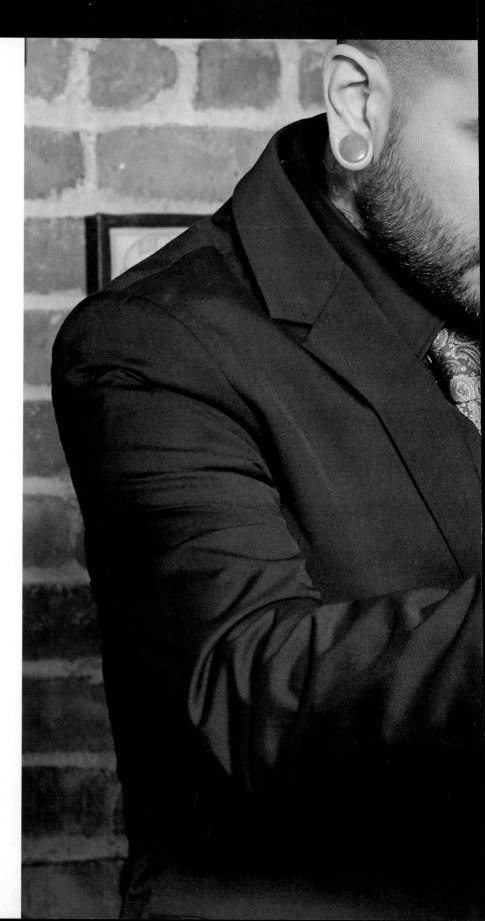

PART 1 ORIENTATION TO BARBERING

1 THE HISTORY
OF BARBERING

2 LIFE SKILLS

3 PROFESSIONAL IMAGE

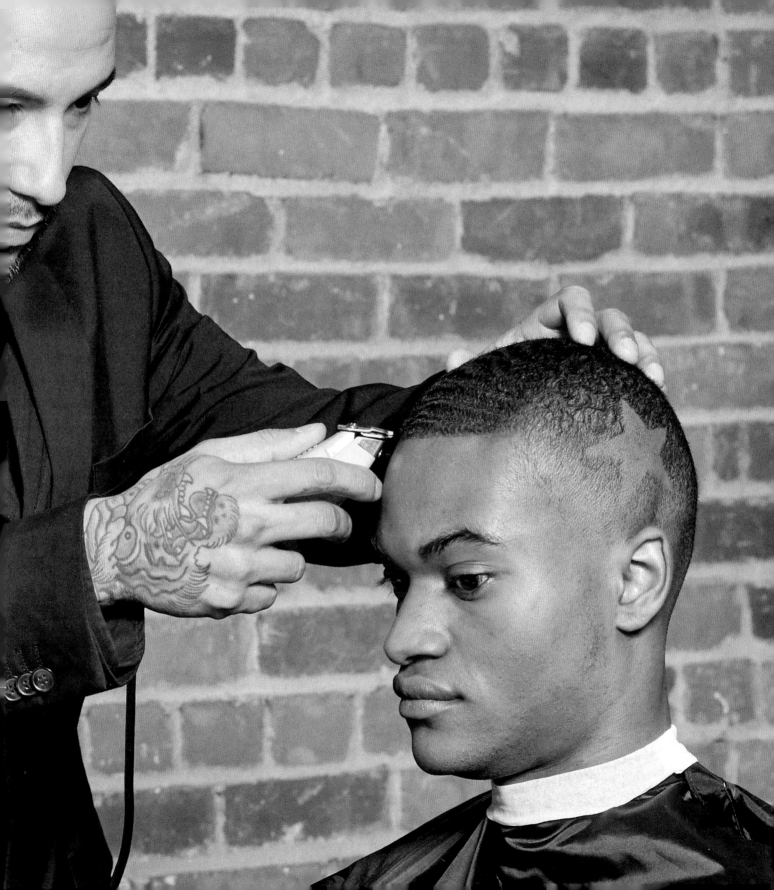

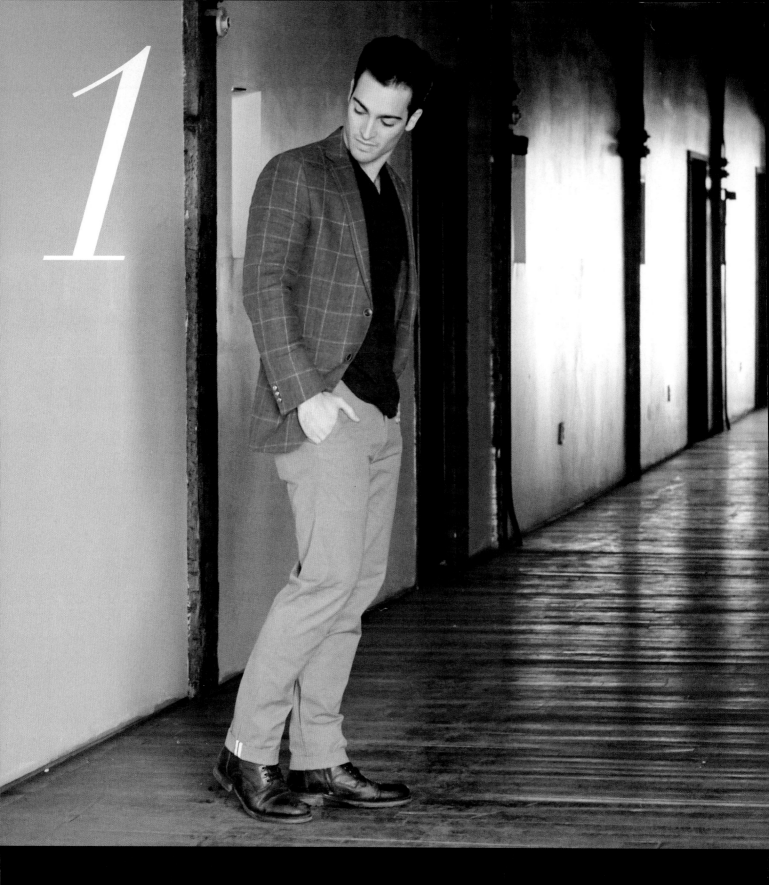

1

THE HISTORY OF
BARBERING

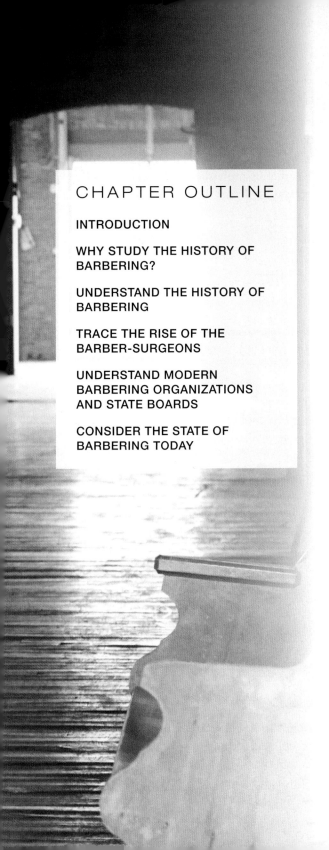

LEARNING OBJECTIVES

After completing this chapter, you will be able to:

LO❶
Discuss the evolution of barbering and the origin of the word *barber*.

LO❷
Describe the practices of the barber-surgeons and the meaning behind the barber pole.

LO❸
Identify the organizations responsible for advancing the barbering profession and explain the function of state barber boards.

LO❹
Recognize the resurgence of barbering in the twenty-first century and the wealth of opportunities available to the new barber.

Introduction

Barbering is one of the oldest professions in the world. Whether from a sense of aesthetics or because of religious conviction, virtually all early cultures practiced some form of beautification and adornment, given the archaeological evidence found in painted pottery, early sculptures, and burial mounds. As civilization advanced, so did the barbering profession, developing from its beginnings as cultural and tribal necessity to the art form it is today.

why study
THE HISTORY OF BARBERING?

Barbers should study and have a thorough understanding of the history of barbering because:

> Barbering is one of the oldest documented professions. Understanding its evolution can provide you with an appreciation of the prominent role it achieved in different cultures throughout the ages.

> Knowing the history of your profession can help you predict and understand upcoming trends.

> Having a clear picture of how modern barbering organizations and regulations developed gives you a better idea of where you fit into the profession at large and what is expected of you as a barber.

Understand the History of Barbering

After reading this section, you will be able to:

LO❶ Discuss the evolution of barbering and the origin of the word *barber*.

Barbering has a rich history, stretching back millennia. Although technological developments—metal shears, clippers, electricity—have certainly advanced the barber's profession, its standing within human civilization has been more significantly influenced through the ages by changing traditions, cultural trends, and shifting political influences.

ANCIENT CULTURES

Archaeological studies from around the world have shown that haircutting and hairstyling were practiced as early as the glacial age. The simple implements used then were shaped from sharpened flints, oyster shells, or bone. Animal sinew or strips of hide were used as adornment or to tie the hair back, and braiding techniques were employed in many cultures.

Many primitive cultures maintained a connection between the body, mind, and spirit. This conviction translated into superstitions and beliefs that merged spirituality, religious rituals, and medical practices together in an integrated relationship. For example, some tribes believed that both good and bad spirits entered the individual through the hairs on the head and that the only way to exorcise bad spirits was to cut the hair. In another similar religious ceremony, long hair was worn loose to allow the evil spirits to exit the individual. Then, after ritual dancing, the barber cut the hair, combed it back tightly against the scalp, and tied it off to keep the good spirits in and the evil spirits out. Belief systems elevated tribal barbers to positions of importance, such as medicine men, shamans, or priests.

The Egyptians are credited with being the first people to cultivate beauty in an extravagant fashion. Excavations from tombs have revealed such relics as combs, brushes, mirrors, cosmetics, scissors, and razors made of tempered copper and bronze (**Figure 1-1**). Coloring agents made from berries, bark, minerals, and other natural materials were used on the hair, skin, and nails. Eye paint was the most popular of all cosmetics, with the use of henna as a coloring agent first recorded in 1500 BC.

The use of barbers by Egyptian noblemen and priests 6,000 years ago is substantiated by Egypt's written records, art, and sculpture (**Figure 1-2**). High-ranking men and women of Egypt had their heads shaved for comfort when wearing wigs and for the prevention of parasitic infestations. Every third day, barbers would shave the priests' entire bodies to ensure their purity before entering the temple. The work of the barber **Meryma'at** (mare-a-mott) was apparently held in particularly high esteem, as his image was sculpted for posterity.

In some African cultures, hair was groomed with intricately carved combs and decorated with beads, clay, and colored bands (**Figure 1-3**). The Masai warriors, for example, wove their front hair into three sections of tiny braids and the rest of the hair into a queue down the back. Braiding was used extensively, with intricate patterns frequently denoting status within the tribe.

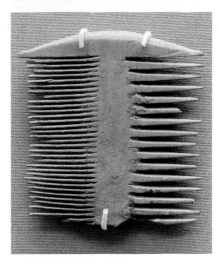

figure 1-1
Ancient Egyptian comb, of the type found in tomb excavations.

figure 1-2
Egyptian engravings depicting soldiers having their hair cut.

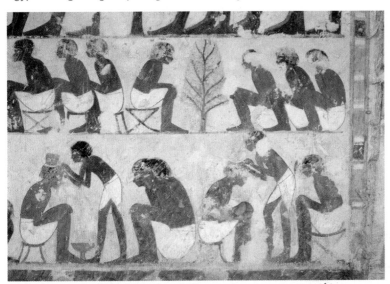

figure 1-3
Africans decorated their hair with beads, clays, colored bands, or braiding, often in intricate patterns.

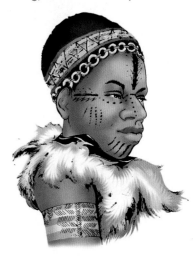

Several Biblical passages give insight into the state of the barber in the Middle East. According to Leviticus, Moses commanded those who had recovered from leprosy to shave all their body hair as part of a ritual cleansing. Ezekiel refers to another ancient shaving custom when he says, "Take thou a barber's razor and cause it to pass upon thy head and upon thy beard." Based on these and other Biblical references, it has been accepted that barbering was available to the general population of the Middle East during the lifetime of Moses (circa 1392 to circa 1272 BC).

Although Greek barbers from Sicily introduced shears to Rome sometime between 800 and 700 BC, barbers were virtually unknown in Rome until 296 BC.

It was in Greece during its golden age (500 to 300 BC) that barbering became a highly developed art. Well-trimmed beards were status symbols—Greek men had their beards trimmed, curled, and scented on a regular basis (**Figure 1-4**). Barbershops became the gathering places for exchanging sporting, social, and political news, while barbers themselves rose in prominence to become leading citizens within the social structure.

The status of the beard in Greece drastically changed in the third century BC, when Alexander the Great's Macedonian troops lost several battles to the Persians as a result of the warriors' beards. The Persians would grab the Macedonian warriors by their beards and drag them to the ground, where they were either speared or beheaded. Alexander issued a decree that all soldiers be clean shaven. Eventually, the general populace adopted the trend, and barbers were kept busy performing shaves and haircuts.

Ticinius Mena (ti-cin-i-us me-nah) of Sicily has been credited with having brought shaving and barbering services to Rome in 296 BC. The men of Rome soon enjoyed tonsorial services such as shaves, haircutting and dressing, massage, and manicuring on a daily basis, with a good portion of their day spent with the barber. While the average citizen patronized the barbers' places of business, rich noblemen engaged private *tonsors* to take care of their hairdressing and shaving needs. The Romans expanded the concept of these personal services to include communal bathing and what became known as the Roman baths.

Clean-shaven faces were the trend until Hadrian came into power in 117 AD. Emperor Hadrian became a trendsetter when he grew his beard to hide scars on his chin (**Figure 1-5**), resulting in the populace following his lead, and the beard was again in fashion. In fact, the word *barber* is derived from the Latin word **barba**, meaning "beard." Another word derived from Latin, **tonsorial** (TON-SORE-ee-ahl) (derived from *tondere*, meaning "to shear"), means the cutting, clipping, or trimming of hair with shears or a razor. It is often used in conjunction with barbering—barbers are sometimes referred to as tonsorial artists.

CUSTOMS AND TRADITIONS

The beliefs, rituals, and superstitions of early civilizations varied from one ethnic group to another, depending on the region and social interactions with other groups. There was a general belief among many groups that hair

figure 1-4
The Golden Age of Greece saw the rise of barbering as an art, along with the well-trimmed, curled, and scented beard.

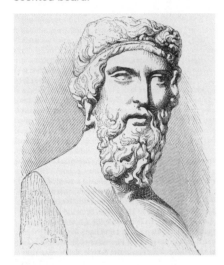

figure 1-5
Roman Emperor Hadrian grew a beard to hide facial scarring, inadvertently bringing the beard back into fashion.

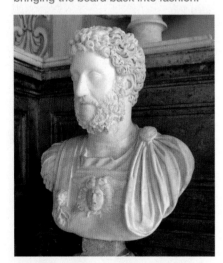

© Marzolino/Shutterstock.com.

© Heritage Images/Contributor/Hulton Archive/Getty Images.

clippings could bewitch an individual. Hence, the privilege of haircutting was reserved for the priest, medicine man, or spiritual leader of the tribe. According to the Greek philosopher and mathematician Pythagoras, the hair was the source of the brain's inspiration, and cutting it decreased an individual's intellectual capacity. The Irish peasantry believed that if hair cuttings were burned or buried with the dead, no evil spirits would haunt the individual. Among some Native American tribes, it was believed that the hair and the body were so linked that anyone possessing a lock of hair of another might work his will on that individual.

In almost every early culture, hairstyles indicated social status. In ancient Greece, boys would cut their hair upon reaching adolescence, while their Hindu counterparts would shave their heads. Following the invasion of China by the Manchu, Chinese men adopted the queue as a mark of dignity and manhood. Noblemen of ancient Gaul indicated their rank by wearing their hair long, until Caesar, upon conquering Gaul, made them cut it, as a sign of submission. At various times in Roman history, slaves would be allowed or disallowed to wear beards, depending on the dictates of the ruler.

Coloring agents were often used to add further dimension. The ancient Britons, extremely proud of their long hair, brightened blond hair with washes composed of tallow, lime, and the extracts of certain vegetables. Darker hair was treated with dyes extracted and processed from plants, trees, and various soils. The Danes, Angles, and Normans dressed their hair for beautification, adornment, and ornamentation before battles with the Britons. In ancient Rome, the color of a woman's hair indicated her class or rank. Noblewomen tinted their hair red, those of the middle class colored their hair blond, and poor women were compelled to dye their hair black. Much later, during the reign of Queen Elizabeth in England, it would become fashionable for men to dye the beard and cut it into a variety of shapes.

In later centuries, religion, occupation, and politics also influenced the length and style of hair as well as the wearing (or not) of beards. Clergymen of the Middle Ages were distinguished by the **tonsure** (TON-shur), a shaved patch on the crown of the head. During the seventh century, Celtic and Roman church leaders disagreed on the exact shape the tonsure should take. The circular tonsure, called the *tonsure of St. Peter*, left only a slight fringe of hair around the head and was preferred in Germany, Italy, and Spain (**Figure 1-6**). The Picts and Scots preferred a semicircular design, known as the *tonsure of St. John*. After much argument, the pope eventually decreed that priests were to shave their beards and mustaches and adopt the tonsure of St. Peter.

Although the edicts of the church maintained some influence over priests and the general populace for several centuries, beards and longer hairstyles had returned by the eleventh century. Priests curled or braided their hair and beards until Pope Gregory issued another papal decree requiring shaved faces and short hair. It was not until 1972 that the Roman Catholic Church finally abolished the practice of tonsure.

Most rulers and monarchs became trendsetters by virtue of their position and power in society. Personal whim, taste, and even physical

figure 1-6
The circular tonsure (tonsure of St. Peter) left only a slight fringe of hair around the head of the clergymen who wore it.

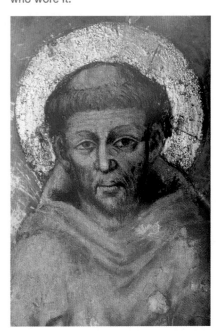

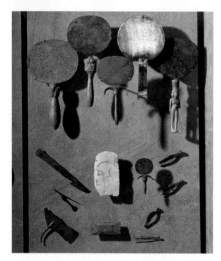

figure 1-7
Selection of ancient Egyptian barbering tools, including mirrors, razors, and tweezers.

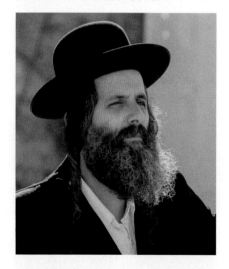

figure 1-8
The beard is a sign of religious devotion for Orthodox Jews.

? DID YOU KNOW?
During Medieval times, tradesmen learned their craft through apprenticeships. Guilds, similar to associations, were formed by tradesmen to control the practice and training of their professions. Trade guilds eventually led to the development of schools and universities.

limitations could become the basis for changes in hairstyles and fashion. For example, in the sixteenth century, when Francis I of France accidentally burned his hair with a torch, his loyal subjects had their hair, beards, and mustaches cut short. During the reign of Louis XIV in the seventeenth century, noblemen wore wigs because the king, who was balding, did so. During the nineteenth century in France, men and women showed appreciation for antiquity by wearing variations of the "Caesar cut," the style of the early Roman emperors.

THE BEARD AND SHAVING

With the razor being such a defining tool for barbering, the history of shaving, as well as caring for the beard in general, deserves a second look. Since the practice of shaving predates the written word, it is difficult to determine just when this form of hair removal began.

Excavations of early stone razors or scrapers from the Upper Paleolithic period (40,000 to 10,000 BC) indicate that early man may have used these tools for hair removal as well as for the skinning of animals. By the time of the Neolithic period (8000 to 5000 BC), early man had created settlements and begun to farm and raise animals. Artwork of this period shows examples of clean-shaven men, but it is unknown how the hair was removed. In Egypt, however, pyramids from around 7000 BC have yielded flint-bladed razors that are known to have been used by the ruling classes to shave their heads as well as their faces, and by 4000 BC, a form of tweezers was also used (see **Figure 1-7**).

It stands to reason that the nomadic nature of many early groups helped spread the practice of shaving throughout the rest of the world. Mesopotamians of 3000 BC were shaving with obsidian blades, and by 2800 BC, the Sumerians were also clean shaven. Likewise, Greek men of 1000 BC are seen in works of art visiting their local barber for shaving services.

In early times, most groups considered the beard to be a sign of wisdom, strength, or manhood. In some cultures, the beard was a sacred symbol. For example, in Rome, a young man's first shave, on his 22nd birthday, constituted a rite of passage from boyhood to manhood and was celebrated with great festivity. To this day, among Orthodox Jews, the beard is a sign of religious devotion, and to cut off one's beard is contrary to Mosaic law (**Figure 1-8**).

Beards have been removed throughout the centuries at the command of rulers and priests. Alexander the Great, as mentioned earlier, ordered his soldiers to shave so their beards could not be seized in battle. The Archbishop of Rouen in France prohibited the wearing of a beard in 1096, spurring the formation of the first-known barber guild in France. Peter the Great encouraged shaving by imposing a tax on beards. During the spread of Christianity, long hair came to be considered sinful and the clergy were directed to shave their beards. Although the shaving of the beard was still forbidden among Orthodox Jews, the use of scissors to trim or shape excess growth was permitted. Muslims took great care in trimming their facial hair after prayer and the removed hair was preserved so that it could be buried with its owner.

Trace the Rise of the Barber-Surgeons

After reading this section, you will be able to:

LO ❷ Describe the practices of the barber-surgeons and the meaning behind the barber pole.

By the Middle Ages, barbers not only provided tonsorial services but also entered the world of medicine, where they figured prominently in the development of surgery as a recognized branch of medical practice. This progress was the result of the barbers' interaction with the religious clerics of the day. As the most learned and educated people of the Middle Ages, monks and priests had become the physicians of the period. One of the most common treatments for curing a variety of illnesses was the practice of bloodletting, and barbers often assisted the clergy in this practice. But in 1163 at the Council of Tours, Pope Alexander III forbade the clergy to act as physicians and surgeons or to draw blood because to do so was contrary to Christian doctrine. Barbers stepped in and took over the duties previously performed by the clergy. They continued the practices of bloodletting, minor surgery, herbal remedies, and tooth pulling. For centuries, dentistry was performed only by barbers, and for more than a thousand years, they were known as **barber-surgeons** (BAR-bur SIR-genz).

The barber-surgeons formed their first organization in France in 1096 AD, and by the 1100s had created a guild of surgeons that specialized in the study of medicine. By the middle of the thirteenth century, these barber companies had also founded the School of St. Cosmos and St. Domain in Paris to instruct barbers in the practice of surgery.

The Worshipful Company of Barbers guild was formed in London, England, in 1308 with the objective of regulating and overseeing the profession. The Barbers' Company was ruled by a master and consisted of two classes of barbers: those who practiced barbering and those who specialized in surgery. By 1368, the surgeons formed their own guild with oversight by the Barbers' Guild, which lasted until 1462 (**Figure 1-9**).

Although competition and antagonism likely existed between the two organizations, a parliamentary act united the two groups in 1450 while it officially separated the practices of each profession. Barbers were limited to bloodletting, cauterization, tooth pulling, and tonsorial services, while surgeons were forbidden to act as barbers. The merged guilds became the Company of Barber-Surgeons (**Figure 1-10**).

In 1540, Henry VIII recombined the barbers and surgeons of London through an Act of Parliament by granting a charter to the Company of Barber-Surgeons. The company commissioned Hans Holbein the Younger, a noted artist of the time, to commemorate the event (**Figure 1-11**).

With the advancement of medicine, the practice of bloodletting became all but obsolete. Although the barber-surgeons' medical practice dwindled in importance, they were still relied upon for dispensing medicinal herbs and pulling teeth. Finally, in 1745, a law was passed in

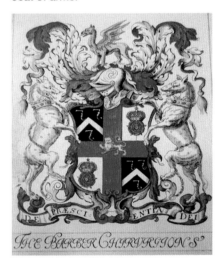

figure 1-9
The Worshipful Company of Barbers' coat of arms.

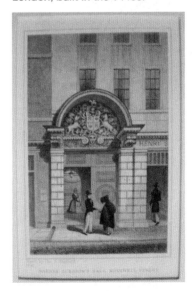

figure 1-10
Nineteenth-century engraving depicting the first Barber-Surgeon's Hall in London, built in the 1440s.

figure 1-11
Henry VIII issuing a charter to the Company of Barber-Surgeons, painted by Hans Holbein.

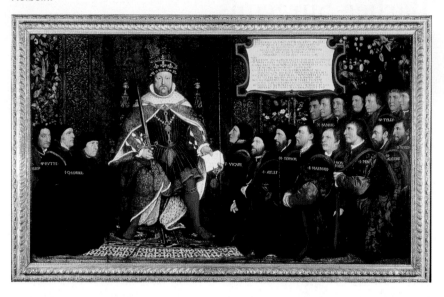

England to separate the barbers from the surgeons and the alliance was completely dissolved.

Barber-surgeons had also flourished in France and Germany. Following the formation of the first French barber guild in 1096, barber-surgeons under the rule of the king's barber formed another guild in 1371, which lasted until about the time of the French Revolution (1789). Ambroise Paré (1510 to 1590) was a particularly noteworthy French barber-surgeon, who went on to become the greatest surgeon of the Renaissance period and the father of modern surgery.

Finally, many Europeans had become so dependent upon the services of the barber-surgeons that Dutch and Swedish settlers brought barber-surgeons with them to America to look after the well-being of the colonists.

THE BARBER POLE

The symbol of the **barber pole** evolved from the technical procedures of bloodletting performed by the barber-surgeons. The pole is thought to symbolize the staff that the patient would hold tightly in order for the veins in the arm to stand out during bloodletting. The bottom end-cap of modern barber poles represents the basin that was used as a vessel to catch the blood during bloodletting. The white stripes on the pole stand for the bandages that were used to stop the bleeding and were hung on the staff to dry. The stained bandages would then twist around the pole in the breeze, forming a red-and-white pattern (**Figure 1-12**).

One interpretation of the colors of the barber pole is that red represented the blood, blue the veins, and white the bandages. Later, when the Company of Barber-Surgeons was formed in England, barbers were required to use blue-and-white poles and surgeons red-and-white poles.

figure 1-12

figure 1-13

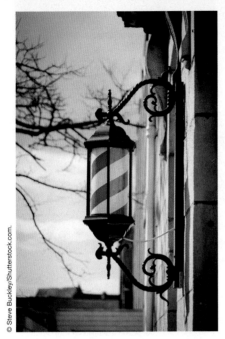

© Steve Buckley/Shutterstock.com.

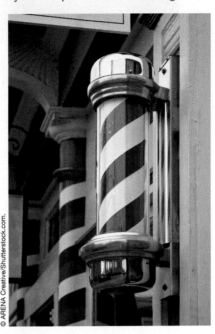

© ARENA Creative/Shutterstock.com.

It is also thought that the red, white, and blue poles displayed in the
United States originated in deference to the nation's flag. Modern barbers
have retained the barber pole as the foremost symbol of the business and
profession of barbering. In fact, display of a barber pole at an establishment
that is not a licensed barbershop employing licensed barbers is prohibited
in some states (Figure 1-13).

Understand Modern Barbering Organizations and State Boards

After reading this section, you will be able to:

LO❸ Identify the organizations responsible for advancing
the barbering profession and explain the function of
state barber boards.

By the end of the nineteenth century, the profession of barbering had completely separated from religion and medicine, emerging as an independent
profession. During the late 1800s, the profession's structure changed and
it began to take new directions. The formation of employer organizations
known as **master barber groups** and employee organizations known as
Journeymen barber groups (JUHR-knee-men BAR-ber GROOPS) was the first
step toward upgrading and regulating the profession. During this era, the
emergence and growth of these organizations helped establish precedents
and standards that are part of today's barbering profession.

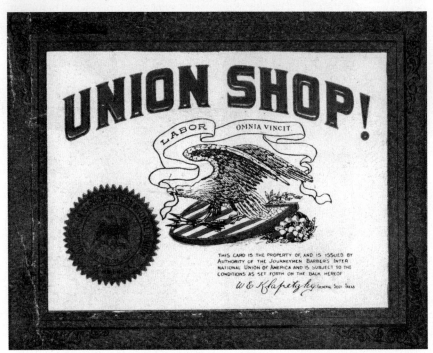

A noteworthy example is the Barbers' Protective Association, organized in 1886. In 1887, it became the Journeymen Barbers' International Union of America at its first convention in Buffalo, New York, affiliated with the American Federation of Labor. By 1963, the name had changed again to the Journeymen Barbers, Hairdressers, Cosmetologists, and Proprietors' International Union of America (Figure 1-14).

Passed in 1897, the first barber-licensing law set standards for sanitation, minimum education, and licensing requirements for barbers and barbershops in the state of Minnesota. The setting of standards was important because at the time it was common for towels, shaving brushes, and other barbering tools to be used on more than one customer without being disinfected in between. These practices provided ample opportunity for bacteria, parasites like headlice, and infections like ringworm and herpes to be spread from one person to another, casting a bad light on barbers and barbershops in general. Similar laws that included hand washing, powdered (rather than stick) astringents, regular floor sweeping, and the disinfection of tools were soon passed in other states in response to the need to protect the public from infectious conditions.

Awareness of the importance of cleaning practices in preventing disease became so widespread that the terminal methods system was enacted in 1916 in New York City. At that time, it was common to see barbershops, beauty shops, and other small business enterprises at the main railway terminals in larger cities. The terminal methods system outlined strict disinfection and cleaning practices, such as boiling tools in view of customers and using airtight storage for disinfected implements. The system soon spread to other shops throughout New York, providing customers with superior, sanitary service.

The Associated Master Barbers of America was established in Chicago, Illinois, in 1924, eventually expanding to include beauty salon owners and managers and changing its name to the **Associated Master Barbers and Beauticians of America (AMBBA)** in 1941. By 1925, its members had established the National Educational Council with the goal of standardizing and upgrading barber training. The council successfully set down the requirements of barber schools and barber instructor training, established a curriculum, and promulgated the passage of state licensing laws.

Working in cooperation with the AMBBA, the National Association of Barber Schools, formed in 1927, developed a program that standardized the operation of the barber schools themselves. In 1929 in St. Paul, Minnesota, the National Association of State Board of Barber Examiners was created to solidify the qualifications required for barber examination applicants and the methods of evaluation to be used. Finally, by 1929, the AMBBA adopted a *barber code of ethics* to promote professional responsibility in the trade and later published its own barbering textbook.

Since 1929, all states have passed laws regulating the practice of barbering and hairstyling. The state boards are primarily concerned with the protection of the health, safety, and welfare of the public. They do this through the maintenance of high educational standards to assure competent and skilled service, the licensing of individuals and shops, and the enforcement of infection control laws. Many of today's state barber boards meet up to twice a year as members of the **National Association of Barber Boards of America (NABBA)**. The NABBA established the month of September as National Barber Month to recognize the contributions of barbers to society. According to the NABBA's website, the organization's mission statement and objectives are as follows:

- The National Association of Barber Boards of America represents over 300,000 barbers and is the icon of the independent business person;

- The tonsorial arts have been a tradition in the United States of America since its inception;

- The time-honored tradition of the neighbor barbershop continues to grow and prosper.

Additionally, the organization proclaims the following objectives:

- To promote the exchange of information between state barber boards and state agencies examining, licensing, and regulating the barber industry.

- To develop standards and procedures for examining barbers.

- To develop standards for licensing and policing the barber industry.

- To develop curriculum for educating barbers.

- To promote continuous education in the barber industry.

- To develop and promote procedures for insuring that the consumer is informed and protected.

Consider the State of Barbering Today

After reading this section, you will be able to:

LO ④ Recognize the resurgence of barbering in the twenty-first century and the wealth of opportunities available to the new barber.

In this chapter we discussed the progression of barbering from prehistory through the regulatory agencies of the twentieth century (Table 1-1). As a profession, barbering has risen from its localized tribal beginnings to provide indispensable haircutting, styling, and shaving services across the globe. Barbers have served as surgeons, dentists, and wigmakers. The profession has been shaped by advances in technology throughout the centuries (see Table 1-2 on page 20), from the earliest shears to the manual clippers of the nineteenth century to the high-quality electric tools and social media available today. Barbers have continuously had to respond to trends and political developments in order to maintain their profession and their livelihoods. Some of these changes have presented challenges—kings who mandated the wearing of wigs, for example—while others have served the profession in beneficial ways. Some noteworthy improvements to barbering over the past century include the following:

- Implementation of regulatory and educational standards
- Improved hygiene and cleaning practices in the barbershop
- Availability and use of better implements and tools
- Mandatory study of anatomy dealing with the head, face, and neck
- Study of products and preparations used in facial, scalp, and hair treatments

As a student of barbering, you are now a member of this profession with its long and established history, the past 50 years of which has experienced more change than what a history of organizations and standards alone suggests.

The 1940s and 1950s represented the heyday for American barbershops, with many men visiting their neighborhood shops every two weeks to maintain a clean-cut appearance. However, February 9, 1964, marked a symbolic but critical turning point in the barbering industry. On that night in New York City, the British boy band The Beatles appeared on *The Ed Sullivan Show*, helping cement the cultural and social bedrock of a long-hair revolution for men in America and the world. This revolution in style also linked various political movements—the hippy subculture, resistance to the Vietnam War—with hair left longer and shaggier. Barbers' services, while still needed during and after the 1960s, were called upon less through the coming decades, as standards of male grooming relaxed and the skills required to cut longer hair were more readily found with hairstylists. Barbershop culture itself also became less attractive to younger generations of men, associated as it was with the conservatism of their parents' generation.

As longer hairstyles became more mainstream and less associated with social or political ideologies, there was a rise of unisex salons starting in the 1980s, which further threatened the livelihood of barbers, pulling clients away with the offer of fast and cheap hair services. On the other end of the spectrum, full-service salons and spas rocketed in popularity in the 1990s, drawing even more men away from barbershops. So diluted did the profession seem to have become around this time that some states chose to move away from barber-specific licenses, in favor of general cosmetology licensing.

However, after the turn of the century, a resurgence in barbering took place: New schools opened in many states, along with new barbershops, both independent and franchised. The salons and spas of the 1990s had lost their attractiveness, and barbershops could offer an atmosphere more geared to the male consumer—though that should not discount the diversity that barbering had been gaining since the 1950s. According to the National Barber Museum, by 1985, over half of all barbering students were women. Even today, the number of female clients continues to climb, with some shops claiming as many as 30 percent of clients being women. Economic fluctuations further helped barbershops rebound in the 2000s. By the recession of 2008, barbershops made up an attractive middle ground for consumers who could no longer afford high-end salons but were interested in more than what lower-end unisex shops offered.

Barbering has received an even stronger boost in recent years from the flourishing of an "art of manliness" and a reconsideration of what male style means. The grunge of the last decades has given way to a return of the dapper aesthetic, the clean lines and controlled styles of the 1940s and 1950s. This change has highlighted the importance of the barbershop in providing necessary upkeep. The year 2010 saw a massive return of beards and beard designs on young men, accompanied by a concern for facial grooming as part of a larger interest in cultivating personal style that includes hair, body art, clothing, and more. Creative young barbers have joined their peers in the profession in increasing numbers, with new barbers up 10 percent in two years. Barbershops have developed to reflect the interests of their barbers and clientele by paying homage to earlier periods and traditions of barbering while integrating advances in technology and new techniques into the shop environment.

The barbering world you are entering is as vibrant, diverse, and culturally relevant as the profession's long history suggests. Barbers are increasingly recognized for their creativity and their craft, and barbershops remain important pillars of their communities, both on the street and online. At the same time, while barbers today actively forge new traditions from old in the pursuit of style, it is important for them to remember their responsibilities—to protect the health, safety, and welfare of the public; to maintain and enhance standards; to continue the quest for knowledge; and to advance this great and lasting industry.

TABLE 1-1

HISTORY OF BARBERING TIMELINE

5000 BC   **2500 BC**   **1000 BC**   **500 BC**

5000 BC Barbering services first performed in Egypt.

1391–1271 BC Barbering becomes available to general populace of the Middle East by Moses' time.

595 BC The Biblical prophet Ezekiel writes of a "barber's razor."

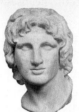

334 BC Alexander the Great prohibits the wearing of beards in battle, so shaving gains popularity.

© Kamira/Shutterstock.com.

1300   **1440**   **1600**

1163 Council of Tours prohibits clergy to draw blood or act as physicians; barber-surgeons assume medical duties of the clergy, including dentistry.

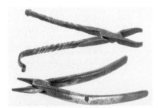

1308 Worshipful Company of Barbers guild founded in London, England; two groups formed: barbers who practiced barbering and those who practiced surgery.

1450 English surgeon and barber guilds merge and become the Company of Barber-Surgeons until 1745; barbers restricted to blood-letting, tooth pulling, cauterization, and tonsorial services.

1540 Henry VIII of England reunites the barbers and surgeons through an Act of Parliament to set up the Company of Barbers and Surgeons of London.

© Science & Society Picture Library/Contributor/SSPL/Getty Images.

1900   **1930**   **1940**

1893 A.B. Moler establishes America's first barber school in Chicago, Illinois.

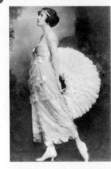

1915 Irene Castle, a well-known dancer, popularizes the "bob cut" for American women. Barbers must quickly meet demand.

1925 Associated Master Barbers of America establishes the National Education Council to improve and standardize barbering education.

1940–1949 Flat top, butch cut, crew cut, and Princeton cut become popular hairstyles.

© FPG/Staff/Archive Photos/Getty Images.

1985   **1988**   **1990**   **2000**

1985 Over 50% of barber students reported to be female.

1988 Ed Jeffers establishes Barber Museum in Canal Winchester, Ohio.

1995 Over 50% of barber students reported to be African American.

2000s Resurgence in barbering takes place; new schools open in many states; new barbershops, both independent and franchised, combine traditional skills with an atmosphere geared to the male consumer.

100 BC | 1 AD | 1000

296 BC According to Pliny, barbering and shaving were introduced to Rome by Ticinius Mena.

100 BC–100 AD Being clean shaven is a rule in Rome.

30–325 Barbers practice shaving throughout Europe and assist the physician-clergy until the twelfth century (1100s).

1096 William, Archbishop of Rouen (France), prohibits wearing of beards; barber-surgeons travel and practice throughout Europe.

1800 | 1850 | 1860

1745 Surgeons again separate from barbers and form the Company of Surgeons (becomes Royal College of Surgeons in 1800); complete separation of barbers from surgeons enacted by law; barbers keep the barber pole as the sign of their profession.

1750–1850 Wigs in vogue in Europe and worn in the American colonies by the upper classes; barbers add wigmaking and maintenance to tonsorial services.

1848 Disappearance of bloodletting equipment from most doctors' satchels.

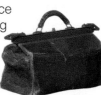

1861–1899 American Civil War (1861 to 1865); beards become popular; barbershops established in towns by English, French, German, and Italian immigrants.

1970 | 1980

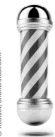

1959 Edmond "Pop" O. Roffler develops the Roffler Sculptur-Kut based on European razor-cutting techniques; still used today.

1964 The Beatles arrive in New York City to appear on *The Ed Sullivan Show*. Social and cultural influences set the stage for the "long-hair revolution" of the 1960s and beyond.

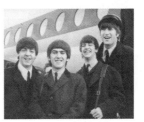

1980s Some states move away from barber-specific licenses in favor of general cosmetology licensing. Unisex salons pull clients away from barbershops, along with popularity of full-service salons and spas in 1990s.

2050

2008 Recession further drives consumers away from high-end spas and to mid-range barbershops; women make up 30% of barber clientele.

2010s Reemergence of beards on young men and investment in art of male upkeep has barbering booming: number of new barbers up by 10% in two years. Large-scale "barber battle" competitions grow in popularity.

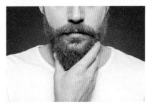

TABLE 1-2

HISTORY OF SHEARS AND CLIPPERS TIMELINE

4000	3000	2000	1000	0

700,000–600,000 BC Stone Age: early cutting tools of bone, flint, antler, and shell are produced.

3000–2000 BC Earliest known scissors appear in Middle East.

3000–1200 BC Bronze Age: the process of smelting is developed.

1300–900 BC Iron Age: smelting processes and metallurgy are refined.

800–700 BC Greek barbers from Messina introduce shears to Rome for cutting hair.

Courtesy Manx National Heritage.

1	1000	1800

1–100 AD Cross-bladed shears developed in Rome.

400–500 Cross-bladed shears developed with center pivot in Rome.

1850–1890 Nikola Bizumic, Serbian barber, invents manual hair clippers.

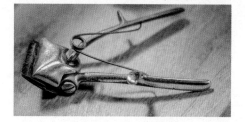

© bookzaa/Shutterstock.com.

1920	1930

1919 Leo J. Wahl invents first practical electric hair clippers; Wahl Clipper Corporation incorporated in 1921.

1921 Matthew Andis Sr. develops own model of an electric clipper and sells it door to door to barbershops; opens Andis Company in 1922.

1924 John Oster markets a hand-driven hair clipper for women's hair; his motorized clipper follows in 1928.

REVIEW QUESTIONS

1. What is the origin of the word *barber*?

2. Which country is credited with being the first to develop barbering as an art?

3. What are the characteristics sometimes associated with the wearing of a beard?

4. What is a *tonsure*?

5. What were the duties of the barber-surgeons?

6. What is the origin of the modern barber pole?

7. What were the names for the barbering employer and employee organizations?

8. Which state was the first to pass a barber's license law, and in what year was it passed?

9. What is the primary function of state barber boards?

10. What is the name of the national organization under which state barber boards function?

CHAPTER GLOSSARY

A.B. Moler	p. 18	in 1893 established America's first barber school in Chicago, Illinois
AMBBA	p. 15	Associated Master Barbers and Beauticians of America
barba	p. 8	Latin for beard
barber pole	p. 12	symbol of Barbering that evolved from the technical procedures of bloodletting performed by barber-surgeons
barber-surgeons (BAR-bur SIR-genz)	p. 11	early practitioners who cut hair, shaved, and performed bloodletting and dentistry
Journeymen barber groups (JUHR-knee-men BAR-bur GROOPS)	p. 13	organizations formed to represent barber employees prior to the establishment of barber licensing laws
master barber groups	p. 13	employer organizations formed prior to the establishment of barber licensing laws
Meryma'at (mare-a-mott)	p. 7	Egyptian barber commemorated with a statue
NABBA	p. 15	National Association of Barber Boards of America
Ticinius Mena (ti-cin-i-us me-nah)	p. 8	Sicilian credited with bringing barbering and shaving to Rome in 296 BC
tonsorial (TON-SORE-ee-ahl)	p. 8	related to the cutting, clipping, or trimming of hair with shears or a razor
tonsure (TON-shur)	p. 9	a shaved patch on the head

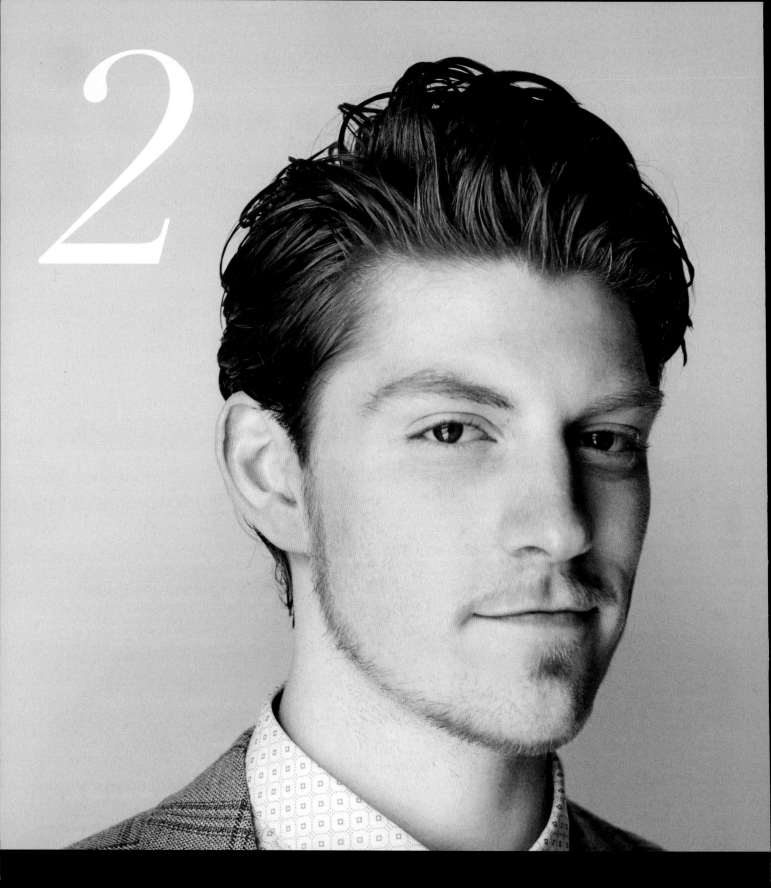

2

LIFE SKILLS

LEARNING OBJECTIVES

After completing this chapter, you will be able to:

LO❶
List the life skills to put into action.

LO❷
List the principles that contribute to personal and professional success.

LO❸
Create a mission statement.

LO❹
Explain long-term and short-term goals.

LO❺
Discuss the most effective ways to manage time.

LO❻
Demonstrate good study habits.

LO❼
Define ethics.

LO❽
List the characteristics of a healthy, positive attitude.

Introduction

While good technical skills are extremely important to master, learning and applying sound life skills is just as important. Barbering is a creative profession, where you are expected to exercise your artistic talent. To be successful in a barbershop environment, you need to have well-developed communication, decision-making, image-building, customer service, self-actualization, goal-setting, and time management skills. These life skills are the foundation of success for students and professionals. In addition, developing effective study skills will help you achieve your educational and professional goals.

why study
LIFE SKILLS?

Barbers should study and have a thorough understanding of life skills because:

> Practicing good life skills will lead to a more satisfying and productive career in the industry. Barbering professionals work with many types of clients and coworkers; having good life skills can help ensure positive interactions with others in any situation.

> The ability to deal with difficult circumstances comes from having well-developed life skills.

> Having good life skills builds self-esteem, which helps individuals achieve their goals.

Life Skills in Action

After reading this section, you will be able to:

LO **1** List the life skills to put into action.

Life skills are those day-to-day actions and skills that help you to be a productive and well-rounded person. Some of the most important life skills for you to remember and practice include the following:

- Being helpful and caring to others
- Making good friends
- Feeling good about yourself
- Having a sense of humor
- Maintaining a cooperative attitude
- Approaching work with a strong sense of responsibility
- Being consistent in your work
- Adapting successfully to different situations

- Sticking to a goal and seeing a job through to completion
- Mastering techniques to become more organized
- Developing sound decision-making skills

Interpret the Psychology of Success

After reading this section, you will be able to:

LO List the principles that contribute to personal and professional success.

Success has been defined in many ways over the years and the definition varies from person to person. What is your definition of success? Take a few minutes to think about your answer and write it down. The process of **self-actualization**, fulfilling one's full potential, requires lifelong commitment. Stay the course and fuel your passion by following proven success-building steps.

ACTION STEPS FOR SUCCESS

Being successful in life requires hard work and effort. Continually focusing on the following action steps will create a solid foundation for achieving your goals:

- **Build self-esteem.** Self-esteem is based on inner strength and begins with trusting your ability to achieve set goals. It is essential that you begin developing high self-esteem while you are in school. Reading positive affirmations is a great way to start building your self-esteem.

- **Visualize success.** Constantly imagine yourself working in your dream shop. You are competently handling clients, loving the job and the environment. The more you practice visualization, the more easily you will turn your vision into reality.

- **Build on your strengths.** Practice doing whatever helps you maintain a positive self-image. If you are good at doing something (e.g., playing the guitar, running, cooking, gardening, or singing), the time you invest in that activity will allow you to feel good about yourself. Remember that there may be things you are good at that you do not realize. You may be a good listener, for instance, or a caring and considerate friend.

- **Be kind to yourself.** This action step may be the hardest but it is the most important one for success. Eliminate self-critical or negative thoughts, which are counterproductive. If you make a mistake, view it as a learning opportunity to improve yourself and get it right the next time.

- **Stay true to yourself.** Be yourself and be professional! It takes too much time and effort to be someone that you are not. Being unique is a valuable asset.

- **Practice new behaviors.** Because achieving success is a skill, you can develop it by practicing positive new behaviors, such as speaking with confidence, standing tall, and using proper grammar.

- **Keep your personal life separate from your work.** Talking about your personal life at work is counterproductive and can cause the whole shop to suffer. Try to separate your work life from your home life and develop a healthy work–life balance.

- **Keep your energy up.** Successful barbers take care of themselves. Get the proper amount of sleep, eat healthy foods, and manage your time wisely. Also, create balance by spending time with family and friends, having hobbies, and enjoying recreational activities (Figure 2-1).

- **Respect others.** Make a conscious effort to respect everyone. Exercise good manners with others by using words such as *please, thank you,* and *excuse me.* Practice being a good listener and remember not to interrupt others when they are speaking.

- **Stay productive.** There are three bad habits that can keep you from maintaining peak performance: (1) procrastination, (2) perfectionism, and (3) lack of a game plan. You will see an almost instant improvement in your productivity when you eliminate these troublesome tendencies.

  1. **Procrastination** (PRO-crass-tin-aye-shun) is putting off until tomorrow what you can do today. (For example, I will study tomorrow instead of today.) This thought process may be attributed to scheduling too many tasks at one time, which is a symptom of faulty organization.
  2. **Perfectionism** (PUR-fek-shun-izm) is an unhealthy compulsion to do things perfectly. Success is not defined as doing everything perfectly. As long as you learn from your mistakes, you will be successful. In fact, someone who never makes a mistake may not be taking the necessary risks for growth and improvement.
  3. Having a **game plan** is the conscious act of planning your life, instead of just letting things happen. While an overall game plan is usually organized into large blocks of time (5 or 10 years), it is just as important to set daily, monthly, and yearly goals. Where do you want to be in your career five years from now? What do you have to do this week, this month, and this year to move closer to that goal?

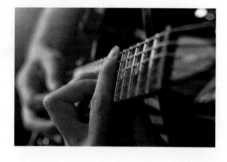

figure 2-1
Make time for your hobbies and personal interests.

MILADYPRO LEARN
Optional info on **goal setting** can be found at MiladyPro.com; keyword: *FutureBarberPro.*

© Danil Nevsky/Shutterstock.com.

MOTIVATION AND SELF-MANAGEMENT

Starting something new can be both exciting and intimidating. For example, many new students feel nervous about starting barbering school. Whatever the emotions you may feel, motivation and self-management skills will help you move to the next level in your career. To achieve success, you need more than an external push; you must feel a sense of personal excitement and have a good reason for staying the course. You are the one in charge of managing your own life and learning. To achieve this goal successfully, use creativity.

YOUR CREATIVE CAPABILITY

Creativity means having a talent such as painting, acting, playing an instrument, writing, or cutting hair (**Figure 2-2**). Creativity is also an unlimited inner resource of ideas and solutions. To enhance your creativity, keep these guidelines in mind:

- **Be positive.** Criticism blocks the creative mind from exploring ideas and discovering solutions to challenges.

- **Look around for creative inspiration.** Tap into the creative energy of art museums, music, hair shows, and magazines.

- **Improve your vocabulary.** Build a positive vocabulary by using active problem-solving words such as *explore, analyze,* and *determine*.

- **Surround yourself with others who share your passion.** In today's hectic and pressured world, many talented people find that they are more creative in an environment where people work together and share ideas. This is where the value of a strong team comes into play.

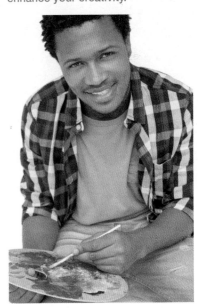

figure 2-2
Painting is one way to express and enhance your creativity.

Design a Mission Statement

After reading this section, you will be able to:

LO **3**   Create a mission statement.

An essential part of business is the **mission statement** (MISH-uhn STATE-ment), which establishes the purpose and values for which an individual or institution lives and works by. It provides a sense of direction by defining guiding principles and clarifying goals, as well as indicating how an organization operates. Often, you will find the mission statement of a company posted for customers to read. Look for a mission statement next time you are in a hotel, fast-food restaurant, or any other service-related business. The mission often becomes more than just a statement. It becomes the cultural pulse for organizations. A well-thought-out sense of purpose in the form of a mission statement will also help individuals on their journey to success.

Create a mission statement by beginning with your interests. We have created a tool, the Interests Self-Test, to help you get started (see **Figure 2-3**).

Next, try to prepare a mission statement in one or two sentences that communicates who you are and what you want for your life. One example of a simple, yet thoughtful, mission statement is: "I am dedicated to pursuing a successful career with dignity, honesty, and integrity." Your mission statement will lead you in the right direction and help you feel secure when things temporarily go off course. For reinforcement, keep a copy of your mission statement where you can see it, and read it frequently.

figure 2-3
The Interests Self-Test.

The Interests Self-Test

Your personality is tied to your interests. As a barber, you may decide to specialize in one or more service areas to build your reputation and clientele. This quick quiz gives you an idea of where your future might lie, based on your personal preferences.

1. Which subject interests you most?
  A. Chemistry   **B.** Geometry   **C.** Accounting

2. Which of the following would you rather do?
  A. Analyze a problem   **B.** Solve a problem   **C.** Read about a problem

3. When you look at a painting, what do you notice first?
  A. Color   **B.** Shape   **C.** Details

4. When it comes to coworkers, would you prefer to:
  A. Work with one other person on a specific problem   **C.** Work alone or tell teammates what to do
  B. Work with a team to get lots of ideas

5. When it comes to shop clients, do you think they:
  A. Know exactly what they want, and that's good   **C.** Probably want a good value
  B. Are open to new ideas and suggestions, which is fun

Instructions: Add up the number of As, Bs, and Cs. Then check below to see what might be of most interest to you.

Mostly As. All of the chemical services, perms, relaxers, and hair coloring involve chemistry, detail work, and solving specific problems, which might be a good choice for you. You will need strong fundamentals and a mind for detail to know how to get from point A (their natural texture or color) to point B (their desired texture or color).

Mostly Bs. Haircutting involves an understanding of geometry, lines, and shapes. Clients may want a certain look but their hair density or texture may not allow it. That's why the ability to gather ideas and make suggestions is important. At the advanced level, there are different elevations and techniques that can be combined to create new styles.

Mostly Cs. Business demands an attention to details, the ability to crunch numbers, and an understanding of the client's desires and consumer trends. While you sometimes work alone, you also have to be able to manage other people, which is an additional consideration. If you like taking responsibility for yourself and others, you might consider focusing on the business aspects of barbershops.

Set Goals

After reading this section, you will be able to:

LO**4** Explain long-term and short-term goals.

DID YOU KNOW?

Real-Life Goal Setting:

Many real-life, daily examples of goal setting can be found at MiladyPro.com.

Do you have direction, drive, desire, and a dream? If so, do you have a reasonable idea of how to go about meeting your goal(s)?

Goal setting is the identification of long-term and short-term goals. When you know what you want, you can draw a circle around your destination and chart the best course to get there. By mapping out your goals, you will see where to focus your attention in order to fulfill your dreams.

HOW GOAL SETTING WORKS

When setting goals, categorize them based on the amount of time it takes to accomplish the goals. An example of a short-term goal is to get through an exam successfully. Another short-term goal is to graduate from barbering school. Short-term goals are usually those that are to be accomplished in a year or less.

Long-term goals are measured in larger increments of time, such as 2, 5, 10 years, or even longer. An example of a long-term goal is becoming a barbershop owner in 5 years.

Once you have organized your thoughts, write them down in short-term and long-term columns and divide each set of goals into workable segments. Now the goals will not seem out of sight or overwhelming. For example, if you are a part-time barbering student, one of your long-term goals should be to become a licensed barber. At first, getting this license might seem to require an overwhelming amount of time and effort. However, when larger aspirations are divided into short-term goals (such as going to class on time, completing homework assignments, and mastering techniques), you would find that accomplishing each short-term goal leads progressively to the accomplishment of the larger goal.

Remember to set feasible goals, to create a plan of action, and to revisit the plan often. While adjusting goals and action plans may be necessary from time to time, successful people know that focusing on their goals will move them toward additional successes (**Figures 2-4** and **2-5**).

+ **FOCUS ON**

The Goal

Determine whether your goal-setting plan is effective by asking yourself these key questions:

- Are there specific skills I will need to learn in order to meet my goals?
- Is the information I need to reach my goals readily available?
- Am I willing to seek out a mentor or a coach to enhance my learning?
- What is the best method or approach that will allow me to accomplish my goals?
- Am I open to finding better ways of putting my plan into practice?

figure 2-4
A sample of how to set and track short-term goals.

HOW TO SET AND TRACK SHORT-TERM GOALS

Number	Goal Setting Checklist	Completion Date	Done
1.	Read this chapter. Action Steps: Read first part at lunch; finish it after dinner.	6/09/2016	✓
2.	Practice speaking to clients in a pleasing voice. Action Steps: Do with family tonight.	6/10/2016	✓
3.	Create my own mission statement. Action Steps: Review sample in this chapter; write my own.	6/15/2016	✓
4.	Start learning trends. Action Steps: Search online, read trade and beauty magazines. Make a five-word "trend list."	6/20/2016	✓
5.	Prepare to pass the Chapter 2 exam. Action Steps: Review what I read, ask instructor any questions, have study session with two friends.	7/10/2016	✓
6.	Practice being on time! Action Steps: Set alarm for 15 minutes earlier. Give self $1 every time I get to class 10 minutes early.	Start 6/20 5 days in a row by 7/20	
7.	Build my vocabulary. Action Steps: Buy book or find website. Learn one new word a day.	Daily	

figure 2-5
Photocopy the template shown and fill in your own goals.

MY GOALS

Number	Goal Setting Checklist	Completion Date	Done
1.			
2.			
3.			
4.			
5.			
6.			
7.			

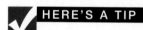
HERE'S A TIP

Real-Life Time Management

In a barbershop environment, it takes team effort to efficiently manage time. Barbershops book appointments based on the types of services being provided, the clientele, and the shop type. Some shops operate without setting appointments, and instead work on a walk-in or first-come-first-serve basis. Both methods require barbers to practice effective communication with fellow barbers and peers.

Making sure that you arrive on time, starting work with your first client as soon as the client arrives, and staying on schedule will take you a long way toward success as a barber. The front desk and shop manager can be a tremendous help if you find yourself falling behind or if you have the opportunity to add on an additional service and need help fitting it into your day. With experience, you will learn to accommodate late clients and add-on services like a pro.

Demonstrate Time Management

After reading this section, you will be able to:

LO❺ Discuss the most effective ways to manage time.

Effectively managing your time will help you reach your goals more quickly. Here are some ways you can be more effective at time management:

- Learn to **prioritize** (PRIH-or-uh-tize) by ordering tasks on your to-do list from most important to least important.

- When designing your time management system, make sure it will work for you. For example, if you are a person who needs a fair amount of flexibility, schedule some blocks of unstructured time.

- Never take on more than you can handle. Learn to say "no" firmly but kindly, and mean it. It will be easier to complete tasks if activities are limited.

- Learn problem-solving techniques that will save you time and needless frustration.

- Give yourself some downtime whenever you are frustrated, overwhelmed, worried, or feeling guilty. You lose valuable time and energy when you are in a negative state of mind. Unfortunately, there may be situations where you cannot get up and walk away. To handle these difficult times, try practicing the technique of deep breathing. Just fill your lungs as much as you can and exhale slowly. After about 5 to 10 breaths, you will usually find that you have calmed down and your inner balance has been restored.

- Have a notepad, organizer, tablet, or any other digital application accessible at all times.

- Make daily, weekly, and monthly schedules that show exam times, study sessions, and any other regular commitments. Plan leisure time around these commitments rather than the other way around (Figure 2-6).

- Identify times during the day when you are energetic and times when you want or need to relax. Plan your schedule accordingly.

- Reward yourself with a special treat or activity for work well done and efficient time management.

- Do not neglect physical activity. Remember that exercise and recreation stimulate clear thinking.

- Schedule at least one block of free time each day. This free time will be your hedge against events that happen unexpectedly, such as car trouble, child-care problems, helping a friend in need, or other unforeseen circumstances.

- Understand the value of to-do lists for the day and the week. These lists help prioritize tasks and activities, a key element to organizing time efficiently (Figure 2-7).

- Make effective time management a habit.

Employ Successful Learning Tools

After reading this section, you will be able to:

LO ❻ Demonstrate good study habits.

Having a successful career as a professional barber begins by employing key learning tools while in school. To realize the greatest benefits education can provide, commit yourself to doing the following:

- Attend all classes.
- Arrive for class early.
- Have all necessary materials ready.
- Listen attentively to your instructor.
- Take notes.
- Highlight important points.
- Pay close attention during summary and review sessions.
- When something is not clear, ask for clarification. If you are still unsure, ask again for assistance (Figure 2-8).

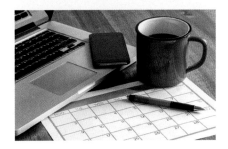
figure 2-6
Schedules help keep track of your commitments—exam times, study sessions, work shifts, and so on.

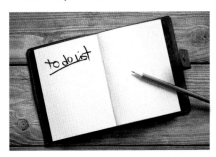
figure 2-7
To-do lists prioritize tasks and activities.

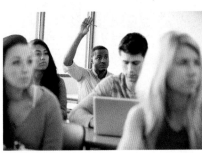
figure 2-8
Do not be afraid to ask for help.

Everyone learns in their own personal and unique ways. Your study skills should utilize the methods or tools that will help you absorb and retain new information. Learning all of the study skills available will help you find what works best for you and make valuable use of your time.

REPETITION

Whether you repeat information in your head, say it out loud, write it down, or practice it hands-on, **repetition** helps your short-term memory secure a firmer grasp on the information, making the information easier to retrieve when you need it.

ORGANIZATION

Organization can be used to process new information for both short-term and long-term memory use. If a new topic seems particularly overwhelming, categorize the information into smaller segments. For example, rather than trying to learn about all the layers of skin at once, study and learn about one skin division at a time.

MNEMONICS

A **mnemonic** (NEW-mon-ick) is a device that helps you remember or recall information; they can be word associations, acronyms, songs or rhymes, or any other form of memory trigger that helps you to recall information.

Word Associations

To promote better long-term memory, try to associate new information with prior knowledge by using word association techniques. For example, the outermost layer of the epidermis is the stratum corneum. It is also known as the horny layer because it consists of tightly packed cells that are similar to an animal's horn or hoof. The outer cells are continually shed and replaced with new cells from the underlying layers of the epidermis. In this example, *corn* in *corneum* rhymes with *horn*, providing an easy way to remember both technical and alternate terminology.

Using word associations can be helpful for remembering most information but be sure to create associations that mean something to you. Meaningful associations will assist you in actually learning the material and make it easier for you to retrieve from your long-term memory when you need it.

Acronyms

Acronyms are created by using the first letters in a series of words (Figure 2-9). For example, the functions of the skin can be remembered by using the word SHAPES—sensation, heat regulation, absorption, protection, excretion, and secretion. SHAPES is a particularly good acronym because the skin also gives shape to the body.

Songs or Rhymes

Songs or rhymes do not have to be complicated. Something as simple as "keep the air and the hair moving when blowdrying" to prevent burning the client's scalp or "rock 'n roll rodding creates a spiral perm" to illustrate a rodding technique can be effective reminders during application procedures.

© Gustov Frazao/Shutterstock.com.

figure 2-9
Acronyms connect related ideas and make them more memorable.

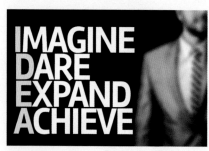

VISUAL STUDY SKILLS

For some, the need to visually lay out thoughts, plans, and ideas is key to retaining information. For these learners, the more visual study skills of mind mapping and note taking can be effective learning tools.

Mind Mapping

Mind mapping (MYND MAP-ing) is a method you can use to create a visual representation of your thoughts, ideas, or class notes (**Figure 2-10**). Here are some basic guidelines for mind mapping a topic:

- Write the main topic or problem in the center of a piece of paper.
- Think about the topic and allow your ideas to flow.
- Write down key words or ideas that come to mind.
- Use lines to connect the key words to the main topic.
- Expand on the key words by creating new connections to additional thoughts or information.
- Use colors and/or symbols to highlight important information.

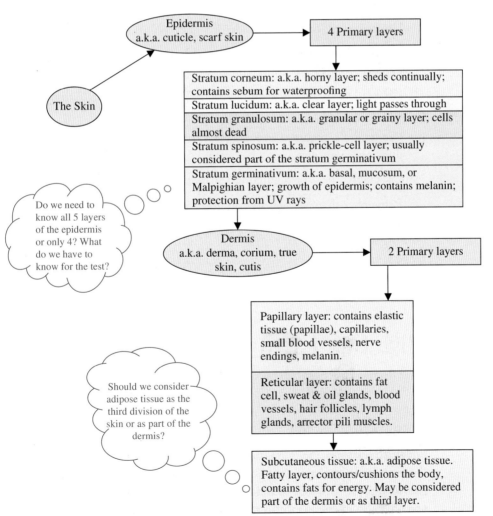

figure 2-10
Mind mapping skin divisions and layers.

Taking Notes

Note taking is a valuable skill to develop for studying and working in the business world. Effective note takers listen carefully and pay attention to verbal cues that alert them to important information. When taking notes, listen and watch for these cues:

- The speaker emphasizes words or phrases.
- You hear a directive, such as "You need to know" or "You might want to remember."
- The speaker uses definitive words such as *main* or *first* that provide the importance or the order of something.
- If it gets written on the board, it is usually important.

Although most of us develop our own way of taking notes, here are some general tips to get you started. Remember, you need to take notes in a way that makes sense to you and that will help you make the most of the process.

- Develop or select a note-taking template that works best for the way you like to organize new information.
- Date and number the note pages for easier organization when you need to review them.
- Listen carefully to lesson introductions and summaries.
- Use key words or phrases to identify main points.
- Use complete and accurate sentences when the instructor says "You need to know …" or "This is important" or when technical definitions are used.
- Use marks or symbols to emphasize important words, definitions, and so on.
- Use symbols, pictures, and diagrams to create visual reminders or to illustrate a concept.
- Use colored pens or highlighters to emphasize important points.

Remember that every effort you make to follow through on your education is an investment in your future. The progress you make with your learning will increase your confidence. In fact, when you have mastered a range of information and techniques, your self-esteem will soar right along with your grades.

Practice Ethical Standards

After reading this section, you will be able to:

LO ⑦ Define ethics.

Ethics (ETH-iks) are the moral principles by which we live and work. In a shop setting, ethical standards should guide your conduct with clients and fellow employees. When your actions are respectful, courteous, and helpful, you are behaving in an ethical manner.

Practice ethical behavior in the barbershop by employing these five professional actions:

- Provide skilled and competent services

- Be honest, courteous, and sincere

- Avoid sharing clients' private matters with others—even your closest friends

- Participate in continuing education and staying on track with new information, techniques, and skills

- Give clients accurate information about treatments and products

PROFESSIONAL ETHICS

To be an ethical person, you need to embody the following qualities:

- **Self-care.** To be helpful to others, it is essential to take care of yourself. Try the Self-Care Test to assess how you are doing (**Figure 2-11**).

- **Integrity.** Maintain your integrity by aligning your behavior and actions to your values. For example, recommending products that clients do not really need is unethical behavior. On the other hand, if you feel that a client would benefit from certain products and additional services, it would be unethical not to give the client that information.

figure 2-11
Self-Care Test.

The Self-Care Test

Some people know intuitively when they need to stop, take a break, or even take a day off. Other people forget when to eat. You can judge how well you take care of yourself by noting how you feel physically, emotionally, and mentally. Here are some questions to ask yourself to see how you rate on the self-care scale.

1. Do you wait until you are exhausted before you stop working?
2. Do you forget to eat nutritious food and substitute junk food on the fly?
3. Do you say you will exercise and then put off starting a program?
4. Do you have poor sleep habits?
5. Are you constantly nagging yourself about not being good enough?
6. Are your relationships with people filled with conflict?
7. When you think about the future are you unclear about the direction you will take?
8. Do you spend most of your spare time watching TV?
9. Have you been told you are too stressed and yet you ignore these concerns?
10. Do you waste time and then get angry with yourself?

Score 5 points for each yes. A score of 0–15 says that you take pretty good care of yourself, but you would be wise to examine those questions you answered yes to. A score of 15–30 indicates that you need to rethink your priorities. A score of 30–50 is a strong statement that you are neglecting yourself and may be headed for high stress and burnout. Reviewing the suggestions in this chapter will help you get back on track.

- **Discretion.** Do not share your personal issues with clients. Likewise, never breach confidentiality by repeating personal information that clients have shared with you.

- **Communication.** Your responsibility to behave ethically extends to your communications with customers and coworkers. Be aware of what you say and how you say it. Also, be conscious of your nonverbal communications, such as facial expressions or body language, which are just as important as verbal communication.

Develop a Positive Personality and Attitude

After reading this section, you will be able to:

LO**8**   List the characteristics of a healthy, positive attitude.

Barbers interact with people from all walks of life—every day, all day. It is useful, therefore, to have a sense of how different personality traits work together. Refer regularly to the following characteristics of a healthy, positive attitude:

- **Diplomacy.** Being assertive is good because it helps people understand your position. However, it is a short step from being assertive to being aggressive or even bullying. Take your attitude temperature to see how well you practice the art of diplomacy. Diplomacy—also known as tact—is the ability to deliver truthful, even sometimes critical or difficult, messages in a kind way.

- **Pleasing tone of voice.** The tone of your voice is a personality trait, but if your natural voice is harsh or if you tend to mumble, you can consciously improve by speaking more softly or more clearly. Another technique is to smile when speaking if it is appropriate. Smiling will help the tone of your voice, so practice it when speaking in person and when talking on the phone.

- **Emotional stability.** Learning how to handle a confrontation and how to share your feelings in a professional manner is important to building emotional stability and control (**Figure 2-12**).

- **Sensitivity.** Being sensitive means being compassionate and responsive to other people.

- **Values and goals.** Values and goals guide our behavior and give us direction.

- **Receptivity.** Be interested in other people and responsive to their opinions, feelings, and ideas. Receptivity involves taking the time to really listen to others. Also, be open minded and willing to work with all personality types.

- **Effective communication skills.** Commit to practicing effective communication through active listening, nonverbal, and verbal skills.

figure 2-12
Emotional stability plays a key part in successfully handling confrontations.

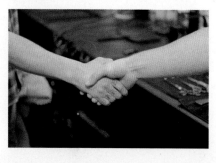

© Dmytro Zinkevych/Shutterstock.com.

REVIEW QUESTIONS

1. What principles contribute to personal and professional success?

2. How do you create a mission statement? Give an example.

3. How do you go about setting long-term and short-term goals?

4. What are some of the most effective ways to manage time?

5. How do you describe good study habits?

6. What are some learning tools you should use while studying?

7. What is the definition of ethics?

8. What are the characteristics of a healthy, positive attitude?

CHAPTER GLOSSARY

ethics (ETH-iks)	p. 34	the moral principles by which we live and work
game plan	p. 26	the conscious act of planning your life, instead of just letting things happen
goal setting	p. 28	the identification of long-term and short-term goals that helps you decide what you want out of your life
mind mapping (MYND MAP-ing)	p. 33	a graphic representation of an idea or problem that helps organize one's thoughts
mission statement (MISH-uhn STATE-ment)	p. 27	a statement that establishes the purpose and values for which an individual or institution lives and works by. It provides a sense of direction by defining guiding principles and clarifying goals, as well as how an organization operates
mnemonic (NEW-mon-ick)	p. 32	any memorization device that helps a person recall information
organization	p. 32	a method used to store new information for short-term and long-term memory
perfectionism (PUR-fek-shun-izm)	p. 26	an unhealthy compulsion to do things perfectly
prioritize (PRIH-or-uh-tize)	p. 30	to make a list of tasks that need to be done in the order of most-to-least important
procrastination (PRO-crass-tin-aye-shun)	p. 26	putting off until tomorrow what you can do today
repetition	p. 32	repeatedly saying, writing, or otherwise reviewing new information until it is learned
self-actualization	p. 25	fulfilling one's full potential

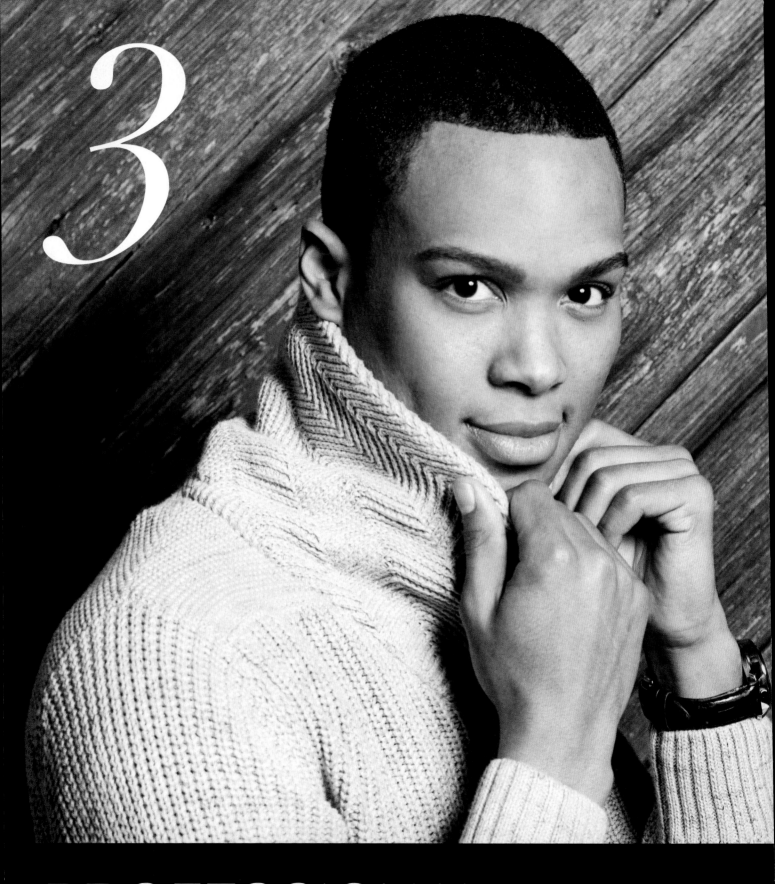

3

PROFESSIONAL
IMAGE

LEARNING OBJECTIVES

After completing this chapter, you will be able to:

LO❶
Name four important personal hygiene habits.

LO❷
Explain the concept of dressing for success.

LO❸
Practice ergonomically correct movement, postures, and principles.

LO❹
Demonstrate an understanding of human relations and communication skills.

figure 3-1
Put your best professional image
forward.

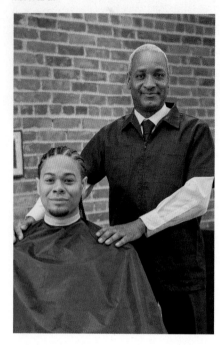

Introduction

Do you believe that first impressions are important? First impressions are often the gateway to obtaining a job interview, getting new customers, or building a professional image. Making a positive impact is essential when working in the business of personal style. Barbers are often held to higher image standards by clients because they view barbers as image experts. For this reason alone, it is vital to look and act your absolute best when in public because the image you project sets the standard for clients and peers in the workplace (Figure 3-1).

There are many factors that help create a professional image. However, for better or worse, how a person looks is often the first clue to determining if that person has what it takes to do the job. From there, professional behavior, a positive attitude, team camaraderie, proper ergonomics, and good communication skills all contribute to your total image.

why study
PROFESSIONAL IMAGE?

Barbers should study and have a thorough understanding of professional image because:

> Clients rely on barbers to look good and be well groomed. Having a professional image helps build trust with clients and leads to repeat business.

> Working in a barbershop whose culture complements your image standards and goals is important for career growth and achievements.

> Understanding ergonomics can help prevent health issues associated with poor working habits and help professionals to stay gainfully employed.

> There are consequences to not maintaining a professional image, including loss of clients, a poor reputation, and loss of income.

Apply Healthful Habits in Your Daily Routine

After reading this section, you will be able to:

LO**1**   Name four important personal hygiene habits.

In accordance with the general concept of a profession that helps others look their best, barbers should strive to present their own best image as well. An important part of this representation is the barber's personal health and physical appearance. To achieve success in this area, it is helpful to follow a set of guidelines that help maintain a healthy body and a healthy mind.

HYGIENE

Basic hygienic practices such as showering or bathing should never be omitted from daily personal care practices. **Personal hygiene** (pur-sun-AL HY-jene) is the daily maintenance of cleanliness by practicing good healthful habits. When working as a barber, you will be in close proximity to clients. One weak moment of drinking coffee right before performing a service, or wearing something that needs laundering because you did not plan ahead, could be disastrous. Rather than telling you that you smell offensive, most clients will simply not return and may tell others about their bad experience.

The following personal habits result in good hygiene throughout the day:

- Wash your hands throughout the day as required, including at the beginning of each service (**Figure 3-2**).

- Perform self-checks, and wash or freshen under the arms as needed.

- Brush and floss your teeth, and use mouthwash or breath mints throughout the day.

- If you smoke cigarettes, *do not* smoke during work hours. Many clients find the lingering smell of smoke offensive. If you smoke during your lunch break, brush your teeth, use mouthwash, and wash your hands afterward.

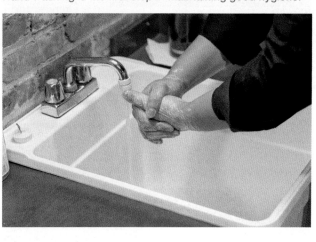

figure 3-2
Hand washing is the first step in maintaining good hygiene.

REST AND RELAXATION

Adequate sleep is essential for good health because without it you cannot function efficiently. The body needs to be allowed to recover from the fatigue of the day's activities and should be replenished with a good night's sleep. The amount of sleep needed to feel refreshed varies from person to person. Some people function well with 6 hours of sleep while others need 8 hours. An average of 7 or 8 hours of sleep each night is recommended by medical professionals. Relaxation is also important as a change of pace from day-to-day routines. Going to a movie or museum, reading a book, watching television, playing sports, or dancing are just some ways to escape and unwind. When you return to work, you should feel refreshed and eager to attend to your duties.

NUTRITION

What you eat affects your health, appearance, personality, and performance on the job. A balanced diet should include foods containing a variety of important vitamins and minerals (**Figure 3-3**). Drink plenty of water daily. Try to avoid sugar, salt, caffeine, and fatty or highly refined and processed foods.

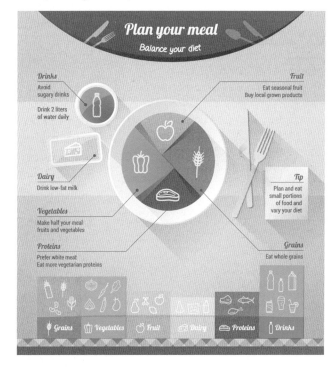

figure 3-3
Meal planning can help maintain a balanced diet.

Plan your meal
Balance your diet

Drinks
Avoid sugary drinks
Drink 2 liters of water daily

Fruit
Eat seasonal fruit
Buy local grown products

Dairy
Drink low-fat milk

Tip
Plan and eat small portions of food and vary your diet

Vegetables
Make half your meal fruits and vegetables

Proteins
Prefer white meat
Eat more vegetarian proteins

Grains
Eat whole grains

Grains   Vegetables   Fruit   Dairy   Proteins   Drinks

MILADYPRO LEARN MORE!

Optional info on **professionalism** can be found at MiladyPro.com; keyword: *FutureBarberPro*.

figure 3-4
Strive for harmony in your life.

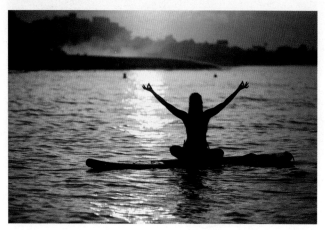

EXERCISE

Exercise and recreation in the form of walking, dancing, sports, and gym activities tend to develop the muscles and help keep the body fit. Regular physical activity benefits the body by improving blood circulation, oxygen supply, and proper organ function.

STRESS MANAGEMENT AND A HEALTHY LIFESTYLE

Stress is the inability to cope with a real or imagined threat that results in a series of mental and physical responses or adaptations. The way in which individuals perform under stressful situations depends on their temperament, physical health, and coping skills. Practice stress management through a combination of rest, relaxation, exercise, and daily routines that provide you with time to calm the body and its systems. Live a life of moderation in which work and other activities are balanced so that you can achieve a sense of harmony in your life (Figure 3-4).

Follow Image-Building Basics

After reading this section, you will be able to:

LO ❷ Explain the concept of dressing for success.

Being well groomed advertises a barber's commitment to the barbering industry. Consider yourself a representative of the profession and make sure to follow personal grooming habits and to practice professional behaviors. If you present a poised and attractive image, your clients will have confidence in you as a professional.

PERSONAL GROOMING

Many barbershop owners and managers view appearance and personality as being just as important as technical knowledge and skills. **Personal grooming** is the process of caring for parts of the body and maintaining an overall polished look. How you dress and how you take care of your hair, skin, and nails reflect your personal grooming habits.

Dress for Success

While working, your wardrobe selection should express a professional image that is consistent with the image of the barbershop (Figure 3-5). Your **professional image** (pruh-FESH-un-ul IM-aje) is the impression you project through both your outward appearance and your conduct in the workplace. Your clothes must be pressed and clean—not simply free of the dirt that you can see, but stain free, an objective that is sometimes difficult to achieve in a barbershop environment. Be mindful about spills and drips when using chemicals, and avoid leaning on counters in the work area—particularly in

⚠ CAUTION

Often barbershops have a no-fragrance policy for staff members because a significant number of people are sensitive or allergic to a variety of chemicals, including perfume oils. Whether or not your barbershop has a no-fragrance policy, cologne and perfume should not be worn at work.

© GaudiLab/Shutterstock.com.

Practice the following guidelines for maintaining a more stress-free standing posture behind the chair:

- Keep your head up and chin parallel to the floor.
- Keep your neck elongated and balanced directly above the shoulders.
- Lift your upper body so that your chest is up and out—do not slouch.
- Hold your shoulders level and relaxed.
- Stand with your spine straight.

Just as there is a mechanically correct posture for standing, there is also a correct sitting posture. Use the following guidelines to learn to sit correctly in a balanced position:

- Keep your hips level and horizontal, not tilted forward or backward.
- Flex your knees slightly and position them over your feet.
- Lower your body smoothly into a chair, keeping your back straight.
- Keep the soles of your feet on the floor directly under your knees.
- Have the seat of the chair even with your knees. This position will allow the upper and lower legs to form a 90-degree angle at the knees.
- Rest the weight of your torso on the thighbones, not on the end of the spine.
- Keep your torso erect.
- When sitting at a desk, make sure it is at the correct height so that the upper and lower parts of your arm form a right angle when you are writing.

BODY MOVEMENT

Your muscles and bones work together as a musculoskeletal system, allowing you to walk, raise your arms, and use your fingers. **Ergonomics** (UR-go-nom-icks) is the science of designing the workplace as well as its equipment and tools to make specific body movements more comfortable, efficient, and safe.

For example, a hydraulic chair can be raised or lowered to accommodate barbers of different heights, allowing each barber to service clients without bending over too far. Certain shears are designed to eliminate hand fatigue when cutting hair because repetitive movements are of particular concern.

Each year, hundreds of barbering professionals report musculoskeletal disorders, including carpal tunnel syndrome (a wrist injury) and back injuries (Figure 3-9). Barbers may have to stand or sit all day and perform repetitive movements, which makes them susceptible to problems of the hands, wrists, shoulders, neck, back, feet, and legs.

Prevention is the key to avoiding problems. An awareness of your posture and movements, coupled with good work habits, proper tools, and equipment, will enhance your health and comfort.

Ergonomics is important to your ability to work and your body's wellness. Repetitive motions have a cumulative effect on the muscles and joints.

figure 3-9
Common posture problems.

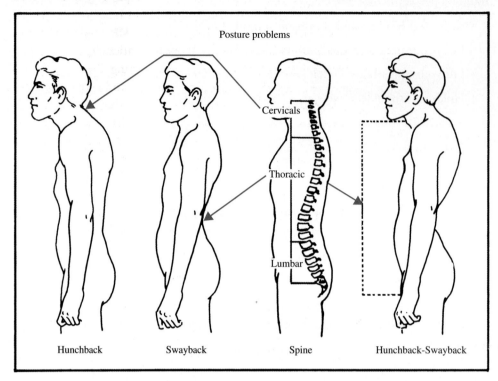

Posture problems

Cervicals

Thoracic

Lumbar

Hunchback   Swayback   Spine   Hunchback-Swayback

To avoid problems and work more effectively, practice some of the following suggestions:

- Do not grip or squeeze tools and implements too tightly.
- Do not bend the wrist up or down constantly when cutting hair or using a blowdryer (Figure 3-10).
- Try to position your arms at less than a 60-degree angle when holding your arms away from your body while working.
- Avoid bending forward and/or twisting your body to get closer to your client.
- Adjust the height of the chair so that the client's head is at a comfortable working level.
- Tilt the client's head as necessary for better access during hair services.

  To avoid ergonomic-related injuries, consider these further guidelines:

- Keep your wrists in a straight or neutral position as much as possible (Figure 3-11).
- Use ergonomically designed implements.
- Keep your back and neck straight.
- Stand on an antifatigue mat.
- When standing to cut hair, position your legs hip-width apart, bend your knees slightly, and align your pelvic area with your abdomen.

figure 3-10
Improper haircutting position.

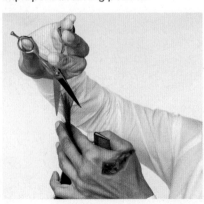

Counter the negative impact of repetitive motions or long periods spent in one position by stretching and walking around at intervals. Always put your well-being first.

figure 3-11
Correct wrist and hand position for haircutting.

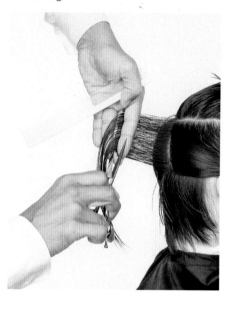

Activity

Practice these quick exercises to help you relieve stress from repetitive movements or from standing or sitting in one position for too long.

For Wrists

1. Stand up straight.
2. Raise both of your arms straight out.
3. Bend your wrists so your fingers point upward and hold for 5 seconds.
4. Hold your wrists steady and turn your hands, so your fingers face the floor and hold for 5 seconds.
5. Repeat the cycle five times.

For Fingers

1. Get a ball the size of a tennis ball or a tension ball.
2. Grip it tightly for a count of five. Release.
3. Repeat five times.

For Shoulders

1. Stand up straight and shrug your shoulders upward.
2. Roll your shoulders back and hold for a count of five.
3. Reverse direction and roll your shoulders forward for a count of five.
4. Repeat five times.

Practice Effective Human Relations and Communication Skills

After reading this section, you will be able to:

LO④ Demonstrate an understanding of human relations and communication skills.

figure 3-12
Treat clients with respect, empathy, and confidence.

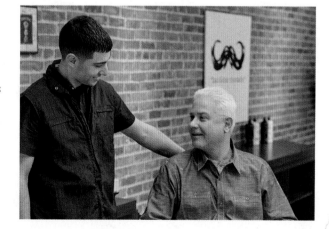

Human relations describes the interactions and relationships between two or more people. Effective human relations skills help you build rapport with clients and coworkers. Rapport involves establishing a close and empathetic relationship that fosters agreement and harmony between individuals. Your professional attitude is expressed through your self-esteem, confidence, and the respect you show others (**Figure 3-12**). Good habits and practices acquired during your education lay the foundation for a successful career in barbering.

The following guidelines for good human relations will help you gain confidence, deal courteously with others, and become a successful professional:

- Always greet clients by name, using a pleasant tone of voice. Address clients by their last name, as in "Mr. Jones" or "Mrs. Smith," unless the client prefers first names or it is customary to use first names in the barbershop.

- Be alert to the client's mood. Some clients prefer quiet and relaxation; others like to talk. Be a good listener and confine the conversation to the client's needs. Never gossip or tell off-color stories.

- Topics of conversation should be carefully chosen. Friendly relations are achieved through pleasant conversations. Let the client guide the topic of conversation. In a business setting, it is best to avoid such controversial topics as religion and politics, personal problems, or issues relating to other people. Never discuss other clients or coworkers, and always maintain an ethical standard of confidentiality. Never discuss personal wages, tips, rent, or tax information.

- Make a good impression by looking the part of the successful barber and by speaking and acting in a professional manner at all times.

- Cultivate self-confidence and project a pleasing personality.

- Show interest in the client's personal preferences and give the client undivided attention.

- Use tact when dealing with problems you may encounter.

- Deal with all disputes and differences in private. Take care of all problems promptly and to the client's satisfaction.

- Be capable and efficient.

- Be punctual. Arrive at work on time and keep appointments on schedule. Plan your day so that you have time to take breaks and enjoy a healthy lunch.

In addition to basic human relations skills, barbering students need to cultivate other aspects of a professional image that can impact their success in the profession. Some desirable qualities for effective client relations are the following:

figure 3-13
Recognize and control your emotions.

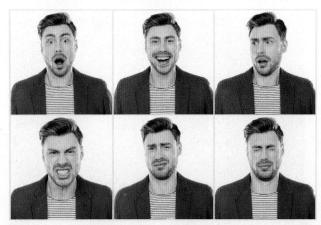

- **Talking less, listening more.** When you practice good listening skills, you are fully attentive to what the other person is saying. If there is something that you do not understand, ask questions to gain understanding.

- **Emotional control.** Learn to control your emotions. Try to respond rather than to react. Do not reveal negative emotions such as anger, envy, and dislike through gestures, facial expressions, or conversation. An even-tempered person is usually treated with respect (Figure 3-13).

- **Positive approach.** Be pleasant and gracious. Be ready with a smile of greeting and a word of welcome for each client and coworker. A good sense of humor is also important in maintaining a positive attitude.

- **Good manners.** Good manners reflect your thoughtfulness toward others. Treating others with respect, exercising care of other people's property, being tolerant and understanding of their shortcomings and efforts, and being considerate of those with whom you work all express good manners. Courtesy is one of the most important keys to a successful career.

- **Mannerisms.** Gum chewing and nervous habits such as tapping your foot or playing with your hair detract from the effectiveness of your image. Yawning, coughing, and sneezing should be concealed with your hand in front of your mouth. Control negative body language—sarcastic or disapproving facial grimaces, for example. Exhibiting pleasant mannerisms and attractive gestures and actions should be your goal at all times.

EFFECTIVE COMMUNICATION SKILLS

Communication is one of the barber's most important human relations skills. Communication includes listening skills, tone, speech, and conversational ability—all of which are necessary to forming satisfying relationships with customers and coworkers.

Effective communication (uh-FEK-tive COM-yun-ik-ay-shun) is the act of successfully sharing information between two people (or groups of people) so that the information is understood (**Figure 3-14**). In the barbershop, effective communication requires sending and receiving messages in order to establish a relationship with the client. The following steps can be used to help you determine your clients' service expectations.

- **Organize your thoughts.** What question or information do you want your client to understand? For example, a client with medium-length hair that covers the top part of the ears says he wants a trim. You will need to determine just what the client's definition of a trim is and may ask if he wants the tops of his ears covered or not.

- **Clarify.** The next step is to clarify what the client is telling you. In the preceding scenario, let's say the client's response to the question is that he wants his hair "over the ears." This answer still does not provide you with the information you need to proceed with the haircut. Why? Because you now have to clarify what the client means by "over the ears." Does it mean covering the tops of the ears or does it mean above and/or around the ears?

figure 3-14
Communication is key to understanding the client's needs and wants.

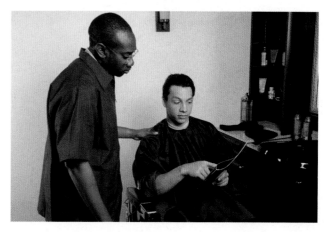

- **Repeat.** Once you have an understanding of the client's definition of "over the ears" or any other description used, repeat to the client your interpretation of what you think he told you. This communication step will provide you with further clarification and the opportunity to make needed changes—in short, to reach an understanding of the client's expectations.

There are many ways in which effective communication skills can impact your professional success. Review the following barbershop activities that benefit from effective communication skills:

- Making contacts and networking
- Meeting and greeting clients
- Understanding a client's service needs, likes, dislikes, desires, and expectations
- Self-promotion and building a clientele
- Selling services and products
- Telephone conversations and appointment bookings
- Conversation and interaction with the shop staff, clients, and vendors

SOCIAL MEDIA

Finally, a frequent form of communication that can easily be misunderstood, yet has serious impact upon your business, is online communication (**Figure 3-15**). Establishing a professional online image is an essential image-building attribute, and not one to be taken lightly. Social-media websites, including photo-sharing sites, can quickly diminish a person's reputation if media etiquette is neglected.

figure 3-15
Social media is a powerful tool when used correctly.

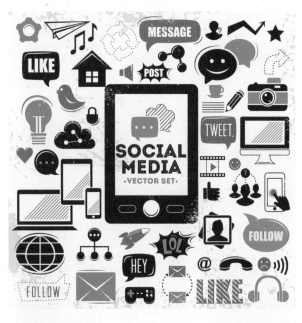

DO
- Manage your personal pages and walls.
- Use social media to communicate with peers and clients.
- Post helpful content.

DON'T
- Use profane language.
- Participate in or entertain arguments online.
- Post nude or embarrassing photographs.
- Forward spam.

Maintaining your professional image online can be a daily process, but it is also an investment of time that can have huge returns for your business. Social media allows you to share your professional image—including proof of your skills, your creativity, and your passion—with an enormous world of potential clients and fellow barbers. It is up to you to make sure that image is your best.

REVIEW QUESTIONS

1. What are the five basic requirements for personal and professional health?

2. What are four important personal hygiene habits?

3. What is the best way to ensure you are dressed for success?

4. What are five ways you can avoid ergonomic-related injuries?

5. What is *rapport*?

6. What are five desirable qualities for effective client relations?

7. What are the three communication steps that help determine a client's service expectations?

8. What are four things not to do when it comes to social media?

CHAPTER GLOSSARY

effective communication (uh-FEK-tive COM-yun-ik-ay-shun)	p. 49	the act of successfully sharing information between two people (or groups of people) so that the information is understood
ergonomics (UR-go-nom-icks)	p. 45	the science of designing the workplace as well as its equipment and tools to make specific body movements more comfortable, efficient, and safe
human relations	p. 47	the interactions and relationships between two or more people
personal grooming	p. 42	the process of caring for parts of the body and maintaining an overall polished look
personal hygiene (pur-sun-AL HY-jene)	p. 41	the daily maintenance of cleanliness by practicing good healthful habits
physical presentation (FIZ-ih-kuhl pres-ent-TAY-shun)	p. 44	your posture, as well as the way you walk and move
professional image (pruh-FESH-un-ul IM-aje)	p. 42	the impression you project through both your outward appearance and your conduct in the workplace

PART 2 GENERAL SCIENCES

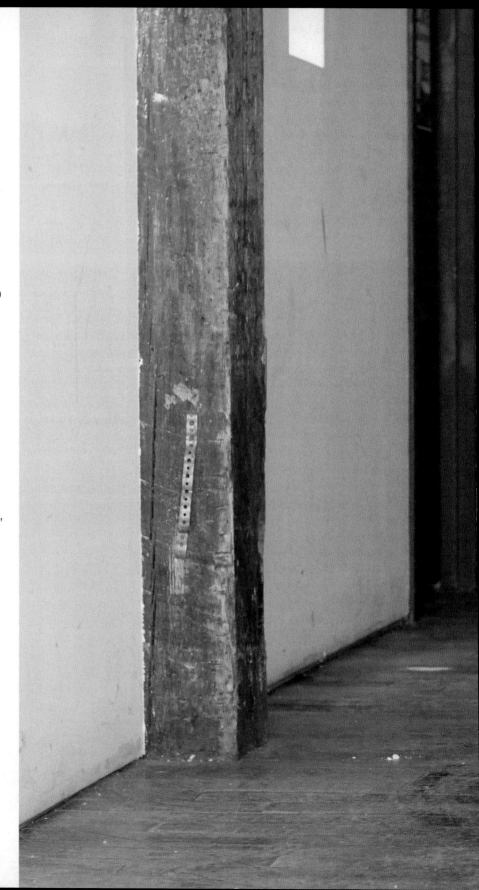

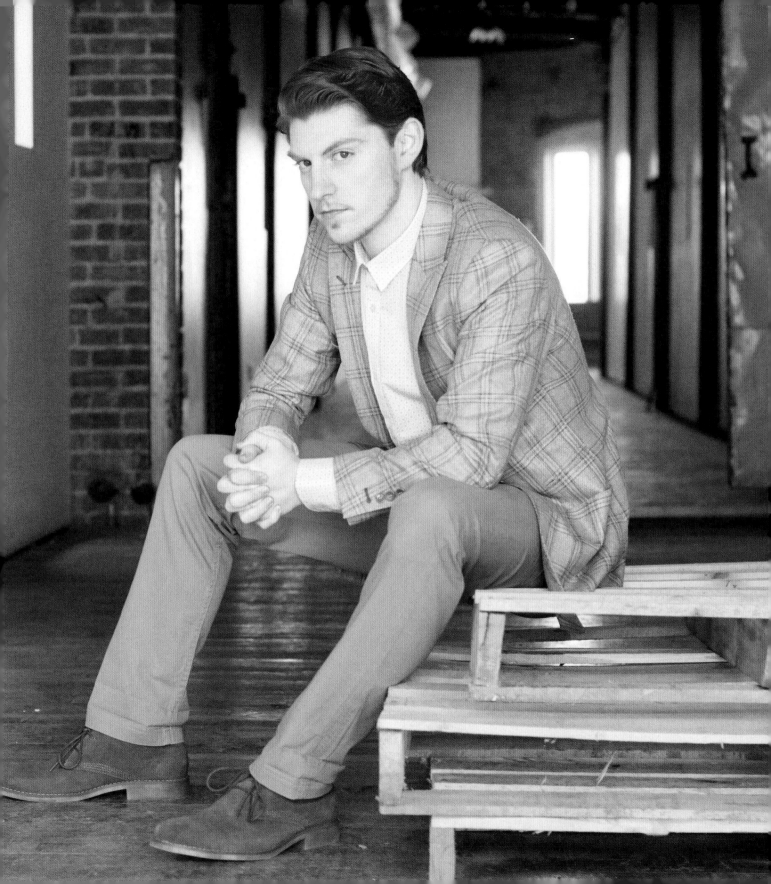

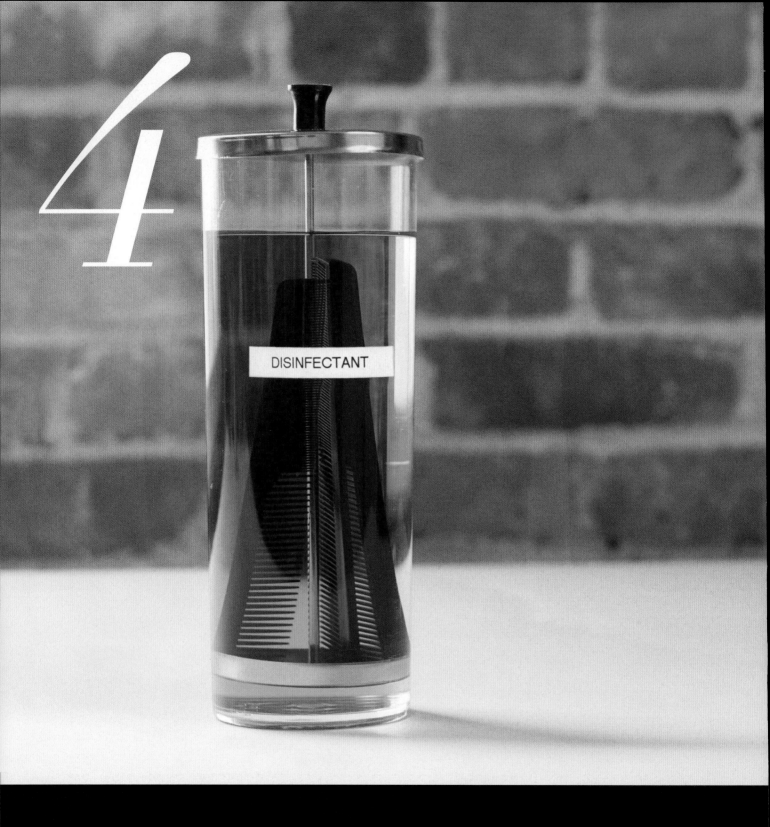

4

INFECTION CONTROL: PRINCIPLES AND PRACTICES

LEARNING OBJECTIVES

After completing this chapter, you will be able to:

LO❶
Discuss federal and state agencies that regulate the practice of barbering.

LO❷
List the types and classifications of bacteria.

LO❸
Define bloodborne pathogens and explain how they are transmitted.

LO❹
Explain the differences between cleaning, disinfecting, and sterilizing.

LO❺
Identify types of disinfectants and antiseptics appropriate for use in barbershops.

LO❻
Discuss Standard Precautions and explain procedures for handling an exposure incident.

LO❼
Discuss safe work practices that help prevent accidents and injuries.

LO❽
List your responsibilities as a professional barber.

Publisher's Note

In the previous edition of this text, the term *sanitation*, also known as *sanitizing*, was used interchangeably to mean, "clean" or "cleaning." You will also find that many commercially available products used in the cleaning and disinfecting process continue to use the words *sanitize* and *sanitizing*. However, the publisher's goal is to clearly define these terms in this book, in textbooks across the industry, and within the glossary.

Before we discuss infection control and safe work practices, the terms *cleaning*, *sanitizing*, *disinfecting*, and *sterilizing* need to be properly differentiated, because of the following factors:

- There is much confusion about and misuse of the terms *cleaning*, *sanitizing*, *disinfecting*, and *sterilizing* within the professional beauty and barbering industry. In an effort to do what we can to clarify these critical terms, Milady opted to consistently use the term *cleaning*, instead of using *cleaning* in one sentence and *sanitizing* in another sentence.

- Professionals in the healthcare and scientific communities (of disease prevention and epidemiology) and associations, such as the Association for Professionals in Infection Control and Epidemiology, generally do not use the terms interchangeably. Instead, it is more common for infection control professionals to use the term *cleaning*. Infection control professionals consider **sanitation** (san-ih-TAY-shun) a layperson's term or a product marketing term (as in *hand sanitizers*).

- The term *cleaning* is defined as a mechanical process (scrubbing) using soap and water or detergent and water to remove all visible dirt, debris, and many disease-causing germs. Cleaning also removes invisible debris that interferes with disinfection. Cleaning is required as a step before disinfecting.

- The term *sanitizing* is defined as a chemical process for reducing the number of disease-causing germs on cleaned surfaces to a safe level.

- The term *disinfecting* is defined as a chemical process for use with nonporous items that uses specific products to destroy harmful organisms (except bacterial spores) on implements and environmental surfaces.

Introduction

State barber boards and other regulatory agencies require that infection control measures and safe work practices be applied while serving the public. Infection control measures help minimize the spread of contagious diseases and skin infections that are caused by the transmission of infectious material from one individual to another. Since transmission can also occur when using contaminated implements, tools, or equipment, the performance of effective infection control procedures must be a top priority in the barbershop.

Safe work practices require that implements, tools, and equipment be used safely and that you be aware of situations that can cause accidents in the barbershop. This chapter provides some helpful guidelines to minimize potential risks and accidents.

It is your responsibility as a professional barber to use proper and effective infection control methods that help safeguard your health and the health of your clients. You are also responsible for employing safe work practices to help prevent accidents and injuries from occurring in the workplace.

why study
INFECTION CONTROL: PRINCIPLES AND PRACTICES?

Barbers should study and have a thorough understanding of infection control: principles and practices because:

> It is important to know about the pathogens you and your clients may be exposed to in the barbershop and their modes of transmission.

> Understanding and practicing proper infection control within the laws and rules will help safeguard your health, the health of your clients, and your business.

> It is important to respect the procedures for handling chemicals used in cleaning and disinfecting by reading labels and following manufacturers' instructions to keep you and your clients safe.

> Practicing safety precautions on a daily basis protects your clients and your license.

> A responsible professional barber is conscientious about infection control and safety.

Meet the Current Regulations for Health and Safety

After reading this section, you will be able to:

LO❶ Discuss federal and state agencies that regulate the practice of barbering.

Many federal and state agencies regulate the practice of barbering. Federal agencies set guidelines for the manufacturing, sale, and use of equipment and chemical ingredients. These guidelines also monitor safety in the workplace and place limits on the types of services you can perform in a barber or styling shop. State agencies regulate licensing, enforcement, and your conduct when you are working in the shop.

FEDERAL AGENCIES

Occupational Safety and Health Administration

The Occupational Safety and Health Administration (OSHA) was created as part of the U.S. Department of Labor to regulate and enforce safety and health standards to protect employees in the workplace. Regulating

WEB RESOURCES
You can find a list of disinfectants approved by the Environmental Protection Agency (EPA) by going to the EPA's website, at http://www.epa.gov and entering a search on the home page for EPA-registered disinfectants. Disinfectants are not listed as "hospital grade" but instead are listed based on the pathogens they are effective against. Products on list D meet the criteria of most states for hospital disinfectants; products on list E meet the criteria of a tuberculocidal in those states where that is required.

employee exposure to potentially toxic substances and informing employees about the possible hazards of materials used in the workplace are key points of the Occupational Safety and Health Act of 1970. This regulation created the Hazard Communication Standard (HCS), which requires that chemical manufacturers and importers assess and communicate the potential hazards associated with their products. The Material Safety Data Sheet (MSDS) was a result of the HCS. In 2012, along with representatives from most of the nations in the United Nations, OSHA agreed to comply with the Globally Harmonized System of Classification and Labeling of Chemicals System (GHS). This initiative was designed to create label standards to be used around the globe and includes the use of specific pictograms to indicate possible safety concerns; the initiative also includes the adoption of a 16-category, standard-format Safety Data Sheet (SDS) to replace the MSDS. The HCS Act in 1983 gave workers the *right to know*, but the new GHS gives workers the *right to understand*.

The standards set by OSHA are important to barbers because of the products they use daily. OSHA standards address issues relating to the handling, mixing, storing, and disposing of products; general safety in the workplace; and your right to know about any potentially hazardous ingredients contained in the products and how to avoid these hazards. Barbers should view OSHA as an agency designed to ensure a safe workplace for all U.S. workers.

Safety Data Sheets (SDS) Replace Material Safety Data Sheets (MSDS)

Both federal and state laws require that manufacturers supply a **Safety Data Sheet** (previously known as *Material Safety Data Sheet* [muh-TEE-ree-uhl SAYF-tee DAY-tuh SHEET]) for all chemical products manufactured and sold (**Figure 4-1**). All SDSs will be organized identically and will contain the following 16 categories of information:

1. **Identification.** Product identifier, manufacturer or distributor with contact information (including emergency phone number), recommended use of the product, and restrictions on use are displayed.

2. **Hazard identification.** All hazards of using the chemical are detailed.

3. **Composition/information on ingredients.** Information on chemical ingredients is included.

4. **First-aid measures.** Important symptoms/effects (acute and delayed) and required treatment are included.

5. **Firefighting measures.** Suitable fire-extinguishing techniques and equipment and the chemical hazards of fire are listed.

6. **Accidental release measures.** Emergency procedures, protective equipment, and proper methods of containment and clean-up are listed.

7. **Handling and storage.** Precautions for safe handling and storage, including incompatibilities, are listed.

8. **Exposure controls/personal protection.** OSHA's permissible exposure limits and personal protective equipment are listed.

9. **Physical and chemical properties.** The chemical's characteristics are listed.

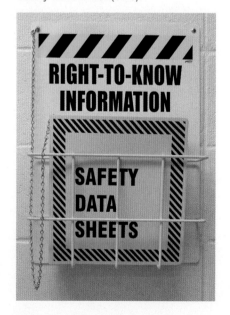

? DID YOU KNOW?

The term *hospital grade* is a term that is not used by the EPA. The EPA does not grade disinfectants; a product either is approved by the EPA for use as a hospital disinfectant or is not.

figure 4-1
Safety Data Sheet (SDS).

RIGHT-TO-KNOW INFORMATION

SAFETY DATA SHEETS

10. **Stability and reactivity.** Chemical stability and possibility of hazardous reactions are detailed.

11. **Toxicology information.** Routes of exposure, related symptoms, and acute and chronic effects are included.

12. **Ecological information.** Effects on wastewater and environment are detailed.

13. **Disposal consideration.** Proper disposal techniques and disposal restrictions are detailed.

14. **Transport information.** Restrictions on transportation are included.

15. **Regulatory information.** Agencies responsible for the regulation of the product are listed.

16. **Revision date.** Original date of document and any revisions are listed.

Source: Adapted from United States Department of Labor. (n.d.) *OSHA QuickCard— Hazard Communication Safety Data Sheets.* Retrieved from http://www.OSHA.gov.

In addition, pictograms that are internationally recognized are used (**Figure 4-2**) to ensure that information is being communicated in easily recognizable formats. When necessary, the SDS can be sent to a medical facility so that a doctor can better assess and treat the patient. Not having SDS information available poses a health risk to anyone exposed to hazardous materials and violates federal and state regulations. OSHA and state

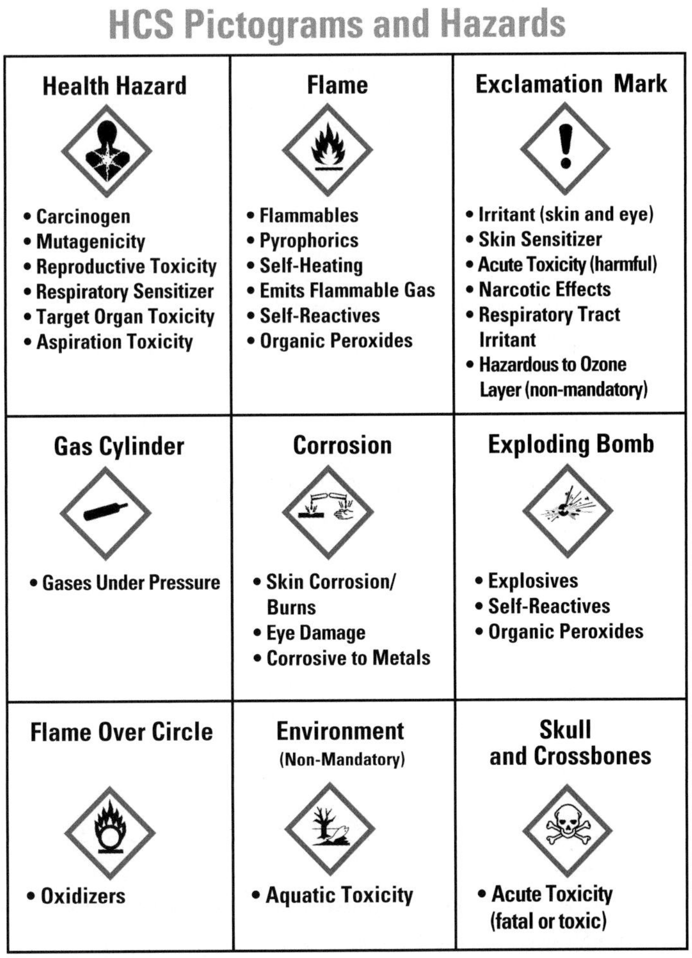

figure 4-2
Pictograms used on SDSs.

HCS Pictograms and Hazards

Health Hazard
- Carcinogen
- Mutagenicity
- Reproductive Toxicity
- Respiratory Sensitizer
- Target Organ Toxicity
- Aspiration Toxicity

Flame
- Flammables
- Pyrophorics
- Self-Heating
- Emits Flammable Gas
- Self-Reactives
- Organic Peroxides

Exclamation Mark
- Irritant (skin and eye)
- Skin Sensitizer
- Acute Toxicity (harmful)
- Narcotic Effects
- Respiratory Tract Irritant
- Hazardous to Ozone Layer (non-mandatory)

Gas Cylinder
- Gases Under Pressure

Corrosion
- Skin Corrosion/Burns
- Eye Damage
- Corrosive to Metals

Exploding Bomb
- Explosives
- Self-Reactives
- Organic Peroxides

Flame Over Circle
- Oxidizers

Environment (Non-Mandatory)
- Aquatic Toxicity

Skull and Crossbones
- Acute Toxicity (fatal or toxic)

regulatory agencies require that SDSs be kept available in the shop for all products used or sold. Both OSHA and state board inspectors can issue fines to establishments not having SDSs readily available.

Federal and state laws require barbers to obtain SDSs from the chemical product manufacturers and/or distributors for each professional product they use. SDSs often can be downloaded from the product manufacturer's or the distributor's website. All workers in the barbershop must read the information included on each SDS and verify that they have read it by adding their signatures to a sign-off sheet for the product. All states require that sign-off sheets must be immediately available to state and federal inspectors upon request.

Environmental Protection Agency (EPA)

The EPA registers all types of disinfectants sold and used in the United States. **Disinfectants** (dis-in-FEK-tents) are chemical products that destroy most bacteria (excluding spores), fungi, and viruses on surfaces. The two types that are used in the barbershop are hospital disinfectants and tuberculocidal disinfectants.

Hospital disinfectants (HOS-pih-tal dis-in-FEK-tents) are effective for cleaning blood and body fluids from nonporous surfaces. By **nonporous** (nahn-POHW-rus), we mean an item made or constructed of a material that has no pores or openings and that cannot absorb liquids. Hospital disinfectants control the spread of **disease** (DIZ-eez). Disease is defined as an abnormal condition of all or part of the body, its systems, or its organs that make the body incapable of carrying on normal functions. The most commonly used disinfectants are the following:

* Quaternary ammonium compounds, commonly known as *quats*, are products made of quaternary ammonium cations and are designed for disinfection of nonporous surfaces. They are appropriate for use in noncritical (noninvasive) environments and are effective against most pathogens of concern in the barbering environment.

* **Tuberculocidal disinfectants** (tuh-bur-kyoo-LOH-syd-ahl dis-in-FEK-tents), often referred to as *phenolics*, are proven to kill the bacterium that causes **tuberculosis** (tuh-bur-kyoo-LOH-sus), in addition to other pathogens destroyed through the use of hospital disinfectants. Tuberculosis is a disease caused by a bacterium that is transmitted through coughing or sneezing. It is passed through inhalation only and is not transmitted by the hands or picked up on surfaces.

Tuberculocidal disinfectants are one kind of hospital disinfectant; however, because these disinfectants are effective against the pathogen does not mean that you should automatically reach for them. Some of these products can be harmful to tools and equipment and they require special methods of disposal. Check the rules of your state to be sure that the product you choose complies with state requirements.

Most pathogens of concern in the barbershop are adequately destroyed by standard EPA-registered disinfectants and do not require tuberculocidal disinfectants; however, some states *do* require tuberculocidal disinfectants, so always check the rules of your state to be sure the product complies with state requirements. There are also some states that require tuberculocidal

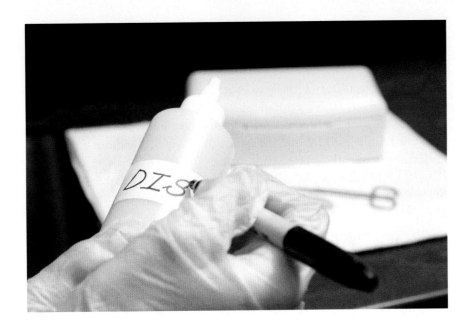

figure 4-3
All products and containers need to be labeled.

disinfectants only when blood contamination has occurred. In those states, you should keep a tuberculocidal disinfectant readily available, but you should use it only when required.

It is against federal law to use any disinfecting product in a way contrary to the use indicated on its label. Before a manufacturer can sell a product for disinfecting surfaces, tools, implements, or equipment, they must obtain an EPA registration number (shown following "EPA Reg. No." near the manufacturer's name) that certifies that the disinfectant, when used correctly, will be effective against the pathogens listed on the label. For example, clipper disinfectants must be approved by the EPA for use with clippers in specific environments (such as a barbershop) or the manufacturer would be breaking federal law by marketing them as clipper disinfectants to the barber market. This also means that if you do not follow the label instructions for mixing, contact time, and the type of surface the disinfecting product can be used on, you are not complying with federal law (**Figure 4-3**). If there were an injury-related lawsuit, you could be held responsible.

STATE REGULATORY AGENCIES

State regulatory agencies exist to protect barbers and their customers' health and safety while they receive services. State regulatory agencies include licensing agencies, state barber boards, commissions, and health departments. Regulatory agencies require that everyone working on consumers in a barbershop follow specific procedures. Enforcement of the rules through inspections and investigations of consumer complaints is also part of an agency's responsibility. An agency can issue penalties against both the shop owner's and the barber's licenses. Penalties vary and include warnings, fines, probation, and suspension or revocation of licenses. It is vital that you understand and follow the laws and rules of your state at all times. Your professional reputation, your license, and your clients' safety depend on it.

> **! CAUTION**
> Remember, barbers are not allowed to treat or recommend treatments for infections, diseases, or abnormal conditions. Customers with such problems should be referred to their physicians.

LAWS AND RULES—WHAT IS THE DIFFERENCE?

Laws are written by both federal and state legislatures that determine the scope of practice (what each license allows the holder to do) and establish guidelines for regulatory agencies to make rules. Laws are also called *statutes*.

Rules and regulations are more specific than laws. The regulatory agency or the state board writes the rules and determines how the law must be applied. Rules establish specific standards of conduct and can be changed or updated frequently. It is the barber's responsibility to be aware of any changes to the rules and regulations and to comply with them. Ignorance of the law is not an acceptable reason or excuse for noncompliance.

Understanding the Principles of Infection

After reading this section, you will be able to:

LO**❷**   List the types and classifications of bacteria.

LO**❸**   Define bloodborne pathogens and explain how they are transmitted.

Being a barber professional is not only rewarding, but it is also a great responsibility. One careless action could cause injury or **infection** (in-FEK-shun), which is the invasion of body tissues by disease-causing pathogens. If your actions result in a client's injury or infection, you could lose your license or ruin the shop's reputation. Fortunately, preventing the spread of infections is easy when you know proper procedures and follow them at all times. Prevention begins and ends with *you*.

Effective infection control in the barbershop also influences the professional image of the establishment. A client's first impression of the shop begins the moment they opens the door; so a clean environment should extend beyond each barber's immediate work area. All of the sights, sounds, smells, and general ambience of the barbershop meld together to form this first impression regardless of how many times a client has previously visited the shop. In essence, this first impression happens over and over again because clients do not see you or the shop daily. A clean and orderly barbershop helps build client confidence and trust that continuous care is being taken to provide a safe and sanitary environment in which to receive their personal services.

INFECTION CONTROL

Infection control (in-FEK-shun CON-trol) refers to the methods used to eliminate or reduce the transmission of **infectious** (in-FEK-shus) organisms. Barbers must understand and remember the following four types of potentially harmful organisms:

- Bacteria
- Viruses
- Fungi
- Parasites

Under certain conditions, many of these organisms can cause infectious diseases. An **infectious disease** (in-FEK-shus DIZ-eez) is caused by pathogenic (harmful) organisms that enter the body. An infectious disease, however, may or may not be spread from one person to another depending on the organism and its method of transmission.

In this chapter, you will learn how to properly clean and disinfect the tools and equipment you use so they are safe for you and your customers.

Cleaning (KLEEN-ing) is a mechanical process (scrubbing) using soap and water or detergent and water to remove all visible dirt, debris, and many disease-causing germs from tools, implements, and equipment.

The process of **disinfection** (dis-in-FEK-shun) involves the use of a chemical to destroy most, but not necessarily all, harmful organisms on environmental surfaces. Disinfection is not effective against **bacterial spores** (bak-TEER-ee-ul SPOORZ), which are bacteria capable of producing a protective coating that allows them to withstand very harsh environments and to shed the coating when conditions become more favorable to them.

Cleaning and disinfecting procedures are designed to prevent the spread of infection and disease. At minimum, disinfectants used in barbershops must be

- **bactericidal** (BAK-TEER-uh-syd-uhl), capable of destroying bacteria;
- **virucidal** (VI-ra-syd-uhl), capable of destroying viruses;
- **fungicidal** (FUN-ji-syd-uhl), capable of destroying molds and fungi.

Remember, in some states, disinfectants must also be effective against tuberculosis (tuberculocidal). Check your state board rules and regulations for compliance information.

Be sure to mix and use these disinfectants according to the instructions on the labels so they are safe and effective.

Contaminated tools and equipment can spread infections between customers if proper disinfection steps are not taken after every service. You have a professional and legal obligation to protect your clients from harm by using proper infection control procedures. If clients are infected or harmed because you did not perform infection control procedures correctly, you may be found legally responsible for their injuries or infections.

BACTERIA

Bacteria (bak-TEER-ee-ah) (singular: bacterium [bak-TEER-ee-uhm]) are single-celled microorganisms that have both plant and animal characteristics. A **microorganism** (my-kroh-OR-gah-niz-um) is any organism of microscopic or submicroscopic size. Some bacteria are harmful and some are harmless. Bacteria can exist almost anywhere: on skin, in water, in the air, in decayed matter, on environmental surfaces, in body secretions, on clothing, or under the free edge of nails. Bacteria are so small they can only be seen with a microscope.

> ✓ **HERE'S A TIP**
>
> This is a quick checklist for a disinfectant label to be in compliance with state and federal regulations:
>
> - The EPA registration number is prominently displayed.
> - The label indicates "hospital grade" and/or if it is bactericidal, virucidal, and fungicidal on label.
> - The label shows the disinfectant's efficacy list—What does it kill? Look for HIV (human immunodeficiency virus), HBV (hepatitis B virus), and MRSA (methicillin-resistant staphylococcus aureus) at the very least.

Types of Bacteria

There are thousands of different kinds of bacteria, which fall into two primary types: pathogenic and nonpathogenic. Most bacteria are **nonpathogenic** (nahn-path-uh-JEN-ik); in other words, they are harmless organisms that may perform useful functions. They are safe to come in contact with since they do not cause disease or harm. For example, nonpathogenic organisms are used to make yogurt, cheese, and some medicines. In the human body, nonpathogenic bacteria help the body break down food, protect against infection, and stimulate the immune system.

Pathogenic (path-uh-JEN-ik) bacteria are harmful microorganisms that can cause disease or infection in humans when they invade the body. Shops and schools must maintain strict standards for cleaning and disinfecting at all times to prevent the spread of pathogenic microorganisms. It is crucial that students learn proper infection control practices while in school to ensure that they understand the importance of following them throughout their career. **Table 4-1** presents terms and definitions related to pathogens.

table 4-1
CAUSES OF DISEASE

Term	Definition
Bacteria	One-celled microorganisms having both plant and animal characteristics. Some are harmful and some are harmless.
Direct Transmission (dy-REKT trans-MISH-uhn)	Transmission of blood or body fluids through touching (including shaking hands), kissing, coughing, sneezing, and talking.
Fungi	Singular: fungus; single-cell organisms that grow in irregular masses that include molds, mildews, and yeasts.
Indirect Transmission (IN-dih-rekt trans-MISH-uhn)	Transmission of blood or body fluids through contact with an intermediate contaminated object, such as a razor, extractor, nipper, or an environmental surface.
Infection	Invasion of body tissues by disease-causing pathogens.
Germs	Nonscientific synonym for disease-producing organisms.
Microorganism	Any organism of microscopic to submicroscopic size.
Pathogens	Harmful microorganisms that enter the body and can cause disease.
Parasites	Organisms that grow, feed, and shelter on or in another organism (referred to as the host) while contributing nothing to the survival of that organism. Parasites must have a host to survive.
Toxins	Various poisonous substances produced by some microorganisms (bacteria and viruses).
Virus	A submicroscopic particle that infects and resides in cells of biological organisms.

Classifications of Pathogenic Bacteria

Bacteria have three distinct shapes that help identify them. Pathogenic bacteria are classified as described below:

- **Cocci** (KOK-sy) are round-shaped bacteria that appear singly (alone) or in groups (**Figure 4-4**):

  - **Staphylococci** (staf-uh-loh-KOK-sy) are pus-forming bacteria that grow in clusters like bunches of grapes. They cause abscesses, pustules, and boils. Some types of staphylococci (or staph, as many call it) may not cause infections in healthy humans, although others may be deadly (**Figure 4-5**).

  - **Streptococci** (strep-toh-KOK-sy) are pus-forming bacteria arranged in curved lines resembling a string of beads. They cause infections such as strep throat and blood poisoning (**Figure 4-6**).

  - **Diplococci** (dip-lo-KOK-sy) are spherical bacteria that grow in pairs and cause diseases such as pneumonia (**Figure 4-7**).

- **Bacilli** (bah-SIL-ee) are short rod-shaped bacteria. They are the most common bacteria and produce diseases such as tetanus (lockjaw), typhoid fever, tuberculosis, and diphtheria (**Figure 4-8**).

- **Spirilla** (spy-RIL-ah) are spiral or corkscrew-shaped bacteria. They are subdivided into subgroups, such as *Treponema pallidum*, which causes syphilis, a sexually transmitted disease, and *Borrelia burgdorferi*, which causes Lyme disease (**Figure 4-9**).

Movement of Bacteria

Different bacteria move in different ways; the term **motility** (MOH-till-it-ee) refers to self-movement. Cocci rarely demonstrate self-movement and are generally transmitted in the air, in dust, or within the substance in which they settle. Bacilli and spirilla are both capable of movement and use slender, hairlike extensions called **flagella** (fluh-JEL-uh) for locomotion (moving about). You may also hear people refer to **cilia** (SIL-ee-uh) in reference to cell movement, but they are much shorter than flagella; bacteria require relatively many more cilia to ensure self-movement. Both flagella and cilia move cells, but they have different types of motion. Bacteria with flagella move in a snakelike motion while those with cilia move in a rowing-like motion.

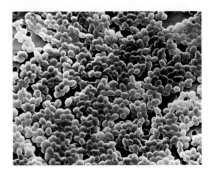

figure 4-4
Cocci.

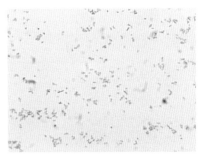

figure 4-5
Staphylococci.

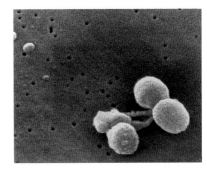

figure 4-6
Streptococci.

figure 4-7
Diplococci.

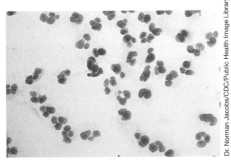

figure 4-8
Bacilli.

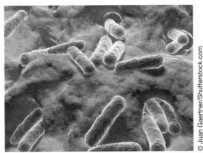

figure 4-9
Spirilla.

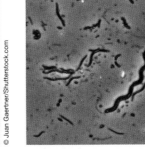

Bacterial Growth and Reproduction

When seen under a microscope, bacteria look like tiny bags. They generally consist of an outer cell wall that contains a liquid called *protoplasm*. Bacterial cells manufacture their own food through what they absorb from the surrounding environment. They give off waste products, grow, and reproduce. The life cycle of bacteria consists of two distinct phases: the active stage and the inactive stage.

Active stage. During the active stage, bacteria grow and reproduce. Bacteria multiply best in warm, dark, damp, or dirty places. When conditions are favorable, bacteria grow and reproduce. When they reach their largest size, they divide into two new cells. This division is called **binary fission** (BY-nayr-ee FISH-un). The cells that are formed as a result of binary fission are called *daughter cells* and are produced every 20 to 60 minutes, depending on the bacteria. For example, the infectious pathogen *Staphylococcus aureus* undergoes cell division every 27 to 30 minutes. When conditions become unfavorable, bacteria either die or become inactive.

Inactive stage (IN-ac-tif STAJE). Certain bacteria, such as the bacteria that cause tetanus and botulism, among others, can form spores by coating themselves with waxlike outer shells during unfavorable conditions. These spores protect the bacteria and enable them to withstand long periods of famine, dryness, and unsuitable temperatures. In this condition, spores can be blown about and are not harmed by disinfectants, heat, or cold. If favorable conditions, such as a moist environment return, the spores can change into the active form and begin to grow and reproduce (**Figure 4-10**).

Bacterial Infections

There can be no bacterial infection without the presence of pathogenic bacteria. Therefore, if pathogenic bacteria are eliminated, clients cannot become infected.

An **inflammation** (in-fluh-MAY-shun) is a condition in which the tissue of the body reacts to injury, irritation, or infection. An inflammation is characterized by redness, heat, pain, and/or swelling.

figure 4-10
Petri dishes with growing cultures.

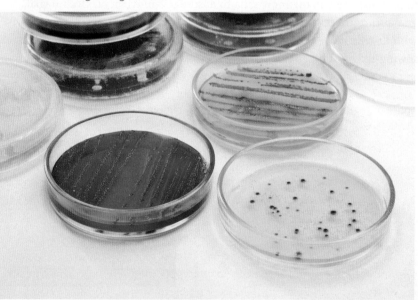

Pus (PUS) is a fluid containing white blood cells, bacteria, and dead cells and is the by-product of the infectious process. The presence of pus is a sign of a bacterial infection. A **local infection** (LOHK-al in-FEK-shun), such as a pimple or abscess (Figure 4-11), is confined to a particular part of the body and appears as a lesion-containing pus. A systemic infection is an infection where the pathogen has distributed throughout the body rather than staying in one area or organ.

Staphylococci are among the most common bacteria that affect humans and are commonly found in our environment, including on our bodies, although most strains do not make us ill. Staph bacteria can be picked up on doorknobs, countertops, and other surfaces, but in the barbershop, they are more frequently spread through skin-to-skin contact (such as shaking hands) or through the use of unclean tools or implements and can be very dangerous.

Staph is responsible for food poisoning and a wide range of diseases, including toxic shock syndrome. Some types of infectious staph bacteria are highly resistant to conventional treatments such as antibiotics. An example is the staph infection called **methicillin-resistant staphylococcus aureus** (METH-eh-sill-en-ree-ZIST-ent staf-uh-loh-KOK-us OR-ee-us). Historically, MRSA occurred most frequently among persons with weakened immune systems or among people who had undergone medical procedures. Today, it has become more common in otherwise healthy people. Clients who appear completely healthy may bring this organism into the shop, where it can infect others. Some people carry the bacteria and are not even aware of their infection, but the people they infect may show more obvious symptoms. MRSA initially appears as a skin infection, presenting as pimples, rashes, or boils that can be difficult to cure. Without proper treatment, the infection becomes systemic and can have devastating consequences that can result in death. Because of these highly resistant bacterial strains, it is important to clean and disinfect all tools and implements used on customers. Also, do not perform services if the client's skin, scalp, or neck shows visible signs of abrasion or infection.

When a disease spreads from one person to another, the disease is said to be a **contagious disease** (kon-TAY-jus DIZ-eez), also known as **communicable** (kuh-MYOO-nih-kuh-bul) disease. Some of the more common contagious diseases that prevent a barber from servicing a client are the common cold, ringworm, conjunctivitis (pinkeye), and viral infections. The most common way these infections spread is through dirty hands, especially under the fingernails and in the webs between the fingers. Be sure to always wash your hands after using the restroom and before eating. Contagious diseases can also be spread by contaminated implements, cuts, infected nails, open sores, pus, mouth and nose discharges, shared drinking cups, telephone receivers, and towels. Uncovered coughing or sneezing and spitting in public also spread germs. Table 4-2 lists terms and definitions that are important for a general understanding of disease.

figure 4-11
Pimples are an example of a local infection.

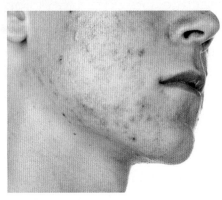

VIRUSES

A **virus** (VY-rus) (plural: viruses) is a submicroscopic particle that infects and resides in the cells of a biological organism. A virus is capable of replication only through taking over the host cell's reproductive function. Viruses are so small that they can only be seen under the most sophisticated and

table 4-2

TERMS RELATED TO DISEASE

Term	Definition
Allergy	Reaction due to extreme sensitivity to certain foods, chemicals, or other normally harmless substances.
Contagious Disease	Also known as *communicable disease*; a disease that is spread from one person to another person. Some of the more contagious diseases are the common cold, ringworm, conjunctivitis (pinkeye), viral infections, and natural nail or toe and foot infections.
Contamination (kun-tam-uh-NAY-shun)	The presence, or the reasonably anticipated presence, of blood or other potentially infectious materials on an item's surface or visible debris or residues such as dust, hair, and skin.
Decontamination	The removal of blood or other potentially infectious materials on an item's surface and the removal of visible debris or residue such as dust, hair, and skin.
Diagnosis (dy-ag-NOH-sis)	Determination of the nature of a disease from its symptoms and/or diagnostic tests. Federal regulations prohibit salon professionals from performing a diagnosis.
Disease	An abnormal condition of all or part of the body or its systems or organs that makes the body incapable of carrying on normal function.
Exposure Incident	Contact with non-intact (broken) skin, blood, body fluid, or other potentially infectious materials that are the result of the performance of an employee's duties.
Infectious Disease	Disease caused by pathogenic (harmful) microorganisms that enter the body. An infectious disease may be spread from one person to another person.
Inflammation	Condition in which the body reacts to injury, irritation, or infection. An inflammation is characterized by redness, heat, pain, and swelling.
Occupational Disease	Illnesses resulting from conditions associated with employment, such as prolonged and repeated overexposure to certain products or ingredients.
Parasitic Disease	Disease caused by parasites, such as lice and mites.
Pathogenic Disease	Disease produced by organisms, including bacteria, viruses, fungi, and parasites.
Systemic Disease	Disease that affects the body as a whole, often due to under-functioning or over-functioning internal glands or organs. This disease is carried through the bloodstream or the lymphatic system.

powerful microscopes. They cause common colds and other respiratory and gastrointestinal (digestive tract) infections. Some of the viruses that plague humans are measles, mumps, chicken pox, smallpox, rabies, yellow fever, hepatitis, polio, influenza, and HIV, which causes AIDS.

One difference between viruses and bacteria is that a virus can live and reproduce only by taking over other cells and becoming part of them, while bacteria can live and reproduce on their own. Another difference is that while bacterial infections can usually be treated with specific antibiotics, viral infections cannot, and viruses are hard to kill without harming the host cells in the process. When available, vaccinations can prevent viruses from growing in the body. There are many vaccines available for viruses, but not all viruses have vaccines. There are vaccines available for hepatitis B and varicella (the virus that causes shingles), and you should strongly consider receiving these vaccines, as well as vaccines for the seasonal flu and pneumonia (Figure 4-12).

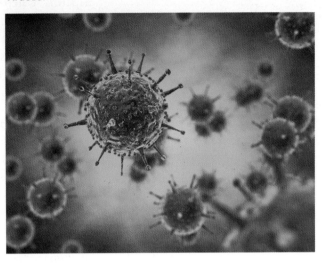

figure 4-12
Viruses.

BIOFILMS

Biofilms are colonies of microorganisms that adhere to environmental surfaces, as well as the human body. They secrete a sticky, hard-to-penetrate, protective coating that cements them together. The biofilm grows into a complex structure, with many kinds of microbes. The sticky matrix substance holds communities together, making them very hard to pierce with antisepsis, antimicrobials, and disinfection. It keeps the body in a chronic inflammatory state that is painful and inhibits healing. One action of the biofilm community is to resist the body's defense mechanisms; we are learning that biofilms play a large role in disease and infection.

Biofilms are usually not visible and must grow very large to be seen without a microscope. Dental plaque is an example of a visible human biofilm. Numerous persistent infections, including periodontal disease, osteomyelitis, cystic fibrosis, otitis media, conjunctivitis, prostatitis, endocarditis, urinary catheter infections, contact lens and corneal infections, and infections associated with medical devices and surgical (and sterile) instruments are associated with biofilms that are not visible. Algae colonies on ponds and slime in drains are examples of environmental biofilms.

Because biofilms are hard to detect, their presence and effects seem to be underestimated. They are one of the most significant scientific discoveries of the past few decades, though we have much more to learn. Conscientiously using infection control precautions, including standard precautions, cleaning, disinfection, and sterilization, is the best method of prevention at the present time.

BLOODBORNE PATHOGENS

Disease-causing microorganisms that are carried in the body by blood or body fluids, such as hepatitis and HIV, are called **bloodborne pathogens** (BLUD-boorn PATH-o-genz). In the barbershop, the spread of bloodborne pathogens is possible during haircutting and shaving services whenever the skin is broken. Use great care to avoid cutting or damaging the customer's skin during any type of service.

Hepatitis

Hepatitis (HEP-uh-tight-is) is a bloodborne virus that causes disease and can damage the liver. In general, it is difficult to contract hepatitis. However, hepatitis is easier to contract than HIV because hepatitis can be present in all body fluids of those who are infected. In addition, unlike HIV, hepatitis can live on a surface outside the body for long periods of time. For this reason, it is vital that all surfaces that a customer comes into contact with are thoroughly cleaned and disinfected.

> **✓ HERE'S A TIP**
>
> There are specific things you should look for on the label of any product you use for disinfection in the barbershop. The label should always have the following:
>
> • List of pathogens it is effective against should include HIV, HBV, and *S. aureus* (including MRSA)
>
> • EPA registration number
>
> • The words *bactericidal*, *virucidal*, and *fungicidal*
>
> • Mixing and changing instructions

© nobeastsofierce/Shutterstock.com.

There are three types of hepatitis that are of concern for barbers: hepatitis A, hepatitis B, and hepatitis C. HBV is the most difficult to kill on a surface, so check the label of the disinfectant you use to be sure that the product is effective against HBV. Hepatitis B and hepatitis C are spread from person to person through blood and, less often, through other body fluids.

HIV/AIDS

The **human immunodeficiency virus** (HYOO-mun ih-MYOO-noh-di-FISH-en-see VY-rus), abbreviated HIV, is the virus that causes **acquired immune deficiency syndrome** (uh-KWY-erd ih-MYOON di-FISH-en-see sin-drohm), abbreviated AIDS. AIDS is a disease that breaks down the body's immune system. HIV is spread from person to person through blood and, less often, through other body fluids, such as semen and vaginal secretions. A person can be infected with HIV for many years without showing symptoms, but testing can determine whether a person is infected within 6 months after exposure to the virus. Sometimes, people who are HIV-positive have never been tested and do not know they have the potential to infect others.

HIV is spread mainly through the sharing of needles by intravenous drug users and by unprotected sexual contact. Less commonly, HIV is spread through accidents with needles in healthcare settings. The virus is less likely to enter the bloodstream through cuts and sores. Holding hands, hugging, kissing, sharing food, or using household items such as the telephone or toilet seats does not spread HIV.

If you accidentally cut a client's skin, the tool will be contaminated with whatever might be in the client's blood, including HIV. You should not continue to use the implement without cleaning and disinfecting it. Continuing to use a contaminated implement without cleaning and disinfecting it puts you and others in the barbershop at risk of infection.

FUNGI

Fungi (FUN-ji) (singular: fungus [FUN-gus]) are single-celled organisms that grow in irregular masses that include molds, mildews, and yeasts. They can produce contagious diseases, such as ringworm. **Mildew** (MIL-doo), another fungus, affects plants or grows on inanimate objects but does not cause human infections in the barbershop.

The most frequently encountered fungal infection resulting from hair services is **tinea barbae** (TIN-ee-uh BAR-bee), also known as barber's itch. Tinea barbae is a superficial fungal infection caused by a variety of dermatophytes (fungi that require keratin for growth) that commonly affects the skin. It is primarily limited to the bearded areas of the face and neck or around the scalp. This infection occurs almost exclusively in older adolescent and adult males. A person with tinea barbae may have deep, inflamed or noninflamed patches of skin on the face or the nape of the neck. Tinea barbae is similar to **tinea capitis** (TIN-ee-uh KAP-ih-tus), a fungal infection of the scalp characterized by red papules, or spots, at the opening of hair follicles.

Barbers must clean and disinfect clipper blades to avoid spreading scalp and skin infections. The risk of spreading skin and scalp infections can be reduced by first removing all visible hair and debris from clippers followed by thorough cleaning and disinfection of the nonelectrical parts. You can use compressed air instead of a stiff brush to remove hair and debris from clippers before cleaning and disinfecting them. Turn the clippers on before applying the air to dislodge as much hair as possible during the procedure.

Always refer to the manufacturer's directions for proper cleaning and disinfecting methods and recommendations.

PARASITES

Parasites (PAYR-uh-sytz) are organisms that grow, feed, and shelter on or inside another organism (referred to as a *host*), while contributing nothing to the survival of that organism. They must have a host to survive. Parasites can live on or inside of humans and animals. They also can be found in food, on plants and trees, and in water. Humans can acquire internal parasites by eating fish or meat that has not been properly cooked. External parasites that affect humans, on or in the skin, include ticks, lice, fleas, and mites. Services should never be performed on a customer with visible signs of a parasitic infestation. Always refer the client to a physician for treatment.

Following are two types of parasites commonly encountered in the barbering environment:

- Head lice (**Figure 4-13**) are a type of parasite responsible for contagious diseases and conditions. One condition caused by an infestation of head lice is called **pediculosis capitis** (puh-dik-yuh-LOH-sis KAP-ih-tus).

- **Scabies** (SKAY-beez) is also a contagious skin disease and is caused by the itch mite, which burrows under the skin.

Contagious diseases and conditions caused by parasites should only be treated by a doctor. Contaminated countertops, tools, and equipment should be thoroughly cleaned and then disinfected with an EPA-registered disinfectant for the time recommended by the manufacturer or with a bleach solution for 10 minutes.

figure 4-13
Head lice.

IMMUNITY

Immunity (im-YOO-net-ee) refers to the ability of the body to destroy and resist pathogens and recognize infection. Immunity against disease can be either natural or acquired and is a sign of good health.

- **Natural immunity** (NATCH-uh-rul im-YOO-net-ee) is partly inherited and partly developed through healthy living.

- **Acquired immunity** (uh-KWY-erd ih-MYOO-nih-tee) is immunity that the body develops after overcoming a disease, through inoculation (such as flu vaccinations), or through exposure to natural allergens (such as pollen, cat dander, and ragweed).

> **⚠ CAUTION**
>
> Pathogenic bacteria, viruses, or fungi can enter the body through the following routes:
>
> - *Skin*: broken or inflamed skin, such as a cut or a scratch, or a bruise (weakened tissue) or a rash, but not through intact skin, which is an effective barrier to infection
>
> - *Mouth*: contaminated water, food, fingers, or objects
>
> - *Nose*: inhaling infectious dust or droplets from a cough or sneeze
>
> - *Eyes or ears*: organisms that reside in water that are commonly transmitted when the person is swimming
>
> - *Genitals*: unprotected sex
>
> The body prevents and controls infections through
>
> - healthy, uncompromised skin—the body's first line of defense;
>
> - body secretions, such as perspiration and digestive juices;
>
> - white blood cells that destroy bacteria;
>
> - antitoxins that counteract **toxins** (various poisonous substances produced by some microorganisms such as bacteria and viruses).

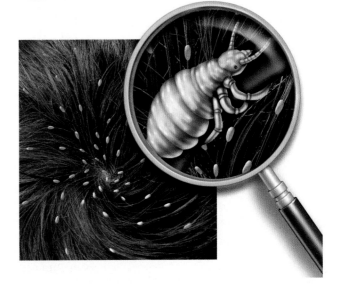

Prevent the Spread of Disease

After reading this section, you will be able to:

LO**4** Explain the differences between cleaning, disinfecting, and sterilizing.

LO**5** Identify types of disinfectants and antiseptics appropriate for use in barbershops.

Proper infection control can prevent the spread of disease caused by exposure to potentially infectious materials on an item's surface. Infection control will also prevent exposure to blood and visible debris or residue such as dust, hair, and skin.

Proper infection control requires two steps: cleaning and then disinfecting with an appropriate EPA-registered disinfectant. When these two steps are followed correctly, virtually all pathogens of concern can be effectively eliminated.

Sterilization (stayr-ih-luh-ZAY-shun), which is the process that destroys all microbial life including spores, is a third step that can be incorporated but it is very rarely mandated. Effective sterilization typically requires the use of an autoclave (**Figure 4-14**)—a piece of equipment that incorporates heat and pressure. For sterilization to be effective, items must be cleaned prior to use and the autoclave must be tested and maintained as instructed in the manufacturer's specifications. The Centers for Disease Control and Prevention (CDC) requires that autoclaves be tested weekly to ensure they are properly sterilizing implements. The accepted method is called a *spore test*. Sealed packages containing test organisms are subjected to a typical sterilization cycle and then sent to a contract laboratory that specializes in autoclave performance testing.

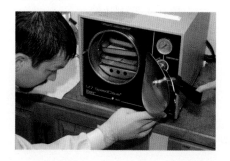

figure 4-14
Autoclave.

STEP 1: CLEANING

As stated, infection control has two steps: cleaning and disinfecting.

Remember that when you clean, you must remove all visible dirt and debris from tools, implements, and equipment by washing them with liquid soap and warm water and by using a clean and disinfected brush to scrub any grooved or hinged portions of the item.

When a surface is properly cleaned, the number of contaminants on the surface is greatly reduced. In turn, this reduces the risk of infection. The vast majority of contaminants and pathogens can be removed from the surfaces of tools and implements through proper cleaning. This is why cleaning is an important part of disinfecting tools and equipment. A surface must be properly cleaned before it can be properly disinfected. Using a disinfectant without cleaning first is like using mouthwash without brushing your teeth—it just does not work properly!

Cleaned surfaces can still harbor small amounts of pathogens, but the presence of fewer pathogens means infections are less likely to be spread (**Figure 4-15**). Applying antiseptics to your skin or washing your hands

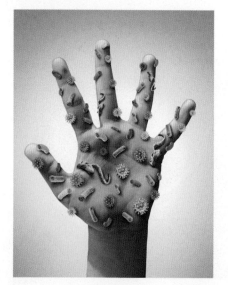

figure 4-15
Unwashed hands can be swarming with pathogens.

© Lightspring/Shutterstock.com.

with soap and water will drastically lower the number of pathogens on your hands. Proper hand cleaning requires rubbing the hands together and using liquid soap, warm running water, a nailbrush, and a clean towel (see Procedure 4-3). Do not underestimate proper cleaning and hand washing. They are the most powerful and important ways to prevent the spread of infection.

There are three ways to *clean* your tools and implements:

- Washing with soap and warm water and then scrubbing them with a clean and properly disinfected nailbrush

- Using an ultrasonic unit

- Using a cleaning solvent (e.g., clipper blade wash)

STEP 2: DISINFECTING

The second step of infection control is disinfection. Remember that disinfection is the process that eliminates most, but not necessarily all, microorganisms on nonporous surfaces. This process, however, is not effective against bacterial spores. In the barbershop, disinfection is extremely effective in controlling microorganisms on surfaces such as shears, clippers, and other **multiuse** (mul-tih-YUS) tools and equipment. A disinfectant used in the shop should carry an EPA registration number, and the label should clearly state the specific organisms the solution is effective against when used according to the manufacturer's product instructions.

Remember that disinfectants are products that destroy most bacteria (not including spores), fungi, and viruses on surfaces. Disinfectants are not for use on human skin, hair, or nails. Never use disinfectants as hand cleaners since this can cause skin irritation and **allergy** (AL-ur-jee), a reaction due to extreme sensitivity to certain foods, chemicals, or other normally harmless substances. All disinfectant manufacturers clearly state on the labels of their products that skin contact should be avoided; this means your skin as well as the client's skin. Do not put your fingers directly into any disinfecting solution. Disinfectants are pesticides and can be harmful if absorbed through the skin. If you mix a disinfectant in a container that is not labeled by the manufacturer, the container must be properly labeled with the contents and the date it was mixed. All concentrated disinfectants must be diluted exactly as instructed by the manufacturer on the product label.

While some customers who know that they have impaired immune systems will share that information with you, many will not because they are embarrassed, they do not know it is important, or they do not know that they have a compromised immune system. These people are at very high risk of infection if they come into contact with pathogens. Because you will not always know who these people are, it is important to practice proper infection control before every customer. One example is a diabetic customer whose immune system does not work effectively and who also has impaired healing. Most type 2 diabetics have been diabetic for 7 years

> ⚠ **CAUTION**
> Read labels carefully. Manufacturers take great care to develop safe and highly effective products. However, when used improperly, many products that are otherwise safe can be rendered dangerous if you do not follow proper guidelines and directions exactly as the label instructs.

> ⚠ **CAUTION**
> Disinfectants must be registered with the EPA. Look for an EPA registration number on the label.

prior to being diagnosed, which means that even if you ask, they may likely say "no" because they have not yet been diagnosed! Another example concerns clients on medication for conditions such as asthma, rheumatoid arthritis, and fibromyalgia—these medications are designed to dull the immune system, making these customers particularly susceptible to infection. Remember, you do not know everybody who sits in your chair, so provide the best in disinfection for everyone.

CHOOSING A DISINFECTANT

You must read and follow the manufacturer's instructions whenever you are using a disinfectant. Mixing ratios (dilution) and contact time (the time as listed on the product label required for the disinfectant to be visibly moist to be effective against pathogens) are very important and can vary widely based on manufacturer and delivery method. For example, most concentrates have a 10-minute contact time, whereas most wipes have a 2-minute contact time. Not all disinfectants have the same concentration, so be sure to mix the correct proportions according to the instructions on the label. If the label does not have the word *concentrate* on it, the product is already mixed and must be used directly from the original container and must not be diluted. All EPA-registered disinfectants, even those sprayed on large surfaces, will specify a contact time in their directions for use. Disinfectants must have **efficacy** (ef-ih-KUH-see) claims on the label. Efficacy is the ability to produce the intended effect. As applied to disinfectant claims, efficacy means the effectiveness with which a disinfecting solution kills organisms when used according to the label instructions.

PROPER USE OF DISINFECTANTS

Implements must be thoroughly cleaned of all visible matter or residue before being placed in disinfectant solution. This is because residue will interfere with the disinfectant and prevent proper disinfection. Properly cleaned implements and tools, free from all visible debris, must be completely immersed in disinfectant solution. Complete immersion means there is enough liquid in the container to cover all surfaces of the item being disinfected, including the handles, for 10 minutes or for the time recommended by the manufacturer (**Figure 4-16**). When using an aerosol disinfectant, you must still look for and adhere to the contact time to ensure that all pathogens on the label are being effectively destroyed.

Disinfectant Tips

- Use disinfectants only on clean, hard, nonporous surfaces.

- Always wear gloves and safety glasses when handling disinfectant solutions.

- Always dilute products according to the instructions on the product label.

- An item must remain submerged in the disinfectant for 10 minutes unless the product label specifies differently.

⚠ **CAUTION**
Improper mixing of disinfectants—to be weaker or more concentrated than the manufacturer's instructions—can significantly reduce their effectiveness. Always add the disinfectant concentrate to the water when mixing and always follow the manufacturer's instructions for proper dilution.

Safety glasses and gloves should be worn while mixing to avoid accidental contact with eyes and skin.

? DID YOU KNOW?
The EPA has recently approved a new disinfectant that can be used in the barbershop and is available in a spray and an immersion form, as well as wipes: accelerated hydrogen peroxide (AHP). This disinfectant includes hydrogen peroxide in the formulation to increase the potency and performance of the product. AHP needs to be changed only every 14 days and is nontoxic to the skin and the environment.

Read the labels of all types of disinfectants closely. Choose the one that is most appropriate for its intended use and is the safest for you and your customers.

- To disinfect large surfaces such as countertops, carefully apply the disinfectant onto the clean surface or use a disinfectant spray and allow it to remain moist for 10 minutes, unless the product label specifies differently.

- If the product label states "complete immersion," the entire implement must be completely immersed in the solution.

- Change the disinfectant according to the instructions on the label. If the liquid is not changed as instructed, it will no longer be effective and may begin to promote the growth of microbes.

TYPES OF DISINFECTANTS

Disinfectants are not all the same. Some are appropriate for use in the shop and some are not. You should be aware of the different types of disinfectants and the ones that are recommended for barbershop use.

Disinfectants Appropriate for Barbershop Use

Quaternary ammonium compounds (KWAT-ur-nayr-ee uh-MOH-nee-um KAHM-powndz), also known as **quats** (KWATZ), are disinfectants that are very effective when used properly. The most advanced type of these formulations is called *multiple quats*. Multiple quats contain sophisticated blends of quats that work together to significantly increase the effectiveness of these disinfectants. Quat solutions usually disinfect implements in 10 minutes. These formulas may contain antirust ingredients, so leaving tools in the solution for prolonged periods can cause dulling or damage. They should be removed from the solution after the specified period, rinsed (if required), dried, and stored in a clean, covered container.

Phenolic disinfectants (fi-NOH-lik dis-in-FEK-tents) are powerful disinfectants, known as *tuberculocidal*. They are a form of formaldehyde, have a very high pH, and can damage the skin and eyes. Phenolic disinfectants can be harmful to the environment if put down the drain. They have been used reliably over the years to disinfect tools; however, they do have drawbacks. Phenol can damage plastic and rubber and can cause certain metals to rust. Extra care should be taken to avoid skin contact with phenolic disinfectants. Phenolics are known carcinogens, and as such should only be used in states that require or permit their use.

Bleach

Household bleach, 5.25 percent **sodium hypochlorite** (soh-DEE-um hy-puh-KLOR-yt), is an effective disinfectant and has been used extensively as a disinfectant in the barbershop. Using too much bleach can damage some metals and plastics, so be sure to read the label for safe use. Bleach can be corrosive to metals and plastics and can cause skin irritation and eye damage.

To mix a bleach solution, always follow the manufacturer's directions. Store the bleach solution away from heat and light. A fresh bleach solution should be mixed every 24 hours or when the solution has been contaminated. After mixing the bleach solution, date the container to ensure that

figure 4-16
Disinfectant.

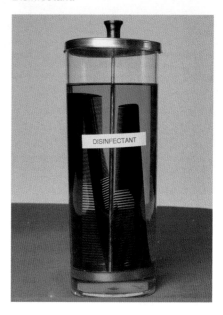

DID YOU KNOW?

Many of the aerosol products for use with clippers have several functions, such as lubricating, cooling, and rust inhibition. As long as "cleaner" and "disinfectant" are indicated on the label, the products are a "one-stop shop" for use between clients! The aerosol action does the cleaning and a disinfectant is added to the mix. Again, it is important to know the contact time for these items and to be sure to brush hair clippings from the blades before spraying.

the solution is not saved from one day to the next, but disposed of daily similar to other disinfectants. Bleach can be irritating to the lungs, so be careful about inhaling the fumes.

Petroleum Distillates

Petroleum distillates have been used by barbers for decades and are generally very similar in chemical structure to kerosene. They are excellent at removing grime and oils from metals, but not all products in this classification are approved for use as disinfectants. It is important that you check the product to ensure that it is bactericidal, virucidal, and fungicidal. The product must also be EPA registered as a disinfectant.

DISINFECTANT SAFETY

Disinfectants are pesticides (a type of poison) and can cause serious skin and eye damage. Some disinfectants appear clear while others, especially phenolic disinfectants, are a little cloudy. Always use caution when handling disinfectants, and follow the safety tips listed below.

Always

- Keep the SDS on hand for the disinfectant(s) you use.
- Wear gloves and safety glasses when mixing disinfectants.
- Avoid skin and eye contact.
- Add disinfectant to water when diluting (rather than adding water to a disinfectant) to prevent foaming, which can result in an incorrect mixing ratio.
- Use tongs, gloves, or a draining basket to remove implements from disinfectants.
- Keep disinfectants out of reach of children.
- Carefully measure and use disinfectant products according to label instructions.
- Follow the manufacturer's instructions for mixing, using, and disposing of disinfectants.
- Carefully follow the manufacturer's directions for when to replace the disinfectant solution in order to ensure the healthiest conditions for you and your client. Replace the disinfectant solution every day— more often if the solution becomes soiled or contaminated.

Never

- Let quats, phenols, bleach, or any other disinfectant come in contact with your skin. If you do get disinfectants on your skin, immediately wash the area with liquid soap and warm water. Then rinse and dry the area thoroughly.
- Place any disinfectant or other product in an unmarked container. All containers should be labeled.
- Mix chemicals together unless specified so in the manufacturer's instructions. (For example, mixing bleach and ammonia together causes toxic vapors and can cause an explosion.)

DISINFECTING CONTAINERS

In the past, jars or containers used to disinfect implements were often incorrectly called wet sanitizers. Disinfectant containers contain disinfectant for disinfecting purposes, not for cleaning. The container you choose must be large enough to contain all items to be disinfected and covered, but not airtight. Remember to clean the container every day and to wear gloves when you do. Always follow the manufacturer's label instructions for disinfecting products (**Figure 4-17**).

DISINFECTING NONELECTRICAL TOOLS AND IMPLEMENTS

State rules require that all multiuse tools and implements be cleaned and disinfected before and after every service—even when they are used on the same person. Mix all disinfectants according to the manufacturer's directions, always adding the disinfectant to the water, not the water to the disinfectant (see Procedure 4-1).

 4-1 **Cleaning and Disinfecting: Nonelectrical Tools and Implements**
pages 86–88

DISINFECTING ELECTRICAL TOOLS AND EQUIPMENT

Hair clippers and other types of electrical equipment have contact points that cannot be completely immersed in liquid. These items should be cleaned and disinfected using an EPA-registered disinfectant designed for use on these devices. Follow the procedures recommended by the disinfectant manufacturer for preparing the solution and follow the item's manufacturer directions for cleaning and disinfecting the device (see Procedure 4-2).

 4-2 **Cleaning and Disinfecting: Clippers and Outliners** *pages 89–92*

DISINFECTING WORK SURFACES

Before beginning a service, all work surfaces must be cleaned and disinfected. Be sure to clean and disinfect tables, stations, shampoo sinks, chairs, armrests, and any other surface that a customer's skin may have touched. Clean doorknobs and handles daily to reduce transfer of germs to your hands.

CLEANING TOWELS, LINENS, AND CAPES

Clean towels, linens, and capes must be used for each client. After a towel, linen, or cape has been used on a client, it must not be used again until it has been properly laundered. To clean towels, linens, and capes, launder according to the directions on the item's label. Be sure that towels, linens, and capes are thoroughly dried. Items that are not dry may grow mildew and bacteria. Store soiled linens and towels in covered or closed containers, away from clean linens and

figure 4-17
Disinfectants.

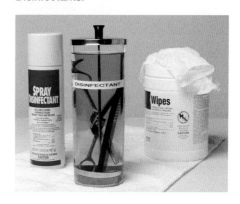

⚠ CAUTION
Electric sterilizers, bead sterilizers, and baby sterilizers should not be used to disinfect or sterilize implements. These devices can spread potentially infectious diseases and should never be used in the barbershop. Also, UV light units will not disinfect or sterilize implements. State rules require that you use liquid disinfecting solutions. Autoclaves are effective sterilizers. If you decide to use an autoclave, be sure that you know how to operate it properly.

figure 4-18
Strop.

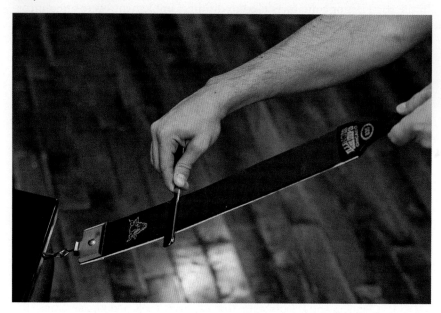

towels, even if your state regulatory agency does not require that you do so. Whenever possible, use disposable towels, especially in restrooms. Do not allow the neckband of capes to touch the client's skin. All states require the use of a barrier such as, disposable neck strips or towels, to prevent the client's skin from touching the neckline of the cape.

STROPS AND LEATHER HOLSTERS

Leather is a **porous** (POHW-rus) material and as such cannot be disinfected. When utilizing a strop or holster, it is important to clean and disinfect the tool or implement after it has come into contact with the leather before using it on a client (**Figure 4-18**). It is also important that you wash your hands prior to using the strop.

Even if you are unlikely to cause a major illness, a "minor" illness spread through improper disinfection can have devastating impacts on your business. A single case of ringworm or folliculitis spread by a dirty comb or razor blade can be quickly publicized in today's social media world where bad news travels faster than good! Do not let your shop be the one posted on the web for dirty practices!

> ⚠️ **CAUTION**
> Products and equipment that do not have the word *disinfectant* on the label are merely cleaners. They do not disinfect. Items must be properly cleaned and disinfected after every use before using them on another client.

MULTIUSE PRODUCTS

When using creams, lotions, gels, or any other product that is dispensed from a multiuse container, it is important not to contaminate the product. Always use a pump or shaker to dispense products when possible. When products are in a tub-type container, always use a clean spatula (disposable or disinfectable) to remove the product—never use your fingers.

HAND WASHING

Properly washing your hands is one of the most important actions you can take to prevent spreading germs from one person to another. Proper hand washing removes germs from the folds and grooves of the skin and from under the free edge of the nail plate by lifting and rinsing germs and contaminants from the surface of your skin. You should wash your hands thoroughly before and after working with each customer. Follow the hand washing procedure described in Procedure 4-3.

Antimicrobial and antibacterial soaps can dry the skin, and medical studies suggest that they are no more effective than regular soaps or detergents. The true benefit of hand washing comes from the friction created by the soap bubbles that can "pull" pathogens off the skin surface. Repeated hand washing can also dry the skin, so using a moisturizing hand lotion after washing is a good practice. Be sure the hand lotion is in a pump container, not a jar.

Avoid using very hot water to wash your hands because this is another practice that can damage the skin. Remember, you must wash your hands thoroughly before and after each service, so do all you can to reduce any irritation that may occur.

Ⓟ 4-3　**Proper Hand Washing** *pages 93–94*

WATERLESS HAND SANITIZERS

Antiseptics (ant-ih-SEP-tiks) are chemical germicides formulated for use on skin and are registered and regulated by the Food and Drug Administration. Antiseptics generally contain a high volume of alcohol and are intended to reduce the numbers and slow the growth of microbes on the skin (**Figure 4-19**). When there is visible dirt/debris on the hands, neither waterless hand sanitizers nor antiseptics will work until the dirt/debris is removed; this can only be accomplished with liquid soap, a soft-bristle brush, and water. Due to the drying effect of alcohol, hand sanitizers should not be overused, but they are an excellent option when hand washing is not possible. Never use an antiseptic to disinfect instruments or other surfaces. They are ineffective for that purpose.

COMMON ANTISEPTICS USED IN THE BARBERSHOP

- Hydrogen peroxide has been used in homes and barbershops virtually forever. It is generally used at 3 percent strength and works well as an antiseptic. However, it should never be used on an open cut as it destroys the cells that begin the healing process in a wound.

- Isopropyl alcohol is effective in cleaning the skin; however, it can be very drying and cause irritation of the skin. Alcohol is not a disinfectant for surfaces or implements and should only be used as a cleaner or antiseptic.

> **⚠ CAUTION**
> When washing hands, use liquid soaps in pump containers. Bacteria can grow in bar soaps.

figure 4-19
Hand sanitizer.

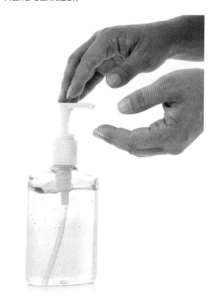

Follow Standard Precautions to Protect You and Your Clients

After reading this section, you will be able to:

LO❻ Discuss Standard Precautions and explain procedures for handling an exposure incident.

Standard Precautions (SP) (STAN-dard PRUH-caw-shuns) are guidelines published by the CDC that require the employer and employee to assume that any human blood and body fluids are potentially infectious. Because it may not be possible to identify customers with infectious diseases, strict infection control practices should be used with all clients. In most instances, clients who are infected with the hepatitis B virus or other bloodborne pathogens are **asymptomatic** (A-symp-toe-mat-ic), which means that they show no symptoms or signs of infection.

OSHA and CDC have set safety standards and precautions that protect employees in situations when they could be exposed to bloodborne pathogens. Precautions include proper hand washing, wearing of gloves, and proper handling and disposing of sharp instruments and any other items that may have been contaminated by blood or other body fluids. It is important that specific procedures be followed if blood or body fluid is present (see Procedure 4-4).

AN EXPOSURE INCIDENT: CONTACT WITH BLOOD OR BODY FLUID

You should never perform a service on any client who comes into the shop with an open wound, a rash, or an abrasion. Sometimes accidents happen while a service is being performed in the barbershop, however.

An **exposure incident** (eks-POH-zhoor in-SI-dent) is contact with non-intact (broken) skin, blood, body fluid, or other potentially infectious materials that is the result of the performance of a worker's duties. Should the client suffer a cut or abrasion that bleeds during a service, follow the steps outlined in Procedure 4-4 for the client's safety, as well as your own.

Ⓟ4-4 **Handling an Exposure Incident** *pages 95–97*

Follow Safe Work Practices and Safety Precautions

After reading this section, you will be able to:

LO❼ Discuss safe work practices that help prevent accidents and injuries.

Most potentially harmful situations in the barbershop can be avoided by being observant and using common sense. Learn to recognize safety hazards to minimize the occurrence of accidents.

Water

- At the shampoo bowl, be careful how you handle the spray hose. Position the client's head for comfort and access, being conscious of your own body position as well. Do not bend or twist from the waist unnecessarily. Wipe up any water spills or leaks immediately.

- If the water temperature reaches a scalding level while in the hot position, turn the thermostat on the hot-water tank down to a more acceptable temperature for application to the skin, scalp, and hair. Water heaters should not be set at higher than 130 degrees Fahrenheit.

- As a precaution, always test the water temperature on the inside of your wrist before applying to a client's hair or scalp. The same procedure may be used to test steam towels for facials and shaves.

Electricity

- Electricity and water do not mix. Make sure that all electrical appliances and tools are stored safely, and preferably unplugged, when in proximity to water.

- Never overload electrical outlets or use extension cords.

- Make sure that electrical outlets located near water sources are ground fault circuit interrupter (GFCI) outlets.

- Have shop wiring checked periodically to ensure a safe, fire-free environment.

- Schedule annual safety and operational check-ups for wiring, hot-water tanks, air conditioners, and ventilation systems.

Tools and Appliances

- Tools and equipment should be strategically placed so that the items are safely stored when not in use, yet are accessible when needed. Smaller tools, such as clippers, trimmers, blowdryers, or curling irons, may be placed in countertop receptacles designed for that purpose. Do not forget to disinfect before and after each use. Larger equipment such as UV-light units (used only for storage of disinfected items) may be mounted under the cabinet, attached to a wall, or set on a shelf. Disinfecting jars and electric latherizers are usually placed on the station countertop, but should be set back toward a wall or partition so as not to interfere with other tools. This also limits the risk of accidental burns from a hot latherizer or the spillage of disinfectant solutions.

- If a tool or implement is dropped on the floor during a service, it must be replaced with a disinfected tool or you must stop the service and properly disinfect the tool that was dropped prior to continuing the service. This is a good reason to keep an extra set of tools that are ready to use handy.

- All tools and implements should be in good working condition. Replace damaged tools immediately, including worn electrical cords, chipped clipper blades, cracked housings, and broken shears. Do not try to repair tools yourself; send them to the manufacturer for service. Never subject yourself or your client to the risks of faulty or broken equipment.

- Barbering tools and implements are designed for specific purposes, so use the right tool for the job. Do not expect a trimmer to do the work of a clipper!

- Electrical cords deserve specific mention because they often become a safety hazard in the shop. Cords to clippers, trimmers, curling irons, and blowdryers tend to become twisted and tangled during use. If the cord is too long, it can get caught on the foot or armrests of a hydraulic chair or even on the foot of a client. Some barbers use cordless trimmers to eliminate the problem altogether. A well-planned workstation with sufficient and conveniently placed outlets can also help minimize the *tangled cord syndrome.*

- Never place any tool or implement in your mouth or pocket.

Equipment and Fixtures

- Keep all hydraulic chairs, headrests, shampoo chairs, heat lamps, and lighting fixtures in good working order. Tighten screws and bolts, grease or oil hinges, and service equipment mechanisms as needed.

- Dust and clean regularly to avoid dust buildup and to maintain clean conditions.

- Maintain lighting fixtures. Change bulbs when necessary to keep workstations well lit.

Ventilation

- Proper ventilation and air circulation are extremely important in today's barbershop. Particles from products such as talc, hair sprays, and disinfectants can be inhaled and may cause allergies or other health problems. Heating and air-conditioning vents should be located to perform their optimum functions without inferring with client services. Vents should be vacuumed or cleaned periodically to prevent any buildup of hair that might impede ventilation. Fumes from chemical applications and nail care products require sophisticated filtration units that cleanse and detoxify the air. Once installed, air filters should be changed or cleaned regularly.

Attire

- Clothing should be comfortable and professional in appearance. Excessively baggy clothes can get in the way of your performance just as *easily as tight clothing can restrict it.*

- Long hair worn in a loose style may easily get caught in blowdryer motor vents and other appliances. Keep hair pulled back or short enough to avoid entanglements.

- Necklaces should be of an appropriate length so as not to get caught on equipment or dangle in a client's face at the shampoo bowl or during a shave. Rings should not be worn on the index and middle fingers as they might interfere with haircutting accuracy. In general, rings with stones and elaborate settings are very hard to keep clean. Watches should be waterproof and shock absorbent.

- Shoes should have nonskid rubber soles with good support.
- Electronic devices that may distract you, such as cell phones or tablets, should be kept stored away and only checked or answered between clients.

Children

- Children can cause serious risk of injury to themselves in the shop environment. Being aware of their inquisitive nature and the speed with which they can move can help prevent accidents from happening.
- Post notices in the reception area that advises patrons that children are not to be left unattended.
- Do not allow children to play, climb, or spin on hydraulic chairs.
- Do not allow children to wander freely around the shop with access to workstations, storage areas, and so forth.
- When cutting a child's hair, try to anticipate the child's sudden moves. Never trust a young child to hold his head still while you approach his head area with shears or other tools. Instead, hold the child's head gently but firmly with one hand while cutting with the other. This technique is especially helpful when cutting around ears and at the nape. When trimming bangs or front hairlines, hold the hair between your fingers at a low elevation, cutting the hair on the inside of your palm, thereby putting the barrier of your fingers between the tool and the child's face.

Adult Clients

- As barbers, many of the things we do to assure client comfort also fall under the category of safety precautions. In the following chapters you will learn proper draping procedures and chemical application methods to ensure client safety and comfort from the standpoint of avoiding skin irritations, burns, wet or soiled clothing, and so forth; however, there are also several common-sense services that should be performed. Using good manners and performing common courtesies will help you gain the reputation of being a safety-conscious and courteous barber.
- Assist clients (especially the elderly) in and out of hydraulic and shampoo chairs. Turn hydraulic chairs so the client may get out of the chair without risk of his feet becoming tangled in any of the cords.
- Always lower the hydraulic chair to its lowest level and lock it in position so that it does not spin before inviting the client to be seated or leave the chair.
- Hold doors open for clients.
- Assist clients in walking whenever necessary.
- Always support the back of the chair, and thus the client, when reclining or raising a chair back.
- Cushion the client's neck with a folded towel in the neck rest at the shampoo bowl. This is especially beneficial for clients with neck injuries such as whiplash.

- Support the client's head whenever appropriate at the shampoo bowl. Do not ask the client to hold his head up for shampooing or rinsing. Instead, gently turn the client's head to the side for easier access to the back and nape areas.

Exits

- Exits should be well marked and identifiable. (Check with your local building inspection office for codes and requirements.)
- Employees should know where exits are located and how to evacuate the building quickly in case of fire or other emergencies. Implement fire drills to practice for this contingency.

Fire Extinguishers

- Fire extinguishers should be placed where they are readily accessible.
- All employees should be instructed in fire extinguisher use.
- It is a law that fire extinguishers be checked periodically. Be guided by the manufacturer's recommendations and state and local ordinances.

Chemicals

- Request an SDS from your supplier(s) for each product purchased for use or sale in the shop, and maintain an SDS notebook. Add to the notebook as new products are brought into the workplace.
- Take the time to study the SDS from the manufacturer so that you will know how and where to store products and what procedures to follow in an emergency.
- There is a correct way to dispose of chemicals such as haircolor tints, chemical relaxers, and bleach. Contact your local hazardous-waste department or agency for disposal guidelines.
- Never mix cleaning products together under any circumstances.
- Never mix leftover chemicals together.
- Do not allow leftover chemicals to stockpile. Dispose of products as often as necessary to maintain a safe environment.
- Check the inventory stock occasionally for plastic bottles with dents or bulges. This swelling of the container indicates that the contents are under pressure and could possibly explode.
- Wear goggles when pouring or mixing products. Add a lab apron and gloves when handling any caustic or skin-irritating material.
- Chemical spills require an absorbent material, such as sawdust, to clean up properly. Be guided by your local hazardous-waste agency.
- Every solution, liquid, cream, powder, paste, gel, and other substance should be properly labeled. This requirement goes beyond labeled products purchased from a supplier and includes spray bottles of water or setting lotions, disinfecting jars, containers of blade wash, and any other substance used in the shop that is not contained within its original packaging.

List Your Professional Responsibilities

After reading this section, you will be able to:

LO⑧ List your responsibilities as a professional barber.

After studying this chapter, it should be clear that your responsibilities as a professional barber far exceed the ability to perform a good haircut; your most important responsibility is to protect your clients' health and safety.

- Never take shortcuts for cleaning and disinfecting. You cannot afford to skip steps or save money when it comes to safety.

- It is your professional and legal responsibility to follow state and federal laws and rules.

- Keep your license current and notify the licensing agency if you move or change your name.

- Check your state's website monthly for any change or update to the rules and regulations.

- Be aware of your environment so that you can identify and eliminate potential hazards to make the barbershop safer for you and your clients.

- Be prepared for emergencies. Every shop should have employee and clientele emergency information available near the telephone.

  - An emergency phone number checklist should include the contact numbers for fire, police, and medical rescue departments; the nearest hospital emergency room; and taxis.

  - Utility service companies, such as electricity, water, heat, air-conditioning, and landlord or custodial numbers are also helpful in an emergency or if something breaks down in the shop. Update this information on an annual basis and you will always be prepared.

- Realize that behavior that stems from a knowledgeable and caring manner is what separates a true professional from a nonprofessional, and being a professional is something you can take pride in.

CLEANING AND DISINFECTING: NONELECTRICAL TOOLS AND IMPLEMENTS

Nonelectrical tools and implements include combs, brushes, shears, clips, hairpins, tweezers, and all other items that can be completely immersed into a disinfectant container.

MATERIALS, IMPLEMENTS, AND EQUIPMENT

- ☐ Covered storage container
- ☐ Disinfectant
- ☐ Disposable gloves
- ☐ Disposable towels
- ☐ Liquid disinfectant

- ☐ Liquid soap
- ☐ Safety glasses
- ☐ Scrub brush
- ☐ Timer
- ☐ Tongs

PROCEDURE

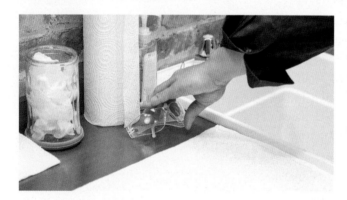

1 It is important to wear safety glasses and gloves while disinfecting nonelectrical tools and implements to protect your eyes from unintentional splashes of disinfectant, to prevent possible contamination of the implements by your hands, and to protect your hands from the powerful chemicals in the disinfectant solution.

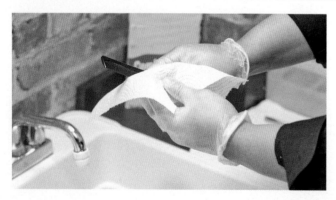

2 Prepare the cleaning solution according to the manufacturer's directions.

3 Remove all visible hair from your tools and implements before washing.

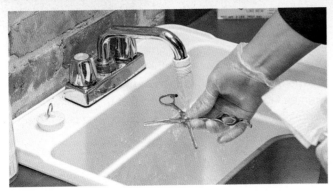

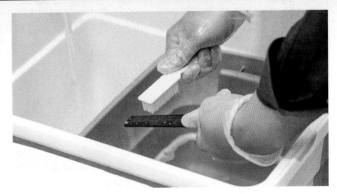

4 Rinse all implements with warm running water.

5 Use a small scrubbing brush to clean them in the cleaning or soap solution.

6 Brush grooved items thoroughly and open hinged implements to scrub the revealed areas clean.

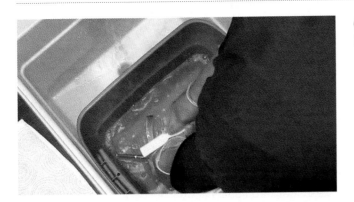

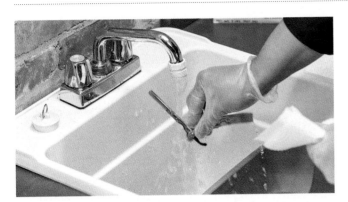

7 Rinse away all traces of solution or soap with warm running water. The presence of soap in most disinfectants will cause them to become inactive. Soap is most easily rinsed off in warm, not hot, water.

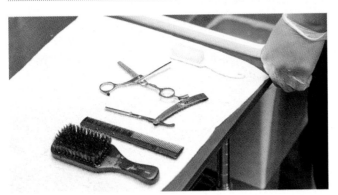

8 Dry implements thoroughly with a clean or disposable towel, or allow them to air dry on a clean towel.

9 Your implements are now properly cleaned and ready to be disinfected.

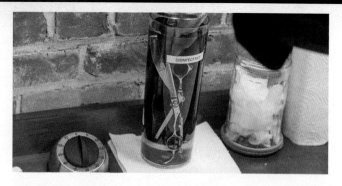

10 Immerse cleaned implements in an appropriate disinfection container holding an EPA-registered disinfectant for the required time (at least 10 minutes or according to the manufacturer's instructions). Remember to open hinged implements before immersing them in the disinfectant. If the disinfectant solution is visibly dirty, or if the solution has been contaminated, it must be replaced.

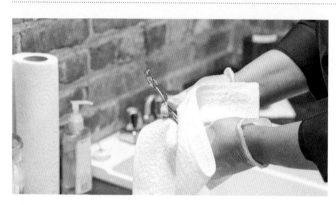

11 After the required disinfection time has passed, remove tools and implements from the disinfectant solution with tongs or gloved hands, rinse the tools and implements well in warm running water, and pat them dry.

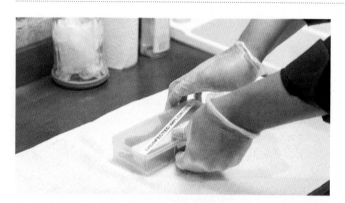

12 Store dry, disinfected tools and implements in a clean, covered container until needed.

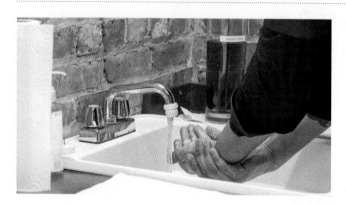

13 Remove gloves and thoroughly wash your hands with warm running water and liquid soap. Rinse and dry hands with a clean fabric or disposable towel.

CLEANING AND DISINFECTING: CLIPPERS AND OUTLINERS

The disinfection of electrical tools, such as clippers and outliners, requires a different approach than that for nonelectric tools and implements. Hair particles and bacteria become trapped between and behind clipper blades; so thorough cleaning and disinfection of these tools is very important. There are a large number of disinfectant choices that work well for clipper blades. Again, it is vital that regardless of what type you choose, the label must be EPA registered as bactericidal, virucidal, and fungicidal, and in some states, even as tuberculocidal. Many of the products that have been used historically do not meet the current requirements of most states, so it is important to know what those requirements are and to follow them, regardless of historical practice.

Setup for Cleaning and Disinfecting Clippers and Outliners

PROCEDURE

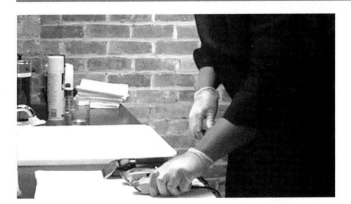

1 Arrange all supplies, products, and tools on a clean surface.

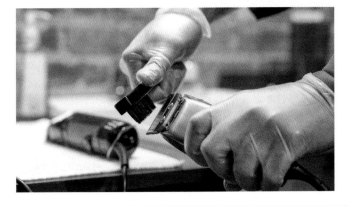

2 Remove hair particles from clipper blades with a stiff brush.

Cleaning and Disinfecting Clippers and Outliners with Nondetachable Blades

3 To clean the blades and prepare them for disinfection, you must follow one of the following two methods.

CLEANING WITH BLADE WASH

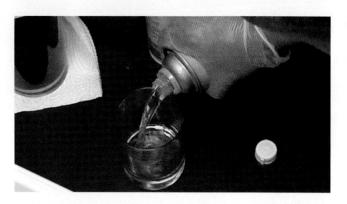

4 Pour blade wash into a glass, plastic, or disposable container wide enough to accommodate the width of the clipper blades to a depth of approximately ½ inch.

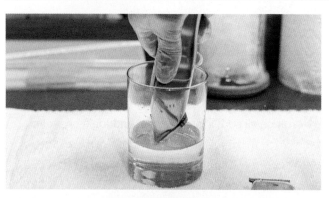

5A For nondetachable blades, submerge only the cutting teeth of the clipper blades into the blade wash and turn the unit on. Run the blades in the solution until no hair particles are seen being dislodged from between the blades.

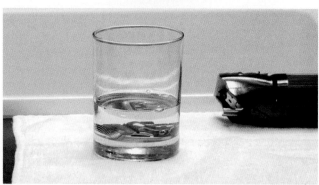

5B For detachable clipper blades, detach the blades and submerge into the blade wash for the manufacturer's recommended time.

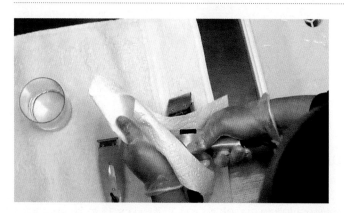

6 Wipe the blades dry with a clean towel.

CLEANING WITH AEROSOL CLEANER

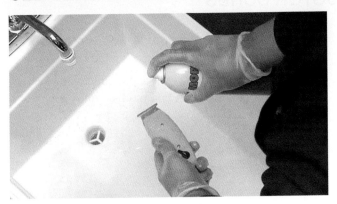

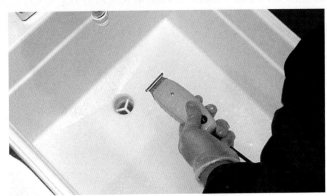

7 Use aerosol spray cleaner as indicated on the label, following the manufacturer's instructions for use. Spray the cleaner until you can see the blades getting wet.

8 Turn the unit on and let the blades run until you see hair being dislodged from the blades.

9 Wipe the blades dry with a clean, dry towel.

Disinfecting Using a Disinfectant Spray

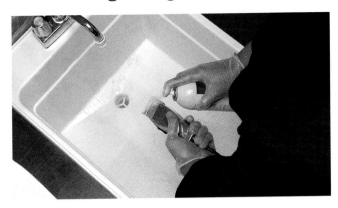

10 Now that your clippers are clean, spray with a clipper disinfectant and allow blades to remain moist for full contact time as mentioned on the manufacturer's label.

Grease or Oil Clippers and Outliners

11 For all of your clippers or outliners, it is important to grease or oil the parts regularly to keep your tools in top shape.

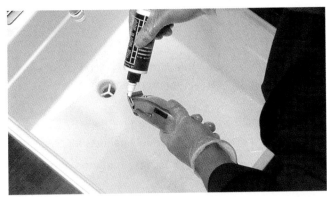

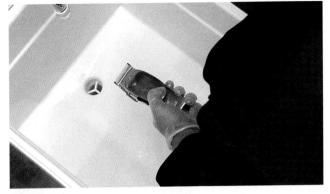

12 To oil the blades, put one drop of clipper oil on each side of the blades.

13 Next, turn the unit on and let it run for 15 to 30 seconds.

14 Turn off the clippers or outliners and unplug.

CLEANING AND DISINFECTING CONDUCTOR CORDS

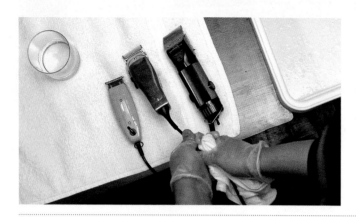

15 Before you begin cleaning the conductor cord, always double-check that it is unplugged.

16 To clean the conductor cord, put soap on a wet towel. Lather up the towel and run the soapy towel down the cord.

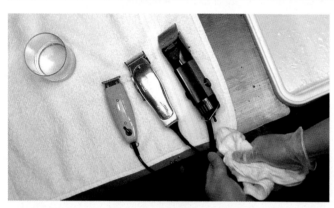

17 Using a wet towel, rinse off the cord by running the towel down the cord.

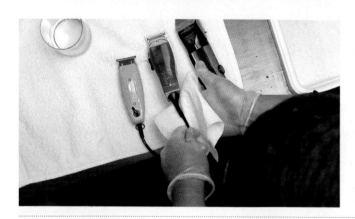

18 With a dry towel, dry the cord completely.

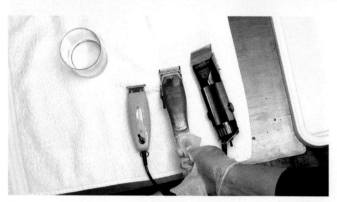

19 Then, wipe down the cord with a disinfectant wipe, ensuring that cord is never dropped to the floor or off of the clean working surface.

20 Store cleaned and disinfected clippers, or outliners, in a clean, covered container until needed for use.

21 Make sure to use one of these methods after each client.

PROPER HAND WASHING

Hand washing is one of the most important procedures in your infection control efforts and is required in every state before beginning any service.

MATERIALS, IMPLEMENTS, AND EQUIPMENT

☐ Disposable paper towels

☐ Liquid soap in a pump container

☐ Nail brush

PROCEDURE

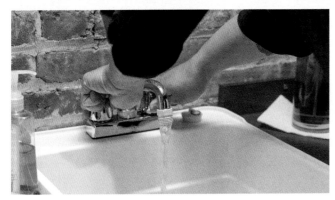

① Turn the water on, wet your hands.

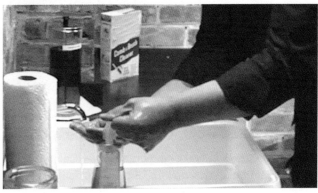

② Pump soap from a pump container onto the palm of your hand.

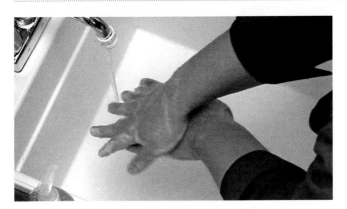

③ Rub your hands together, all over and vigorously, until a lather forms. Continue for a minimum of 20 seconds.

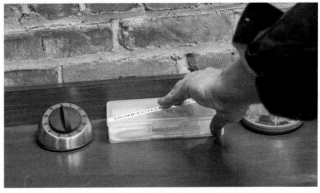

④ Choose a clean and disinfected nail brush.

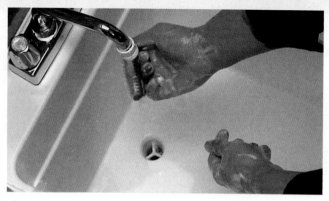

5 Wet the nail brush, and pump soap on to the bristles.

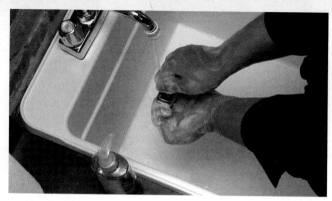

6 Brush your nails horizontally back and forth under the free edges.

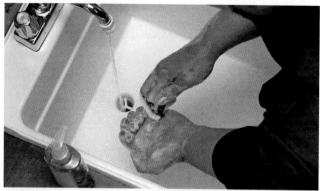

7 Change the direction of the brush to vertical and move the brush up and down along the nail folds of the fingernails. The process for brushing both hands should take about 60 seconds to finish.

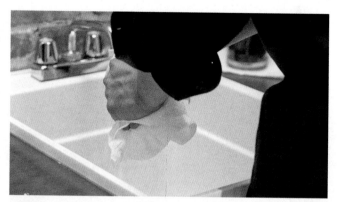

8 Rinse hands in running warm water.

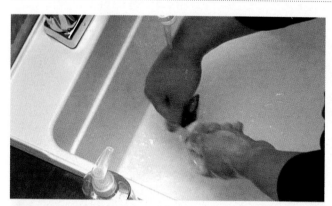

9 Use a clean cloth or paper towel for drying your hands, according to the barbershop's policies or state rules and regulations.

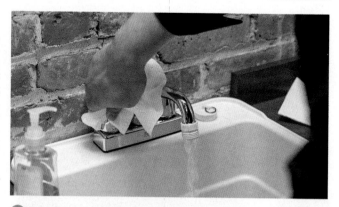

10 After drying your hands, turn off the water with the towel. Use the towel to open the door and then dispose of the towel. Touching a doorknob with your bare fingers can recontaminate your hands.

HANDLING AN EXPOSURE INCIDENT

☐ Antiseptic

☐ Bandages

☐ Cotton

☐ Disposable gloves

☐ Disposable paper towels

☐ Liquid soap

☐ Plastic bag

PROCEDURE

Should you accidentally cut a client, calmly take the following steps:

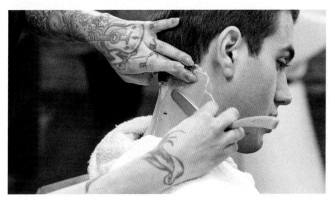

1 Stop the service immediately.

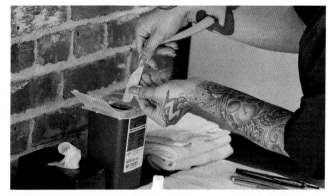

2 Dispose of the blade in a sharps container and place the razor in a container designated for cleaning and disinfection.

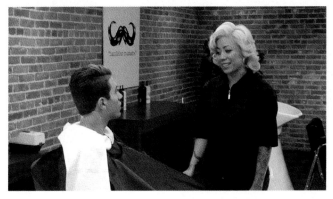

3 Face your client and calmly apologize for the incident.

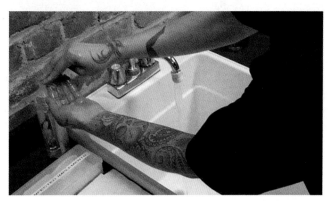

4 Excuse yourself to go wash your hands.

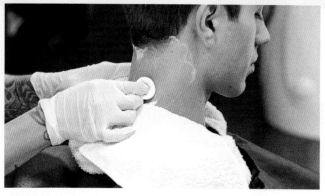

5 Once your hands are clean, immediately put on gloves.

6 Apply slight pressure to the area with a moistened cotton round to stop the bleeding.

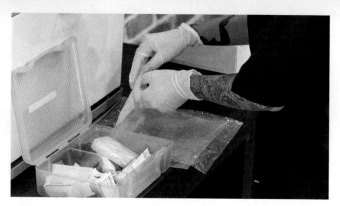

7 Dispose of the used cotton round in a plastic storage bag.

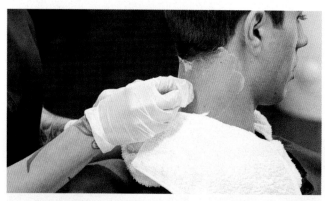

8 Then gently clean with an antiseptic and have the client wash the area if appropriate.

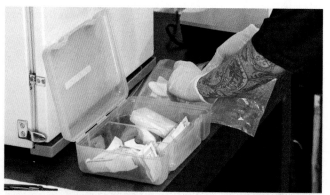

9 Dispose of the antiseptic wipe in the plastic storage bag.

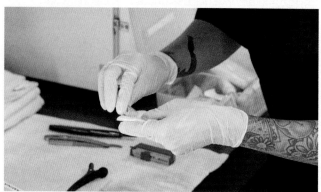

10 Dispense styptic powder onto a cotton round and use a cotton swab to apply it to the injury to stop any residual bleeding.

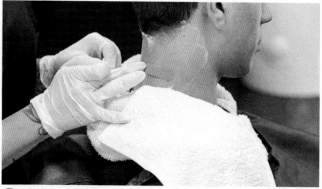

11 Apply an adhesive bandage to completely cover the wound.

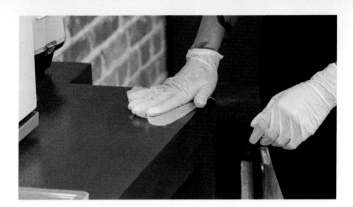

12 Clean and disinfect the workstation, as necessary.

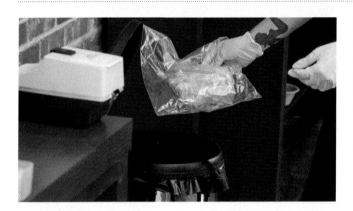

13 Discard all single-use, contaminated objects such as wipes or cotton balls in a plastic bag and then place in a trash bag. Deposit sharp disposables in a sharps box. Dispose of double-bagged items and sharps containers as required by state or local law. Information on these laws may be found on your local board website or through the OSHA website. In general, all of these items (except sharps) may go into the regular trash.

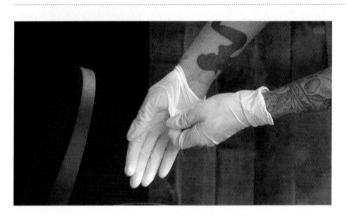

14 Remember, before you remove your gloves, all tools and implements that have come into contact with blood or other body fluids must be thoroughly cleaned and completely immersed in an EPA-registered hospital disinfectant solution designed for 10 minutes. Blood may carry pathogens, so you should never touch an open sore or a wound. Gloves should be removed with caution to avoid touching the contaminated surface of the glove. Remove one glove by holding it in other gloved hand, sliding your finger under the glove at the base of the glove, and pulling it over the other contaminated glove—never allowing either glove to come into contact with your skin.

15 Wash your hands with soap and warm water before returning to the service. Recommend that the client see a physician if any signs of redness, swelling, pain, or irritation develop.

REVIEW QUESTIONS

1. What is the primary purpose of regulatory agencies?

2. What is an SDS? Where can they be obtained?

3. List the four types of microorganisms that are pertinent to a barber.

4. What is a contagious disease?

5. Is HIV a risk in the barbershop? Why or why not?

6. What is the difference between cleaning, disinfecting, and sterilizing?

7. What is complete immersion?

8. List at least nine safety tips to follow when using disinfectants.

9. What are the characteristics of items that can be disinfected?

10. What does porous mean? Name two porous items that can be cleaned and disinfected in between use on clients.

11. What are Standard Precautions?

12. What is an exposure incident?

13. Describe the procedure for handling an exposure incident on a client in the barbershop.

14. List the four things that must be on a disinfectant label for approved use in all states.

CHAPTER GLOSSARY

acquired immune deficiency syndrome (uh-KWY-erd ih-MYOON di-FISH-en-see sin-drohm)	p. 70	abbreviated AIDS; a disease that breaks down the body's immune system; AIDS is caused by the human immunodeficiency virus (HIV)
acquired immunity (uh-KWY-erd ih-MYOO-nih-tee)	p. 71	immunity that the body develops after overcoming a disease, through inoculation (such as flu vaccinations), or through exposure to natural allergens (such as pollen, cat dander, and ragweed)
allergy (AL-ur-jee)	p. 73	reaction due to extreme sensitivity to certain foods, chemicals, or other normally harmless substances
antiseptics (ant-ih-SEP-tiks)	p. 79	chemical germicide formulated for use on skin; registered and regulated by the Food and Drug Administration
asymptomatic (A-symp-toe-mat-ic)	p. 80	showing no symptoms or signs of infection
bacilli (bah-SIL-ee)	p. 65	short rod-shaped bacteria; they are the most common bacteria and produce diseases such as tetanus (lockjaw), typhoid fever, tuberculosis, and diphtheria
bacteria (bak-TEER-ee-ah)	p. 63	single-celled microorganisms that have both plant and animal characteristics; some bacteria are harmful; some are harmless
bacterial spores (bak-TEER-ee-ul SPOORZ)	p. 63	bacteria capable of producing a protective coating that allows them to withstand very harsh environments and to shed the coating when conditions become more favorable to them
bactericidal (bak-TEER-uh-syd-uhl)	p. 63	capable of destroying bacteria
binary fission (BY-nayr-ee FISH-un)	p. 66	the division of bacterial cells into two new cells called *daughter cells*
biofilms	p. 69	colonies of microorganisms that adhere to environmental surfaces, as well as the human body

bloodborne pathogens (BLUD-boorn PATH-o-genz)	p. 69	disease-causing microorganisms carried in the body by blood or body fluids, such as hepatitis and HIV
cilia (SIL-ee-uh)	p. 65	hairlike extensions that protrude from cells and help sweep away fluids and particles
cleaning (KLEEN-ing)	p. 63	a mechanical process (scrubbing) using soap and water or detergent and water to remove all visible dirt, debris, and many disease-causing germs; cleaning also removes invisible debris that interferes with disinfection; cleaning is what barbers are required to do before disinfecting
cocci (KOK-sy)	p. 65	round-shaped bacteria that appear singly (alone) or in groups; the three types of cocci are staphylococci, streptococci, and diplococci
communicable (kuh-MYOO-nih-kuh-bul)	p. 67	able to be communicated; transferable by contact from one person to another as in a communicable disease
contagious disease (kun-TAY-jus DIZ-eez)	p. 67	also known as *communicable disease*; disease that is spread from one person to another person; some of the more contagious diseases are the common cold, ringworm, conjunctivitis (pinkeye), viral infections, and natural nail or toe and foot infections
contamination (kun-tam-uh-NAY-shun)	p. 68	the presence, or the reasonably anticipated presence, of blood or other potentially infectious materials on an item's surface or visible debris or residues such as dust, hair, and skin
diagnosis (dy-ag-NOH-sis)	p. 68	determination of the nature of a disease from its symptoms and/or diagnostic tests; federal regulations prohibit salon professionals from performing a diagnosis
diplococci (dip-loh-KOK-sy)	p. 65	spherical bacteria that grow in pairs and cause diseases such as pneumonia
direct transmission (dy-REKT trans-MISH-uhn)	p. 64	transmission of blood or body fluids through touching (including shaking hands), kissing, coughing, sneezing, and talking.
disease (DIZ-eez)	p. 60	an abnormal condition of all or part of the body, or its systems or organs, that makes the body incapable of carrying on normal function
disinfectants (dis-in-FEK-tents)	p. 60	chemical products approved by the EPA designed to destroy most bacteria (excluding spores), fungi, and viruses on surfaces
disinfection (disinfecting) (dis-in-FEK-shun)	p. 63	a chemical process that uses specific products to destroy harmful organisms (except bacterial spores) on environmental surfaces
efficacy (ef-ih-KUH-see)	p. 74	the ability of a product to produce the intended effect; on a disinfectant label, it indicates specific pathogens destroyed or disabled when used properly
exposure incident (eks-POH-zhoor in-SI-dent)	p. 80	contact with non intact (broken) skin, blood, body fluid, or other potentially infectious materials, which is the result of the performance of an employee's duties
flagella (fluh-JEL-uh)	p. 65	slender, hairlike extensions used by bacilli and spirilla for locomotion (moving about); may also be referred to as *cilia*
fungi (FUN-ji)	p. 70	single-celled organisms that grow in irregular masses and include molds, mildews, and yeasts; they can produce contagious diseases such as ringworm
fungicidal (FUN-ji-syd-uhl)	p. 63	capable of destroying molds and fungi
hepatitis (hep-uh-TY-tus)	p. 69	a bloodborne virus that causes disease and can damage the liver
hospital disinfectants (HOS-pih-tal dis-in-FEK-tents)	p. 60	disinfectants that are effective for cleaning blood and body fluids on nonporous surfaces
human immunodeficiency virus (HYOO-mun ih-MYOO-noh-di-FISH-en-see VY-rus)	p. 70	abbreviated HIV; virus that causes HIV disease and acquired immune deficiency syndrome (AIDS)

immunity (im-YOO-net-ee)	p. 71	the ability of the body to destroy and resist infection; immunity against disease can be either natural or acquired and is a sign of good health
Inactive stage (IN-ac-tif STAJE)	p. 66	also known as *spore-forming stage*; the ability of some bacteria to form a protective coating around themselves to protect them from harsh environments during the inactive stage
indirect transmission (IN-dih-rekt trans-MISH-uhn)	p. 64	transmission of blood or body fluids through contact with an intermediate contaminated object such as a razor, extractor, nipper, or an environmental surface
infection (in-FEK-shun)	p. 62	the invasion of body tissues by disease-causing pathogens
infection control (in-FEK-shun CON-trol)	p. 62	the methods used to eliminate or reduce the transmission of infectious organisms
infectious (in-FEK-shus)	p. 62	caused by or capable of being transmitted by infection
infectious disease (in-FEK-shus DIZ-eez)	p. 63	disease caused by pathogenic (harmful) microorganisms that enter the body; an infectious disease may or may not be spread from one person to another person
inflammation (in-fluh-MAY-shun)	p. 66	a condition in which the body reacts to injury, irritation, or infection, characterized by redness, heat, pain, and swelling
local infection (LOHK-al in-FEK-shun)	p. 67	an infection, such as a pimple or abscess, that is confined to a particular part of the body and appears as a lesion containing pus
methicillin-resistant staphylococcus aureus (METH-eh-sill-en-ree-ZIST-ent staf-uh-loh-KOK-us OR-ee-us)	p. 67	abbreviated MRSA; a type of infectious bacteria that is highly resistant to conventional treatments such as antibiotics
microorganism (my-kroh-OR-gah-niz-um)	p. 63	any organism of microscopic or submicroscopic size
mildew (MIL-doo)	p. 70	a type of fungus that affects plants or grows on inanimate objects but does not cause human infections in the barbershop
motility (MOH-till-it-ee)	p. 65	self-movement
multiuse (mul-tih-YUS)	p. 73	also known as *reusable*; items that can be cleaned, disinfected, and used on more than one person, even if the item is accidentally exposed to blood or body fluid
natural immunity (NATCH-uh-rul im-YOO-net-ee)	p. 71	immunity that is partly inherited and partly developed through healthy living
nonpathogenic (nahn-path-uh-JEN-ik)	p. 64	harmless microorganisms that may perform useful functions and are safe to come in contact with since they do not cause disease or harm
nonporous (nahn-POHW-rus)	p. 60	an item that is made or constructed of a material that has no pores or openings and cannot absorb liquids
occupational disease	p. 68	illness resulting from conditions associated with employment, such as prolonged and repeated overexposure to certain products or ingredients
parasites (PAYR-uh-sytz)	p. 71	organisms that grow, feed, and shelter on or inside another organism (referred to as the *host*), while contributing nothing to the survival of that organism. Parasites must have a host to survive
parasitic disease	p. 68	disease caused by parasites, such as lice and mites
pathogenic (path-uh-JEN-ik)	p. 64	harmful microorganisms that can cause disease or infection in humans when they invade the body
pathogenic disease	p. 68	disease produced by organisms, including bacteria, viruses, fungi, and parasites

pediculosis capitis (puh-dik-yuh-LOH-sis KAP-ih-tus)	p. 71	infestation of the hair and scalp with head lice
phenolic disinfectants (fi-NOH-lik dis-in-FEK-tents)	p. 75	tuberculocidal disinfectants that are a form of formaldehyde, have a very high pH, and can damage the skin and eyes
porous (POHW-rus)	p. 78	made or constructed of a material that has pores or openings; porous items are absorbent
pus (PUS)	p. 67	a fluid created by infection
quaternary ammonium compounds (KWAT-ur-nayr-ee uh-MOH-nee-um KAHM-powndz)	p. 75	commonly known as *quats* are products made of quaternary ammonium cations and are designed for disinfection of nonporous surfaces; they are appropriate for use in noncritical (noninvasive) environments and are effective against most pathogens of concern in the barbershop environment
Safety Data Sheet (SAYF-tee DAY-tuh SHEET)	p. 58	abbreviated SDS; required by law for all products sold. SDSs include safety information about products compiled by the manufacturer, including hazardous ingredients, safe use and handling procedures, proper disposal guidelines, and precautions to reduce the risk of accidental harm or overexposure
sanitation (san-ih-TAY-shun)	p. 56	also known as *sanitizing*; a chemical process for reducing the number of disease-causing germs on cleaned surfaces to a safe level
scabies (SKAY-beez)	p. 71	a contagious skin disease that is caused by the itch mite, which burrows under the skin
sodium hypochlorite (soh-DEE-um hy-puh-KLOR-yt)	p. 75	common household bleach; an effective disinfectant for the barbershop
spirilla (spy-RIL-ah)	p. 65	spiral or corkscrew-shaped bacteria that cause diseases such as syphilis and Lyme
Standard Precautions (STAN-dard PRUH-caw-shuns)	p. 80	are guidelines published by the CDC that require the employer and employee to assume that any human blood and body fluids are potentially infectious
staphylococci (staf-uh-loh-KOKS-sy)	p. 65	pus-forming bacteria that grow in clusters like a bunch of grapes. They cause abscesses, pustules, and boils
sterilization (stayr-ih-luh-ZAY-shun)	p. 72	the process that completely destroys all microbial life, including spores
streptococci (strep-toh-KOK-sy)	p. 65	pus-forming bacteria arranged in curved lines resembling a string of beads. They cause infections such as strep throat and blood poisoning
tinea barbae (TIN-ee-uh BAR-bee)	p. 70	also known as *barber's itch*, a superficial fungal infection that commonly affects the skin; it is primarily limited to the bearded areas of the face and neck or around the scalp
tinea capitis (TIN-ee-uh KAP-ih-tus)	p. 70	a fungal infection of the scalp characterized by red papules, or spots, at the opening of the hair follicles
toxins	p. 71	various poisonous substances produced by some microorganisms (bacteria and viruses)
tuberculocidal disinfectants (tuh-bur-kyoo-LOH-syd-ahl dis-in-FEK-tents)	p. 60	often referred to as phenolics, are proven to kill the bacterium that cause tuberculosis, in addition to other pathogens destroyed through the use of hospital disinfectants
tuberculosis (tuh-bur-kyoo-LOH-sus)	p. 60	a disease caused by bacteria that are transmitted through coughing or sneezing
virucidal (VI-ra-syd-uhl)	p. 63	capable of destroying viruses
virus (VY-rus)	p. 67	a parasitic submicroscopic particle that infects and resides in cells of biological organisms. A virus is capable of replication only through taking over the host cell's reproductive function

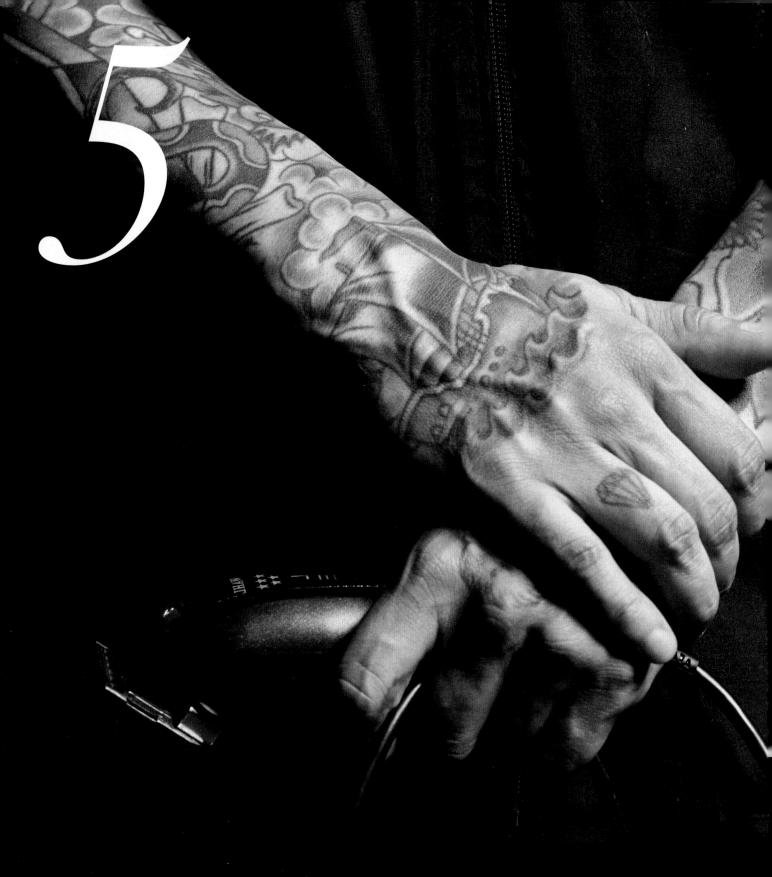

5

IMPLEMENTS, TOOLS, AND EQUIPMENT

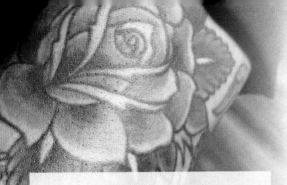

LEARNING OBJECTIVES

After completing this chapter, you will be able to:

LO **1**
List the principal tools of the trade used in barbering.

LO **2**
Describe when to use different combs and brushes.

LO **3**
Discuss and identify the types of haircutting shears.

LO **4**
Identify the parts of haircutting shears.

LO **5**
Show how to properly hold shears for haircutting.

LO **6**
Show how to palm the shears and comb.

LO **7**
Describe two types of clippers.

LO **8**
Identify the main parts of a clipper.

LO **9**
Show different ways to hold clippers for haircutting.

LO **10**
Name two types of straight razors.

LO **11**
Identify the different parts of a straight razor.

LO **12**
Show how to hold a straight razor for shaving, honing, and stropping.

LO **13**
Show how to hold a straight razor for haircutting.

LO⑭
Describe the functions of hones and strops.

LO⑮
Show how to hone and strop a conventional blade straight razor.

LO⑯
Identify the types of equipment and supplies used in barbering.

LO⑰
Identify ways to remove hair clippings.

LO⑱
Show how to perform two towel-wrapping methods.

Introduction

The practice of barbering requires a variety of implements, tools, and equipment. You should strive to purchase high-quality items that will perform effectively and safely to get the job done. This does not mean that you have to purchase the most expensive items, but beware of "bargains." For example, it is unlikely that a comb that can be bent between your thumb and index finger will actually comb through the hair. Low-quality implements, tools, and equipment are a waste of time and money and can end up costing more to replace than what you would have spent in the first place. When taken care of properly, well-made implements and tools will provide years of dependable service. Since the variety of choices can be confusing, ask your instructor or an experienced barber to assist you when selecting and purchasing new implements, tools, or equipment.

why study
IMPLEMENTS, TOOLS, AND EQUIPMENT?

Barbers should study and have a thorough understanding of implements, tools, and equipment because:

> Understanding the purpose and capabilities of your implements and tools will help you select the right tool for the job.

> Knowing the parts of your implements, tools, and equipment will help you understand instructions given during practical work, to comply with infection control procedures, and to know when an item may need repair or replacement.

> Understanding how to hold and use your implements and tools is critical to achieving desired results.

> Using barbering equipment correctly and safely is important to your safety and the comfort and safety of your clients.

Learn about Implements and Tools Used in Barbering

After reading this section, you will be able to:

LO **1** List the principal tools of the trade used in barbering.

As a barber, your principal *tools of the trade* are combs, brushes, shears, clippers, outliners, and razors. In addition, you will use appliances such as blowdryers and thermal styling tools to perform finishing and styling work on your clients. Choosing the right implement or tool for the job will depend on your understanding of the item's functions and characteristics and how to use it in an effective and safe manner.

Identify Different Types of Combs and Brushes

After reading this section, you will be able to:

LO **2** Describe when to use different combs and brushes.

KNOW YOUR COMB BASICS

Combs are made from various materials in different shapes and sizes. A good quality comb is just slightly flexible with smooth, rounded teeth that will comb through the hair without snagging individual strands. Most of the combs used in haircutting measure between 7 and 8 inches long with a shape that may be straight, tapered, or handled. The materials used in the construction of the comb determine its characteristics or qualities:

* Hard rubber combs are slightly flexible and durable but can deteriorate if left in a disinfectant over an extended time.

* Combs made from carbon materials are antistatic, stiff, and heat and chemical resistant.

* Graphite combs are less rigid than carbon material combs and are heat and chemical resistant.

* Metal combs can retain heat to help set-in a hairstyle. Made from tempered aluminum or other metals, metal combs may corrode in reaction to chemicals, such as hydrogen peroxide.

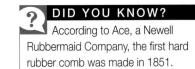

DID YOU KNOW?
According to Ace, a Newell Rubbermaid Company, the first hard rubber comb was made in 1851.

The Comb Teeth

The spacing between the teeth of a comb varies with the style of comb. Many combs are designed with fine or narrow (close together) teeth at one end and coarse or wide (farther apart) teeth at the other end. Other comb styles have uniformly spaced teeth for the entire length of the comb.

figure 5-1
Assorted all-purpose combs.

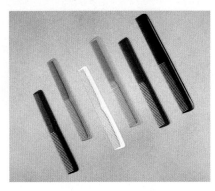

The spacing of the teeth is important because the thickness and distribution of the hair strands that flow through the comb can affect your cutting or styling outcomes. For example, combing through a section of hair with the narrow end of the comb merges the hair strands closer together than the wide end of the comb does; thus, the narrow end allows for better control of the hair and more precise haircutting.

Generally speaking, combination combs give you the ability to adapt to different densities within the hair without switching combs. Narrow-toothed combs can be useful for combing and cutting fine hair textures or when performing detail work. Wide-toothed combs are preferable for detangling, creating styling effects, or for distributing product through the hair.

figure 5-2
Taper combs.

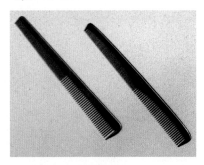

Comb Styles

Given all the different types of combs available, the most appropriate or best comb to use ultimately depends on the procedure to be performed, the client's hair texture, and the barber's personal preference.

- A styling or all-purpose comb, usually constructed of both narrow and wide-spaced teeth, is used for general haircutting and styling (Figure 5-1).

- A **taper comb** (TAY-pur KOM) can be used for cutting hair in those areas where a gradual blending of the hair is required. The tapered end is especially useful when working in tight areas or for trimming mustaches, for tapering necklines, or for blending around the ears (Figure 5-2).

figure 5-3
Wide-tooth combs.

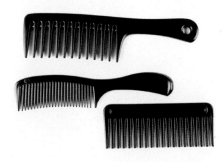

- A flat handle comb with evenly spaced teeth works best to achieve a flat-top style and is also an option to use in clipper-over-comb cutting.

- Wide-toothed combs can be used to control larger amounts of hair, spread relaxer cream, detangle hair, or comb through curly hair textures (Figure 5-3).

- The tail comb is the best choice for sectioning longer hair or when making partings to create subsections, for wrapping the hair on rods or rollers, or for color applications (Figure 5-4).

- A hair pick is an effective choice for combing through textured or tightly curled hair (Figure 5-5).

? DID YOU KNOW?
Using a light-colored comb on dark hair or a dark-colored comb on light hair provides greater contrast between the comb and the hair, which can help you simplify and perfect your work.

figure 5-4
Tail combs.

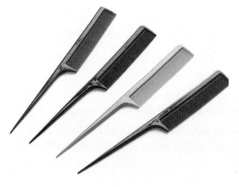

figure 5-5
Pick combs.

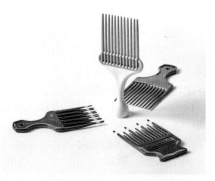

figure 5-6
Proper comb holding position.

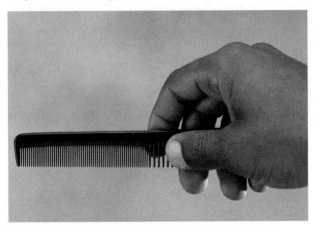

figure 5-7
Improper comb holding position.

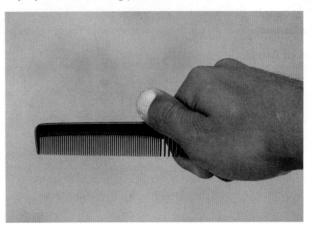

figure 5-8
Proper shear-over-comb position.

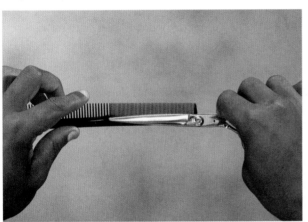

figure 5-9
Improper shear-over-comb position.

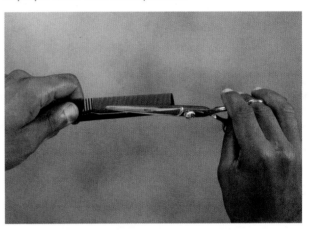

Holding the Comb

The correct manner in which to hold the comb will be dictated by the type of comb used, the service being performed, and the dexterity and comfort of the barber. **Figures 5-6** through **5-9** show correct and incorrect holding positions with a styling comb. Be guided by your instructor and practice, practice, practice!

KNOW YOUR BASIC BRUSHES

Styling brushes are used to control, smooth, wave, or add fullness to hair or to stimulate the scalp. The choice of bristle texture, spacing, and material will depend on the hair texture, the hairstyle to be achieved, and the barber's personal preference. Most hairbrushes are manufactured with plastic, rubber, wood, or metal bases with natural, synthetic, combined, or metal bristles (**Figure 5-10**). Hairbrushes are available in a variety of shapes and sizes for different purposes (**Table 5-1**).

figure 5-10
Assorted brushes.

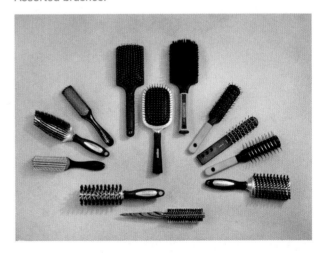

sh	Characteristics	Use(s)
Synthetic bristle brush	Flexible or rigid nylon bristles set into a cushioned, plastic, or cushioned base.	General brushing and detangling.
Natural bristle brush	Typically made of boar bristles, set into a cushioned or rigid base; traps particles and polishes the hair by distributing sebum through the strands.	General brushing and detangling on fine, delicate, and relaxed hair types.
Mixed bristle brush	Combination of boar and synthetic bristles set into a cushioned or rigid base.	General brushing and detangling.
Paddle brush	Available with all bristle and base types in a rectangular or oval shape.	General brushing and detangling.
Round brush	Available with all bristle types in metal or plastic bases in different diameters.	Creates volume and/or curl in blowdry styling.
Vented brush	Rigid base has openings or "vents" to facilitate quicker drying.	General drying and styling work.
Wet brush	Stiff bristles designed to avoid snagging wet hair.	Detangling wet hair.

Know about Haircutting Shears

After reading this section, you will be able to:

LO**3**   Discuss and identify the types of haircutting shears.

LO**4**   Identify the parts of haircutting shears.

Your haircutting shears are one of the most important tools you will use when performing barbering services. Therefore, your understanding of shears and your ability to select the right type, style, and size that will fit you comfortably is vital to your future success as a barber.

RECOGNIZE SHEAR STYLES

There are two basic styles of shears generally used by barbers: the French style with a finger rest or tang for the little finger and the German style without a tang. Barbers often choose the French-style shear because the tang helps to ensure balance and control during cutting (Figure 5-11).

Cast versus Forged Shears

Professional haircutting shears are either cast or forged during manufacture.

Cast shears are made by heating steel to a liquid form for pouring into a mold. As the metal cools, it expands; this process produces a more porous and weaker steel that does not retain its sharpness, is more brittle, and is likely to chip or break. Because cast shears are less expensive to produce than forged shears, they are also usually less expensive to purchase.

figure 5-11
Haircutting shears.

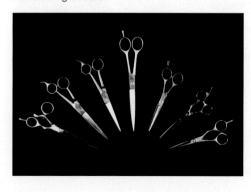

Forged shears (FORJed SHEERZ) are made by working heated metal into a finished shape through the processes of hammering or compression. In today's shear manufacturing, the metal is either dropped on to a mold to be pounded into the desired shape or is hydraulically pressed into a die mold. The heating and cooling processes are repeated until the desired density, hardness, and shape of the implement has been achieved.

A forged shear may be constructed in one or two pieces and is more durable, stays sharp longer, and is of higher quality than a cast shear.

KNOW THE BASIC PARTS OF HAIRCUTTING SHEARS

Haircutting shears are composed of two blades called the moving blade and the still blade that are fastened with a tension screw or adjustment knob. Other basic parts of the shears include the points (tips), cutting edges, shanks, bumper, finger grip, thumb grip, and finger rest (tang) (**Figure 5-12**). Let's take a closer look at these features and other important information you need to know.

- **Shear blades.** The cutting edge is the part of the blade that does the cutting. The *grind* refers to the inside construction of the blade and the way it is cut in preparation for sharpening and polishing. The flat grind is traditionally associated with beveled shears, while hollow-ground blades are typically a feature of convex shears. There are also shear designs with replaceable blades that eliminate the need for sharpening.

- **Blade edges.** The cutting edges may be convex, beveled, or semi-convex in design (see **Table 5-2** and **Figure 5-13**).

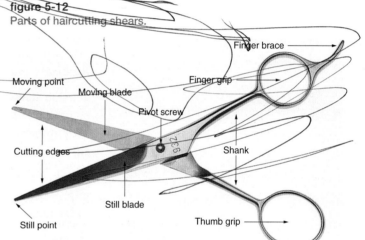

figure 5-12
Parts of haircutting shears.

Finger brace
Moving point
Moving blade
Finger grip
Pivot screw
Cutting edges
Shank
Still blade
Still point
Thumb grip

table 5-2

COMPARE BLADE EDGES

Convex Edge	Beveled Edge
Very sharp edges	Usually has serrated edges
Glides through hair easily	Holds hair on blade edge; reduces slippage
Cuts hair shaft cleanly	Grips hair shaft for cutting
Less tension used when cutting	More tension used when cutting
Good for dry, wet, and slide cutting	Not intended for slide cutting
Reduced noise while cutting	Serrations create some noise while cutting
More subject to nicks than beveled blade	Durable; stays sharp longer than convex blade
Sharpen every 4 to 6 months	Sharpen every 9 to 12 months

figure 5-13
Convex and beveled edges.

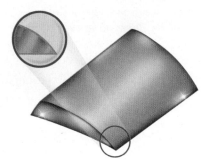

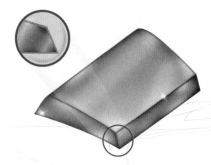

- The outside of a *convex* blade edge has a clamshell or half-moon shape and the inside is concave or hollow-ground. This arrangement produces a smoother and sharper cutting blade that requires more frequent sharpening than beveled edges.
- A *beveled* edge means there is an angle on the cutting surface of the blade. Beveled edges can be plain-ground with smooth, polished, or razor-edged surfaces. Beveled shears usually have one plain and one corrugated (serrated) blade. The design of the corrugations helps to hold the hair in place and to prevent it from sliding on the blade while it is being cut. A beveled edge will stay sharper longer than a convex blade but tends to require more tension when cutting hair.
- A semi-convex blade consists of a convex blade that has a bevel ground onto the blade edge. This design reduces production costs and extends the time in-between sharpening.

- **Set.** The **set of the shears** refers to the angle of the blade from its tip to the ride and the alignment of the blades in relation to each other. This alignment is just as important as the grind of the blades because even shears with the finest cutting edges will be inferior cutting tools if the blades are not set properly. Tension also affects the set and alignment of the blades and should be checked frequently.

- **Tension screw.** The tension screw or knob, also called a pivot screw, controls the distance between the blades. Refer to the Maintain Your Shears section later in this chapter to learn how to perform an adjustment.

- **Shank.** The *shank* is located between the ride and the base of the finger grip. When the ring finger is positioned properly in the finger grip, the index and middle fingers will rest on the shank.

- **Finger grip and tang.** The *finger grip* or *ring* is the part of the still blade of the shears where you will position your ring finger between the first and second knuckle. To use your shears properly and to maintain control, do not use your middle finger or allow the finger grip to slide past the second knuckle of your ring finger. The *finger tang* is where your little finger can rest for greater control of the shears and to relieve pressure on your nerves and tendons.

- **Thumb grip.** The *thumb grip* or *ring* is a part of the moving blade of the shears. Your thumb will control the moving blade and should rest no lower than your cuticle within the grip.

- **Bumper.** The *bumper* (not pictured in **Figure 5-12**) is usually positioned on the thumb grip to prevent the grips from touching when the shears are completely closed.

- **Size.** Shears are available in a variety of lengths and are measured in inches and half inches. Convex shears are measured from the tip (points) to the end of the finger ring where it joins the finger rest (**Figure 5-14**). Beveled shears are measured from the tip to the end of the finger rest. Most barbers prefer shears that are 6½″ to 7½″ in length because they facilitate shear-over-comb cutting better than shorter shears (**Figure 5-15**).

DID YOU KNOW?
You can reduce the diameter of a finger or thumb grip for a more comfortable fit by inserting a shear ring or guard into the grip.

figure 5-14
Convex shears are measured from the tip to the end of the finger ring.

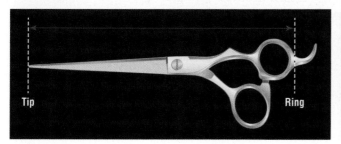

figure 5-15
Beveled shears are measured from the tip to the end of the finger rest.

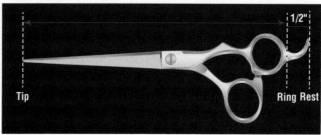

figure 5-16
Opposing handle design.

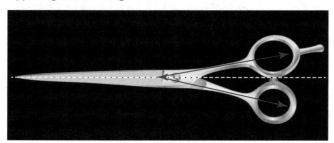

figure 5-17
Offset handle design.

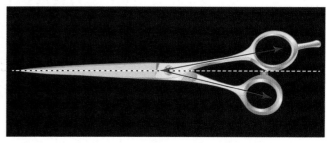

- **Handle designs**. Three standard handle designs are the opposing grip, the offset grip, and the crane grip. In the opposing handle design, the finger and thumb grips are positioned directly across from each other (**Figure 5-16**). The offset handle design has a shorter thumb shank to reduce overextension and is considered to be more ergonomically correct than the opposing design (**Figure 5-17**). The crane handle also has offset grips but the angle of the finger grip is less in relation to the center of the shears and the thumb grip (**Figure 5-18**). This reduces pressure and stress in the hand and thumb. Refer to **Figures 5-16** to **5-18** to compare handle designs.

figure 5-18
Crane handle design.

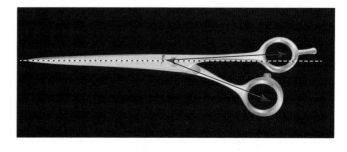

DESCRIBE TEXTURIZING, THINNING, AND BLENDING SHEARS

Texturizing (TEKS-churyz-ing), **thinning** (THIN-ing), and blending shears are designed with blades that have teeth of varying widths and distances between them (**Figure 5-19**). The wider the spacing of the teeth, the more hair is removed during cutting. The greater the number of teeth, the more finely the hair strands can be cut without leaving noticeable cut marks. Although the terms *texturizing shears*, *thinning shears*, and *blending shears* tend to be used interchangeably within the industry, there are some differences in their designs. Refer to **Table 5-3** for a summary of these differences.

figure 5-19
Thinning or texturizing shears.

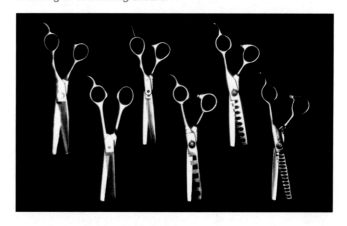

table 5-3

COMPARE TEXTURIZING, THINNING, AND BLENDING SHEARS

Texturizing Shears	Thinning and Blending Shears
Chunking shears: 5 to 9 widely spaced teeth; creates patterns and texture in hair. Texturizing shears: 14 to 28 medium width teeth; differences in hair lengths are visible; adds texture and volume.	Thinning and blending shears: 30 to 50 thin, narrowly spaced teeth that eliminate visible lines in hair; may be designed with teeth on one or both blades; used for blending hair ends and removing bulk or weight.

Show How to Hold the Shears and Comb

After reading this section, you will be able to:

LO⑤ Show how to properly hold shears for haircutting.

LO⑥ Show how to palm the shears and comb.

figure 5-20
Correct finger placement 1.

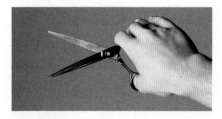

figure 5-21
Correct finger placement 2.

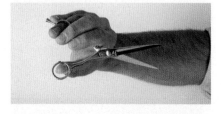

figure 5-22
Incorrect finger placement.

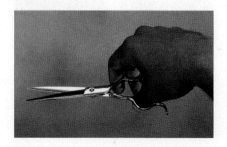

Holding your tools properly will give you the most control and best results when cutting hair and helps to avoid muscle strain in your hands, arms, neck, and back. Haircutting shears are designed to be held and manipulated differently than basic household scissors, so the position of your fingers and hand may feel awkward at first. This is to be expected but a little practice will have you being comfortable with it in no time.

During a haircut, you will be holding the comb and shears at the same time throughout the entire cut. Doing this properly requires that you learn how to palm the shears and comb safely. Knowing how to palm the shears and comb will also help you avoid setting the tool down during a cut, which not only wastes time but also requires that the item be disinfected before you can use it again. Review the following sections and practice, practice, practice!

HOLDING THE SHEARS

The following points indicate the procedure for holding the shears.

1. Insert your ring finger into the finger grip (still blade) approximately halfway between the first and second knuckle with the little finger resting on the finger brace. Do not allow the finger grip to slide past the second knuckle or you will lose control of the shears. To ensure proper balance, rest the index and second fingers on the shank of the still blade.

2. Simultaneously, insert the tip of your thumb into the thumb grip (moving blade) no further than your cuticle, which is about halfway between the end of your thumb and the first knuckle. Do not allow the thumb grip to slide below the first knuckle or you will lose control of the cutting blade. See **Figures 5-20** and **5-21** for the correct finger placement and holding position of the shears. Incorrect finger placement is shown in **Figure 5-22**.

3. Practice opening and closing the shears, using only the thumb to manipulate the moving blade of the shears. To gain more control during practice, rest the tip of the shears on the first finger of your other hand to steady the still blade while you open and close the moving blade with your thumb.

HOLDING THE SHEARS AND COMB

For safety, shears need to be closed and resting in the palm while you comb the hair; this is called **palming the shears** (PAHM-ing THE SHEERZ). Transferring the comb to the opposite hand after combing to facilitate haircutting is called **palming the comb** (PAHM-ing THE KOM).

1. Palming the shears. To palm the shears, slip your thumb out of the thumb grip and simply pivot the shears into the palm of your hand (**Figure 5-23**).

2. Transferring and palming the comb. Once the shears have been palmed, hold the comb between the thumb and first two fingers of the same hand to comb through the hair (**Figure 5-24**). After the hair section has been combed, transfer the comb into the palm of the opposite hand between the thumb and the base of the index finger (**Figure 5-25**). This procedure allows the first two fingers of that hand to be free to control the hair while the shears hand is free to cut the hair section (**Figure 5-26**).

RIGHT-HANDED VERSUS LEFT-HANDED SHEARS

There is a difference between right-handed and left-handed shears. Not only are the blade designs different, but the assembly of left-handed shears is reversed during manufacture. Simply switching hands or turning right-handed shears over does not make it a functional tool for left-handed barbers.

MAINTAINING YOUR SHEARS

It is important to maintain your shears on a regular basis to keep them in good working order. Use the following as a guide to protect the investment you have made in your shears.

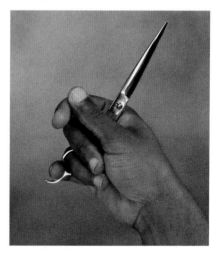
figure 5-23
Palming shears.

figure 5-24
Holding comb and shears.

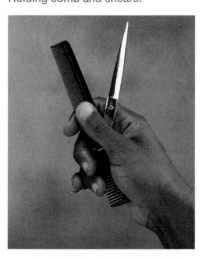

figure 5-25
Palming the comb.

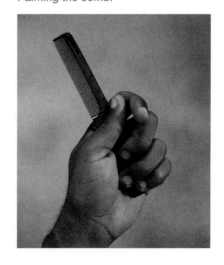

figure 5-26
Correct palming of comb while cutting.

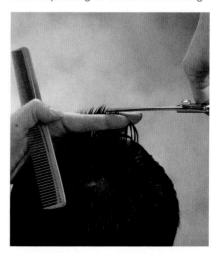

- Clean and disinfect the blades after each use according to state board regulations and manufacturer's directions.
- Adjust the tension screw daily or as needed to maintain proper functioning using the following steps:
  1. Hold the shears horizontally by the thumb grip (moving blade) between the thumb and index finger of the left hand with the tension screw facing you.
  2. Raise the finger grip (still blade) to an open position with the thumb and index finger of the right hand. Release the still blade. The blade should drop 25 percent to 35 percent of the way closed before stopping, depending on the quality and style of the shears. If the blades do not drop at all, the tension is too tight and you will feel resistance while opening or closing them. If the blades close completely, they are too loose and will end up bending the hair over the blades, rather than cutting it.
  3. To adjust a slotted tension screw, close the shears and place the blades flat on a hard surface. Hold the shears securely and use the appropriate size screwdriver to turn the screw in gradual increments, checking the tension after each adjustment.
  4. To adjust a knob tension screw, turn the knob to the right one increment at a time and recheck the tension after each adjustment.

Dos and Don'ts for Handling Your Shears:

- Avoid dropping shears. Even one drop on a hard surface can ruin the set or damage the blades.
- Protect shears in a sheath or holder during transport.
- Never cut anything but human hair with haircutting shears! Use a less expensive shear on mannequin hair and save your finest tools for client services.
- Never force shear blades through a section of hair. If there is resistance, section off a thinner parting for cutting.
- Avoid prolonged immersion of shears in corrosive chemicals including permanent waving lotions, oxidizers, and certain disinfectants.
- Gently place shears into disinfectant containers to avoid damaging the tips.

DID YOU KNOW?

The term *shears* is used to describe a haircutting tool that is longer than 6 inches.

The term *scissors* is used when describing a cutting tool measuring less than 6 inches.

Know about Clippers and Outliners

After reading this section, you will be able to:

LO**7** Describe two types of clippers.

LO**8** Identify the main parts of a clipper.

Clippers (KLIP-uhrz) and outliners are two of the most important tools used in barbering. Clippers can be used for a variety of cutting techniques, from blending to texturizing. Outliners, also known as **trimmers** (TRIM-uhrz) or edgers, are essential tools for finish and detail work. Today's barber has a vast array of clipper styles from which to choose. Function, style, weight, contour, power, and single-speed or two-speed options are just some of the factors that should be considered when purchasing a clipper.

The two main types of clippers are detachable-blade clippers and adjustable-blade clippers. Detachable-blade clippers utilize removable blades in a variety of sizes to achieve different hair lengths. Blade changes are easily accomplished by removing and attaching blades while the clipper is running. Adjustable-blade clippers have adjustable blades that are affixed to the unit with screws. The blades are opened or closed by the adjustment lever on the side of the unit. Clipper guards fit over the blades to extend the length of the hair beyond that left with the blades fully opened, which is about ⅛ inches depending on the manufacturer. Check online or with your local supplier for the latest clipper models and styles.

KNOW THE PARTS OF A CLIPPER

The visible parts of a clipper vary depending on whether the unit is a detachable-blade clipper or an adjustable-blade clipper and whether it is corded or rechargeable. Some detachable clipper models have separate oil reservoirs and carbon brush cover screws that are accessible at the side of the unit and others do not. At the minimum, the visible parts of a detachable clipper are the detachable still and moving blade assembly, on-off switch, hanger loop, and conducting cord. The visible parts of a typical adjustable-blade clipper are the cutting blade, still blade, heel, on-off switch, blade adjustment lever, set or power screw, hanger loop, and the conducting cord (**Figure 5-27**). Electric clippers are driven by one of three basic motor types: rotary, pivot, or magnetic (vibratory). Refer to **Figures 5-28** to **5-30** and **Table 5-4** to compare the features of different types of motors.

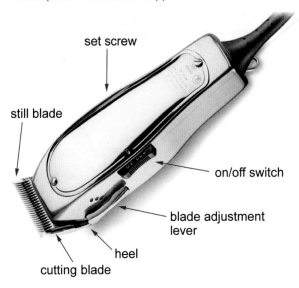

figure 5-27
Visible parts of an electric clipper.

set screw

still blade

on/off switch

blade adjustment lever

heel

cutting blade

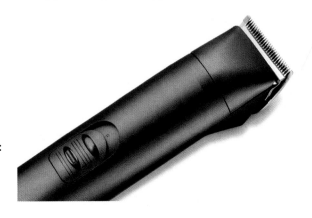

figure 5-28
Rotary (universal) motor clippers.

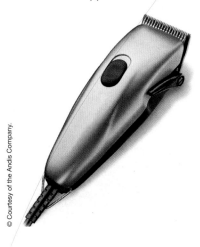

figure 5-29
Pivot motor clippers.

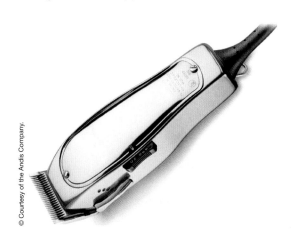

figure 5-30
Magnetic motor clippers.

table 5-4

COMPARE CLIPPER MOTORS

Type of Motor	Power	Blade Speed	Characteristics	Hair Types
Rotary (universal)	High	High	Heavy-duty use; more frequent replacement of parts	All types, damp or dry
Pivot	High	Lower	Blades pulled in both directions; quiet, cool running	Thick, coarse, or damp
Magnetic	Reliable	High	Alternating spring and magnet mechanism; pulls blades in one direction; long lasting	Tapering and general cutting; dry cutting on fine textures

OUTLINERS

An outliner uses a magnetic or pivot motor. Outliners have very fine cutting blades that require very little pressure against the skin to be effective cutting tools. Using too much pressure can cause skin irritations, abrasions, and even ingrown hairs, so use a light hand and let the tool do the work.

- The cutting blade is usually available in two styles: a straight trimmer blade (**Figure 5-31**) and a T-shaped blade (**Figure 5-32**).

- The versatility and utility of the T-blade when trimming rounded or difficult areas makes it the first choice of many barbers and stylists.

- Outliners are essential tools for detail, precision design, and fine finish work on haircuts and facial hair trims, including the eyebrows.

Cordless Clippers and Outliners

A number of manufacturers have produced clippers and outliners that do not have a conducting cord attached directly to the unit. Instead, these tools are designed to rest in a charging unit when not in use. Cordless clippers are an important innovation for barbers because they are easily maneuverable and portable; however, they may not have the same power as corded models.

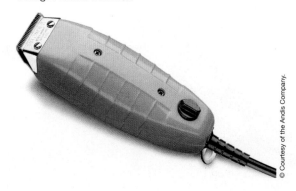

figure 5-31
Straight-blade trimmer.

© Courtesy of the Andis Company.

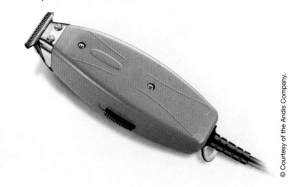

figure 5-32
T-shaped blade trimmer.

© Courtesy of the Andis Company.

DESCRIBE BLADES AND GUARDS

Clipper **blades** (BLAYDZ) are usually made of high-quality carbon steel or ceramic and are available in a variety of styles and sizes. Some styles are designed for use with detachable-blade clippers; others serve as replacement blades for specific adjustable-blade clipper models.

Following are the considerations to keep in mind about clipper blades and guards:

- Detachable-blade sizes can differ from one manufacturer to another and may not always indicate the same cutting length; so be careful when purchasing these items. Visit manufacturers' websites for photos and size charts.

- A detachable 00000 blade produces the closest cut. Most adjustable-blade clippers have a blade length range from a 000 in the closed position to a 1 in the open position.

- Follow the manufacturer's recommendations for the style and size of clipper blades that are appropriate for their clipper models.

- Manufacturers are constantly improving their clipper blades to permit faster and more precise haircutting, so be on the lookout for the newest in haircutting tools (**Figure 5-33**).

Clipper **guards**, also known as attachment combs, are made of plastic, hard rubber, or steel for both detachable-blade and adjustable-blade clippers.

- The purpose of a clipper guard is to allow the hair to be left longer than what might be achieved from using clipper blades alone against the scalp surface.

- Although guards can help to ensure uniformity within the cut, they may also require more passes over a section because they cannot grip the hair the way steel blades do. This can result in lost tension and slippage that may cause steps or gaps in the hair, requiring repeated passes with the clipper. Remember, guards do not do the actual cutting and should not be confused with the clipper blades; they are simply supplemental implements you may choose to use in haircutting services (**Figure 5-34**).

Show How to Hold Clippers and Trimmers

After reading this section, you will be able to:

LO⑨ Show different ways to hold clippers for haircutting.

The technique used by barbers to hold the clipper is most often determined by the section of the head they are working on. For example, cutting the back section will necessitate holding the clippers differently than when

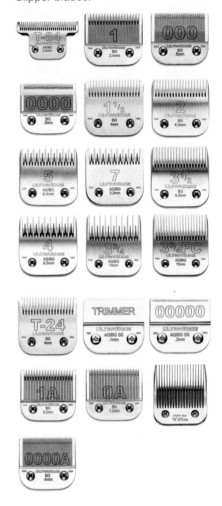

figure 5-33
Clipper blades.

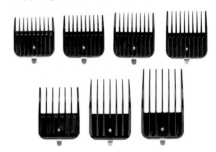

figure 5-34
Clipper guards.

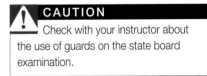

> ⚠ **CAUTION**
> Check with your instructor about the use of guards on the state board examination.

© Courtesy of the Andis Company.

DID YOU KNOW?

When using clippers, the amount of hair that remains on the head depends on whether the hair is cut *with* the grain or *against* the grain. Cutting against the grain cuts the hair shorter than cutting with the grain.

⚠ CAUTION

Never adjust outliner blades flush to each other. Doing so can create a cutting edge so sharp that it may cut the skin or cause skin irritations and ingrown hairs.

- Blades should only be set as recommended by the manufacturer.
- Typically, the top or front blade should rest between $\frac{1}{16}$ and $\frac{1}{32}$ inches below the back blade, depending on the tool.
- If the client requests a closer cut than what the clipper blade will produce, recommend a head shave.

DID YOU KNOW?

Manufacturer's cleaning and maintenance directions should be followed carefully to ensure optimal performance and to maintain product warranties.

---

cutting the top section. A general rule to follow is to hold the clippers in a manner that permits free wrist movement while providing the best access to the area being cut. Four holding positions are explained as follows, but be guided by your instructor for alternative methods.

- Place the thumb on top of the clipper with the fingers supporting it from the underside (**Figure 5-35**). This position is usually comfortable for tapering in the nape or side areas of a haircut or when the clipper is switched to the left hand while cutting hair sections from a different direction.

- An alternative method is to place the thumb on the left side of the unit, at the switch, and the fingers on the right side, with the blades pointing up (**Figure 5-36**). Depending on the style and weight of the clippers, you may find that this position limits the range of your wrist action.

- **Figures 5-37** and **5-38** show alternative underhand positions that may be used when working haircut sections from side-view and back-view positions.

figure 5-35
Clipper holding position 1.

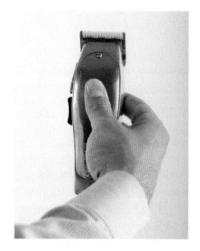

figure 5-36
Clipper holding position 2.

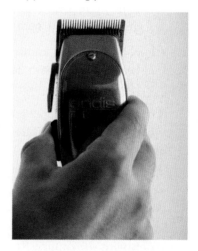

figure 5-37
Clipper holding position 3.

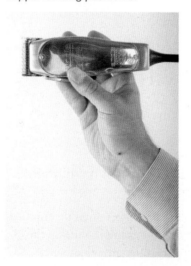

figure 5-38
Clipper holding position 4.

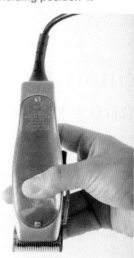

Know about Straight Razors

After reading this section, you will be able to:

LO ⑩   Name two types of straight razors.

LO ⑪   Identify the different parts of a straight razor.

As the sharpest and closest cutting tool, razors are used for facial shaves, head shaves, neck shaves, finish work around the sideburn and behind-the-ear areas, and haircutting. The razor of choice for professional barbering is the straight razor; safety razors are not used to perform barbering services in the barbershop.

The two types of straight razors used in barbering are the **changeable-blade straight razor** (CHAYNJE-able BLAYD STRAYT RAY-zor) and the **conventional straight razor** (kun-VEN-shun-ul STRAYT RAY-zor). Both may be purchased with a razor guard for use in razor-cutting the hair (see Chapter 13).

Selecting the right kind of razor is a matter of personal choice. The best guides for buying high-quality razors are as follows:

- Consult with a reliable company representative or salesperson who can recommend the type of razor best suited to your work.

- Consult with more experienced barbers about which razors they have found best for shaving and haircutting.

- Experiment with a variety of razors to determine the style and type most comfortable for you based on the service to be performed. For example, you may prefer a longer blade razor when performing a facial shave and a shorter blade razor for arching around the ears during a haircut.

- Avoid judging a razor simply on color or design. Neither one of these characteristics provides a true indication of the razor's caliber as a cutting tool.

IDENTIFY THE PARTS OF A STRAIGHT RAZOR

The structural parts of conventional and changeable-blade straight razors are basically the same except in the blade area; the conventional razor has a blade and the changeable-blade razor has a blade holder for the blade. Therefore, the structural parts of a straight razor are the head, back, shoulder, tang, shank, heel, edge, point, blade or blade holder, pivot, and handle (**Figure 5-39**).

DESCRIBE CHANGEABLE-BLADE STRAIGHT RAZORS

The changeable- (or disposable-) blade straight razor closely resembles a conventional straight razor in its overall design. This type of razor tends to be used almost exclusively in the barbershop because its disposable blade eliminates honing and stropping, saves time, and helps to maintain infection control standards (**Figure 5-40**).

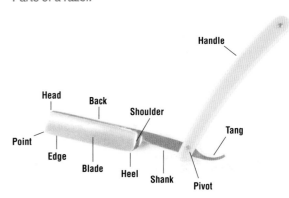

figure 5-39
Parts of a razor.

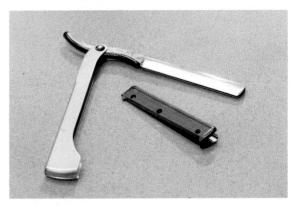

figure 5-40
Changeable-blade razor.

figure 5-41
Razor shaper.

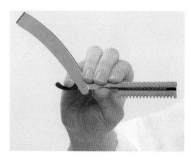

Razor Shapers

There are a variety of razor shapers (also known as hair shapers) available on the market today. One style made of lightweight metal with a pivot and open-handle construction leaves the majority of the blade visible (Figure 5-41). This type of razor is not recommended for facial shaving because the blade size and shape can make it challenging to safely shave smaller areas, such as above the upper lip. Other hair shaper designs do not have a pivot and consist of a stationary handle with a finger rest (Figure 5-42). Both styles use a changeable-blade system and come with a guard.

FOLLOW MANUFACTURER'S DIRECTIONS FOR CHANGING THE BLADE

There are several changeable-razor models available and each will have its own design for holding the blade in place; therefore, the method for replacing the blade will vary depending on the model.

figure 5-42
Hair razor.

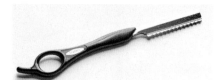

Show How to Hold a Straight Razor

After reading this section, you will be able to:

LO⑫ Show how to hold a straight razor for shaving, honing, and stropping.

LO⑬ Show how to hold a straight razor for haircutting.

LO⑭ Describe the functions of hones and strops.

LO⑮ Show how to hone and strop a conventional blade straight razor.

figure 5-43
Stroke with razor.

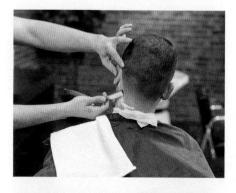

HOLDING THE STRAIGHT RAZOR

How you hold the straight razor will depend on the procedure to be performed, the type of razor you use, and the positioning that gives you the most control of the razor. Refer to Figures 5-43 to 5-47 and the following section to consider several holding techniques.

- Shaving: The ball of the thumb and first two fingers are positioned on the flat side of the shanks with the handle pivoted up to allow the little finger to rest on the tang. This positions the razor at a better angle while providing more control over the razor (Figure 5-43).

- Honing and stropping: The ball of the thumb and first two fingers are positioned on the flat sides of the shank with the handle in a straight position (Figures 5-44).

- Haircutting: The ball of the thumb supports the razor at the bottom of the shank and the little finger rests on the tang, with the first two or three fingers at the top of the shank (Figure 5-45). Or, the razor handle is in a straightened position with the thumb and first two fingers almost touching at the shank (Figure 5-46).

- Holding the comb and razor: To palm the razor for hair combing, simply roll the razor into your hand with the blade facing away from the comb. Hold the comb between the thumb and first two fingers (Figure 5-47). Keep a firm grip on the razor to prevent it from slipping and cutting your hand during combing.

LEARN ABOUT CONVENTIONAL STRAIGHT RAZORS

The conventional straight razor requires honing and stropping to maintain its cutting edge. This razor is composed of a hardened steel blade attached to a handle by means of a pivot. The handle may be constructed of hard rubber, plastic, metal, or new polymer materials.

Consider Razor Quality

In order to determine the quality of a razor, you must consider the following factors: razor balance, temper, grind, finish, size, and style.

Razor Balance

Razor balance refers to the weight and length of the blade relative to that of the handle. A straight razor is properly balanced when the weight of the blade and handle are equal. Proper balance of the razor allows for greater ease and safety in handling the razor during shaving. Opening the razor and resting it on the index finger at the pivot will test the balance of the razor. If the head of the razor moves up or down, the razor is not well balanced.

Razor Temper

Tempering the razor refers to a special heat treatment included in the manufacturing process. When a razor is properly tempered, it acquires the degree of hardness required for a good cutting edge. Razors can be purchased with a hard, soft, or medium temper. The barber should select the temper that produces the most satisfactory shaving results. While hard-tempered razors will hold an edge longer, they are difficult to sharpen; conversely, soft-tempered razors are easier to sharpen, but the sharp edge does not last long. For those reasons, many barbers prefer a medium-tempered razor.

Razor Grind

The grind of a razor is the shape of the blade after it has been ground. There are two general types: the concave grind and the wedge grind (Figure 5-48).

- *Concave grind:* The concave grind (often referred to as the hollow ground) is available in full concave, one-half concave, and one-quarter concave forms. The back and edge of the razor looks hollow, being slightly thicker between the hollow part and the extreme edge. Many barbers prefer the hollow-ground razor since the resistance of a beard can be felt more easily and alerts the barber to check the sharpness of the cutting edge. Although the one-half and one-quarter concave grinds are less hollow than the full concave, the outside dimensions of the blade appear the same.

- *Wedge grind:* The wedge grind is neither hollow nor concave. Both sides of the blade form a sharp angle at the extreme edge of the razor. Most older razors were made with a wedge grind. Although learning how to sharpen a wedge grind may be a challenge, once mastered, this grind produces an excellent shave. It is especially preferred for men with coarse, heavy beards.

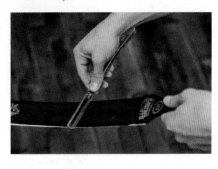

figure 5-44
Razor strop.

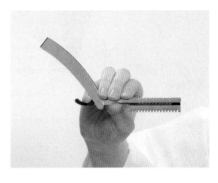

figure 5-45
Holding the razor shaper properly.

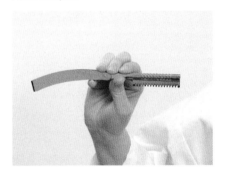

figure 5-46
Alternate method of holding the razor shaper.

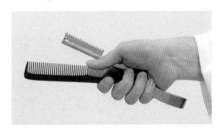

figure 5-47
Palming the razor and comb.

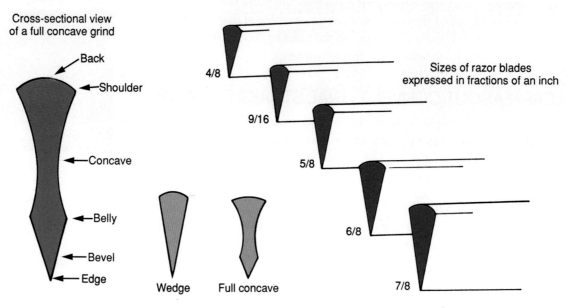

figure 5-48
Razor grinds.

Cross-sectional view
of a full concave grind

Back
Shoulder
Concave
Belly
Bevel
Edge

Wedge   Full concave

4/8
9/16
5/8
6/8
7/8

Sizes of razor blades
expressed in fractions of an inch

Razor Finish

The finish of a razor is the polish of its surface. This finish may be plain, crocus (polished steel), or plated with nickel or silver. Of these types, the crocus finish is usually the choice of the discriminating barber. Although the crocus finish is more costly, it lasts longer and does not rust as easily as other finishes. Metal-plated razors are undesirable because the finish wears off quickly and may hide poor-quality steel.

Razor Size

The size of the razor is measured by the length and width of the blade. The width of the razor is measured either in eighths or sixteenths of an inch, such as 4⁄8 inches, 5⁄8 inches, 6⁄8 inches, 7⁄8 inches, and 9⁄16 inches. Two of the most common sizes are the 5⁄8 inches and 9⁄16 inches, the 5⁄8 inches being the more popular.

Razor Style

The style of a razor indicates its shape and design. Modern razors have such features as a back and edge that are straight and parallel to each other; a round heel; a square point; and a flat or slightly round handle. To avoid scratching the skin, the barber usually rounds off the square point of the razor slightly by drawing the point of the razor along the edge of the hone.

Razor Care

Razors will maintain their quality if care is taken to prevent corrosion of the extremely fine edge. After use, a razor should be cleaned, stropped, and a little oil applied to the cutting edge. Be careful not to drop the razor as doing so may damage the blade. When closing the razor, be careful that the cutting edge does not strike the handle. If the cutting edge strikes the handle when closing the razor, it may indicate that the handle is warped or that the pivot is too tightly riveted. The barber's tool kit should include several high-grade razors so that a damaged razor can be replaced immediately.

IDENTIFY ACCESSORIES USED WITH CONVENTIONAL STRAIGHT RAZORS

There are two vital accessories used with conventional straight razors: the hone and the strop. A **hone** (HOHN) is an abrasive material that has the ability to cut steel. It is used to grind the steel and impart an effective cutting edge to the razor's blade. A **strop** is a leather and canvas accessory that is used to smooth and align the cutting teeth of the razor edge and polish the blade. Honing and stropping techniques must be mastered to prepare a conventional straight razor for shaving.

HONES

There are various types of hones available for the purpose of sharpening razors. Hones are manufactured in a rectangular block shape, without or with an attached handle, for ease of blade placement on the surface. Since the abrasive material of the hone is harder than steel, it will cut or file the edge on the blade of the razor.

Students should practice with a slow-cutting hone, while experienced practitioners generally use a faster-cutting hone.

There are three main types of hones: natural, synthetic, and combination.

- Natural hones are cut from natural rock formations. The two types of natural hones are the water hone and the Belgium hone. These hones have a slow cutting action that can produce a fine, long-lasting edge when used with water or shaving lather to lubricate the stone before sharpening.

- Synthetic hones, such as the carborundum hone, are manufactured products. These hones cut faster than water hones, producing a keen cutting edge in less time and may be used wet or dry, although you need to take care not to over-hone the razor.

- Combination hones consist of both a water hone and a synthetic hone. The synthetic side is used first to develop a good cutting edge and the natural side is used to produce a fine finished edge.

Choosing a Hone

When selecting a hone, remember that the finer the abrasive, the slower its action. Many barbers use combination hones; however, it is advisable to be familiar with the other types of hones and to understand the benefits of each. The type of steel in the razor also makes some difference as to whether a good edge can be obtained with a particular type of hone. Be guided by your instructor, personal experimentation with different hones, and razor manufacturer's recommendations.

Care of Hones

Always clean the hone before use. Use water and a pumice stone to remove the tiny steel particles that accumulate on the surface of the hone. If a new hone is very rough, the same method can be used to work it into shape.

When wet honing is done, always wipe the hone dry after use. This aids the cleaning process and also wipes away the particles of steel that adhere to the cutting surface. Always disinfect the hone according to the manufacturer's directions.

Honing Guidelines

Review the following guidelines before practicing the honing techniques in Procedure 5-1.

- Position the index finger along the top of the shank to ensure even pressure against the blade while honing.
- Make sure your fingertips do not project above the edge of the hone to avoid injury.
- The razor is stroked *edge-first* diagonally across the hone. This produces teeth with a cutting edge.
- The edge blade should be kept flat on the hone, with no rocking or lifting from the surface.
- Stroke the blade with equal pressure from heel to point and from side to side.
- An equal number of strokes should be made on both sides of the blade.
- The angle at which the blade is stroked must be the same for both of its sides.
- As the blade edge is sharpened, gradually lighten the pressure and test frequently.
- The number of strokes required in honing depends on the condition of the razor's edge.

Testing a Honed Blade

A honed blade is tested by lightly passing it over a thumbnail moistened with water or lather (**Figure 5-49**). You should feel one of the following sensations as the blade edge passes over your nail:

- A keen edge has fine teeth and tends to dig into the nail with a smooth, steady grip.
- A blunt or dull razor edge passes over the nail smoothly without any cutting power.
- A coarse razor edge digs into the nail with a jerky feeling.
- A coarse or over-honed edge has large teeth that stick to the nail and produce a harsh, grating sound.
- A nick in the razor produces the feeling of a slight gap or unevenness when drawn across the nail.

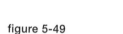

figure 5-49
Testing a honed razor.

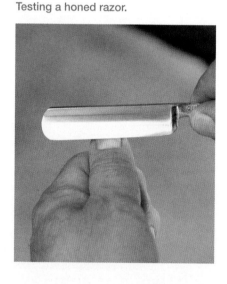

> ⚠️ **CAUTION**
> This testing technique requires a great deal of practice and experience. Be very cautious of the amount of pressure and speed with which the test is performed. Touch the razor's edge lightly, and note the sensation you feel. A dull edge does not produce a drawing sensation. A proper cutting edge will have a sharp drawing sensation. If the razor's edge yields a smooth feeling upon testing, finish it again on the canvas strop, followed by a few more strokes on the leather strop.

Ⓟ 5-1   **Honing the Razor** *pages 133–134*

STROPS

Unlike hones, which are designed to grind the edge of a razor into a sharp cutting edge, strops are used to remove small metal particles from the blade, to smooth the edge, and to polish the razor. A good strop is made of durable and flexible material with the proper thickness and texture and shows a smooth, finished surface. Some barbers like a thin strop; others prefer a thick, heavy strop.

Strops are generally classified as leather or canvas. Cowhide and horsehide are the most common leathers used to manufacture a strop. The four types of strops covered in this chapter are the combination, canvas, Russian, and shell strops.

DID YOU KNOW?

Finer-quality strops are usually "broken in" by the manufacturer, thereby requiring less breaking in and preparation by the barber.

- The combination strop is the type of strop most commonly used in the barbershop because it is an all-in-one accessory for preparing the razor after honing. This strop is actually made of two strops—a canvas strop and a leather strop—that have been riveted together at the attachment end of the strop.

- A **canvas strop** (can-viss strohp), or the canvas side of a combination strop, should be made of high-quality linen or silk, woven into a fine or coarse texture. A fine-textured canvas strop is desirable for removing any metal burrs or imbrications that remain after honing. To obtain the best results, a new canvas strop should be thoroughly broken in. Consult manufacturer's instructions for recommended products and directions to prepare and maintain a canvas strop.

- The **Russian strop** (RUSH-an strohp) was originally imported from Russia and still bears the name even though it may be manufactured elsewhere. The name simply implies that the Russian method of tanning was used to prepare the leather. Russian strops are usually made from cowhide and are considered to be one of the best. Consult the manufacturer's instructions for recommended products and directions to prepare and maintain a Russian strop.

- A **shell strop** is a high-quality strop taken from the muscular rump area of a horse. Although shell strops can be expensive, they are considered to be one of the best strops for barbers as they tend to remain smooth and require very little, if any, breaking in. As with other strops, consult the manufacturer's instructions for recommended products and directions to prepare and maintain your shell strop.

DID YOU KNOW?

If a strop is labeled "Russian shell strop," it indicates that the strop is made from the rump area of a horse and that the Russian tanning method was used in its manufacture.

Strop Dressing

Strop dressing cleans the leather strop, preserves its finish, and also improves its draw and sharpening qualities. Refer to the manufacturer's directions for proper application methods, timing in between applications, and follow-up procedures.

DID YOU KNOW?

The direction of the razor's edge used in stropping is the reverse of the direction used in honing.

STROPPING THE RAZOR

From a technical standpoint, the razor may be stropped from the barber's hand toward the chair or from the chair to the hand. When performed correctly, both methods can achieve the same results; however, your state barber board may have a preferred method. Be sure to check the rules, regulations, and exam performance requirements in your state.

Stropping Guidelines

Review the following guidelines before practicing the stropping techniques in Procedure 5-2.

- The strop is attached to the arm of the barber chair by a closed clip.

- Hold the end of the strop firmly in your nondominant hand so it cannot sag and on a slight diagonal from the chair at a comfortable height.

- When holding the razor, the index finger is on the shank, the subsequent fingers are on the handle, and the thumb rests at the pivot. The index finger of your dominant hand should rest along the edge of the strop.

- The direction of the blade edge in stropping is the reverse of that used in honing; therefore, the back of the razor will lead each stroke, rather than the blade edge.

- Stropping the razor requires being able to roll the razor on its back after completing a stroke to position it for the next one. With the thumb on the side of the shank closest to you and the first two fingers braced on the other side of the shank, use your thumb to roll the blade up and over for the next stroke.

- Strokes should be made in a single, slightly diagonal stroke against the strop, with even pressure from the heel to the point of the razor.

- The blade edge needs to be flat against the surface to avoid cutting or nicking the strop.

- Bear down just enough to feel the razor draw against the strop.

- Do not worry about speed; a moderate pace is preferred.

- Strokes should be repeated as necessary to finish the razor edge.

> ⚠ **CAUTION**
> When testing the razor's edge on the moistened tip of the thumb, a proper cutting edge will have a sharp drawing sensation. Use minimal pressure and speed to perform the test safely.

Ⓟ 5-2 **Stropping the Razor** *page 135*

Learn about Equipment and Supplies Used in Barbering

After reading this section, you will be able to:

LO⑯ Identify the types of equipment and supplies used in barbering.

In addition to your tools and implements, you will need certain equipment and supplies to perform barbering services. Review the following descriptions to become familiar with some common items used in the barbershop.

KNOW THE FEATURES OF A BARBER CHAIR

The barber chair (**Figure 5-50**) is an essential piece of equipment for performing barbering services and should not be confused with a *styling* chair. Styling chairs are typically smaller in design and do not usually have a headrest. Conversely, barber chairs are larger in size, have a headrest, either

figure 5-50
A hydraulic barber chair.

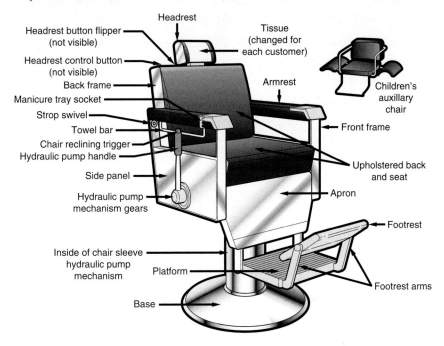

removable or built-in, and are designed to enable clients to fully recline when receiving shaving and facial services.

Barber chairs are available with either hydraulic or motorized bases; both types provide easy height adjustment of the chair. The circumference of the base should be large and heavy enough to accommodate a man's weight without tipping when the customer is in a fully reclined position.

IDENTIFY TYPES OF DRAPES AND CAPES

The two main types of drapes used are shampoo capes and haircutting capes (also known as chair cloths).

- *Shampoo capes* are typically waterproof drapes made of vinyl used to protect the client's skin and clothing from water, liquids, and chemical processes.

- *Haircutting capes* are made of nylon or other synthetic materials. These draping fabrics are usually more comfortable for the client because they do not hold in as much body heat as vinyl capes.

MAINTAIN A SUFFICIENT SUPPLY OF TOWELS AND LINENS

The two types of towels generally used in the barbershop are 100 percent cotton cloth towels and disposable paper towels, especially designed for the profession.

- Cotton towels are available in different weaves and textures. Terry cloth–type towels may be preferred for shampooing and chemical services because of their absorbent qualities; these towels also hold heat and moisture well for steaming the face or scalp.

- Some professionals prefer the type of cotton towel that is traditionally known as a barber towel. This towel has a tighter, flatter weave that is an excellent choice when terry cloth towels are too bulky.

- Disposable paper towels are extra large and measure at least 12 × 24 inches. These multipurpose towels are soft, lint-free, and commonly used as a

  - barrier at the neck instead of a neck strip;
  - wiping paper during shaves;
  - towel wrap for product application or hair removal purposes;
  - sanitary surface on work stations for tools or implements;
  - drawer liner.

In addition to using towels for services or draping purposes, you should know the correct way to towel-wrap your hand to perform the following activities:

- Cleansing and drying the face

- Applying products to the face

- Removing all traces of product, lather, or loose hair from the face, neck, ear areas, and forehead

Practice Procedure 5-3 to master the towel-wrapping methods used when performing barbering services.

- Neck strips are flexible, disposable paper strips used to provide a barrier between the neckband of the cape and the client's neck. Neck strips and hair wrapping strips are not the same thing! Good quality neck strips should be soft and give a little when stretched; hair wrapping strips are usually wider and made of stiffer material that may scratch the skin. See Chapter 11 for the correct way to apply and secure a neck strip.

 5-3 **Towel Wrapping** *pages 136–137*

DESCRIBE THE APPLIANCES USED IN BARBERING SERVICES

Appliances used in the barbershop typically include hot towel cabinets, electric latherizers, blowdryers, massagers, and thermal styling tools. Other appliances, such as high frequency and galvanic machines, may be used to provide advanced skin and scalp care services if permissible in your state.

Hot Towel Cabinet
The hot towel or steam towel cabinet is the ideal appliance for maintaining a ready supply of warm towels for barbering services. Warm towels are used during facials and shaves, but they are also appreciated during a manicure, scalp treatment, or after a neck shave (**Figure 5-51**).

Latherizers
Lather receptacles are containers used to hold, heat, or dispense lather for shaving. The most basic and commonly used types are the electric latherizer, the press-button can latherizer, and the lather mug with paper lining.

An *electric latherizer* is a lather-making device that is commonly seen in barbershops. This appliance is sanitary, convenient, easy to operate, and

figure 5-51
Hot towel cabinet.

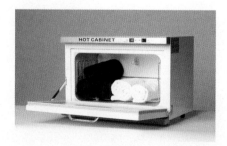

produces rich, warm lather for shaving services (**Figure 5-52**). Follow the manufacturer's directions for proper use and care.

Press-button can latherizers are convenient and sanitary, but they are not as professional as electric latherizers and do not provide warm lather.

Lather mugs are lather receptacles made out of glass, pottery, rubber, or metal (**Figure 5-53**). When the lather mug is used, shaving soap and warm water are mixed thoroughly with the aid of a lather brush. Since the lather mug can harbor bacteria, it requires thorough cleaning and disinfection before and after each use. Disposable paper liners for the shaving mug are also available and help to ensure a sanitary environment. Check your state barber board rules and regulations regarding the use of lather mugs and brushes.

Lather brushes are used to apply the soap lather used to soften the beard. Most barbers favor the number 3 size of lather brush. The vulcanized type is the most durable, since its bristles will not fall apart in hot water. To guard against contaminated brushes, many states have laws requiring that brushes made from animal hair be free of anthrax germs at the time of purchase. These brushes must contain the imprint "Sterilized." Lather brushes must be cleaned and disinfected after each use. *Shaving soaps* can be purchased in various forms and shapes. These soaps usually contain animal and vegetable oils, alkaline substances, and water. The presence of coconut oil improves the lathering qualities of the shaving soap, which helps to keep the hair erect while the alkalinity of the soap softens the hair for shaving.

- Hard shaving soaps include those sold in cake, stick, or powdered form.

- Soft soap is available as shaving cream in a tube, jar, or press-button container.

- Liquid cream soap is used in electric latherizers.

Blowdryers

A blowdryer is an electrical appliance designed for drying and styling hair in a single operation. Standard parts include a handle, directional nozzle (concentrator), small fan, heating element, and speed/heat controls (**Figure 5-54**). Comb, brush, and diffuser attachments are also available with some models.

To keep your blowdryer in safe working order, make sure the unit and air intake at the back are kept clean at all times. A buildup of dirt, hair, or oils can cause the elements to burn out prematurely.

Since there are many different models available, try out several dryers before buying one. You will want to be sure the dryer fits your hand comfortably with the right balance and weight for easy use. Then, review the warranty and service agreements to protect your investment.

The following *blowdryer safety* precautions should be observed:

- Apply a protective blowdrying agent to the hair to shield it from the heat of the dryer.

- Check the comb teeth and brush bristles on attachments for sharp points.

- Test the temperature controls.

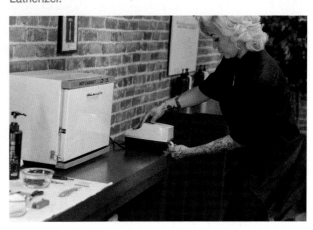
figure 5-52
Latherizer.

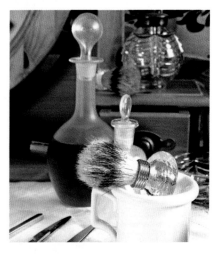
figure 5-53
Lather mug.

⚠ CAUTION
Check your state barber board rules and regulations concerning the use and disinfection of lather mugs and brushes.

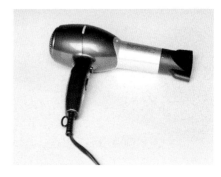
figure 5-54
Blowdryer.

- Keep the air and the hair moving to prevent burns. Do not concentrate dryer heat too close to the scalp.
- Follow the styling brush or comb with the blowdryer, working in the direction of the desired style, blowing damp air onto dry hair.
- Avoid dropping the dryer.
- Never use the dryer near water.

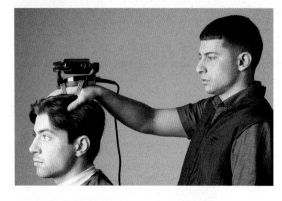

figure 5-55
Electric massager.

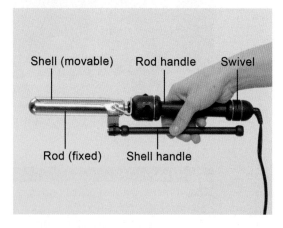

figure 5-56
The parts of a thermal iron.

Shell (movable)   Rod handle   Swivel

Rod (fixed)   Shell handle

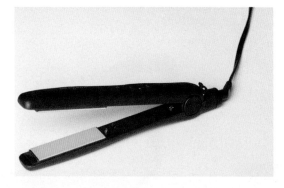

figure 5-57
Flat iron.

Electric Massager

The massager (vibrator) is an electric appliance used in facial, scalp, and shoulder massage services. This device generates vibrations that travel through the barber's fingers to the client's scalp, face, or neck. Some massager units are heavy and may be uncomfortable or difficult for smaller hands to control. Always try one on for size before purchasing (Figure 5-55).

Thermal Styling Tools

Thermal styling tools (THUR-mul STYL-ing TOOLS) create heat that is used to wave, curl, or press hair into another shape or form. Any form of styling performed with a heated tool or appliance may be considered a form of thermal styling. This includes the use of Marcel irons, stoves, hot rollers, flat irons, and other heated tools. Although thermal hairstyling tools are used most often in women's hairstyling, the ability to use these tools correctly is an important aspect of the barber's training. Review Procedure 5-4 on manipulating thermal irons.

- **Thermal irons.** Thermal irons are available in a variety of styles, sizes, and weights, with small to large barrel diameters, and may be electric or require heating on a stove. The four basic parts of thermal irons are the rod handle, shell handle, barrel, and shell (Figure 5-56).
- Electric curling irons are available with or without a vaporizing action feature and can be purchased with a stationary or rotating handle.
- Electric flat irons are used to temporarily straighten curly or wavy hair. They can also be used to give direction to straighter hair textures while imparting a glossy, finished look to the hair. Flat irons are available in many sizes, from mini-irons for short hair lengths or tight styling areas to larger irons suitable for long-hair styling (Figure 5-57).
- The *conventional (Marcel) iron* requires the use of a stove to heat it (Figure 5-58). *Pressing combs* also require the use of a stove and are used for straightening or pressing hair. Electric pressing combs are also available. Both types of combs are constructed of high-quality steel or brass.
- The *electric stove* is used to heat conventional irons and metal pressing combs. Stoves become very hot and must be handled carefully (Figure 5-59).

- **Testing thermal irons.** The temperature of the iron must be tested before applying it to the hair. Use the following guidelines for testing a heated iron:
  - Clamp the iron closed on tissue paper or toweling and hold for 5 seconds.
  - If the paper scorches or turns brown, the iron is too hot.
  - Allow an overheated iron to cool before applying it to the hair.
  - Remember that fine, lightened, or badly damaged hair withstands less heat than normal hair.
- **Maintaining thermal irons.** Since the materials used to make irons can vary greatly, keep your irons clean and functioning properly by always following the manufacturer's directions.
- **Using thermal irons safely.** Consider the following precautions for using thermal irons:
  - Use thermal irons only after receiving instructions on their use.
  - Keep irons clean and do not overheat them.
  - Always test the iron temperature before using it on a client's hair.
  - Handle heated tools carefully and put them in a safe place to cool.
  - Do not place heated stoves near the station mirror as the heat can cause breakage.
  - Place a hard rubber comb between the client's scalp and the iron. Never use a metal comb.

(P) 5-4 **Manipulating Thermal Irons** *pages 138–139*

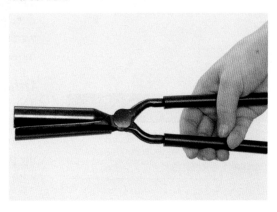

figure 5-58
Marcel iron.

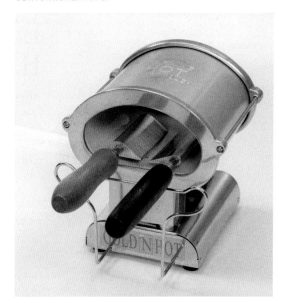

figure 5-59
Electric heater for pressing combs and conventional irons.

LEARN ABOUT ELECTROTHERAPY AND LIGHT THERAPY MACHINES

Electrotherapy and light therapy machines are important equipment items for performing skin care services in many men's spas and high-end, full service shops. Most manufacturers provide special classes to prepare you to use their equipment in a safe and effective manner. Although some basic applications are covered in this textbook, it is recommended that you acquire training in the use of specific machines before performing electrotherapy or light therapy services on clients.

High-Frequency Machine

A **high-frequency machine** (HY-FREE-kwen-see muh-SHEEN) uses electricity to produce a high rate of oscillation within glass electrodes that are used in facial and scalp treatments. Discovered by Nikola Tesla, high-frequency applications warm the skin tissues to stimulate blood flow and to allow for better product absorption. Refer to Chapter 8 for more information.

Galvanic Machine

The galvanic machine is an apparatus with attachments designed to produce galvanic current. The main function of the machine is to introduce water-soluble products into the skin during a facial. Refer to Chapter 7 for more information.

Other Accessories

Two additional accessories you may find in the barbershop are the comedone extractor and tweezers. A **comedone extractor** (KAHM-uh-dohn eks-TRAK-tur) is a metallic implement with a screw on attachment at each end. A fine needle point or lancet is situated at one end; the opposite end has a blunt prong with a hole in the center that is used to press out blackheads.

A *tweezer* is a metallic implement with two blunt prongs at one end that is used to pluck unsightly or ingrown hair. To remove a hair, position the tweezer close to the skin surface, grasp the hair, and pull it out in the direction from which it grows. For added comfort, the area can be pre-steamed to open the hair follicle for easier extraction.

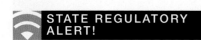

STATE REGULATORY ALERT!

Be guided by your state barber board rules and regulations regarding the use of comedone extractors.

Learn How to Remove Hair Clippings

After reading this section, you will be able to:

LO⑰ Identify ways to remove hair clippings.

LO⑱ Show how to perform two towel-wrapping methods.

Hair removal methods have changed over the years. The neck duster, once a traditional implement in barbershops, is no longer considered a safe and sanitary option for loose hair removal unless it is cleaned and disinfected after each use. Since a number of states prohibit the use of hair dusters, other methods are now used to remove loose hair and clippings. Some methods that are in compliance with state and local health codes are the following:

- A paper or cloth towel folded around the barber's hand

- Paper neck strips, although these may not facilitate a thorough dusting

- Vacuum systems, provided you clean and disinfect the nozzle attachment after each use and empty the container as hair accumulates within it

To complete this section, practice Procedure 5-3 to become proficient in two towel-wrapping methods used in the performance of barbering services.

HONING THE RAZOR

MATERIALS, IMPLEMENTS, AND EQUIPMENT

☐ Conventional straight razor
☐ Hone

☐ Shaving lather
☐ Water

PROCEDURE

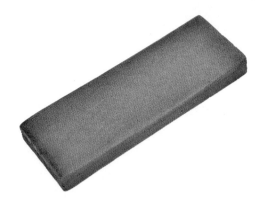

1 Position the hone by placing it firmly and flatly on a hard, smooth surface.

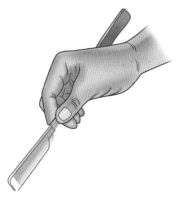

2 Grasp the razor handle comfortably in your dominant hand as follows:
a. Rest the index finger on top of the side part of the shank.
b. Rest the ball of the thumb at the joint.
c. Place the second finger at the back of the razor near the edge of the shank.
d. Fold the remaining fingers around the handle to permit easy turning of the razor.

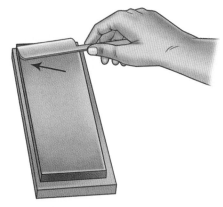

3 *First position and stroke:* Place the razor on its back on the upper far left corner of the hone.

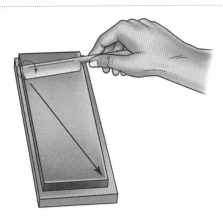

4 Roll the razor, using the thumb and index finger to position the blade edge flat against the hone and facing toward you. Draw the blade diagonally across the hone from heel to point.

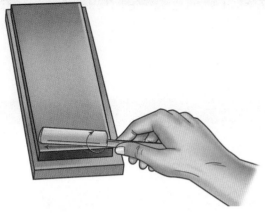

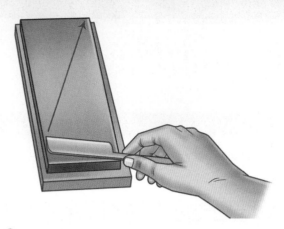

5 Turn the razor on its back and slide it toward the bottom left corner of the hone to position it for the second position and stroke.

6 *Second position and stroke:* Begin at lower left corner of the hone with the blade edge flat against the hone and facing away from you.

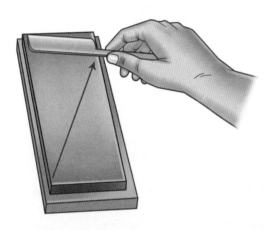

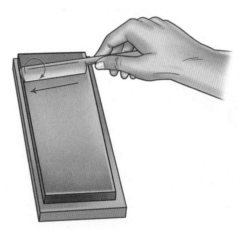

7 Stroke the blade diagonally toward the upper right corner of the hone.

8 Turn the razor on its back, slide it toward the upper left corner of the hone, and roll it into position for the next stroke.

9 Repeat the strokes in a slow and rhythmic manner with equal pressure. If the razor is very dull, use firm pressure during the first honing strokes and then decrease the pressure as the razor takes an edge.

10 Test the edge by lightly passing it over a thumbnail moistened with water or lather.

STROPPING THE RAZOR

MATERIALS, IMPLEMENTS, AND EQUIPMENT

☐ Barber chair

☐ Combination strop

☐ Conventional straight razor

PROCEDURE

1 Clip the strop onto the arm of the barber chair. Hold the end of the strop firmly in the left hand on a slight diagonal from the chair and as high as is comfortable.

2 Grasp the razor firmly in the right hand with the thumb and index finger at the shank and the handle in your palm.

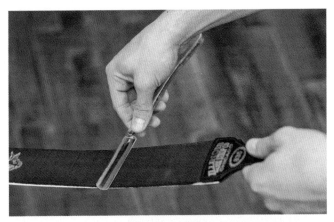

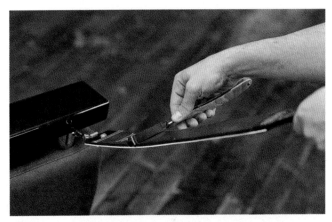

3 *First stroke:* Start the stroke at the top edge of the strop closest to the hand. Using a long, diagonal stroke with even pressure from the heel to the point, draw the razor perfectly flat, with back leading, straight over the surface. Bear down just heavily enough to feel the razor draw.

4 *Second stroke:* When the first stroke is completed, turn the razor on the back of the blade by rolling it between the fingers without turning the hand.

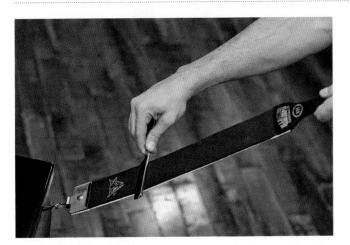

5 Draw the razor away from the chair toward you to complete the second stroke. Repeat strokes as necessary.

6 Make a final test of the razor prior to shaving on the moistened tip of the thumb.

TOWEL WRAPPING

MATERIALS, IMPLEMENTS, AND EQUIPMENT

☐ 100 percent cotton terry cloth or barber towel
☐ Disposable 12" × 24" professional paper towels

PROCEDURE: CLOTH TOWEL WRAP

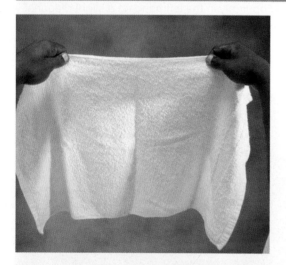

1 Grasp the towel lengthwise.

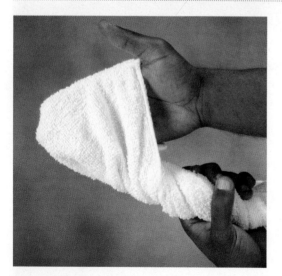

2 Holding your right hand in front of you, draw the upper edge of the towel across the palm of the hand; then grasp the towel ends and twist.

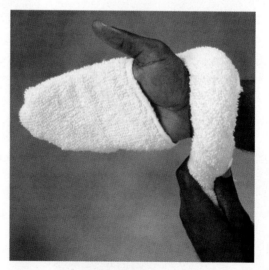

3 Wrap the twisted ends of the towel around the back of the hand and bring over the inside of the wrist.

PROCEDURE: PAPER TOWEL WRAP

4 Hold the ends of the towel while in use to prevent them from flapping in the client's face.

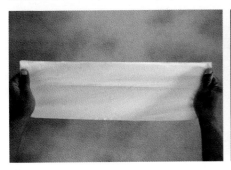

5 Grasp the towel lengthwise.

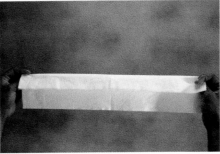

6 Fold down the top third of the towel toward you.

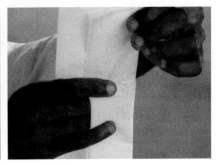

7 Holding the towel at one end, insert the two middle fingers into the fold; maintain your grip on the towel with the thumb, index finger, and fourth finger.

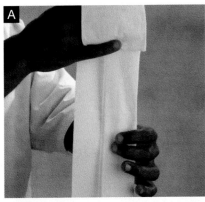

8 Bring the top edge around the back of the hand and secure with the fourth finger.

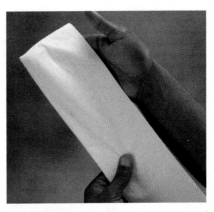

9 Grasp the towel end and shift to a diagonal position.

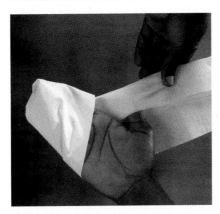

10 Wrap the remaining towel length around the back of the hand and insert thumb into the fold.

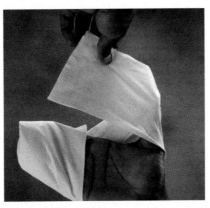

11 Continue wrapping motion around the thumb.

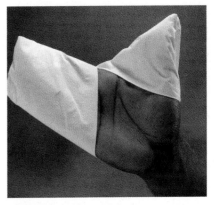

12 Tuck the towel end into wrap at the back of the hand.

MANIPULATING THERMAL IRONS

□ Comb

□ Electric curling iron

□ Mannequin head and stand

PROCEDURE

1 Part off and comb a section of hair for curling.

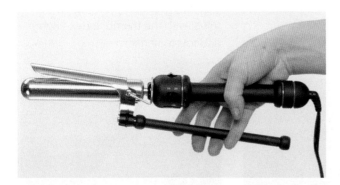

2 Grasp the handle with your dominant hand and open the clamp with your little finger.

3 Guide the iron so the hair section lies in between the clamp and the barrel of the iron.

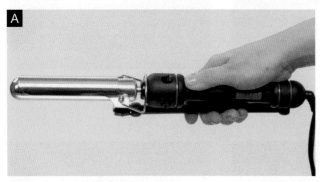

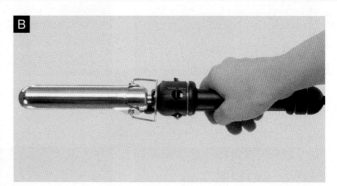

4 Shift your thumb to the top of the iron, close the clamp, and make a one-quarter turn downward.

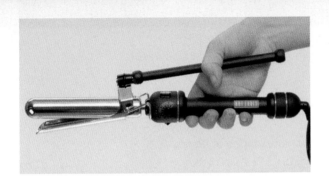

5 Use your thumb to open the clamp slightly to continue rotating the iron to a half turn and close the clamp.

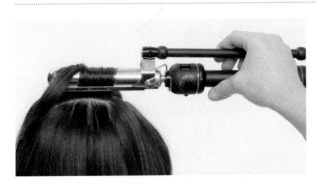

6 Rotate the iron as you continue to open and close the clamp until you have completed a full turn of the iron.

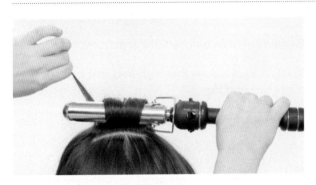

7 Guide the remaining hair section into the center of the curl by opening and closing the clamp while rotating the iron.

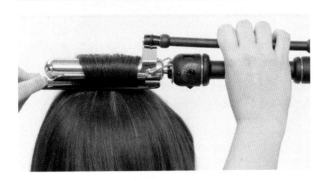

8 Use a comb to secure the section while opening the clamp slightly to slide the iron out of the curl.

REVIEW QUESTIONS

1. List the principal *tools of the trade* used in barbering.

2. What style of comb is generally used for haircutting?

3. Taper combs are especially effective for performing which three services?

4. Identify the parts of haircutting shears.

5. What is the difference between German and French shears?

6. How are the lengths of shears usually measured? Which sizes are used most often?

7. Hollow-ground blades are features of what type of shear?

8. What are thinning and blending shears used for?

9. List three types of clipper motors.

10. List the visible parts of an adjustable-blade electric clipper.

11. Identify the detachable clipper blade size that produces the closest cut.

12. Why should you never set outliner blades flush with each other?

13. Name two types of straight razors.

14. List the basic parts of a straight razor.

15. Explain the purpose of a hone.

16. List three types of hones.

17. Explain the first and second positions and strokes used to hone a razor.

18. Explain the purpose of a strop.

19. What type of strop is considered the best for stropping a conventional straight razor?

20. Explain the first and second strokes used to strop a razor.

21. List three methods of removing loose hair from a client's face and neck other than a neck brush.

22. What does the word *thermal* mean?

23. Explain the main function of the galvanic machine.

24. Identify two services that high-frequency machines might be used for.

25. What is the function of a comedone extractor?

CHAPTER GLOSSARY

blades (BLAYDZ)	p. 117	the cutting parts of the clippers, usually manufactured from high-quality carbon steel and available in a variety of styles and sizes
canvas strop (can-viss strohp)	p. 125	usually one side of a combination strop made of linen or silk, woven into a fine or coarse texture that removes metal burrs or imbrications left after honing
cast shears	p. 108	shears that have been made by heating steel to a liquid form for pouring into a mold
changeable-blade straight razor (CHAYNJE-able BLAYD STRAYT RAY-zor)	p. 119	a type of straight razor that uses changeable, disposable blades
clippers (KLIP-uhrz)	p. 114	electric haircutting tools with a single adjustable-blade or detachable-blade system
comedone extractor (KAHM-uh-dohn eks-TRAK-tur)	p. 132	an implement used to extract blackheads

conventional straight razor (kun-VEN-shun-ul STRAYT RAY-zor)	p. 119	a razor made of a hardened steel bla___ ping to produce a cutting edge
forged shears (FORJed SHEERZ)	p. 109	shears that have been made by ___ shape through the processes o___
guards	p. 117	plastic or hard rubber comb ___ minimize the amount of hai___ applied over a haircutting ___
high-frequency machine (HY-FREE-kwen-see muh-SHEEN)	p. 131	a machine that produces a hi___ purpose of stimulating scalp, facial, ___
hone (HOHN)	p. 123	a sharpening block manufactured from rock or syn___ used to create a cutting edge on conventional straight ra___
palming the comb (PAHM-ing THE KOM)	p. 113	the technique used to hold the comb in the hand opposite of the ___ that is cutting with the shears
palming the shears (PAHM-ing THE SHEERZ)	p. 113	the technique used to hold shears in a safe manner while combing through or otherwise working with hair
Russian strop (RUSH-an strohp)	p. 125	a type of cowhide strop that is considered to be one of the best and that requires breaking in
set of the shears	p. 110	the manner in which the blades and shanks of the shears align with each other and are joined at the tension screw or rivet
shell strop	p. 125	a type of horsehide strop made from the muscular rump area of the horse and considered to be the best strop for use by barbers
strop	p. 123	an elongated piece of leather or other materials used to finish the edge of conventional straight razors to a smooth, whetted cutting edge
taper comb (TAY-pur KOM)	p. 106	used for cutting or trimming hair when a gradual blending from short to longer is required within the haircut
texturizing shears (TEKS-churyz-ing SHEERZ)	p. 111	shears with 14 to 28 medium width teeth that produce visible differences in hair lengths to add texture and volume
thermal styling tools (THUR-mul STYL-ing TOOLS)	p. 130	refers to tools that produce heat for hairstyling purposes
thinning shears (THIN-ing SHEERZ)	p. 111	also known as blending shears; shears with 30 to 50 thin, narrowly spaced teeth that eliminate visible lines in the hair, used for blending hair ends and removing bulk or weight
trimmers (TRIM-uhrz)	p. 114	small clippers, also known as outliners and edgers, used for detail, precision design, and fine finish work after a haircut or beard trim

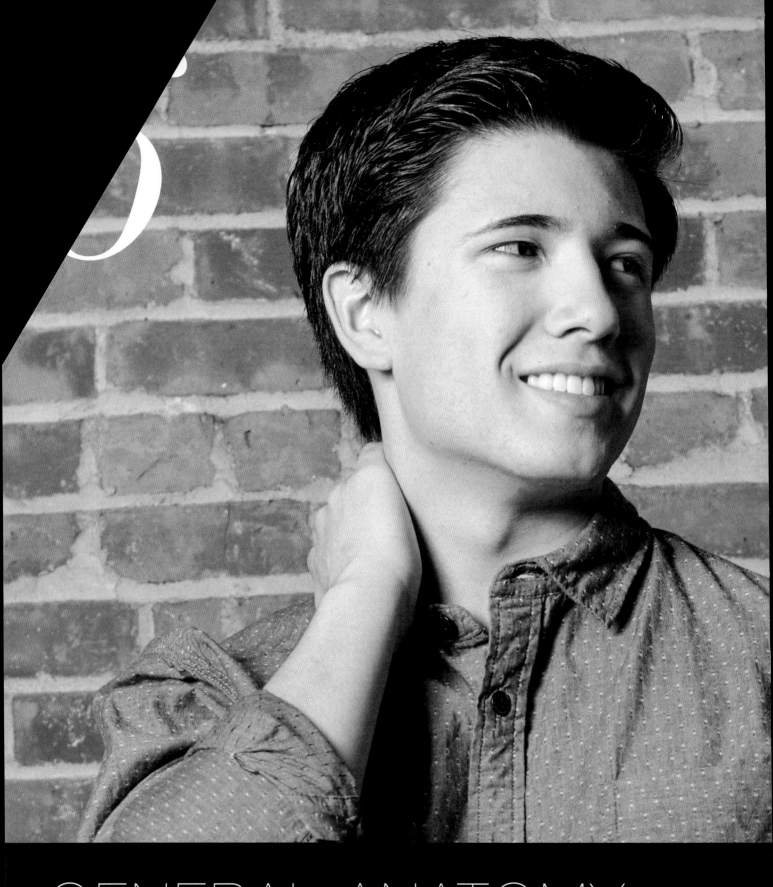

GENERAL ANATOMY
AND PHYSIOLOGY

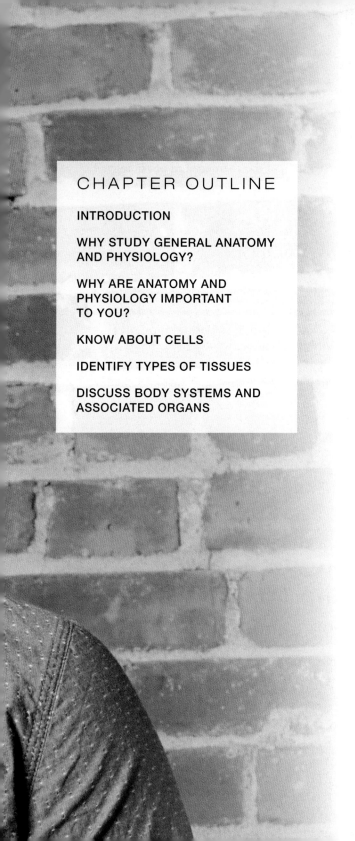

LEARNING OBJECTIVES

After completing this chapter, you will be able to:

LO ❶
Define and explain the importance of anatomy, physiology, and histology to the barbering profession.

LO ❷
Describe cells, their structure, and their reproduction.

LO ❸
Identify and define the types of tissues found in the body.

LO ❹
Define organs and body systems.

LO ❺
Name the main body systems and explain their basic functions.

Introduction

Barbers are licensed to touch and perform services on clients in ways that are not permitted in many other occupations. This is an important responsibility, and as a barber, you should consider it an honor to be able to aid others in achieving a greater sense of well-being. To earn this responsibility, you need to have a solid understanding of the anatomy and physiology of the human body.

why study
GENERAL ANATOMY AND PHYSIOLOGY?

Barbers should study and have a thorough understanding of general anatomy and physiology because:

> Understanding how the human body functions as an integrated whole is a key component in understanding how a client's hair and skin may react to various treatments and services.

> Being able to recognize the difference between what is considered normal and what is considered abnormal in the body will assist you in knowing what requires referral to a physician.

> Understanding the bone, muscle, and nerve structure of the human body will help you determine how to provide services that are appropriate for your client.

Why Are Anatomy and Physiology Important to You?

After reading this section, you will be able to:

LO❶ Define and explain the importance of anatomy, physiology, and histology to the barbering profession.

This high-level overview of human anatomy and physiology will provide you with a basic knowledge of the structure and functions of the human body to assist your performance in the barbering field. This chapter focuses on the anatomy and physiology that is pertinent to the practice of barbering, such as the anatomical structure of the head that provides a foundation for designing haircut and beard styles or performing a proper shave. This chapter will provide you with the definitions and "map" of the human body as a point of reference to be used when you discuss specific services later in the text.

Anatomy (ah-NAT-ah-mee) is the study of the human body structures that can be seen with the naked eye and how the body parts are organized; it is the science of the structure of organisms or of their parts.

Physiology (fiz-ih-OL-oh-gee) is the study of the functions and activities performed by the body's structures. The ending *-ology* means "study of."

Barbers should be aware of the ways in which massage manipulations, heat, or absorptive products used in the practice of barbering might affect physiological activities of the body, such as increasing the circulation. Barbers should also be aware of certain physiological stresses caused by prolonged standing or repetitive movements that may affect their own skeletal or circulatory systems, as well as the preventative measures that can help minimize the occurrence of associated occupational disorders (see Chapter 3).

DID YOU KNOW?

Histology (his-TAHL-uh-jee), also known as *microscopic anatomy* (mi-kroh-SKAHP-ik ah-NAT-ah-mee), is the study of tiny structures found in living tissues.

Know about Cells

After reading this section, you will be able to:

LO❷ Describe cells, their structure, and their reproduction.

Cells (SELLZ) are the basic units of all living things, from bacteria to plants to animals, including human beings. Without cells, life does not exist. As a basic functional unit, the cell is responsible for carrying on all life processes. There are trillions of cells in the human body, and they vary widely in size, shape, and purpose.

BASIC STRUCTURE OF THE CELL

The cells of all living things are composed of a substance called **protoplasm** (PROH-toh-plaz-um), a colorless jellylike substance found inside cells in which food elements such as proteins, fats, carbohydrates, mineral salts, and water are present. You can visualize the protoplasm of a cell as being similar to raw egg white. In addition to protoplasm, most cells also include a nucleus, cytoplasm, and the cell membrane (**Figure 6-1**).

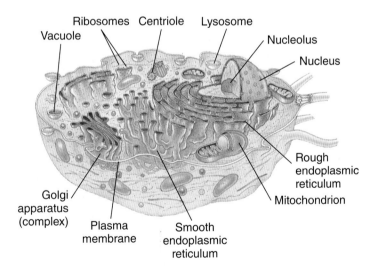

figure 6-1
Basic structure of the cell.

The **nucleus** (NOO-klee-us) is the dense, active protoplasm found in the center of the cell; it plays an important part in cell reproduction and metabolism. You can visualize the nucleus as the yolk in the middle of a raw egg.

The **cytoplasm** (sy-toh-PLAZ-um) is the watery fluid that surrounds the nucleus of the cell and is needed for growth, reproduction, and self-repair. It is part of the protoplasm of the cell.

The **cell membrane** (SELL mem-brain) is the cell wall that encloses the protoplasm and permits soluble substances to enter and leave the cell.

CELL REPRODUCTION AND DIVISION

Cells have the ability to reproduce, thus providing new cells for the growth and replacement of worn or injured ones. **Mitosis** (my-TOH-sis) is the usual process of cell reproduction of human tissues that occurs when the cell divides into two identical cells called *daughter cells*. Two small structures near the nucleus called **centrioles** (SEN-tree-olz) move to each side during the mitosis process to help divide the cell. As long as conditions are favorable, the cell will grow and reproduce. Favorable conditions include an adequate supply of food, oxygen, and water; suitable temperatures; and the ability to eliminate waste products. If conditions become unfavorable, the cell will become impaired or may die. Unfavorable conditions include toxins (poisons), disease, and injury (**Figure 6-2**).

figure 6-2
Phases of mitosis.

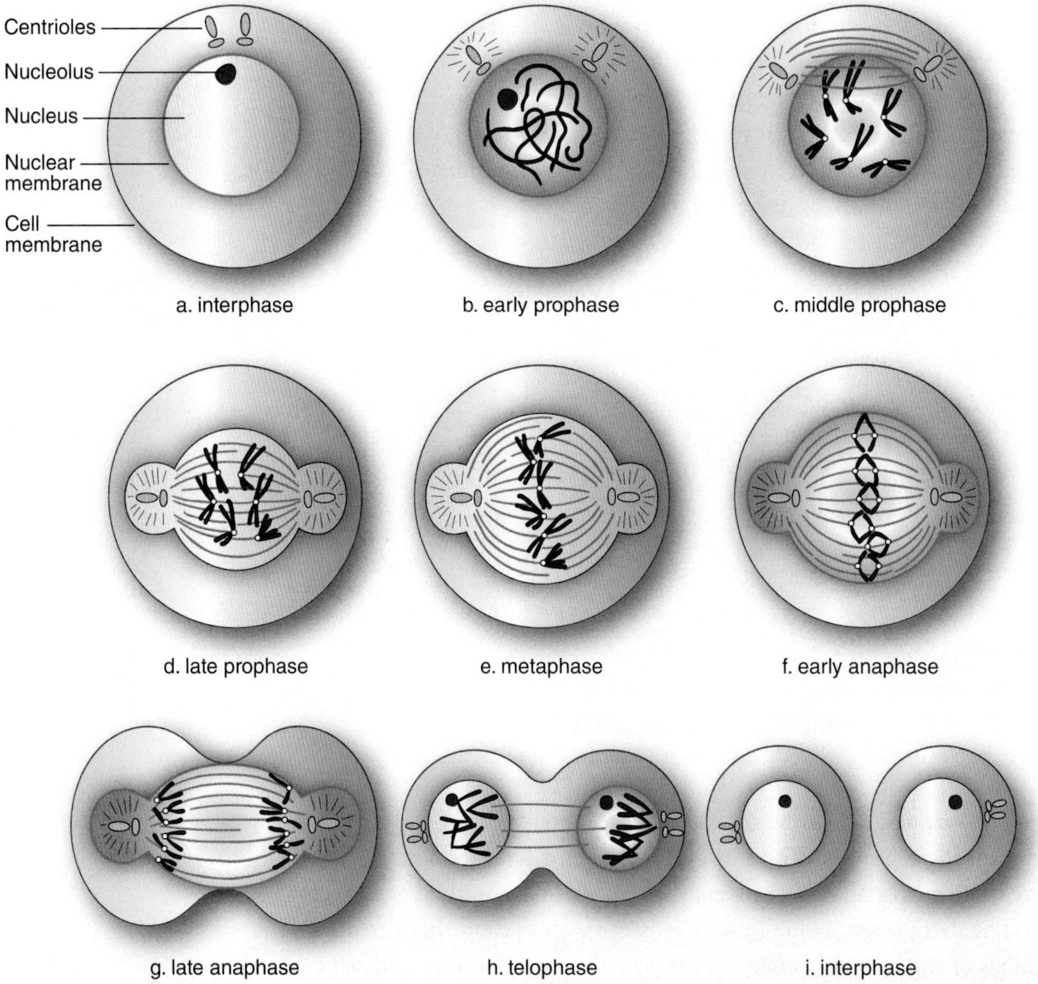

Centrioles
Nucleolus
Nucleus
Nuclear membrane
Cell membrane

a. interphase

b. early prophase

c. middle prophase

d. late prophase

e. metaphase

f. early anaphase

g. late anaphase

h. telophase

i. interphase

Identify Types of Tissues

After reading this section, you will be able to:

LO③ Identify and define the types of tissues found in the body.

Tissue (TISH-oo) is a collection of similar cells that perform a particular function. Each kind of tissue has a specific function and can be recognized by its characteristic appearance. Body tissues are composed of large amounts of water, along with various other substances. There are four types of tissue in the body:

- **Connective tissue** (kuh-NEK-tiv TISH-oo) is fibrous tissue that binds together, protects, and supports the various parts of the body. Examples of connective tissue are bone, cartilage, ligaments, tendons, blood, lymph, and **adipose tissue** (ADD-ih-pohz TISH-oo), a technical term for fat. Adipose tissue gives smoothness and contour to the body.

- **Epithelial tissue** (ep-ih-THEE-lee-ul TISH-oo) is a protective covering on body surfaces, such as skin, mucous membranes, the tissue inside the mouth, the lining of the heart, digestive and respiratory organs, and the glands.

- **Muscle tissue** contracts and moves various parts of the body.

- **Nerve tissue** carries messages to and from the brain and controls and coordinates all bodily functions. Nerve tissue is composed of special cells known as *neurons* that make up the nerves, brain, and spinal cord.

Discuss Body Systems and Associated Organs

After reading this section, you will be able to:

LO④ Define organs and body systems.

LO⑤ Name the main body systems and explain their basic functions.

Organs are structures composed of specialized tissues designed to perform specific functions in plants and animals. During the development of a fetus, tissues are "assigned" to specific functions in the body and they develop specifically for those functions. For example, lung tissue would not work as a part of the brain as it is designed to serve a specific function in the lungs. **Body systems** (BAHD-ee SYS-tums), also known as *systems*, are groups of body organs acting together to perform one or more functions (**Figure 6-3**). **Table 6-1** outlines the body systems, indicating the functions of the system and the major organs that are associated with that system.

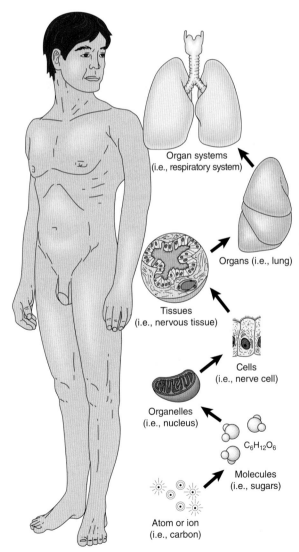

figure 6-3
Life is built from the carbon atom.

Organ systems
(i.e., respiratory system)

Organs (i.e., lung)

Tissues
(i.e., nervous tissue)

Cells
(i.e., nerve cell)

Organelles
(i.e., nucleus)

$C_6H_{12}O_6$

Molecules
(i.e., sugars)

Atom or ion
(i.e., carbon)

table 6-1

THE ELEVEN BODY SYSTEMS, THEIR FUNCTIONS, AND MAJOR ORGANS

Body Systems	Function	Major Organs
Circulatory	Controls movement of blood throughout the body	Heart, blood vessels
Digestive (dy-JES-tiv) (gastrointestinal)	Breaks down food into nutrients or waste for nutrition or excretion	Stomach, intestines, salivary and gastric glands
Endocrine	Controls hormone levels that determine growth, development, sexual function, and health of entire body	Endocrine glands, hormones
Excretory (EKS-kruh-toh-ree)	Eliminates waste from the body reducing buildup of toxins	Kidneys, liver, skin, large intestines, lungs
Integumentary	Provides protective covering and regulates body temperature	Skin, oil and sweat glands, hair, nails
Immune (lymphatic)	Protects the body from disease by developing immunity and destroying pathogens and toxins	Lymph, lymph nodes, thymus gland, spleen
Muscular	Covers, shapes, and holds the skeleton in place. Muscles contract to allow for movement of body structures.	Muscles, connective tissues
Nervous	Coordinates with all other body systems, allowing them to work efficiently and react to the environment	Brain, spinal cord, nerves, eyes
Reproductive	Produces offspring and allows for transfer of genetic material. Differentiates between the sexes	Female: ovaries, uterus, vagina Male: testes, prostate, penis
Respiratory (RES-puh-rah-tor-ee)	Makes blood and oxygen available to body structures through respiration; eliminates carbon dioxide	Lungs, air passages
Skeletal	Forms the physical foundation of the body: 206 bones that are connected by movable and immovable joints	Bones, joints

? DID YOU KNOW?
You have over 230 movable and semi-movable joints in your body.

REVIEW THE SKELETAL SYSTEM

The **skeletal system** (SKEL-uh-tul SIS-tum) forms the physical foundation of the body and is composed of 206 bones that vary in size and shape and are connected by movable and immovable joints. **Osteology** (ahs-tee-AHL-oh-jee) is the study of the anatomy, structure, and function of the bones. **Os** (AHS) means "bone." It is used as a prefix in many medical terms, such as osteoarthritis, a joint disease.

Except for the tissue that forms the major part of the teeth, bone is the hardest tissue in the body. It is composed of connective tissue consisting of about one-third organic matter, such as cells and blood, and two-thirds minerals, mainly calcium carbonate and calcium phosphate.

The primary functions of the skeletal system are to:

- Give shape and support to the body.
- Protect various internal structures and organs.
- Serve as attachments for muscles and act as levers to produce body movement.

- Help produce both white and red blood cells (one of the functions of bone marrow).
- Store most of the body's calcium supply, as well as phosphorus, magnesium, and sodium.

? DID YOU KNOW?
People often complain of joint pain; however, the pain is usually caused by inflammation of the tissue surrounding the joint and not by the joint itself.

A **joint** is the connection between two or more bones of the skeleton. There are two types of joints: movable, such as elbows, knees, and hips, and immovable, such as the joints found in the pelvis and skull, which allow little or no movement. There are exceptions to this condition such as childbirth, where special hormones allow for flexibility of the pelvic joints.

Bones of the Skull

The skull is the skeleton of the head and is divided into two parts:

- **Cranium** (KRAY-nee-um). An oval, bony case that protects the brain.
- **Facial skeleton** (FAY-shul skell-uh-tin). The framework of the face that is composed of 14 bones.

Bones of the Cranium

The following are the eight bones of the cranium (**Figure 6-4**):

- **Occipital bone** (ahk-SIP-it-ul BOHN). Hindmost bone of the skull, below the parietal bones; forms the back of the skull above the nape.
- **Parietal bones** (puh-RY-ate-ul BOHNZ). Bones that form the sides and top of the cranium. There are two parietal bones.
- **Frontal bone** (FRUNT-ul BOHN). Bone that forms the forehead.
- **Temporal bones** (TEM-puh-rul BOHNZ). Bones that form the sides of the head in the ear region. There are two temporal bones.
- **Ethmoid bone** (ETH-moyd BOHN). Light spongy bone between the eye sockets; forms part of the nasal cavities.
- **Sphenoid bone** (SFEE-noyd BOHN). Bone that joins all of the bones of the cranium together.

The ethmoid and sphenoid bones are not affected when performing services or giving a massage.

figure 6-4
Bones of the cranium and the face.

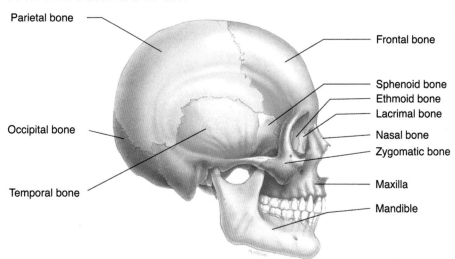

Bones of the Face

There are 14 bones of the face, but those listed below are the most involved in the practice of barbering:

- **Nasal bones** (NAY-zul BONZ). Bones that form the bridge of the nose. There are two nasal bones.
- **Lacrimal bones** (LAK-ruh-mul BONZ). Small, thin bones located at the front inner wall of the orbits (eye sockets). There are two lacrimal bones.
- **Zygomatic bones** (zy-goh-MAT-ik BONZ), also known as *malar bones* or *cheekbones*. Bones that form the prominence of the cheeks. There are two zygomatic bones.
- **Maxillae** (mak-SIL-ee) (singular: maxilla [mak-SIL-uh]). Bones of the upper jaw. There are two maxillae.
- **Mandible** (MAN-duh-bul). Lower jawbone; largest and strongest bone of the face.

Bones of the Neck

The main bones of the neck are the following:

- **Hyoid bone** (HY-oyd BOHN). U-shaped bone at the base of the tongue that supports the tongue and its muscles.
- **Cervical vertebrae** (SUR-vih-kul VURT-uh-bray). The seven bones of the top part of the vertebral column, located in the neck region (**Figure 6-5**).

Bones of the Chest, Shoulder, and Back

The **thorax** (THOR-aks), or chest, is an elastic, bony cage consisting of the sternum, clavicle, scapula, and 12 pairs of ribs. This framework serves as a protective covering for the heart, lungs, and other delicate internal organs.

figure 6-5
Bones of the neck, shoulders, and back.

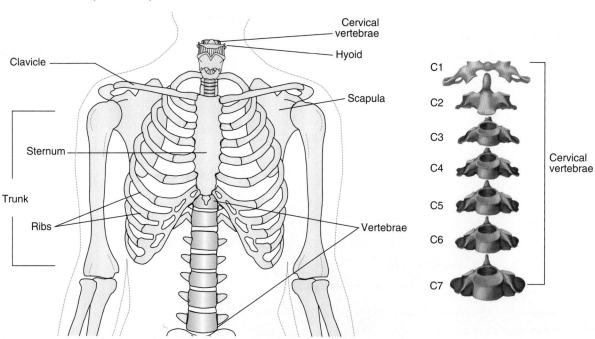

Bones of the Shoulder, Arm, and Hand

Some of the major causes of chronic pain for barbers are related to the repetitive action of the shoulders, arms, and hands. The important bones of the shoulders, arms, and hands that barbers should know about include the following (**Figures 6-6** and **6-7**):

- The **humerus** (HYOO-muh-rus) is the largest bone of the arm and extends from the shoulder to the elbow.

- The **ulna** (UL-nuh) is the inner and larger bone of the forearm, forms the elbow, and is located along the same side of the arm as the little finger.

- The **radius** (RAY-dee-us) is the smaller bone on the thumb side of the forearm.

- The **carpus** (KAR-pus) or wrist is a flexible joint composed of eight small, irregular bones held together by ligaments.

- The **metacarpals** (met-uh-KAR-pulz) are the bones of the palm, consisting of five slender bones between the carpus and the phalanges.

- The **phalanges** (FA-lanj-eez) are the bones of the fingers, consisting of three in each finger and two in the thumb, totaling 14 bones in each hand.

REVIEW THE MUSCULAR SYSTEM

The **muscular system** (MUS-kyuh-lur SIS-tum) covers, shapes, and supports the skeleton, and its function is to help produce movement within the body. **Myology** (my-AHL-uh-jee) is the study of the structure, functioning, and diseases of the muscles.

The muscular system consists of over 600 large and small muscles that comprise 40 to 50 percent of the body's weight. Muscles are composed of contractile, fibrous tissues that stretch and contract to facilitate the action of various body movements. The muscular system relies upon the skeletal and nervous systems for its activities and proper operation.

There are three types of muscular tissues:

1. Striated (striped) or voluntary muscles contain nerves, are attached to bones, and are controlled by will. For example, the face consists of many voluntary muscles that facilitate expression.

2. Nonstriated (smooth) or involuntary muscles function without the action of the will. These muscles are found in the internal organs of the body, such as the stomach and intestines.

3. Cardiac muscle is the heart itself. An involuntary muscle with striations and centrally located nuclei, it is not duplicated anywhere else in the body.

Muscle Structure

When a muscle contracts and shortens, one of its attachments usually remains fixed and the other one moves. A muscle has three parts (**Figure 6-8**):

- **Origin** (OR-ih-jin). The part of the muscle that does not move and is attached closest to the skeleton.

- **Belly** (BELL-ee). The middle part of the muscle.

- **Insertion** (in-SUR-shun). The part of the muscle that moves and is farthest from the skeleton.

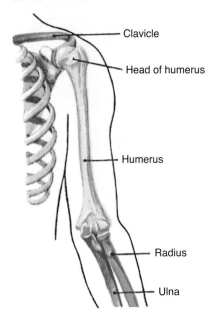

figure 6-6
Bones of the arm.

Clavicle
Head of humerus
Humerus
Radius
Ulna

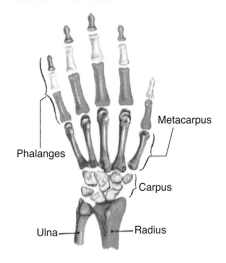

figure 6-7
Bones of the hand.

Metacarpus
Phalanges
Carpus
Ulna
Radius

figure 6-8
Muscle origin and insertion.

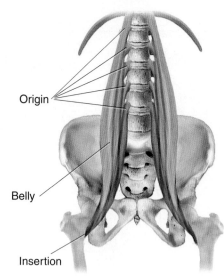

Origin

Belly

Insertion

Stimulation of Muscles

Muscular tissue can be stimulated by:

- Massage (hand, electric vibrator, or water jets).
- Electrical therapy current. (See Chapter 8, Basics of Electricity, for additional information on types of electrical therapy current.)
- Infrared light.
- Dry heat (heating lamps or heating caps).
- Moist heat (steamers or moderately warm steam towels).
- Nerve impulses (through the nervous system).
- Chemicals (certain acids and salts).

Muscles of the Scalp, Face, and Neck

The performance of professional services such as scalp, facial, and neck massages requires barbers to know the location of the voluntary muscles of the head, face, and neck and the functions these muscles control (**Figures 6-9** and **6-10**).

Muscles of the Scalp

The four muscles of the scalp are the following:

- **Epicranius** (ep-ih-KRAY-nee-us), also known as *occipitofrontalis* (ahk-SIP-ih-toh-frun-TAY-lus). Broad muscle that covers the top of the skull and consists of the occipitalis and frontalis.
- **Occipitalis** (ahk-SIP-ih-tahl-is). Back (posterior) portion of the epicranius; the muscle that draws the scalp backward.
- **Frontalis** (frun-TAY-lus). Front (anterior) portion of the epicranius; the muscle of the scalp that raises the eyebrows, draws the scalp forward, and causes wrinkles across the forehead.
- **Epicranial aponeurosis** (ep-ih-KRAY-nee-al ap-uh-noo-ROH-sus). Tendon that connects the occipitalis and frontalis muscles (**Figure 6-9**).

figure 6-9
Muscles of the head, face, and neck.

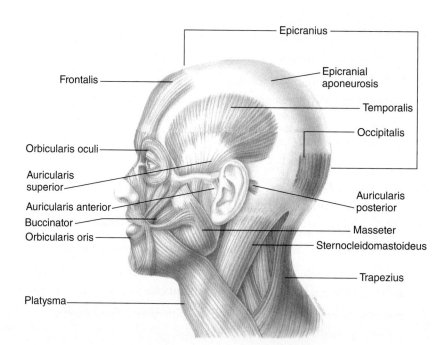

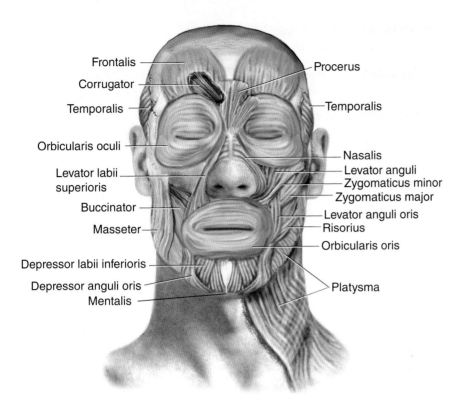

figure 6-10
Muscles of the face.

Frontalis — | — Procerus
Corrugator —
Temporalis — | — Temporalis
Orbicularis oculi —
Levator labii superioris — | — Nasalis
 — Levator anguli
 — Zygomaticus minor
 — Zygomaticus major
Buccinator —
Masseter — | — Levator anguli oris
 — Risorius
 — Orbicularis oris
Depressor labii inferioris —
Depressor anguli oris — | — Platysma
Mentalis —

Muscles of the Ear

The three muscles of the ear are the following:

- **Auricularis superior** (aw-rik-yuh-LAIR-is soo-PEER-ee-ur). Muscle above the ear that draws the ear upward.

- **Auricularis anterior** (aw-rik-yuh-LAIR-is an-TEER-ee-ur). Muscle in front of the ear that draws the ear forward.

- **Auricularis posterior** (aw-rik-yuh-LAIR-is poh-STEER-ee-ur). Muscle behind the ear that draws the ear backward.

Muscles of Mastication (Chewing)

The main muscles of mastication, also known as the *chewing muscles*, are the following:

- **Masseter** (muh-SEET-ur).

- **Temporalis** (tem-poh-RAY-lis).

These muscles coordinate to open and close the mouth and bring the jaw forward or backward, assisted by the *pterygoid* (THER-ih-goyd) muscles.

Muscles of the Neck

The two major muscles of the neck are the following:

- The **platysma** (plah-TIZ-muh) is a broad muscle extending from the chest and shoulder muscles to the side of the chin and is responsible for depressing the lower jaw and lip.

- The **sternocleidomastoideus** (STUR-noh-KLEE-ih-doh-mas-TOYD-ee-us) is the muscle extending from the collar and chest bones to the temporal bone at the back of the ear; this muscle bends and rotates the head.

Muscles of the Eye

The eye muscles include the following:

- **Orbicularis oculi muscle** (or-bik-yuh-LAIR-is AHK-yuh-lye MUS-uhl). Ring muscle of the eye socket; enables you to close your eyes.

- **Corrugator muscle** (KOR-uh-gayt-or MUS-uhl). Muscle located beneath the frontalis and orbicularis oculi muscle that draws the eyebrow down and wrinkles the forehead vertically.

- **Levator palpebrae superioris muscle** (lih-VAYT-ur PAL-puh-bree soo-peer-ee-OR-is MUS-uhl). Thin muscle that controls the eyelid and can be easily damaged during massage or makeup application.

Muscles of the Nose

- The **procerus** (proh-SEE-rus) covers the top of the nose, depresses the eyebrow, and causes wrinkles across the bridge of the nose. The other nasal muscles are small muscles around the nasal openings, which contract and expand the opening of the nostrils.

Muscles of the Mouth

The important muscles of the mouth are the following:

- **Buccinator muscle** (BUK-sih-nay-tur MUS-uhl). Thin, flat muscle of the cheek between the upper and lower jaw that compresses the cheeks and expels air between the lips.

- **Depressor labii inferioris muscle** (dee-PRES-ur LAY-bee-eye in-FEER-ee-or-us MUS-uhl), also known as *quadratus labii inferioris muscle* (kwah-DRAY-tus LAY-bee-eye in-FEER-ee-or-us MUS-uhl). Muscle surrounding the lower lip; lowers the lower lip and draws it to one side, as in expressing sarcasm.

- **Levator anguli oris muscle** (lih-VAYT-ur ANG-yoo-ly OH-ris MUS-uhl), also known as *caninus muscle* (kay-NY-nus MUS-uhl). Muscle that raises the angle of the mouth and draws it inward.

- **Levator labii superioris muscle** (lih-VAYT-ur LAY-bee-eye soo-peer-ee-OR-is MUS-uhl), also known as *quadratus labii superioris muscle* (kwah-DRAY-tus LAY-bee-eye soo-peer-ee-OR-is MUS-uhl). Muscle surrounding the upper lip; elevates the upper lip and dilates the nostrils, as in expressing distaste.

- **Mentalis muscle** (men-TAY-lis MUS-uhl). Muscle that elevates the lower lip and raises and wrinkles the skin of the chin.

- **Orbicularis oris muscle** (or-bik-yuh-LAIR-is OH-ris MUS-uhl). Flat band of muscle around the upper and lower lips that compresses, contracts, puckers, and wrinkles the lips.

- **Risorius muscle** (rih-ZOR-ee-us MUS-uhl). Muscle of the mouth that draws the corner of the mouth out and back, as in grinning.

- **Triangularis muscle** (try-ang-gyuh-LAY-rus MUS-uhl). Muscle extending alongside the chin that pulls down the corner of the mouth.

- **Zygomaticus major muscles** (zy-goh-MAT-ih-kus MAY-jor MUS-uhlz). Muscles on both sides of the face that extend from the zygomatic bone to the angle of the mouth. These muscles pull the mouth upward and backward, as when you are laughing or smiling.

- **Zygomaticus minor muscles** (zy-goh-mat-ih-kus MY-nor MUS-uhlz). Muscles on both sides of the face that extend from the zygomatic bone to the upper lips. These muscles pull the upper lip backward, upward, and outward, as when you are smiling.

Muscles That Attach the Arms to the Body

The muscles that attach the arms to the body are the following:

- **Latissimus dorsi** (lah-TIS-ih-mus DOR-see). Large, flat, triangular muscle covering the lower back. It helps extend the arm away from the body and rotate the shoulder.

- **Pectoralis major** (pek-tor-AL-is MAY-jor) and **pectoralis minor** (located under the pectoralis major) are muscles of the chest that assist the swinging movements of the arm.

- **Serratus anterior** (ser-RAT-us an-TEER-ee-ur). Muscle of the chest that assists in breathing and in raising the arm.

- **Trapezius** (truh-PEE-zee-us). Muscle that covers the back of the neck and the upper and middle region of the back; rotates and controls swinging movements of the arm (**Figures 6-11** and **6-12**).

Muscles of the Shoulder and Arm

There are three principal muscles of the shoulders and upper arms (**Figure 6-13**):

- **Bicep** (BY-sep). Muscle that produces the contour of the front and inner side of the upper arm; lifts the forearm and flexes the elbow.

- **Deltoid** (DEL-toyd). Large, triangular muscle covering the shoulder joint that allows the arm to extend outward and to the side of the body.

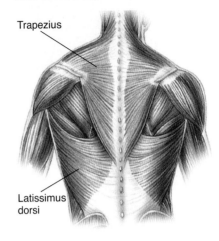

figure 6-11
Muscles of the back that attach the arms to the body.

Trapezius

Latissimus dorsi

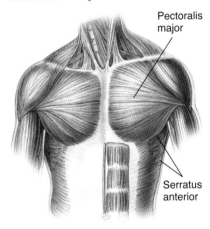

figure 6-12
Muscles of the chest that attach the arms to the body.

Pectoralis major

Serratus anterior

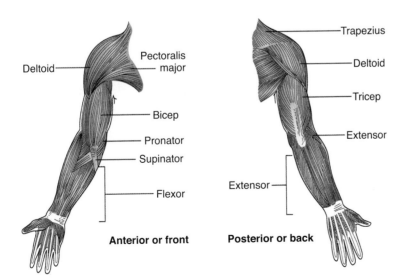

Deltoid

Pectoralis major

Bicep

Pronator

Supinator

Flexor

Anterior or front

Trapezius

Deltoid

Tricep

Extensor

Extensor

Posterior or back

figure 6-13
Muscles of the anterior and posterior shoulder and arm.

- **Tricep** (TRY-sep). Large muscle that covers the entire back of the upper arm and extends the forearm.

The forearm is made up of a series of muscles and strong tendons. As a barber, you will be concerned with the following muscles of the forearm:

- **Extensors** (ik-STEN-surs). Muscles that straighten the wrist, hand, and fingers to form a straight line.

- **Flexor** (FLEK-sur). Extensor muscle of the wrist involved in flexing the wrist.

- **Pronator** (proh-NAY-tohr). Muscle that turns the hand inward so that the palm faces downward.

- **Supinator** (SOO-puh-nayt-ur). Muscle of the forearm that rotates the radius outward and the palm upward.

Muscles of the Hand

The hand is one of the most complex parts of the body, with many small muscles that overlap from joint to joint and provide the flexibility and strength to open and close the hand and fingers. Important muscles to know include the following (**Figure 6-14**):

figure 6-14
Muscles of the hand.

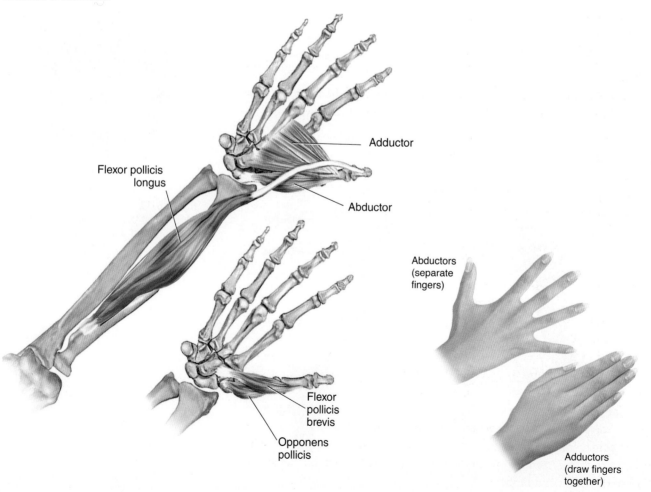

Flexor pollicis longus

Adductor

Abductor

Flexor pollicis brevis

Opponens pollicis

Abductors (separate fingers)

Adductors (draw fingers together)

- **Abductors** (ab-DUK-turz). Muscles that draw a body part, such as a finger, arm, or toe, away from the midline of the body or of an extremity. In the hand, abductors separate the fingers.

- **Adductors** (ah-DUK-turz). Muscles that draw a body part, such as a finger, arm, or toe, inward toward the median axis of the body or of an extremity. In the hand, adductors draw the fingers together.

REVIEW THE NERVOUS SYSTEM

Neurology is the study of the structure, function, and pathology of the nervous system. The nervous system is one of the most important systems of the body. It controls and coordinates the functions of all the other systems and makes them work harmoniously and efficiently. Every square inch of the human body is supplied with fine fibers known as *nerves*.

An understanding of how nerves work will help barbers perform the massage services associated with shampoos, scalp treatments, and facials. It will also help increase awareness of the effects these treatments can have on the skin, the scalp, and on the body as a whole.

Divisions of the Nervous System

The principal components of the nervous system are the brain, the spinal cord, and the nerves themselves. The nervous system is divided into two main subdivisions: the central nervous system and the peripheral nervous system (**Figure 6-15**).

1. The **central nervous system (CNS)** (SEN-trul NUR-vus SIS-tum) consists of the brain, cranial nerves, spinal cord, and spinal nerves. It controls consciousness and all mental activities, the functions of the five senses, and voluntary muscle actions, including all body movements and facial expressions.

2. The **peripheral nervous system (PNS)** (puh-RIF-uh-rul NUR-vus SIS-tum) is made up of sensory and motor nerve fibers that extend from the brain and spinal cord to all parts of the body. Their function is to carry impulses, or messages, to and from the central nervous system. Subdivisions of the peripheral nervous system are the autonomic and somatic nervous systems, which control involuntary and voluntary functions and actions.

The Brain and Spinal Cord

The **brain** (BRAYN) is the part of the central nervous system contained in the cranium. It is the largest and most complex organization of nerve tissue and controls sensation, muscles, activity of glands, and the power to think, sense, and feel. On average, the brain weighs a little less than three pounds. It sends and receives messages through 12 pairs of cranial nerves that originate in the brain and reach various parts of the head, face, and neck.

The **spinal cord** (SPY-nal KORD) is the portion of the central nervous system that originates in the brain and extends down to the lower extremity of the trunk. It is protected by the spinal column. Thirty-one pairs of spinal nerves extending from the spinal cord are distributed to the muscles and skin of the trunk and limbs.

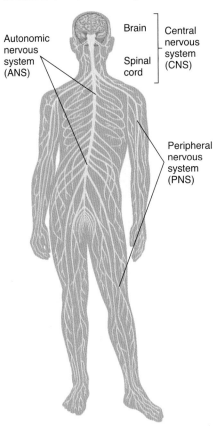

figure 6-15
Divisions of the nervous system.

Autonomic nervous system (ANS)

Brain

Central nervous system (CNS)

Spinal cord

Peripheral nervous system (PNS)

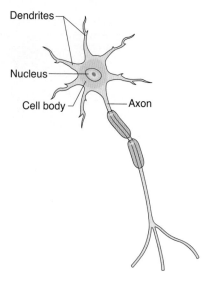

figure 6-16
A neuron or nerve cell.

Dendrites

Nucleus

Cell body — Axon

Nerve Cell Structure and Function

A **neuron** (NOO-rahn), also known as *nerve cell*, is the primary structural unit of the nervous system, consisting of the cell body, nucleus, dendrites, and the axon.

Dendrites (DEN-dryts) are treelike branchings of nerve fibers extending from the nerve cell that carry impulses toward the cell and receive impulses from other neurons. The **axon** (AK-sahn) and **axon terminal** (AK-sahn TER-min-al) are extensions of a neuron through which impulses are sent away from the cell body to other neurons, glands, or muscles (**Figure 6-16**).

Nerves are whitish cords made up of bundles of nerve fibers held together by connective tissue, through which impulses are transmitted. Nerves have their origin in the brain and spinal cord and send their branches to all parts of the body.

Types of Nerves

There are two types of nerves:

- **Sensory nerves**, also known as *afferent nerves* (AAF-eer-ent NURVZ), carry impulses or messages from the sense organs, where sensations such as touch, cold, heat, sight, hearing, taste, smell, pain, and pressure are experienced. Sensory nerve endings called *receptors* are located close to the surface of the skin. Impulses pass from the sensory nerves to the brain and back through the motor nerves to the muscles; the muscles move as a result of the completed circuit.

- **Motor nerves** (MOH-tur NURVZ), also known as *efferent nerves* (EF-uh-rent NURVZ), carry impulses from the brain to the muscles or glands. These transmitted impulses produce movement.

A **reflex** (REE-fleks) is an automatic reaction to a stimulus that involves the movement of an impulse from a sensory receptor along the sensory nerve to the spinal cord. A responsive impulse is sent along a motor neuron to a muscle, causing a reaction (e.g., the quick removal of your hand from a hot object). Reflexes do not have to be learned; they are automatic.

Activity

There are sensory nerve endings all over the body. Try gently pinching a small piece of skin on your arm. You feel a slight pressure, right? That is the sensory nerve endings sending a message from your arm to your brain that something is happening to your arm.

Nerves of the Head, Face, and Neck

There are 12 pairs of cranial nerves. All are connected to a part of the brain surface. They emerge through openings on the sides and base of the cranium and reach various parts of the head, face, and neck. The largest of the cranial nerves is the **fifth cranial nerve** (FIFTH KRAY-nee-ul NURV), also known as *trifacial nerve* (try-FAY-shul NURV) or *trigeminal nerve* (try-JEM-un-ul NURV). It is the chief sensory nerve of the face and serves as the motor nerve of the muscles that control chewing. It consists of three branches:

- **Ophthalmic nerve** (ahf-THAL-mik NURV). Supplies impulses to the skin of the forehead, upper eyelids, and interior portion of the scalp, orbit, eyeball, and nasal passage.

- **Mandibular nerve** (man-DIB-yuh-lur NURV). Affects the muscles of the chin, lower lip, and external ear.

- **Maxillary nerve** (MAK-suh-lair-ee NURV). Supplies impulses to the upper part of the face (**Figure 6-17**).

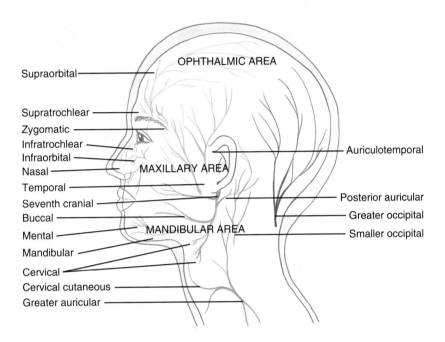

figure 6-17
Nerves of the head, face, and neck.

The following are the branches of the fifth cranial nerve that are affected by massage (**Figure 6-18**):

- **Auriculotemporal nerve** (aw-RIK-yuh-loh-TEM-puh-rul NURV). Affects the external ear and skin above the temple, up to the top of the skull.

- **Infraorbital nerve** (in-fruh-OR-bih-tul NURV). Affects the skin of the lower eyelid, side of the nose, upper lip, and mouth.

- **Infratrochlear nerve** (in-frah-TRAHK-lee-ur NURV). Affects the membrane and skin of the nose.

- **Mental nerve** (MEN-tul NURV). Affects the skin of the lower lip and chin.

- **Nasal nerve** (NAY-zul NURV). Affects the tip and lower side of the nose.

- **Supraorbital nerve** (soo-pruh-OR-bih-tul NURV). Affects the skin of the forehead, scalp, eyebrow, and upper eyelid.

- **Supratrochlear nerve** (soo-pruh-TRAHK-lee-ur NURV). Affects the skin between the eyes and upper side of the nose.

- **Zygomatic nerve** (zy-goh-MAT-ik NURV). Affects the muscles of the upper part of the cheek.

The **seventh cranial nerve** (SEV-AHNTH CRAN-ee-ahl NURV), also known as the *facial nerve*, is the chief motor nerve of the face (**Figure 6-19**). Its divisions

figure 6-18
Fifth cranial nerve.

figure 6-19
Seventh cranial nerve.

figure 6-20
Eleventh cranial nerve.

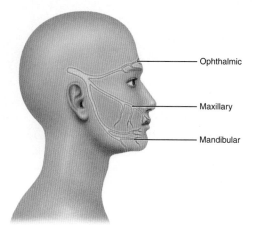

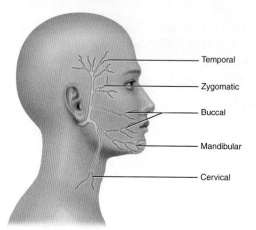

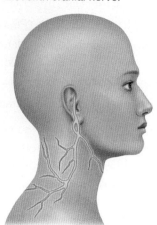

and their branches supply and control all the muscles of facial expression. It emerges near the lower part of the ear and extends to the muscles of the neck. The following are the most important branches of the facial nerve:

- **Posterior auricular nerve** (poh-STEER-ee-ur aw-rik-yuh-lur NURV). Affects the muscles behind the ear at the base of the skull.

- **Temporal nerve** (TEM-poh-rul NURV). Affects the muscles of the temple, side of the forehead, eyebrow, eyelid, and upper part of the cheek.

- Zygomatic nerve (upper and lower). Affects the muscles of the upper part of the cheek.

- **Buccal nerve** (BUK-ul NURV). Affects the muscles of the mouth.

- **Marginal mandibular nerve** (MAR-jin-ul man-DIB-yuh-lur NURV). Affects the muscles of the chin and lower lip.

The **eleventh cranial nerve** (ee-LEV-unth CRAY-nee-ul NURV), also known as *accessory nerve*, is a motor nerve that controls the motion of the neck and shoulder muscles (**Figure 6-20**). This nerve is important to barbers because it is affected during facials, primarily when you are giving a massage to your client.

Cervical Nerves

The cervical or spinal nerves originate at the spinal cord. Their branches supply the muscles and scalp at the back of the head and neck as follows:

- The **greater occipital nerve** (GRAY-tur ahk-SIP-ut-ul NURV) is located at the back of the head and affects the scalp as far up as the top of the head.

- The **smaller** (lesser) **occipital nerve** (SMAWL-ur ahk-SIP-ut-ul NURV) is located at the base of the skull and affects the scalp and muscles of this region.

- The **greater auricular nerve** (GRAYT-ur aw-RIK-yuh-lur NURV) is located at the side of the neck and affects the external ears and the areas in front and back of the ears.

- The **cervical cutaneous nerve** (SUR-vih-kul kyoo-TAY-nee-us NURV) is located at the side of the neck and affects the front and sides of the neck as far down as the breastbone.

REVIEW THE CIRCULATORY SYSTEM

The **circulatory system** (SUR-kyool-ah-tohr-ee SIS-tum), also known as *cardio-vascular system* (KAHRD-ee-oh-VAS-kyoo-lur SIS-tum) or *vascular system*, controls the steady circulation of the blood through the body by means of the heart and blood vessels. The circulatory system consists of the heart, arteries, veins, and capillaries that distribute blood throughout the body.

The Heart

The **heart** (HART) is a muscular, cone-shaped organ that keeps the blood moving within the circulatory system. It is often referred to as the *body's pump*.

The heart is approximately the size of a closed fist, weighs about nine ounces, and is located in the chest cavity. A normal adult heart beats about 60 to 80 times per minute, but it can beat as high as 100 times per minute when necessary and as low as 50 beats per minute in very physically fit individuals. Heart rate norms vary with age and fitness.

The blood is in constant and continuous circulation from the time that it leaves the heart, is distributed throughout the body to deliver nutrients and oxygen, and then returns to the heart to be replenished with oxygen. Two systems are important to this circulation (**Figure 6-21**):

- **Pulmonary circulation** (PUL-muh-nayr-ee sur-kyoo-LAY-shun). Takes deoxygenated blood to the lungs for oxygenation and waste removal and then returns that blood to the heart (left atrium) so oxygen-rich blood can be delivered to the body.

- **Systemic circulation** (sis-TEM-ik sur-kyoo-LAY-shun), also known as **general circulation**. Carries the oxygen-rich blood from the heart throughout the body and returns deoxygenated blood back to the heart.

Blood Vessels

The **blood vessels** are tubelike structures that include the arteries, arterioles, capillaries, venules, and veins. The function of these vessels is to transport blood to and from the heart and then to various tissues of the body. The types of blood vessels found in the body are:

- **Arteries** (AR-tuh-reez). Thick-walled, muscular, flexible tubes that carry oxygenated blood away from the heart to the arterioles. The largest artery in the body is the **aorta** (ay-ORT-uh).

- **Arterioles** (ar-TEER-ee-ohls). Small arteries that deliver blood to capillaries.

- **Capillaries** (KAP-ih-lair-eez). Tiny, thin-walled blood vessels that connect the smaller arteries to venules. Capillaries bring nutrients to the cells and carry away waste materials.

- **Venules** (VEEN-yools). Small vessels that connect the capillaries to the veins. They collect blood from the capillaries and drain it into the veins.

- **Veins** (VAYNS). Thin-walled blood vessels that are less elastic than arteries; veins contain cuplike valves that keep blood flowing in one direction to the heart and prevent blood from flowing backward. Veins carry blood containing waste products back to the heart and lungs for cleaning and to pick up oxygen. Veins are located closer to the outer skin surface of the body than arteries.

figure 6-21
Drawing of blood flow through the heart.

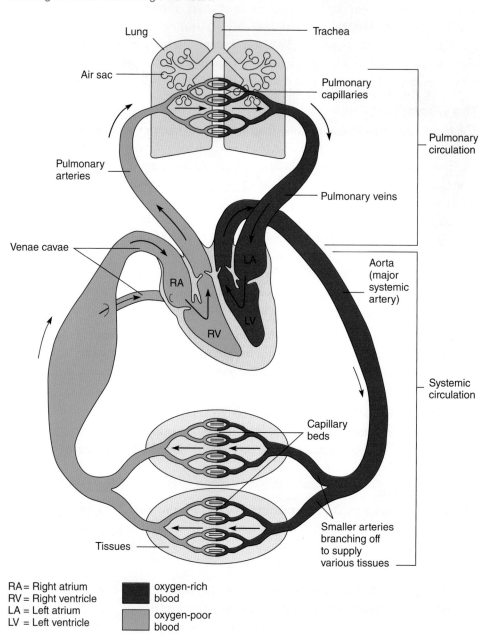

RA = Right atrium
RV = Right ventricle
LA = Left atrium
LV = Left ventricle

oxygen-rich blood

oxygen-poor blood

Blood

Blood (BLUD) is a nutritive fluid circulating through the circulatory system (heart and blood vessels) to supply oxygen and nutrients to cells and tissues and to remove carbon dioxide and waste from them. There are approximately 8 to 10 pints of blood in the human body, which contribute about 1/20th of the body's weight. Blood is approximately 80 percent water. It is sticky and salty, with a normal temperature of 98.6 degrees Fahrenheit. It is bright red in the arteries (except for the pulmonary artery) and dark red in the veins. The color change occurs with the exchange of carbon dioxide for oxygen as the blood passes through the lungs, and again with the exchange of oxygen for carbon dioxide as the blood circulates throughout the body.

Chief Functions of the Blood

Blood performs the following critical functions:

- Carries water, oxygen, and food to all cells and tissues of the body

- Carries away carbon dioxide and waste products to be eliminated through the lungs, skin, kidneys, and large intestines

- Helps equalize the body's temperature, thus protecting the body from extreme heat and cold

- Works with the immune system to protect the body from harmful toxins and bacteria

- Seals leaks found in injured blood vessels by forming clots, thus preventing further blood loss

Arteries of the Head, Face, and Neck

The **common carotid arteries** (KAHM-un kuh-RAHT-ud ART-uh-rees) are the main arteries that supply blood to the head, face, and neck. They are located on both sides of the neck, and each artery is divided into an internal and external branch.

The **internal carotid artery** (in-TUR-nul kuh-RAHT-ud ART-uh-ree) supplies blood to the brain, eyes, eyelids, forehead, nose, and internal ear. The **external carotid artery** supplies blood to the anterior (front) parts of the scalp, ears, face, neck, and sides of the head (**Figure 6-22**).

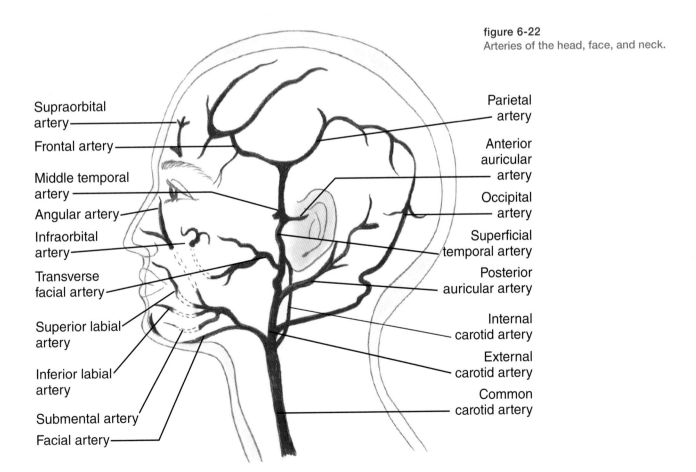

figure 6-22
Arteries of the head, face, and neck.

Supraorbital artery

Frontal artery

Middle temporal artery

Angular artery

Infraorbital artery

Transverse facial artery

Superior labial artery

Inferior labial artery

Submental artery

Facial artery

Parietal artery

Anterior auricular artery

Occipital artery

Superficial temporal artery

Posterior auricular artery

Internal carotid artery

External carotid artery

Common carotid artery

Two branches of the internal carotid artery that are important to know are the following:

- **Supraorbital artery** (soo-pruh-OR-bih-tul AR-tuh-ree). Supplies blood to the upper eyelid and forehead.

- **Infraorbital artery** (in-fruh-OR-bih-tul ARE-ter-ee). Supplies blood to the muscles of the eye.

There are four branches of the external carotid artery—the facial artery, the superficial temporal artery, the occipital artery, and the posterior auricular artery.

The **facial artery** (FAY-shul ART-uh-ree), also known as the *external maxillary artery* (eks-TUR-nul MAK-sah-lair-ee ART-uh-ree), supplies blood to the lower region of the face, mouth, and nose. Some of the important facial artery branches include:

- **Submental artery** (sub-MEN-tul AR-tuh-ree). Supplies blood to the chin and lower lip.

- **Inferior labial artery** (in-FEER-ee-ur LAY-bee-al ART-ur-ee). Supplies blood to the lower lip.

- **Angular artery** (ANG-yoo-lur ART-ur-ee). Supplies blood to the side of the nose.

- **Superior labial artery** (soo-PEER-ee-ur LAY-bee-ul AR-tuh-ree). Supplies blood to the upper lip and region of the nose.

The **superficial temporal artery** (soo-pur-FISH-ul TEM-puh-rul AR-tuh-ree) is a continuation of the external carotid artery and supplies blood to the muscles of the front, side, and top of the head. Some of the important superficial temporal artery branches include:

- **Frontal artery** (FRUNT-ul ART-uh-ree). Supplies blood to the forehead and upper eyelids.

- **Parietal artery** (puh-RY-ate-ul ART-uh-ree). Supplies blood to the side and crown of the head.

- **Transverse facial artery** (tranz-VURS FAY-shul AR-tuh-ree). Supplies blood to the skin and masseter muscle.

- **Middle temporal artery** (MID-ul TEM-puh-rul ART-uh-ree). Supplies blood to the temples.

- **Anterior auricular artery** (an-TEER-ee-ur aw-RIK-yuh-lur ART-ur-ee). Supplies blood to the front part of the ear.

The **occipital artery** (ahk-SIP-it-ul AR-tuh-ree) supplies blood to the skin and muscles of the scalp and back of the head up to the crown.

The **posterior auricular artery** (poh-STEER-ee-ur aw-RIK-yuh-lur AR-tuh-ree) supplies blood to the scalp, the area behind and above the ear, and the skin behind the ear.

Veins of the Head, Face, and Neck

The blood returning to the heart from the head, face, and neck flows on each side of the neck in two principal veins:

- The **internal jugular vein** (in-TUR-nul JUG-yuh-lur VAYN) is located at the side of the neck to collect blood from the brain and parts of the face and neck.

- The **external jugular vein** (eks-TUR-nul JUG-yuh-lur VAYN) is located at the side of the neck and carries blood returning to the heart from the head, face, and neck.

The most important veins of the face and neck are parallel to the arteries and take the same names as the arteries.

REVIEW THE LYMPHATIC/IMMUNE SYSTEM

The **lymphatic/immune system** (lim-FAT-ik/ih-MYOON SIS-tum) is made up of lymph, lymph nodes, the thymus gland, the spleen, and lymph vessels. The lymphatic/immune system carries waste and impurities away from the cells and protects the body from disease by developing immunity and destroying disease-causing microorganisms. **Lymph** (LIMF) is a clear fluid that circulates in the lymph spaces (lymphatics) of the body. Lymph helps carry wastes and impurities away from the cells before it is routed back to the circulatory system. The lymphatic/immune system drains the tissue spaces of excess **interstitial fluid** (in-tur-STISH-al FLOO-id), which is blood plasma found in the spaces between tissue cells. The lymphatic/immune system is closely connected to the cardiovascular system. They both transport streams of fluids, like rivers throughout the body. The difference is that the lymphatic/immune system transports lymph, which eventually returns to the blood where it originated.

Lymphatic vessels start as tubes that are closed at one end. They can occur individually or in clusters that are called **lymph capillaries**, blind-end tubes that are the origin of lymphatic vessels. The lymph capillaries are distributed throughout most of the body (except the nervous system). **Lymph nodes** are glandlike structures found inside lymphatic vessels. Lymph nodes filter the lymphatic vessels, which helps fight infection.

The primary functions of the lymphatic/immune system are to:

- Carry nourishment from the blood to the body cells.

- Act as a defense against toxins and bacteria, and remove by-products of infection such as pus and dead tissue.

- Remove waste material from the body cells to the blood.

- Provide a suitable fluid environment for the cells.

REVIEW THE INTEGUMENTARY SYSTEM

The **integumentary system** (in-TEG-yuh-ment-uh-ree SIS-tum) consists of the skin and its accessory organs, such as the oil and sweat glands, sensory receptors, hair, and nails. It is a very complex system that serves as a protective covering and helps regulate the body's temperature (**Figure 6-23**).

The word *integument* means "a natural covering." So you can think of the skin as a protective overcoat for your body against the outside elements that you encounter every day, such as germs, chemicals, and sun exposure. Skin is also water resistant.

figure 6-23
Structures of the skin.

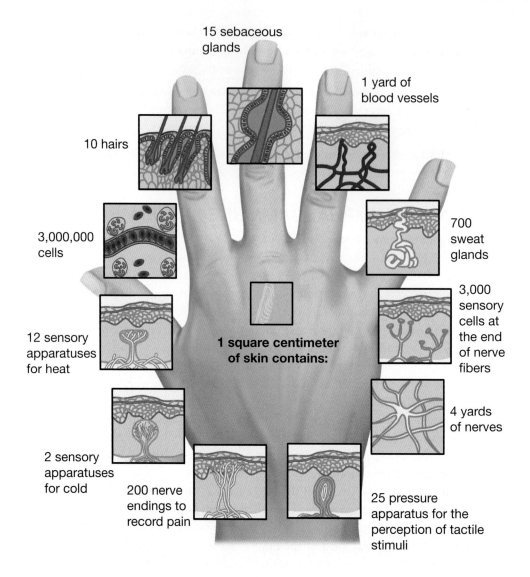

15 sebaceous glands

1 yard of blood vessels

10 hairs

3,000,000 cells

700 sweat glands

12 sensory apparatuses for heat

3,000 sensory cells at the end of nerve fibers

1 square centimeter of skin contains:

2 sensory apparatuses for cold

4 yards of nerves

200 nerve endings to record pain

25 pressure apparatus for the perception of tactile stimuli

Skin structure and growth are discussed in detail in Chapter 9, The Skin—Structures, Disorders, and Diseases.

REVIEW THE ENDOCRINE SYSTEM

The **endocrine system** (EN-duh-krin SIS-tum) is a group of specialized glands that affect the growth, development, sexual functions, and health of the entire body. **Glands** are secretory organs that remove and release certain elements from the blood to convert them into new compounds (**Figure 6-24**).

There are two main types of glands:

* **Endocrine glands**, also known as *ductless glands*, such as the thyroid and pituitary glands, release hormonal secretions directly into the bloodstream.

* **Exocrine glands** (EK-suh-krin GLANDZ), also known as *duct glands*, such as sweat and oil glands of the skin, produce a substance that travels through small, tubelike ducts.

? DID YOU KNOW?

Every minute, you shed about 30,000 to 40,000 dead skin cells from your body. That can total up to about 40 pounds of skin in your lifetime!

- **Hormones** (HOR-mohnz) are secretions, such as insulin, adrenaline, and estrogen, that stimulate functional activity or other secretions in the body. Hormones influence the welfare of the entire body.

figure 6-24
Endocrine glands and other body organs.

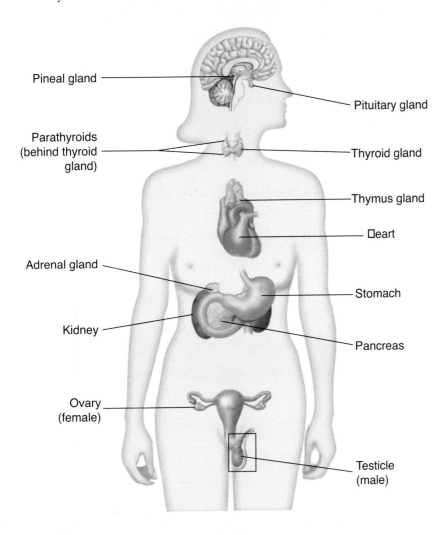

Pineal gland

Pituitary gland

Parathyroids
(behind thyroid
gland)

Thyroid gland

Thymus gland

Heart

Adrenal gland

Stomach

Kidney

Pancreas

Ovary
(female)

Testicle
(male)

REVIEW THE REPRODUCTIVE SYSTEM

The **reproductive system** (ree-proh-DUK-tiv SIS-tum) includes the ovaries, uterine tubes, uterus, and vagina in the female and the testes, prostate gland, penis, and urethra in the male. This system performs the function of producing offspring and passing on the genetic code from one generation to another.

The reproductive system produces hormones—primarily estrogen in females and primarily testosterone in males. These hormones affect and change the skin in several ways. Acne, loss of scalp hair, facial hair growth and color, and darker skin pigmentations are some of the results of changing or fluctuating hormones.

REVIEW QUESTIONS

1. Define *anatomy*, *physiology*, and *histology*.

2. Identify the anatomical parts of the body that barbers will be most concerned with.

3. What is a cell?

4. Define *mitosis*.

5. Describe the composition of body tissues.

6. What is an *organ*?

7. List eight important organs of the body.

8. What are *systems*?

9. Name the 11 body systems and their main functions.

10. List the primary functions of the skeletal system.

11. Name the two parts of the skull and the number of bones in each.

12. List the bones in the cranium.

13. Identify the bone that joins all the cranial bones together.

14. List the bones in the facial skeleton with their locations and functions.

15. Where is the *hyoid bone* located?

16. Describe the function and composition of muscles.

17. List and describe the parts of a muscle.

18. List the ways in which muscles may be stimulated.

19. List the scalp, facial, and neck muscles with their locations and functions.

20. List and describe the functions of the two main divisions of the nervous system.

21. List and describe the two types of nerves found in the human body.

22. List the ways in which nerves may be stimulated.

23. Give an example of nerve reflex.

24. Name the cranial nerves most important in massage services and their functions.

25. What is the function of the heart? What does it look like?

26. List three kinds of vessels found in the circulatory system.

27. Identify and describe the two main types of glands in the human body.

28. What structures (appendages) are included in the integumentary system?

CHAPTER GLOSSARY

abductors (ab-DUK-turz)	p. 157	muscles that draw a body part, such as a finger, arm, or toe, away from the midline of the body or of an extremity
adductors (ah-DUK-turz)	p. 157	muscles that draw a body part, such as a finger, arm, or toe, inward toward the median axis of the body or of an extremity
adipose tissue (ADD-ih-pohz TISH-oo)	p. 147	a technical term for fat; gives smoothness and contour to the body
anatomy (ah-NAT-ah-mee)	p. 144	the science of the structure of organisms and of their parts
angular artery (ANG-yoo-lur ART-ur-ee)	p. 164	artery that supplies blood to the sides of the nose
anterior auricular artery (an-TEER-ee-ur aw-RIK-yuh-lur ART-ur-ee)	p. 164	artery that supplies blood to the front part of the ear
aorta (ay-ORT-uh)	p. 161	largest artery in the body

Term	Page	Definition
arteries (AR-tuh-rees)	p. 161	thick-walled, muscular, flexible tubes that carry oxygenated blood away from the heart to the arterioles
arterioles (ar-TEER-ee-ohls)	p. 161	small arteries that deliver blood to capillaries
auricularis anterior (aw-rik-yuh-LAIR-is an-TEER-ee-ur)	p. 153	muscle in front of the ear that draws the ear forward
auricularis posterior (aw-rik-yuh-LAIR-is poh-STEER-ee-ur)	p. 153	muscle behind the ear that draws the ear backward
auricularis superior (aw-rik-yuh-LAIR-is soo-PEER-ee-ur)	p. 153	muscle above the ear that draws the ear upward
auriculotemporal nerve (aw-RIK-yuh-loh-TEM-puh-rul NURV)	p. 159	nerve that affects the external ear and skin above the temple, up to the top of the skull
axon (AK-sahn) and **axon terminal** (AK-sahn TER-min-al)	p. 158	extensions of a neuron through which impulses are sent away from the cell body to other neurons, glands, or muscles
belly (BELL-ee)	p. 151	middle part of a muscle
bicep (BY-sep)	p. 155	muscle that produces the contour of the front and inner side of the upper arm; lifts the forearm and flexes the elbow
blood (BLUD)	p. 162	nutritive fluid circulating through the circulatory system that supplies oxygen and nutrients to cells and tissues and removes carbon dioxide and waste from them
blood vessels	p. 161	tubelike structures that include the arteries, arterioles, capillaries, venules, and veins; function is to transport blood to and from the heart and then to various tissues of the body
body systems (BAHD-ee SIS-tums)	p. 147	groups of body organs acting together to perform one or more functions
brain (BRAYN)	p. 157	largest and most complex nerve tissue; part of the central nervous system contained within the cranium
buccal nerve (BUK-ul NURV)	p. 160	nerve that affects the muscles of the mouth
buccinator muscle (BUK-sih-nay-tur MUS-uhl)	p. 154	thin, flat muscle of the cheek between the upper and lower jaws
capillaries (KAP-ih-lair-eez)	p. 161	tiny, thin-walled blood vessels that connect the smaller arteries to venules and bring nutrients to the cells and carry away waste materials
carpus (KAR-pus)	p. 151	the bones of the wrist
cell membrane (SELL mem-brain)	p. 146	part of the cell that encloses the protoplasm; permits soluble substances to enter and leave the cell
cells (SELLZ)	p. 145	basic units of all living things
central nervous system (CNS) (SEN-trul NUR-vus SIS-tum)	p. 157	division of nervous system consisting of the brain, spinal cord, spinal nerves, and cranial nerves
centrioles (SEN-tree-olz)	p. 146	two small structures near the nucleus that move to each side during the mitosis process to help divide the cell
cervical cutaneous nerve (SUR-vih-kul kyoo-TAY-nee-us NURV)	p. 160	nerve located at the side of the neck; affects the front and sides of the neck to the breastbone
cervical vertebrae (SUR-vih-kul VURT-uh-bray)	p. 150	seven bones that form the top part of the spinal column in the neck region

circulatory system (SUR-kyoo-lah-tohr-ee SIS-tum)	p. 161	system that controls the steady circulation of blood through the body by means of the heart and blood vessels
common carotid arteries (KAHM-un kuh-RAHT-ud ART-uh-rees)	p. 163	arteries that supply blood to the head, face, and neck
connective tissue (kuh-NEK-tiv TISH-oo)	p. 147	fibrous tissue that binds together, protects, and supports the various parts of the body; examples include bone, cartilage, ligaments, tendons, blood, lymph, and adipose tissue
corrugator muscle (KOR-uh-gayt-or MUS-uhl)	p. 154	facial muscle that draws eyebrows down and wrinkles the forehead vertically
cranium (KRAY-nee-um)	p. 149	an oval, bony case that protects the brain
cytoplasm (sy-toh-PLAZ-um)	p. 145	is the watery fluid that surrounds the nucleus of the cell and is needed for growth, reproduction and self-repair.
deltoid (DEL-toyd)	p. 155	a large, triangular muscle covering the shoulder joint that allows the arm to extend outward and to the side of the body
dendrites (DEN-dryts)	p. 158	treelike branchings of nerve fibers extending from the nerve cell that carry impulses toward the cell and receive impulses from other neurons
depressor labii inferioris muscle (dee-PRES-ur LAY-bee-eye in-FEER-ee-or-us MUS-uhl)	p. 154	muscle surrounding the lower lip
digestive system (dy-JES-tiv SIS-tum)	p. 148	the mouth, stomach, intestines, and salivary and gastric glands that change food into nutrients and wastes
eleventh cranial nerve (ee-LEV-unth CRAY-nee-ul NURV)	p. 160	spinal nerve branch that affects the muscles of the neck and back
endocrine glands	p. 166	also known as *ductless glands*; release hormonal secretions directly into the bloodstream, for example, thyroid and pituitary glands
endocrine system (EN-duh-krin SIS-tum)	p. 166	group of specialized glands that affect growth, development, sexual function, and general health
epicranial aponeurosis (ep-ih-KRAY-nee-al ap-uh-noo-ROH-sus)	p. 152	a tendon that connects the occipitalis and frontalis muscles
epicranius (ep-ih-KRAY-nee-us)	p. 152	also known as *occipitofrontalis* (ahk-SIP-ih-toh-frun-TAY-lus) broad muscle that covers the top of the skull and consists of the occipitalis and frontalis
epithelial tissue (ep-ih-THEE-lee-ul TISH-oo)	p. 147	a protective covering on body surfaces, such as skin, mucous membranes, the tissue inside the mouth, the lining of the heart, digestive and respiratory organs, and the glands
ethmoid bone (ETH-moyd BOHN)	p. 149	a light, spongy bone between the eye sockets forming part of the nasal cavities
excretory system (EKS-kruh-toh-ree SIS-tum)	p. 148	group of organs including the kidneys, liver, skin, large intestine, and lungs that purify the body by the elimination of waste matter
exocrine glands (EK-suh-krin GLANDZ)	p. 166	also known as *duct glands*; produce a substance that travels through small, tubelike ducts; for example, sweat and oil glands of the skin
extensors (ik-STEN-surs)	p. 156	muscles that straighten the wrist, hand, and fingers to form a straight line
external carotid artery	p. 163	artery that supplies blood to the anterior parts of the scalp, face, neck, and side of the head

Term	Page	Definition
external jugular vein (eks-TUR-nul JUG-yuh-lur VAYN)	p. 165	vein located at the side of the neck that carries blood returning to the heart from the head, face, and neck
facial artery (FAY-shul ART-uh-ree)	p. 164	artery that supplies blood to the lower region of the face, mouth, and nose
facial skeleton (FAY-shul skell-uh-tin)	p. 149	two nasal bones; two lacrimal bones; two zygomatic bones; two maxillae; the mandible; two turbinal bones; two palatine bones; and the vomer
fifth cranial nerve (FIFTH KRAY-nee-ul NURV)	p. 158	chief sensory nerve of the face; controls chewing
flexor (FLEK-sur)	p. 156	extensor muscle of the wrist involved in flexing the wrist
frontal artery (FRUNT-ul ART-uh-ree)	p. 164	artery that supplies blood to the forehead and upper eyelids
frontal bone (FRUNT-ul BOHN)	p. 149	bone that forms the forehead
frontalis (frun-TAY-lus)	p. 152	anterior or front portion of the epicranius; muscle of the scalp
general circulation	p. 161	see systemic circulation
glands	p. 166	specialized organs varying in size and function that have the ability to remove certain elements from the blood and to convert them into new compounds
greater auricular nerve (GRAYT-ur aw-RIK-yuh-lur NURV)	p. 160	nerve at the sides of the neck affecting the face, ears, and neck
greater occipital nerve (GRAY-tur ahk-SIP-ut-ul NURV)	p. 160	nerve located at the back of the head, affecting the scalp
heart (HART)	p. 161	muscular, cone-shaped organ that keeps blood moving through the circulatory system
histology (his-TAHL-uh-jee)	p. 145	the study of the minute structure of the various tissues and organs that make up the entire body of an organism
hormones (HOR-mohnz)	p. 167	secretions that stimulate functional activity or other secretions in the body, for example, insulin, adrenaline, and estrogen
humerus (HYOO-muh-rus)	p. 151	uppermost and largest bone in the arm
hyoid bone (HY-oyd BOHN)	p. 150	U-shaped bone at the base of the tongue at the front part of the throat
inferior labial artery (in-FEER-ee-ur LAY-bee-al ART-ur-ee)	p. 164	artery that supplies blood to the lower lip
infraorbital artery (in-fruh-OR-bih-tul ARE-ter-ee)	p. 164	artery that supplies blood to the eye muscles
infraorbital nerve (in-fruh-OR-bih-tul NURV)	p. 159	nerve that affects the skin of the lower eyelid, side of the nose, upper lip, and mouth
infratrochlear nerve (in-frah-TRAHK-lee-ur NURV)	p. 159	nerve that affects the membrane and skin of the nose
insertion (in-SUR-shun)	p. 151	the part of the muscle that moves and is furthest from the skeleton
integumentary system (in-TEG-yuh-ment-uh-ree SIS-tum)	p. 165	the skin and its appendages—glands, sensory receptors, nails and hair
internal carotid artery (in-TUR-nul kuh-RAHT-ud ART-uh-ree)	p. 163	artery that supplies blood to the brain, eyes, eyelids, forehead, nose, and ear

internal jugular vein (in-TUR-nul JUG-yuh-lur VAYN)	p. 165	vein located at the side of the neck; collects blood from the brain and parts of the face and neck
interstitial fluid (in-tur-STISH-al FLOO-id)	p. 165	blood plasma found in the spaces between tissue cells
joint	p. 149	the connection between two or more bones of the skeleton
lacrimal bones (LAK-ruh-mul BONZ)	p. 150	small bones located in the wall of the eye sockets
latissimus dorsi (lah-TIS-ih-mus DOR-see)	p. 155	a large, flat, triangular muscle covering the lower back; helps extend the arm away from the body and rotate the shoulder
levator anguli oris muscle (lih-VAYT-ur ANG-yoo-ly OH-ris MUS-uhl)	p. 154	muscle that raises the angle of the mouth and draws it inward
levator labii superioris muscle (lih-VAYT-ur LAY-bee-eye soo-peer-ee-OR-is MUS-uhl)	p. 154	muscle surrounding the upper lip
levator palpebrae superioris muscle (lih-VAYT-ur PAL-puh-bree soo-peer-ee-OR-is MUS-uhl)	p. 154	a thin muscle that controls the eyelid
lymph (LIMF)	p. 165	colorless, watery fluid that circulates in the lymphatic system; carries waste and impurities from cells
lymph capillaries	p. 165	blind-end tubes occurring individually or in clusters that are the origin of lymphatic vessels
lymph nodes	p. 165	glandlike structures found inside lymphatic vessels that filter lymph
lymphatic/immune system (lim-FAT-ik/ih-MYOON SIS-tum)	p. 165	consists of lymph, lymph nodes, the thymus gland, the spleen, and lymph vessels that act as an aid to the blood system
mandible (MAN-duh-bul)	p. 150	lower jawbone
mandibular nerve (man-DIB-yuh-lur NURV)	p. 159	branch of the fifth cranial nerve that affects the muscles of the chin, lower lip, and external ear
marginal mandibular nerve (MAR-jin-ul man-DIB-yuh-lur NURV)	p. 160	affects the muscles of the chin and lower lip
masseter (muh-SEET-ur)	p. 153	one of the jaw muscles used in chewing
maxillae (mak-SIL-ee)	p. 150	bones of the upper jaw
maxillary nerve (MAK-suh-lair-ee NURV)	p. 159	supplies impulses to the upper part of the face
mental nerve (MEN-tul NURV)	p. 159	nerve that affects the skin of the lower lip and chin
mentalis muscle (men-TAY-lis MUS-uhl)	p. 154	muscle that elevates the lower lip and raises and wrinkles the skin of the chin
metacarpals (met-uh-KAR-pulz)	p. 151	the bones of the palm, consisting of five slender bones between the carpus and the phalanges
middle temporal artery (MID-ul TEM-puh-rul ART-uh-ree)	p. 164	artery that supplies blood to the temples
mitosis (my-TOH-sis)	p. 146	cells dividing into two new cells (daughter cells)
motor nerves (MOH-tur NURVZ)	p. 158	nerves that carry impulses from the brain to the muscles

muscle tissue	p. 147	contracts and moves various parts of the body
muscular system (MUS-kyuh-lur SIS-tum)	p. 151	body system that covers, shapes, and supports the skeletal tissue
myology (my-AHL-uh-jee)	p. 151	study of the structure, function, and diseases of the muscles
nasal bones (NAY-zul BONZ)	p. 150	bones that form the bridge of the nose
nasal nerve (NAY-zul NURV)	p. 159	nerve that affects the point and lower sides of the nose
nerve tissue	p. 147	type of tissue that carries messages to and from the brain and controls and coordinates all bodily functions
nerves	p. 158	whitish cords made up of bundles of nerve fibers held together by connective tissue, through which impulses are transmitted
neuron (NOO-rahn)	p. 158	also known as *nerve cell*; the primary structural unit of the nervous system, consisting of the cell body, nucleus, dendrites, and the axon
nucleus (NOO-klee-us)	p. 145	dense, active protoplasm found in the center of a cell; important to reproduction and metabolism
occipital artery (ahk-SIP-it-ul AR-tuh-ree)	p. 164	artery that supplies the scalp and back of the head up to the crown
occipital bone (ahk-SIP-it-ul BOHN)	p. 149	hindmost bone of the skull; located below the parietal bones
occipitalis (ahk-SIP-ih-tahl-is)	p. 152	back of the epicranius; muscle that draws the scalp backward
ophthalmic nerve (ahf-THAL-mik NURV)	p. 159	supplies impulses to the skin of the forehead, upper eyelids, and interior portion of the scalp, orbit, eyeball, and nasal passage
orbicularis oculi muscle (or-bik-yuh-LAIR-is AHK-yuh-lye MUS-uhl)	p. 154	ring muscle of the eye socket
orbicularis oris muscle (or-bik-yuh-LAIR-is OH-ris MUS-uhl)	p. 154	flat band around the upper and lower lips
organs	p. 147	structures composed of specialized tissues performing specific functions
origin (OR-ih-jin)	p. 151	more fixed part of a muscle that does not move
os (AHS)	p. 148	means "bone"; it is used as a prefix in many medical terms
osteology (ahs-tee-AHL-oh-jee)	p. 148	the study of the anatomy, structure, and function of the bones
parietal artery (puh-RY-ate-ul ART-uh-ree)	p. 164	artery that supplies blood to the side and crown of the head
parietal bones (puh-RY-ate-ul BONZ)	p. 149	bones that form the sides and top of the cranium
pectoralis major (pek-tor-AL-is MAY-jor) and **pectoralis minor**	p. 155	muscles of the chest that assist the swinging movements of the arm
peripheral nervous system (PNS) (puh-RIF-uh-rul NUR-vus SIS-tum)	p. 157	made up of sensory and motor nerve fibers that extend from the brain and spinal cord to all parts of the body. Their function is to carry impulses or messages to and from the CNS.
phalanges (FA-lanj-eez)	p. 151	bone of the fingers or toes
physiology (fiz-ih-OL-oh-gee)	p. 144	study of the functions or activities performed by the body's structures
platysma (plah-TIZ-muh)	p. 153	broad muscle extending from the chest and shoulder muscles to the side of the chin that is responsible for depressing the lower jaw and lip

posterior auricular artery (poh-STEER-ee-ur aw-RIK-yuh-lur AR-tuh-ree)	p. 164	artery that supplies blood to the scalp, behind and above the ear
posterior auricular nerve (poh-STEER-ee-ur aw-rik-yuh-lur NURV)	p. 160	nerve that affects the muscles behind the ear at the base of the skull
procerus (proh-SEE-rus)	p. 154	muscle that covers the bridge of the nose, depresses the eyebrows, and wrinkles the nose
pronator (proh-NAY-tohr)	p. 156	muscle that turns the hand inward so that the palm faces downward.
protoplasm (PROH-toh-plaz-um)	p. 145	a colorless jellylike substance found inside cells in which food elements such as proteins, fats, carbohydrates, mineral salts, and water are present
pulmonary circulation (PUL-muh-nayr-ee sur-kyoo-LAY-shun)	p. 161	takes deoxygenated blood to the lungs for oxygenation and waste removal and then returns that blood to the heart so oxygen-rich blood can be delivered to the body
radius (RAY-dee-us)	p. 151	smaller bone in the forearm on the same side as the thumb
reflex (REE-fleks)	p. 158	automatic nerve reaction to a stimulus
reproductive system (ree-proh-DUK-tiv SIS-tum)	p. 167	body system responsible for processes by which plants and animals produce offspring
respiratory system (RES-puh-rah-tor-ee SIS-tum)	p. 148	consists of the lungs and air passages; enables breathing
risorius muscle (rih-ZOR-ee-us MUS-uhl)	p. 154	muscle of the mouth that draws the corner of the mouth out and back as in grinning
sensory nerves	p. 158	nerves that carry impulses or messages from the sense organs to the brain
serratus anterior (ser-RAT-us an-TEER-ee-ur)	p. 155	muscle of the chest that assists in breathing and in raising the arm
seventh cranial nerve (SEV-AHNTH CRAN-ee-ahl NURV)	p. 159	chief motor nerve of the face
skeletal system (SKEL-uh-tul SIS-tum)	p. 148	physical foundation of the body; composed of bones and movable and immovable joints
smaller occipital nerve (SMAWL-ur ahk-SIP-ut-ul NURV)	p. 160	nerve that affects the scalp and muscles behind the ear
sphenoid bone (SFEE-noyd BOHN)	p. 149	bone that connects all the bones of the cranium
spinal cord (SPY-nal KORD)	p. 157	portion of the central nervous system that originates in the brain and runs downward through the spinal column
sternocleidomastoideus (STUR-noh-KLEE-ih-doh-mas-TOYD-ee-us)	p. 153	muscle of the neck that depresses and rotates the head
submental artery (sub-MEN-tul AR-tuh-ree)	p. 164	artery that supplies blood to the chin and lower lip
superficial temporal artery (soo-pur-FISH-ul TEM-puh-rul AR-tuh-ree)	p. 164	artery that supplies blood to the muscles of the front, sides, and top of the head

superior labial artery (soo-PEER-ee-ur LAY-bee-ul AR-tuh-ree)	p. 164	artery that supplies blood to the upper lip and lower region of the nose
supinator (SOO-puh-nayt-ur)	p. 156	muscle of the forearm that rotates the radius outward and the palm upward
supraorbital artery (soo-pruh-OR-bih-tul AR-tuh-ree)	p. 164	artery that supplies blood to the upper eyelid and forehead
supraorbital nerve (soo-pruh-OR-bih-tul NURV)	p. 159	nerve that affects the skin of the forehead, scalp, eyebrows, and upper eyelids
supratrochlear nerve (soo-pruh-TRAHK-lee-ur NURV)	p. 159	nerve that affects the skin between the eyes and the upper side of the nose
systemic circulation (sis-TEM-ik sur-kyoo-LAY-shun)	p. 161	carries the oxygen-rich blood from the heart throughout the body and returns deoxygenated blood back to the heart
temporal bones (TEM-puh-rul BONZ)	p. 149	bones that form the sides of the head in the ear region
temporal nerve (TEM-poh-rul NURV)	p. 160	nerve that affects the muscles of the temple, side of the forehead, eyelid, eyebrow, and upper cheek
temporalis (tem-poh-RAY-lis)	p. 153	muscle that aids in opening and closing the mouth and chewing
thorax (THOR-aks)	p. 150	the chest
tissue (TISH-oo)	p. 147	collections of similar cells that perform a particular function
transverse facial artery (tranz-VURS FAY-shul AR-tuh-ree)	p. 164	artery that supplies blood to the skin and the masseter
trapezius (truh-PEE-zee-us)	p. 155	muscle that covers the back of the neck and upper and middle region of the back
triangularis muscle (try-ang-gyuh-LAY-rus MUS-uhl)	p. 154	muscle that extends alongside the chin and pulls down the corner of the mouth
tricep (TRY-sep)	p. 156	large muscle that covers the entire back of the upper arm and extends the forearm
ulna (UL-nuh)	p. 151	inner and larger bone of the forearm
veins (VAYNS)	p. 161	thin-walled blood vessels that are less elastic than arteries; veins contain cuplike valves that keep blood flowing in one direction to the heart and prevent blood from flowing backward. Veins carry blood containing waste products back to the heart and lungs for cleaning and to pick up oxygen.
venules (VEEN-yools)	p. 161	small vessels that connect the capillaries to the veins; they collect blood from the capillaries and drain it into the veins
zygomatic bones (zy-goh-MAT-ik BONZ)	p. 150	bones that form the prominence of the cheeks
zygomatic nerve (zy-goh-MAT-ik NURV)	p. 160	affects the muscle of the upper part of the cheek
zygomaticus major muscles (zy-goh-MAT-ih-kus MAY-jor MUS-uhlz)	p. 155	muscle extending from the zygomatic bone to the angle of the mouth; pull the mouth upward and backward as in laughing
zygomaticus minor muscles (zy-goh-mat-ih-kus MY-nor MUS-uhlz)	p. 155	muscles on both sides of the face that extend from the zygomatic bone to the upper lips; pull the upper lip backward, upward, and outward, as when you are smiling

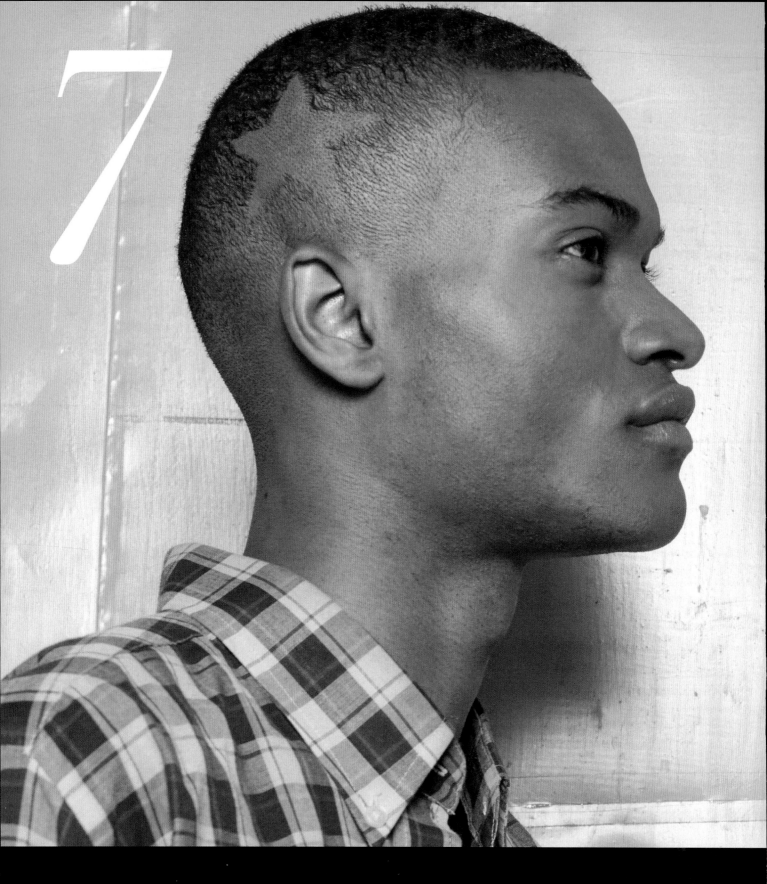

7

BASICS OF CHEMISTRY

LEARNING OBJECTIVES

After completing this chapter, you will be able to:

LO❶
Define *organic* and *inorganic chemistry*.

LO❷
Define the properties of *matter*.

LO❸
Discuss the physical and chemical properties of matter.

LO❹
Explain oxidation-reduction reactions.

LO❺
Describe emulsions, suspensions, and solutions.

LO❻
Define *pH* and describe the pH scale.

LO❼
Explain how product pH levels affect the hair and skin.

LO❽
Name nine types of shampoos.

LO❾
List four classifications of conditioners.

LO❿
Recognize other cosmetic preparations used in barbering services.

Introduction

This chapter provides an overview of basic chemistry so that you will understand its applications to the field of barbering. Barbers use chemical products on a daily basis and it is important that you know how to use these preparations safely and effectively in the performance of your work.

One of the most important uses of chemicals in the barbershop is the application of cleaners and disinfectants to maintain an effective infection control program. Products are usually more economical if purchased in concentrated form and will require you to mix the solutions; others will be used straight from the container. Always follow the manufacturer's directions for mixing and/or use. Hair care and skin care products are also chemical preparations that are used daily in the barbershop. Since the ingredients in these products can vary greatly, it is important that you understand their properties so that you can make informed selections for your clients' services.

Chemical preparations are necessary when a permanent change to the hair structure is desired. Certain haircolor formulations, permanent waving lotions, and chemical hair-relaxing products all create permanent changes within the hair; in fact, without chemicals, a permanent change in the hair is not possible!

why study
BASICS OF CHEMISTRY?

Barbers should study and have a thorough understanding of the basics of chemistry as it applies to barbering because:

> An understanding of chemistry will enable you to use professional products effectively and safely.

> Chemicals are common ingredients found in the products used in the barbershop and in barbering services.

> An understanding of chemical preparations and their effect on the hair and skin will help you select the best products to achieve the desired outcome.

> An understanding of chemical preparations and their effect on the hair and skin will help you prevent or solve problems that can occur during product applications.

Understand Basic Chemistry

After reading this section, you will be able to:

LO❶ Define *organic* and *inorganic chemistry*.

LO❷ Define the properties of *matter*.

LO❸ Discuss the physical and chemical properties of matter.

LO❹ Explain oxidation-reduction reactions.

LO❺ Describe emulsions, suspensions, and solutions.

EXPLAIN THE DIFFERENCES BETWEEN ORGANIC AND INORGANIC CHEMISTRY

Chemistry (KEM-is-tree) is the science that deals with the composition, structure, and properties of matter and how matter changes under different chemical conditions. The field is divided into two areas: organic and inorganic chemistry.

Organic chemistry (or-GAN-ik KEM-is-tree) is the study of substances that contain the element carbon; all living things are made of compounds that contain carbon. The term *organic* applies to all living things and those things that were once alive. Gasoline, synthetic fabrics, plastics, and pesticides are all considered organic because they are manufactured from natural gas and oil, which are the remains of plants and animals that died millions of years ago. Most organic substances will burn.

Inorganic chemistry (in-or-GAN-ik KEM-is-tree) is the study of substances that do not contain carbon but may contain hydrogen. Inorganic substances are not, and never were, alive; therefore, they will not burn. Metals, minerals, water, air, and ammonia are inorganic substances.

DEFINE MATTER

Matter (MAT-ur) is defined as anything that occupies space (volume) and has mass (weight). All matter has physical and chemical properties and exists in the form of a solid, liquid, or gas.

Matter has *physical* properties we can touch, taste, smell, or see, but not everything is matter. For example, we can see visible light and electrical sparks, but light and electricity are forms of energy and energy is not matter because it does not have mass; in fact, energy can be defined as the ability to change or put matter into motion. The *chemical* properties of matter can only be seen or measured when a chemical change or chemical reaction occurs.

Elements

An **element** (EL-uh-ment) is the simplest form of chemical matter and contains only one type of atom. It cannot be broken down into a simpler substance without a loss of identity. Refer to **Figure 7-1** as you read through the following:

- There are 118 different elements known to science today with 98 of these occurring naturally on Earth. The remaining elements, known as *synthetic elements*, are produced artificially or through synthesis.

figure 7-1
Periodic table information for carbon.

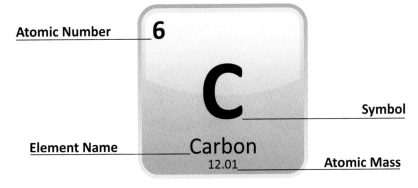

Atomic Number — **6**

C

Symbol

Element Name — Carbon

12.01 — Atomic Mass

figure 7-2
Atom.

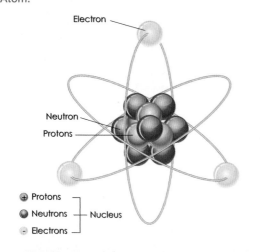

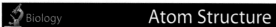

- All the matter in the known universe is made up of elements that have their own distinct physical and chemical properties. Each element is given a letter symbol such as O for oxygen, S for sulfur, or H for hydrogen.

- Elements are made up of atoms. The atomic number of an element indicates how many protons are in one atom of that element. If the number of protons changes, the element changes.

- The complete Periodic Table of Elements can be found in chemistry textbooks or by searching the Internet.

Atoms

Atoms (AT-umz) are the basic building blocks of all matter and are the smallest particle of an element that has the chemical identity of the chemical. At the center of an atom is the nucleus that is made up of subatomic particles of protons (P), with a positive charge, and neutrons (N), with no charge. The nucleus is orbited by electrons (E) with a negative charge (**Figure 7-2**). As the basic unit of matter, atoms cannot be divided into simpler substances by ordinary chemical means.

Molecules

A **molecule** is formed when two or more atoms combine chemically in definite (fixed) proportions. For example, hydrogen (H_2) contains two atoms of hydrogen. The air, or atmospheric gases, we breathe is primarily made up of nitrogen, oxygen, carbon dioxide, argon, and water vapor. The oxygen in air is an example of an elemental molecule. **Elemental molecules** (EL-uh-ment-uhl MAHL-uh-kyoolz) consist of two or more atoms of the same element in fixed proportions; in this case, two atoms of the element oxygen, which is written as O_2. Ozone (O_3), a major component of smog, is another elemental molecule but contains three atoms of oxygen (**Figure 7-3**).

   Compound molecules (KAHM-pownd MAHL-uh-kyoolz) are chemical combinations of two or more atoms of different elements. Sodium chloride, or common table salt, is a compound molecule that is a chemical combination of one atom of sodium (Na) and one atom of chlorine (Cl). Other examples of compound molecules you will recognize are water (H_2O), carbon dioxide (CO_2), and hydrogen peroxide (H_2O_2) (**Figure 7-4**).

figure 7-3
Elemental molecules.

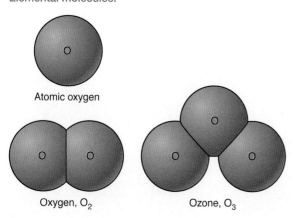

figure 7-4
Compound molecules.

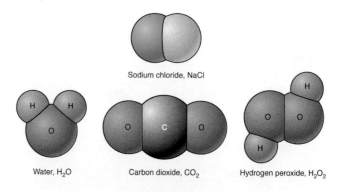

IDENTIFY THE STATES OF MATTER

All matter exists in one of three different physical forms: solid, liquid, or gas (Figure 7-5). When energy is added through increased temperature or pressure, or taken away through decreased temperature or pressure, changes in the states of matter occur. For example, water is a chemical compound that can exist in all three states of matter depending on its temperature. Consider how temperature changes create physical changes in water without changing its chemical properties:

- When water freezes, it turns to ice. As ice, water is in a solid state with definite shape and volume.

- When ice melts, it turns back into water. In its liquid state, water has volume, but no definite shape.

- When water boils, it turns to steam (vapor); when the steam cools, it turns back into water. As steam, water is a liquid that has evaporated into a gaslike state that does not have volume or shape.

UNDERSTAND THE PHYSICAL AND CHEMICAL PROPERTIES OF MATTER

Every substance has unique properties that allow us to identify it. The two types of properties are *physical* and *chemical*.

Physical properties (FIZ-ih-kuhl PRAH-ur-teez) are characteristics that can be determined without a chemical reaction and that do not involve a chemical change in the substance. Physical properties include, but are not limited to, color, solubility, odor, density, weight, melting point, boiling point, and hardness.

Chemical properties (KEM-uh-kul PRAH-ur-teez) are characteristics that can only be determined by a chemical reaction and that cause a change in the identity of the substance. Rusting iron and burning wood are examples of a change in chemical properties. In both these examples, the chemical reaction of oxidation creates a chemical change in the substance: iron is changed to rust, and wood is changed to ash.

Physical and Chemical Changes

Matter can be changed in two different ways: Physical forces cause physical changes and chemical reactions cause chemical changes.

- A **physical change** (FIZ-ih-kuhl CHAYNJ) is a change in the form or physical properties of a substance without a chemical reaction or the creation of a new substance. Therefore, no chemical reactions are involved in physical change and no new chemicals are formed (Figure 7-6). An example of physical change is ice melting to water. Temporary haircolor is another example of physical change because it physically adds color to the surface of the hair, but does not create a chemical change in the hair's structure or color.

A **chemical change** (KEM-uh-kul CHAYNJ) is a change in the chemical composition or makeup of a substance, as in the iron-to-rust example. This change is caused by chemical reactions that create new chemical substances, usually by combining or subtracting certain elements, that will have

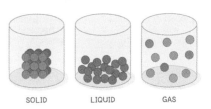

? DID YOU KNOW?
Hydrogen is the most common element found in the known universe.

figure 7-5
Arrangement of particles in solid, liquid, and gaseous state.

SOLID   LIQUID   GAS

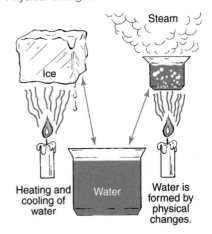

figure 7-6
Physical changes.

Steam

Ice

Heating and cooling of water

Water

Water is formed by physical changes.

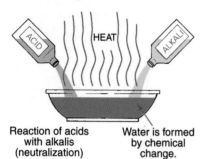

figure 7-7
Chemical changes.

Reaction of acids with alkalis (neutralization)

Water is formed by chemical change.

different physical and chemical properties (**Figure 7-7**). An example of a chemical change is the oxidation of haircolor products. Oxidation refers to a chemical reaction that combines a substance with oxygen to produce an oxide. Permanent haircolor creates chemical changes in the hair when oxidation takes place to develop the dye in the color. In hair lightening processes, hydrogen peroxide oxidizes the melanin pigments in hair, leaving the hair a lighter color.

EXPLAIN OXIDATION-REDUCTION REACTIONS

Oxidation (ahk-sih-DAY-shun) can be defined as either the addition of oxygen or the loss of hydrogen. Oxidation is a chemical reaction that combines an element or compound with oxygen to produce an oxide. When oxygen is chemically combined with a substance, the substance is *oxidized*.

Oxidizing agents are substances that release oxygen. Hydrogen peroxide (H_2O_2) contains an extra oxygen atom that makes it an oxidizing agent. Different forms of hydrogen peroxide are commonly used in haircoloring, hair lightening, and chemical texture services. **Reduction** (ree-DUK-shun) refers to either the loss of oxygen or the addition of hydrogen. When oxygen is chemically removed from a substance, the substance is *reduced*.

REDOX REACTIONS

Oxidation and reduction always occur simultaneously and are referred to as a **redox** (REE-dux) reaction. In a redox reaction, the oxidizing agent is always reduced and the reducing agent is always oxidized. Oxidation cannot occur without reduction. For example, when hydrogen peroxide (in the form of a developer) is mixed with an oxidation haircolor product (demi-permanent or permanent), the haircolor product gains oxygen and is oxidized. At the same time, the hydrogen peroxide loses oxygen and is reduced. In this example, the haircolor product is the reducing agent (**Table 7-1**).

Redox reactions also occur in another way that involves oxidation resulting from the loss of hydrogen and reduction that results from the addition of hydrogen. The permanent waving process is a good example of this type of redox reaction.

table 7-1

OXIDATION-REDUCTION REACTIONS

Product	Oxidation + Oxygen or – Hydrogen	Reduction – Oxygen or + Hydrogen
Oxidation Haircolor	Haircolor gains oxygen from H_2O_2	H_2O_2 loses oxygen
Permanent Wave Solution	Waving solution is oxidized	Adds hydrogen atoms to hair
Permanent Wave Neutralizer	Hair is oxidized by removing hydrogen	Neutralizer is reduced by losing oxygen
Exothermic Perm Activator	Adds oxygen to waving solution; creates heat	H_2O_2 loses oxygen

- Certain permanent waving solutions contain ammonium thioglycolate acid.

- The waving solution breaks the disulfide bonds in the hair through a reduction reaction that adds hydrogen atoms (H) to the hair. In this reaction, the hair is reduced and the permanent waving solution is oxidized.

- After processing and rinsing, the neutralizer is used to oxidize the hair by removing the hydrogen that was previously added with the waving solution. When the hair is oxidized, the neutralizer is reduced (Table 7-1).

Exothermic Reactions

When certain chemical reactions release energy in the form of heat, it is called an **exothermic reaction**. An example of this is the heat produced after mixing the activator and waving lotion in an exothermic permanent wave product. When the activator, which contains hydrogen peroxide, is added to the waving lotion, an oxidation reaction occurs that produces heat (Table 7-1). The mixing of these chemicals produces a more rapid form of oxidation than the slower oxidation that occurs with permanent wave neutralizers or oxidation haircolor products. In most cases, you can expect to feel a slight warming of the container after mixing the activator with the waving lotion.

Endothermic Reactions

An **endothermic reaction** is a chemical reaction that requires the absorption of energy or heat from an external source for the reaction to actually occur. Melting ice is an example of an endothermic reaction because if it was not absorbing heat from its surroundings, it would not be melting! Another example is a permanent waving lotion that requires the application of heat from a hood dryer to activate it for processing rather than processing at room temperature; these are called *endothermic waves*.

DEFINE PURE SUBSTANCES AND MIXTURES

All matter can be classified as either a pure substance or a physical mixture (blend) (Figure 7-8).

A **pure substance** (PYOOR SUB-stantz) is a chemical combination of matter that has a fixed chemical composition, definite proportions, and distinct properties. Elements and chemical compounds are pure substances. Aluminum foil is an example of a pure substance because it is composed only of atoms of the element, aluminum.

A **physical mixture** (FIZ-ih-kuhl mix-CHUR) is a combination of two or more substances united physically in any proportions without a fixed composition. Concrete is an example of a physical mixture because it is composed of water, sand, gravel, and dry cement. It is a mixture that has its own functions, yet does not lose the characteristics of the individual

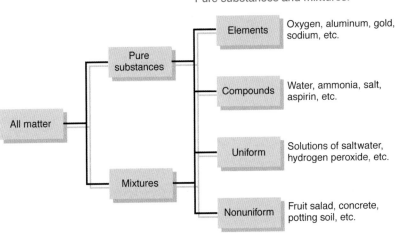

figure 7-8
Pure substances and mixtures.

ingredients. Powder is another good example of a physical mixture because it consists of a uniform mixture of insoluble inorganic, organic, and colloidal substances that have been properly blended.

IDENTIFY CHEMICAL COMPOUNDS

Chemical compounds (KEM-uh-kul KAHM-powndz) are combinations of two or more atoms of different elements united chemically with fixed chemical composition, definite proportions, and distinct properties. Chemical compounds are the result of a chemical reaction in which the elements that are united give up their own chemical identity and properties, for example, water is a chemical compound consisting of two atoms of hydrogen and one atom of oxygen. Table 7-2 summarizes the differences between pure substances, physical mixtures, and chemical compounds.

As a barber, learning about chemical compounds will help your understanding of potential hydrogen and the pH scale. Chemical compounds are classified as follows:

1. **Oxides** are compounds of any element combined with oxygen. For example, one part carbon and two parts oxygen create carbon dioxide. One part carbon and one part oxygen create carbon monoxide.

2. **Acids** are compounds of hydrogen, a nonmetal such as nitrogen, and, sometimes, oxygen. For example, hydrogen, sulfur, and oxygen combine to form sulfuric acid. Acids turn blue litmus paper red, providing a quick way to test a compound.

3. **Bases**, also known as **alkalis** (AL-kuh-lyz), are compounds of hydrogen, a metal, and oxygen. For example, sodium, oxygen, and hydrogen form sodium hydroxide, which is used in the manufacture of soap. Bases will turn red litmus paper blue.

4. **Salts** are compounds that are formed by the reaction of acids and bases, with water also being produced by the reaction. Two common salts are sodium chloride (table salt), which contains sodium and chloride, and magnesium sulfate (Epsom salts), which contains magnesium, sulfur, hydrogen, and oxygen.

table 7-2

PURE SUBSTANCES, PHYSICAL MIXTURES, AND CHEMICAL COMPOUNDS

Pure Substances	Physical Mixtures	Chemical Compounds
Matter with a fixed chemical composition; elements, compounds, and elemental molecules	Two or more substances united physically with no fixed composition	Two or more different elements united chemically with a fixed chemical composition
Composition does not vary	Each substance retains its own identity and properties	Chemical reaction changes the chemical properties of the elements
Definite proportions	Mixed in any proportion	Definite proportions
Examples: oxygen, aluminum, gold	Examples: saltwater solution, pure air, concrete, powders	Examples: water (H_2O), salt (NaCl), ammonia

DEFINE SOLUTIONS, SUSPENSIONS, AND EMULSIONS

Solutions, suspensions, and emulsions are physical mixtures of two or more different substances. The differences between these mixtures are determined by the types of substances, the size of the particles, and the solubility of the substances. The *solubility* of a substance is defined as the amount of a substance that will dissolve in a given amount of another substance. For our purposes, we will define solubility to be the degree to which a solute (substance) dissolves in a solvent to make a solution.

All liquids are either miscible or immiscible. Miscible liquids, such as water and alcohol, are mutually soluble. This means they can be mixed together to form stable solutions. Conversely, immiscible liquids, such as water and oil, do not mix well together, are not capable of forming stable solutions, and will separate if left to sit for any time.

Solutions

A **solution** is a stable, uniform mixture of two or more mixable substances that is made by dissolving a solid, liquid, or gaseous substance in another substance. A **solute** is any substance that is dissolved into a solvent to form a solution. A **solvent** is any substance, usually a liquid, that dissolves the solute to form a solution. For example, dissolving salt (solute) into water (solvent) creates a saltwater solution. The components of a solution are illustrated in **Figure 7-9**. When a gas or a solid is dissolved in a liquid, the gas or solid is the solute and the liquid is the solvent.

figure 7-9
Components of a solution.

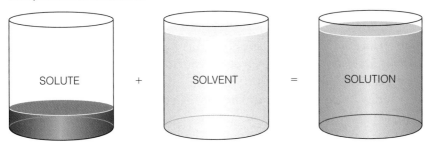

SOLUTE + SOLVENT = SOLUTION

Suspensions

Suspensions (sus-PEN-shunz) are unstable uniform mixtures of two or more substances. The particles in suspensions can be seen with the naked eye because they are larger than the particles in solutions.

- Suspensions are not usually transparent, may be colored, and tend to separate over time.

- Many of the products used by barbers, such as hair tonics, are suspensions and should be shaken or mixed well before use. Calamine lotion and paint are also examples of suspensions.

Emulsions

An **emulsion** is a physical mixture of two immiscible liquids held together by an emulsifying agent. An emulsion is a suspension of one liquid dispersed in another. Although emulsions tend to separate over

table 7-3

SOLUTIONS, SUSPENSIONS, AND EMULSIONS

Solutions	Suspensions	Emulsions
Miscible	Slightly miscible	Immiscible
No surfactant	No surfactant	Surfactant
Small particles	Larger particles	Largest particles
Usually clear	Usually cloudy	Usually a solid color
Stable mixture	Unstable mixture	Limited stability
Witch hazel	Calamine lotion	Shampoos and conditioners

time, with proper formulation and storage an emulsion may remain stable for at least 3 years.

- Mayonnaise is an oil-in-water emulsion of two immiscible liquids. The egg yolk in mayonnaise emulsifies the oil droplets and disperses them uniformly in the water. Mayonnaise should not separate upon standing. Review Table 7-3 for a summary of the differences between solutions, suspensions, and emulsions.

- Shampoos and conditioners are examples of emulsions used in barbering services.

- Cosmetic emulsions should be used within one year of purchase.

Surfactants

A **surfactant** (sur-FAK-tant) (or base detergent) is a substance that allows oil and water to mix or emulsify by reducing surface tension. The term *surfactant* is a contraction for *surface active agent*.

A surfactant molecule has two distinct parts: the head of the molecule is hydrophilic (water-loving) and the tail is lipophilic (oil-loving) (Figure 7-10). Since "like dissolves like," the hydrophilic head dissolves in water and the lipophilic tail dissolves in oil. This configuration allows the surfactant molecule to mix and dissolve in both water and oil to join together to form an emulsion.

- In an oil-in-water (O/W) emulsion, droplets of oil are dispersed in water, where they are surrounded by surfactants. The lipophilic surfactant tails point inward with the hydrophilic heads pointing outward, which keeps the oil dispersed in the water. Most of the emulsions used in the barbershop are O/W emulsions and do not feel as greasy as water-in-oil preparations.

figure 7-10
Surfactant molecules.

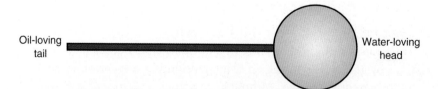

Oil-loving
tail

Water-loving
head

- In a water-in-oil (W/O) emulsion, droplets of water are dispersed in oil, where they are surrounded by surfactants. The surfactant tails point outward and the heads point inward, which keeps the water dispersed in the oil. Cold cream is an example of a W/O emulsion.

Discuss the Properties of Water and pH

After reading this section, you will be able to:

LO ⑥ Define *pH* and describe the pH scale.

LO ⑦ Explain how product pH levels affect the hair and skin.

Water (H_2O) is the most abundant and important of all chemicals, composing about 71 percent of the earth's surface and an average of about 65 percent of the human body. Water is known as the *universal solvent*, because it dissolves more substances than any other liquid. Distilled or demineralized water is used as a nonconductor of electricity, while water containing certain mineral substances is an excellent conductor of electricity.

Water is purified through boiling, filtration, or distillation.

- Boiling water at 212 degrees Fahrenheit destroys most microbes and renders it suitable for drinking.

- During filtration, water passes through a porous substance, such as filter paper or charcoal, to remove organic material.

- Distillation is the process whereby water is heated to a vapor in a closed vessel. The vapors are captured and passed off through a tube into another vessel, where they are cooled and condensed to a liquid. This type of purified water is used in the manufacturing of cosmetics.

Soft water is rainwater or chemically treated water that has low levels of mineral substances such as calcium and magnesium salts. This type of water not only allows soaps and shampoos to lather freely but can also leave the hair and skin feeling too slick even after thorough rinsing.

Conversely, hard water contains mineral substances, such as calcium and magnesium salts, that can interfere with the lathering and foaming process. Hard water may be softened by distillation, water-softening units, or by adding sodium carbonate (washing soda); however, today's hair products and modern filtration systems have helped eliminate some of the problems associated with hard water in the past. If you are in doubt about the quality of the water in the barbershop, use a test kit designed to measure both the water hardness and pH level.

LEARN ABOUT WATER AND pH (POTENTIAL HYDROGEN)

A basic understanding of ions is important to an understanding of pH. An **ion** (EYE-ahn) is an atom or molecule that carries an electrical charge. **Ionization** (eye-ahn-ih-ZAY-shun) is the separation of a substance into ions

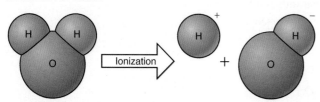

figure 7-11
Ionization of water.

Ionization

that have opposite electrical charges. A negatively charged ion is called an *anion*, and a positively charged ion is called a *cation*.

In pure water, some of the water molecules ionize naturally into hydrogen ions and hydroxide ions. The pH scale measures those ions. The hydrogen ion is acidic and the hydroxide ion is alkaline.

- The ionization of water is what makes pH possible because only aqueous (water) solutions have pH. Nonaqueous solutions, such as alcohol or oil, do not have pH.

- In pure water, every water molecule that ionizes produces one hydrogen ion and one hydroxide ion (**Figure 7-11**). Pure water contains the same number of hydrogen ions as hydroxide ions, which makes it neutral, as denoted by the number 7 on the pH scale. This means that pure water is 50 percent acidic and 50 percent alkaline.

- The letters **pH** (P-H) denote **potential hydrogen**, which is the relative degree of acidity or alkalinity of a substance. The **pH scale** (P-H SKAYL) measures the concentration of hydrogen ions in acidic and alkaline *water-based* solutions. Notice that pH is written with a small *p*, which represents quantity, and a capital *H*, which represents the hydrogen ion.

The pH Scale

The pH values are arranged on a scale ranging from 0 to 14. A pH below 7 indicates an acidic solution, a pH of 7 is a neutral solution, and a pH above 7 indicates an alkaline solution (**Figure 7-12**).

The pH scale is a logarithmic scale, which means that a change of one whole number represents a 10-fold change in pH. For example, a pH of 8 is 10 times more alkaline than a pH of 7. A change of two whole numbers indicates a change of 10 times 10, or a 100-fold change. Therefore, a pH of 9 is 100 times more alkaline than a pH of 7.

The pH range of hair and skin is 4.5 to 5.5, with an average of 5, on the pH scale. That means that pure water is 100 times more alkaline than hair and skin, even though it has a neutral pH. In fact, pure water can cause the hair to swell up to 20 percent.

figure 7-12
The pH scale.

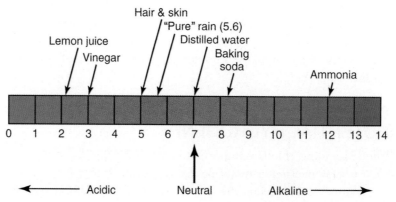

Acids and Alkalis

All acids owe their chemical reactivity to the hydrogen ion (H^+).

- Acids have a pH below 7.0, taste sour, and turn litmus paper from blue to red.
- Acidic solutions tend to contract and harden the hair (**Figure 7-13**). As toners or skin fresheners, they also tighten the skin.

All alkalis owe their chemical reactivity to the hydroxide (OH^-) ion. The terms *alkalis* and *bases* are interchangeable.

- Alkalis have a pH above 7.0, taste bitter, feel slippery on the skin, and turn litmus paper from red to blue.
- Alkalis soften and swell the hair (**Figure 7-13**). Sodium hydroxide (lye) is a very strong alkali used in chemical drain cleaners and chemical hair relaxers.

Figure 7-13
The effect of pH on hair.

Solution	Effect on Hair		Important Features
Very Strong Acid (pH 0.0—1.0)	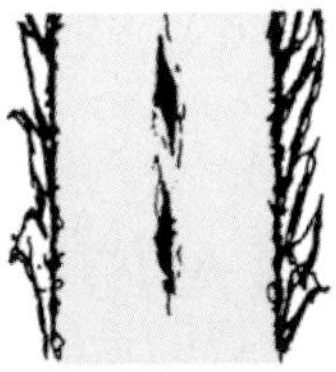	Dissolves hair completely.	Must not be applied to hair or scalp.
Strong to Mild Acid (pH 1.0—4.5)	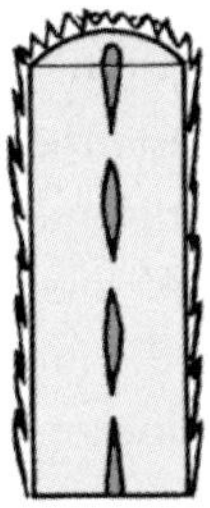	Hair shrinks and hardens. Body is increased. Cuticle imbrications close up. Porosity is reduced. Sheen of hair is improved. Soap residues are removed. Neutralizes traces of alkalis.	Acid or cream rinses restore body to bleached, porous hair. Conditioners and fillers overcome the excess porosity of damaged hair. Special shampoos reduce tangling and matting of hair and prevent color loss. Hair creams increase sheen. Color rinses provide temporary effect. Neutralizers remove residual waving lotion.
Neutral (pH 4.5—5.5)	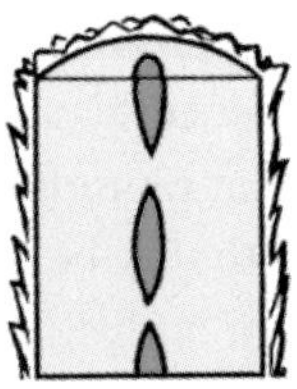	Hair is normal diameter. Texture and luster standard.	Neutral solutions are designed to prevent excess swelling of normal and damaged hair. Mild shampoos for normal cleaning and manageability of hair.
Mild Alkali (pH 5.5—10.0)	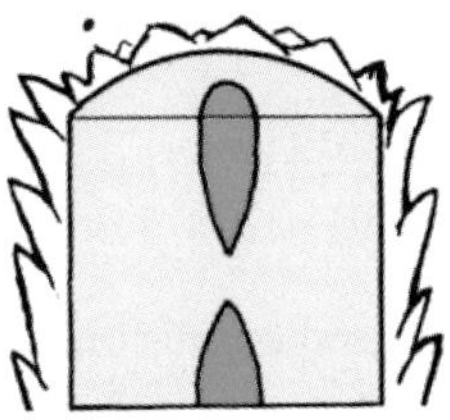	Hair swells. Porosity increases as imbrications open. Hair has a dry, drab appearance.	Tints and bleaches penetrate easier and chemical action increases. Cold wave solutions for resistant hair. Soap shampoos to overcome acidity of tap water. Activators for hydrogen peroxide.
Stronger Alkali (pH 10.0—14.0)	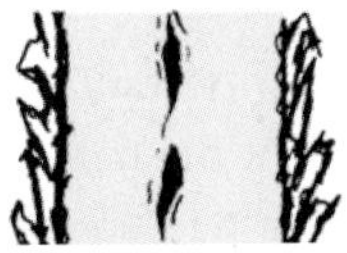	Dissolves hair completely.	Must not be applied to hair or scalp unless used as relaxers or depilatories.

Acid–Alkali Neutralization Reactions

When acids and alkalis are mixed together in equal proportions, they neutralize each other to form water and a salt. For example, because hydrochloric acid is a strong acid and sodium hydroxide is a strong alkali, they will neutralize each other when mixed in equal amounts and form a solution of pure water and table salt (refer to **Figure 7-7**). Acid-balanced shampoos and normalizing lotions associated with hydroxide hair relaxers work to create a similar acid–alkali neutralization reaction.

Identify Cosmetic Preparations Used in Barbering

After reading this section, you will be able to:

LO**8** Name nine types of shampoos.

LO**9** List four classifications of conditioners.

LO**10** Recognize other cosmetic preparations used in barbering services.

LEARN ABOUT SHAMPOOS AND CONDITIONERS

Most shampoo products are emulsions, and there are many different types on the market. As a professional barber, you will need to become skilled at selecting products that best serve the condition of the client's hair and scalp. Make it a standard operating procedure to read the manufacturer's labels so that an informed choice can be made. In addition, display and use the barbershop's retail products at the workstation or shampoo sink back bar. Doing so not only promotes product sales but also demonstrates to clients that you endorse the product and its effectiveness inside and outside the barbershop.

To be effective, a **shampoo** (sham-POO) must remove all dirt, oil, perspiration, and skin debris, without adversely affecting either the scalp or the hair. The hair collects dust particles, natural oils from the sebaceous glands, perspiration, and dead skin cells that can accumulate on the scalp. This accumulation creates a breeding ground for disease-producing bacteria, which can lead to scalp disorders. The hair and scalp should be thoroughly shampooed as frequently as is necessary to keep it clean, healthy, and free from bacteria.

An effective shampoo product should:

- cleanse the hair of oils, debris, and dirt.

- work efficiently in hard as well as soft water.

- not irritate the eyes or skin.

- leave the hair and scalp in their natural condition.

Shampoo Chemistry

The acidity or alkalinity of a shampoo is important because it influences how the product will affect various layers of the hair and skin. Acidic solutions (below pH 7.0) shrink, constrict, and harden the cuticle scales of the hair shaft. An alkaline solution (above pH 7.0) softens, swells, and expands the cuticle scales. Remember, the lower the pH of a solution, the greater the degree of acidity; the higher the pH of a solution, the greater the degree of alkalinity. (See **Figure 7-12**.)

Shampoo emulsions usually range between 4.5 and 7.5 on the pH scale. Since the normal pH range for hair and skin is 4.5 to 5.5, mild or more acidic shampoos are found closer to this range. Conversely, stronger or more alkaline shampoos are found beyond 6.0 on the pH scale.

Shampoo Molecules

Shampoos consist of two main ingredients: water and surfactants. Next to water, surfactants are the second most common ingredients found in shampoos and act as cleansing, emulsifying, or foaming agents. Shampoo molecules are created by combining water and at least one surfactant. In a shampoo molecule, the tail attracts dirt, grease, debris, and oil, but repels water. The head of the shampoo molecule attracts water, but repels dirt. Working together, both parts of the molecule effectively cleanse the hair (**Figures 7-14 to 7-17**).

The base surfactant or combination of surfactants determines the classification of a shampoo. These classifications include *anionic, cationic,*

figure 7-14
The tail of the shampoo molecule is attracted to oil and dirt.

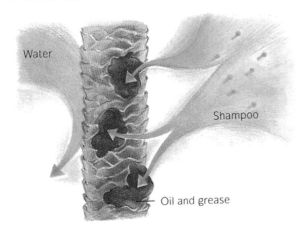

figure 7-15
Shampoo causes oil to run up into small globules.

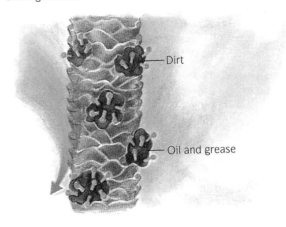

figure 7-16
During rinsing, the heads of the shampoo molecules attach to water molecules and cause debris to roll off.

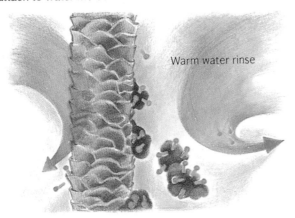

figure 7-17
Thorough rinsing washes away debris and excess shampoo.

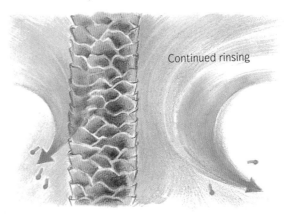

table 7-4

CLASSIFICATIONS OF SHAMPOOS

Base Surfactant(s)	Common Ingredients	Actions	Features
Anionics	Sodium lauryl sulfate	Relatively harsh cleanser; produces rich foam	Rinses easily
	Sodium laureth sulfate	Less alkaline than lauryl	Less drying to hair shaft
Cationics	Quaternary ammonium compounds	Antibacterial action	Used in dandruff shampoos
Nonionics	Cocamide (DEA, MEA)	Mild cleansing action	Low incidences of irritation
Amphoterics	Amphoteric I-20	Behaves as anionic or cationic depending on pH; clings to hair for manageability	Nonstinging to eyes; used in baby shampoos

nonionic, and *amphoteric* surfactants. Most manufacturers use detergents from more than one classification. It is customary to use a secondary surfactant to complement, or offset, the negative qualities of the base surfactant. For example, an amphoteric that is nonirritating to the eyes can be added to a harsh anionic to create a product that is more comfortable to use.

Additional ingredients in the forms of moisturizers, preservatives, foam enhancers, perfumes, and others are added to create a variety of shampoo formulations. Along with water and base surfactants, these ingredients are listed on product labels in descending order according to the percentage of each ingredient in the shampoo. Refer to **Table 7-4** to review the properties associated with different shampoo classifications.

IDENTIFY TYPES OF SHAMPOOS

Shampoo products account for the highest dollar expenditure by consumers in hair care products. Shampoo products are available in liquid, liquid-dry, and dry (powder) formulations to meet the needs of all types of hair and scalp conditions. There are shampoos for dry, oily, normal, fine, coarse, limp, or chemically treated hair. There are shampoos that add a slight amount of color to hair and those that cleanse the hair of mineral deposits and product buildup. Many manufacturers have become more "hair condition conscious" so that even medicated shampoos are less drying to the hair and scalp.

A visit to your local barber supply will introduce you to a wide variety of products for use in the barbershop. Be sure to read the label for the product's recommended use and refer to **Table 7-4** to become familiar with base surfactants.

- Most of the shampoo products you use will be in a cream or clear liquid form. Generally speaking, cream shampoos contain more emollients than clear shampoos.

- **Liquid-dry shampoos** are used for cleansing the scalp and hair when the client is prevented from having a regular shampoo. Typically, these shampoos have an astringent quality that allows the product to evaporate quickly.

- **Dry or powder shampoos** can be used when the client's health or condition will not permit a wet shampoo. The powder is sprinkled onto the hair, where it picks up dirt and oils as it is brushed through the hair. Always follow the manufacturer's directions and never give a dry shampoo prior to a chemical service.

Most of today's shampoos can be classified as belonging to one of the following shampoo types.

pH-Balanced Shampoos

pH-balanced shampoos, also known as *acid-balanced shampoos*, are balanced to the pH level of hair and skin and usually contain citric, lactic, or phosphoric acid. These shampoos are mild formulations designed to prevent the stripping of haircolor from the hair. They have a low alkaline content, which makes them a good choice for normal, chemically treated, and fragile hair. Follow the manufacturer's directions, but most pH-balanced shampoos can be used daily.

Balancing Shampoos

Balancing shampoos are designed for oily hair and scalps. These shampoos wash away excess oiliness while keeping the hair from drying out.

Clarifying Shampoos

Clarifying shampoos contain an active chelating agent that binds to metals (such as iron and copper) and removes them from the hair. They also provide thorough cleansing and cut through product buildup that can coat and flatten hair. For these reasons, clarifying shampoos are recommended for preparing the hair for chemical services or to remove medication or hard-water minerals from the hair.

Color-Enhancing Shampoos

Color-enhancing shampoos are created by combining the surfactant with basic colors. They are attracted to porous hair and provide only slight color changes, which are removed with plain shampooing. Color shampoos are used to brighten the hair, add slight color, and eliminate unwanted color tones.

Conditioning Shampoos

Conditioning shampoos (KAHN-dish-shun-ing sham-POOZ), also known as *moisturizing shampoo*, are mild cream shampoos that contain moisturizing agents (*humectants*) designed either to "lock in" the moisturizing properties of the product or to draw moisture into the hair. They are formulated to make the hair smooth and shiny and to avoid damaging chemically treated hair. Protein and biotin are conditioning agents that help restore moisture and elasticity, strengthen the hair shaft, and add volume. Like pH-balanced shampoos, moisturizing shampoos are non-stripping shampoos and do not remove artificial color from the hair.

Medicated Shampoos

Medicated shampoos contain antifungal agents such as pyrithione zinc, selenium sulfide, or ketoconazole, which help control dandruff by suppressing the growth of malassezia, the fungus that causes dandruff. These shampoo products are available for all hair types and are gentle enough for daily use.

Therapeutic medicated shampoos (thayr-uh-PYOOT-ik MED-ih-kayt-ud sham-POOZ) contain special chemicals or drugs that are very effective in reducing excessive dandruff. These are prescribed shampoos that must include instructions from the client's physician for their application and use.

Neutralizing Shampoos

A **neutralizing shampoo** helps to rebalance and restore the pH level of the hair by neutralizing any alkali or unwanted residues that remain in the hair after chemically relaxing the hair. Some manufacturers call their neutralizing shampoo, *balancing* shampoo; be sure to read labels carefully to avoid confusing this type of balancing shampoo with a balancing shampoo intended for oily hair and scalp.

Sulfate-Free Shampoos

Sulfates, such as sodium laureth sulfate, are surfactants used in shampoos and other products for their thickening and lathering capabilities. A **sulfate-free shampoo** is formulated with little to no sulfates and is generally a good choice for color-treated and chemically treated hair because it does not strip natural oils from the hair.

Shampoos for Hair Replacements and Wigs

Wig and hair replacement shampoos are specially prepared products for cleaning hair systems. You should always use the manufacturer's recommended cleaning product because some hair systems require the use of a cleaning solvent rather than the mild shampoo that may be appropriate for other hair replacement products. Always follow the manufacturer's instructions carefully.

IDENTIFY TYPES OF CONDITIONERS

Conditioners are special chemical agents that are applied to hair to deposit protein or moisture to help restore the hair's strength and body or to protect against possible damage. Conditioners typically range from 3.0 to 5.5 on the pH scale. They are a temporary remedy for hair that feels dry or appears damaged. As such, conditioners cannot actually repair damaged hair nor can they increase or improve the quality of new hair growth.

Excessive use of conditioners, or using the wrong type of conditioner, can lead to a heavy or oily buildup of product on the hair. For this reason, you need to be able to select the right product for your client, for example, an instant conditioner for detangling or a repair conditioner for damaged hair.

There are three basic types of conditioners: instant (or rinse-out), treatment or repair, and leave-in. As a barber, you must decide the type to use based on the texture and condition of your client's hair and the desired results.

- **Instant conditioners** (IN-stant KAHN-dish-uhn-uhrz), also known as *rinse-out conditioners*, are applied to freshly shampooed hair and rinsed out after being worked through the hair. These conditioners usually have a lower pH than the hair, which helps close the cuticle scales. The typical instant conditioner does not penetrate into the hair shaft but may add oils, moisture, and sometimes protein to the cuticle scales. Detangling rinses, basic conditioners, and finishing rinses are examples of instant conditioners.

- **Treatment or repair conditioners** are deep, penetrating formulations that help restore moisture and protein in the hair. These conditioners sometimes require longer processing time or the application of heat before being rinsed out.

- **Leave-in conditioners** (LEEV-in KAHN-dish-uhn-uhrz), such as thermal protectors or blowdrying sprays, are applied to hair and not rinsed out. Some of these conditioners are designed for use with thermal tools, while others may be included with permanent wave products to help equalize the porosity of the hair shaft.

- **Medicated conditioners**, or rinses, are formulated to help control minor dandruff and scalp conditions. A dandruff rinse is a commercial product that usually works in conjunction with an antidandruff shampoo to help control dandruff. Always follow the manufacturer's directions.

Conditioner Ingredients

Most conditioners contain a large amount of fatty materials and a small amount of surfactant. In fact, without surfactants, conditioners could not be rinsed from the hair. In addition, conditioners contain the following types of ingredients:

- Protein and protein derivatives consist of hydrolyzed protein that can pass through the cuticle and penetrate into the cortex of the hair. Concentrated protein conditioners are used to increase the tensile strength of the hair and to temporarily close split ends. They also improve texture, equalize porosity, and help increase elasticity in the hair. Deep-conditioning treatments, also known as *hair masks* or *conditioning packs*, are chemical mixtures of concentrated protein in the heavy cream base of a moisturizer. Be sure to rinse the hair thoroughly prior to cutting, setting, or drying, as excess conditioner may coat or weigh down the hair.

- Fatty materials are the basic ingredients of many conditioners and include fatty alcohols, silicones, humectants, and moisturizers.

  - *Fatty alcohols* consist of nonvolatile oils, fats, or waxes that contain an alcohol group. Some examples are cetyl alcohol, glycerol, and stearyl alcohol.
  - *Humectants* are chemical compounds that attract and retain moisture from the atmosphere. For example, moisturizing conditioners contain humectants that help seal moisture inside the hair by coating the cuticle.
  - *Moisturizers* frequently refer to oily substances that coat the hair or skin and prevent water loss by evaporation. Lanolin, mineral oils, and cholesterol are examples of water-trapping additives found in many conditioners.
  - *Silicones* are oils that contain a repeating silicon-oxygen chain that is superior to plain oils because they are less greasy and form a breathable film over the hair or skin.

It is the barber's responsibility to be knowledgeable about the products used in the shop or salon. Basic product knowledge can be easily obtained from product labels, distributors, trade show demonstrations, and manufacturer representatives. See Table 7-5 for shampoo and conditioning products suitable for different hair types.

table 7-5
MATCHING PRODUCTS TO HAIR TYPES

Hair type	Fine	Medium	Coarse
Straight	Volumizing shampoo Detangler, if necessary Protein treatments Fine-hair shampoo	pH-balanced shampoo Finishing rinse Protein treatments	Moisturizing shampoo Leave-in conditioner Moisturizing treatments
Wavy, Curly, Extremely Curly	Light leave-in conditioner Protein treatments Spray-on thermal protectors	pH-balanced shampoo Leave-in conditioner Moisturizing treatments	Leave-in conditioner Protein and moisturizing treatments
Dry and Damaged (perms, color-treated, relaxers, blowdrying, sun, hot irons)	Gentle cleansing shampoo Light leave-in conditioner Protein and moisturizing repair treatments Spray-on thermal protection	Shampoo for chemically treated hair Moisturizing conditioner Protein and moisturizing repair treatments	Deep-moisturizing shampoo for damaged hair Leave-in conditioner Deep-conditioning treatments and hair masks

Scalp Conditioners

Scalp conditioners are topical preparations designed to maintain or improve the condition of the scalp. These products are available in a variety of formulations for different purposes; however, none will make the hair "grow."

- Cream-based products with moisturizers and emollients are usually used to soften and improve the health of the scalp.

- Medicated scalp lotions or ointments are products that promote healing of the scalp and may be prescribed by a physician.

- Astringent scalp tonics help remove oil accumulation on the scalp and can be used after a scalp treatment.

BECOME FAMILIAR WITH STYLING AIDS

Styling aids are available in a variety of formulations that include hair sprays, hair creams, tonics, waxes, gels, mousses, molding pastes and clays, to name but a few. The main thing to remember about using these products is to become familiar with their properties so that you can select the right product for the job. Some products will provide too much control and others not enough. For example, while a hair spray may be effective for holding a finished style in place, your client may prefer a light cream product that allows his or her hair to move more freely. With practice and experience you will identify the products that best meet your clients' needs.

Hair Tonics

Hair tonics are liquid or cream preparations, generally considered to be grooming or styling aids, that have been a part of the barbershop environment for decades. Depending on the formula, these products are used to stimulate the surface circulation of the scalp; remove loose dandruff; or impart manageability, shine, and control to the hair. Hair tonics are leave-in products that are available in oil-based, water-based, and alcohol-based formulations. Be sure to read the label carefully to select the right product for the intended purpose.

REVIEW OTHER COSMETIC PREPARATIONS

As a barber, you will use a variety of cosmetic preparations as you perform services on clients. The following section provides a brief description of some of the other products that you should become familiar with in preparation for working in a barbershop.

- *Astringents* may have an alcohol content of up to 35 percent. Astringents cause contraction of tissues and may be used to remove oil accumulation on the skin or to close the pores after a facial or shave. Due to the high alcohol content of astringent lotions, some skin types may be sensitive and react with a slight swelling or redness of the skin. Discontinue use if either of these symptoms appears. Skin tonics or toners and fresheners are milder forms of astringents.

  - *Skin tonics or toners* usually have an alcohol content of 4 to 15 percent, which positions them between fresheners and astringents in terms of alcohol content. Most toners are designed for use on normal and combination skin types.

  - *Fresheners,* also known as *skin freshening lotions*, have the lowest alcohol content (0 to 4 percent) in the group of astringents. They are designed for dry, mature, and sensitive skin types. The formulation of a freshener typically includes some or all of the following: witch hazel, alcohol and camphorated alcohol, citric acid, boric acid, lactic acid, phosphoric acid, aluminum salts, menthol, chamomile, and floral scents.

- *Cleansing creams* are used during facials and shaves in the barbershop. The action of a cleansing cream is caused in part by the oil content of the cream, which has the ability to dissolve other greasy substances. Older formulas, such as cold cream, contain relatively few ingredients that may include vegetable or mineral oil, beeswax, water, preservatives, and emulsifiers. The newer cleansing formulations are more skin condition–specific and may contain additional degreasers such as lemon juice, synthetic surfactants, emollients, or humectants.

- *Cleansing lotions* serve the same purposes as cleansing creams but are of a lighter consistency and are usually water-based emulsions. They are available in dry-, normal-, and oily-skin formulations. Some ingredients common to cleansing lotions are cetyl alcohol, cetyl palmitate, and sorbitol; perfumes and colorings are added to enhance lotions' marketing value.

- *Depilatories* are preparations used for the temporary removal of superfluous hair by dissolving it at the skin line. Depilatories contain detergents to strip the sebum from the hair and adhesives to hold the chemicals to the hair shaft for the 5 to 10 minutes necessary to remove the hair. During the short processing time, swelling accelerating agents such as urea or melamine expand the hair, helping break the hair bonds. Finally, chemicals such as sodium hydroxide, potassium hydroxide, thioglycolic acid, or calcium thioglycolate destroy the disulfide bonds. These chemicals turn the hair into a soft, jellylike mass of hydrolyzed protein that can be scraped from the skin. Although depilatories are not commonly used in barbershops, knowing about them is necessary because your customers may use them at home.

- *Epilators* remove hair by pulling it out of the follicle. Two types of wax are currently used for professional epilation: cold and hot. Both products are made primarily of resins and beeswax. Beeswax has a relatively high incidence of allergic reaction; therefore, it is advisable to do a small patch test of the product to be used. Recently, an electrical apparatus made for the home hair-removal market has become available.

- *Hair spray* is used to hold the finished style. Many new formulations for hair spray contain a variety of polymers, such as acrylic/acrylate copolymer, vinyl acetate, crotonic acid copolymer, PVM/MA copolymer, and polyvinylpyrrolidone (PVP), and plasticizers such as acetyl triethyl citrate, benzyl alcohol, and silicones as stiffening agents. Additional ingredients might include silicone, shellac, perfume, lanolin or its derivatives, vegetable gums, alcohol, sorbitol, and water.

- *Hairdressings,* such as pomades, creams, and lotions, give shine and manageability to dry or curly hair. They may be applied to either wet or dry hair and typically consist of lanolin or its derivatives, petrolatum, oil emulsions, fatty acids, waxes, mild alkalis, and water.

- *Masks* and *packs* are available to serve many purposes and skin conditions, including deep cleansing, pore reduction, tightening, firming, moisturizing, and wrinkle reduction. Clay masks typically contain varying combinations of kaolin (china clay), bentonite, purified siliceous (fuller's) earth or colloidal clay, petrolatum, glycerin, proteins, specially denatured (SD) alcohol, and water. The primary ingredients typically found in peel-off masks are SD alcohol 40, polysorbate-20, and polymers such as polyvinyl alcohol or vinyl acetate.

- *Massage creams* are used to help the hands glide over the skin. They contain formulations of cold cream, lanolin or its derivatives, and sometimes casein (a protein found in cheese).

- *Medicated lotions* are available by prescription for skin problems such as acne, rashes, or other eruptions.

- *Moisturizing creams* are designed to treat dryness. They contain humectants, which create a barrier that allows the natural water and oil of the skin to accumulate in the tissues. This barrier also works to protect the skin from air pollution, dirt, and debris. Moisturizers contain a variety of emollients ranging from simple ingredients such as peanut, coconut, or a variety of other oils to more complex chemical compounds such as cetyl alcohol, cholesterol, dimethicone, or glycerin derivatives.

- *Ointments* are semisolid mixtures of organic substances, such as lard, petrolatum, or wax, and a medicinal agent. No water is present. For the ointment to soften, its melting point should be below body temperature (98.6 degrees Fahrenheit). Ointments are prepared by melting an organic substance and then mixing it with a medicinal agent.

- *Pastes* are soft, moist cosmetics with a thick consistency that are used as a styling aid. They are bound together with the aid of gum, starch, and water. If oils and fats are present, water is absent.

- *Scalp lotions* and ointments usually contain medicinal agents for active correction of a scalp condition such as itching or flakiness. An astringent lotion may be applied to the scalp before shampooing to control oiliness as well as the itching and flakiness of dry scalp conditions. Medicated lotions and ointments for severe scalp conditions must be prescribed by a physician.

- *Soaps* are compounds that are made by mixing plant oils or animal fats with strong alkaline substances. Glycerin is also formed in the process. Potassium hydroxide produces a soft soap, whereas sodium hydroxide forms a hard soap. A mixture of the two alkalis will yield a soap of intermediate consistency. A good soap does not contain excess free alkali and is made from pure oils and fats. Soaps used in the industry may be categorized as deodorant soaps, beauty soaps, medicated soaps, and shaving soaps.

- *Styling aids*, such as gels and mousses, typically consist of polymer and resin formulations that are designed to give the hair body and texture. Many incorporate the same ingredients found in hair sprays but add moisturizers and humectants, such as cetyl alcohol, panthenol, hydrolyzed protein, quats, or a variety of oils to the ingredient list.

- *Suntan lotions* are designed to protect the skin from the harmful ultraviolet rays of the sun. They are rated with a sun protection factor (SPF) that enables sunbathers to calculate the time they can remain in the sun before the skin begins to burn. Suntan lotions are emulsions that might contain para-aminobenzoic acid (PABA), a variety of oils, petrolatum, sorbitan stearate, alcohol, ultraviolet inhibitors, acid derivatives, preservatives, and perfumes.

- *Wrinkle treatment creams* are designed to conceal lines on aging skin either via a crease-filling capacity or through a "plumping up" of the tissues. Among the many possible ingredients in these treatments are hormones and collagen. Some are made of herbs and other natural ingredients while others are entirely synthetic.

REVIEW THE UNITED STATES PHARMACOPEIA

The *United States Pharmacopeia* (USP) is a public health organization that sets standards for food ingredients, healthcare products, and drugs sold or manufactured in the United States and used by the public. Some of the most common chemical ingredients used in the formulation of hair and skin products are as follows:

- *Alcohol* is a colorless liquid obtained from the fermentation of starch, sugar, and other carbohydrates. Isopropyl (rubbing) and ethyl (beverage or grain) alcohol are both volatile (readily evaporated) alcohols. These alcohols function as solvents and can be found in shampoos, conditioners, hair colorants, hair sprays, tonics, and styling aids. Fatty alcohols, such as cetyl and cetearyl alcohol, are nonvolatile oils that are used as conditioners. The alcohols most often used in the barbershop are ethyl alcohol and isopropyl alcohol. Fifty to sixty percent isopropyl alcohol is an effective antiseptic that can be applied to the skin.

- *Alkanolamines* (al-kan-all-AM-eenz) are substances used to neutralize acids or raise the pH of hair products. They are often used in place of ammonia because there is less odor associated with their use. Alkanolamines are used as alkalizing agents in hair lighteners and permanent wave solutions.

- *Alum* is aluminum potassium or ammonium sulfate supplied in the form of crystals or powder; it has a strong astringent action. For this reason, alum is found in some skin tonics and is also used to make styptic powder or liquid to stop the bleeding of small nicks and cuts. Check with your state barber board before using styptic in any form.

- *Ammonia*, a colorless gas composed of hydrogen and nitrogen, has a pungent odor. Ammonia is used to raise the pH in permanent waving, haircoloring, and lightening substances. Ammonium hydroxide and ammonium thioglycolate are examples of ammonia compounds that are used to raise solution pH levels for better penetration into the hair.

- *Formaldehyde* is a colorless gas manufactured by an oxidation process of methyl alcohol. It is used as a disinfectant, fungicide, germicide, and preservative as well as an embalming solution. In the cosmetics industry, small amounts of formaldehyde are used in soaps, cosmetics, and nail hardeners and polishes. Formaldehyde and its derivatives, such as formalin, should be used with caution because the National Cancer Institute studies indicate that it is toxic, can lead to DNA damage, and is known to react with other chemicals to become a carcinogen.

- *Glycerin* is a sweet, colorless, odorless, oily substance formed by the decomposition of oils, fats, or fatty acids. It is used as a solvent and as a skin moisturizer in cuticle oils and facial creams.

- *Hydrogen peroxide* is a compound of hydrogen and oxygen. It is a colorless liquid with a characteristic odor and a slightly acidic taste. Organic matter, such as silk, hair, feathers, and nails, is bleached by hydrogen peroxide because of its oxidizing power. A hydrogen peroxide solution is used as a bleaching agent for the hair in solutions of 20 to 40 volume. A 3 to 5 percent solution of hydrogen peroxide possesses antiseptic qualities.

- *Petrolatum*, commonly known as Vaseline, petroleum jelly, or paraffin jelly, is a yellowish to white, semisolid, greasy mass that is almost insoluble in water. It is used in wax epilators, eyebrow pencils, lipsticks, protective creams, cold creams, and many other cosmetics for its ability to soften and smooth the skin.

- *Quaternary ammonium compounds* (quats) are found in many antiseptics, surfactants, preservatives, sanitizers, and germicides. Quats are synthetic derivatives of ammonium chloride. Although quats can be toxic, they are considered safe in the proportions used in the industry.

- *Silicones* are a special type of oil used in hair conditioners and as water-resistant lubricants for the skin. Silicones are less greasy than plain oils and have the ability to form a "breathable" film that does not cause comedones.

- *Witch hazel* is a solution of alcohol, water, and powder ground from the leaves and twigs of *Hamamelis virginiana*. It works as an astringent and skin freshener. Because of the alcohol content, it should not be applied directly to an open wound or near the eyes.

REVIEW QUESTIONS

1. Define organic and inorganic chemistry.

2. List the three states of matter.

3. Compare elements and atoms, compounds, and mixtures.

4. Explain the two ways in which matter can be changed.

5. Explain oxidation-reduction (redox) reactions.

6. Name the four classifications of chemical compounds.

7. Describe the differences between solutions, suspensions, and emulsions.

8. Define *pH* and draw a pH scale.

9. Explain oxidation and reduction reactions. Give an example of each.

10. Why is it important to know the acidity or alkalinity of a shampoo product?

11. What effect do acidic solutions have on hair?

12. What effect do alkaline solutions have on hair?

13. Identify the parts and functions of the shampoo molecule.

14. List three types of shampoo formulations.

15. List four types of conditioners.

CHAPTER GLOSSARY

acids	p. 184	solutions that have a pH below 7.0
alkalis (AL-kuh-lyz)	p. 184	solutions that have a pH above 7.0
atoms (AT-umz)	p. 180	are the basic building blocks of all matter and are the smallest particle of an element that has the chemical identity of the chemical
balancing shampoos	p. 193	are designed for oily hair and scalps. These shampoos wash away excess oiliness while keeping the hair from drying out
bases	p. 184	see alkalis
chemical change (KEM-uh-kul CHAYNJ)	p. 181	change in the chemical composition of a substance by which new substances are formed
chemical compounds (KEM-uh-kul KAHM-powndz)	p. 184	combinations of two or more atoms of different elements united chemically with fixed chemical composition, definite proportions, and distinct properties
chemical properties (KEM-uh-kul PRAH-ur-teez)	p. 181	characteristics that can only be determined with a chemical reaction
chemistry (KEM-is-tree)	p. 179	the science that deals with the composition, structure, and properties of matter
clarifying shampoos	p. 193	shampoo with an active chelating agent that binds to and helps remove metals from the hair; also provides thorough cleansing and cuts through product buildup
color-enhancing shampoos	p. 193	created by combining surfactant bases with basic dyes
compound molecules (KAHM-pownd MAHL-uh-kyoolz)	p. 180	two or more atoms of different elements united chemically with fixed chemical composition, definite proportions, and distinct properties

conditioners	p. 194	chemical agents used to deposit protein or moisturizers in the hair
conditioning shampoo (KAHN-dish-shun-ing sham-POO)	p. 193	also known as *moisturizing shampoos*, are mild cream shampoos that contain moisturizing agents (*humectants*) designed either to "lock in" the moisturizing properties of the product or to draw moisture into the hair
dry or powder shampoos	p. 193	shampoos that cleanse the hair without water
element (EL-uh-ment)	p. 179	is the simplest form of chemical matter and contains only one type of atom
elemental molecules (EL-uh-ment-uhl MAHL-uh-kyoolz)	p. 180	molecules consisting of two or more atoms of the same element in fixed proportions, for example, oxygen O_2
emulsions	p. 185	mixtures of two or more immiscible substances united with the aid of a binder or emulsifier
endothermic reaction	p. 183	a chemical reaction that requires the absorption of energy or heat from an external source for the reaction to actually occur
exothermic reaction	p. 183	the release of energy in the form of heat through certain chemical reactions
hair tonics	p. 196	grooming aids designed to stimulate the surface circulation of the scalp, remove loose dandruff, or to impart manageability, shine, and control to the hair
inorganic chemistry (in-or-GAN-ik KEM-is-tree)	p. 179	is the study of substances that do not contain carbon but may contain hydrogen
instant conditioners (IN-stant KAHN-dish-uhn-uhrz)	p. 194	conditioners that typically remain on the hair from 1 to 5 minutes and are rinsed out; also known as *rinse-out conditioners*
ion (EYE-ahn)	p. 187	an atom or molecule that carries an electrical charge
ionization (eye-ahn-ih-ZAY-shun)	p. 187	the separating of a substance into ions
leave-in conditioners (LEEV-in KAHN-dish-uhn-uhrz)	p. 195	conditioners and thermal protectors that can be left in the hair without rinsing
liquid-dry shampoos	p. 192	liquid shampoos that evaporate quickly and do not require rinsing
matter (MAT-ur)	p. 179	is defined as anything that occupies space (volume) and has mass (weight)
medicated conditioners	p. 195	conditioners formulated to control minor dandruff and scalp conditions
medicated shampoos	p. 193	shampoos containing medicinal agents for controlling dandruff and other scalp conditions
molecule	p. 180	two or more atoms joined chemically
neutralizing shampoo	p. 194	helps to rebalance and restore the pH level of the hair by neutralizing any alkali or unwanted residues that remain in the hair after chemically relaxing the hair
organic chemistry (or-GAN-ik KEM-is-tree)	p. 179	the study of substances that contain carbon
oxidation (ahk-sih-DAY-shun)	p. 182	either the addition of oxygen or the loss of hydrogen; a chemical reaction that combines an element or compound with oxygen to produce an oxide

oxides	p. 184	compounds of any element combined with oxygen
pH (potential hydrogen) (P-H)	p. 188	relative degree of acidity or alkalinity of a substance
pH-balanced shampoos	p. 193	shampoos that are balanced to the pH of hair and skin (4.5 to 5.5); also known as *acid-balanced shampoos*
pH scale (P-H SKAYL)	p. 188	a measure of the concentration of hydrogen ions in acidic and alkaline solutions
physical change (FIZ-ih-kuhl CHAYNJ)	p. 181	change in the form of a substance without the formation of a new substance
physical mixture (FIZ-ih-kuhl mix-CHUR)	p. 183	combination of two or more substances united physically
physical properties (FIZ-ih-kuhl PRAH-ur-teez)	p. 181	characteristics of matter that can be determined without a chemical reaction
pure substance (PYOOR SUB-stantz)	p. 183	matter that has a fixed chemical composition, definite proportions, and district properties
redox (REE-dux)	p. 182	term used for an oxidation-reduction reaction
reduction (ree-DUK-shun)	p. 182	the subtraction of oxygen from, or the addition of hydrogen to, a substance
salts	p. 184	compounds that are formed by the reaction of acids and bases
scalp conditioners	p. 196	cream-based products and ointments used to soften and improve the health of the scalp
shampoo (sham-POO)	p. 190	removes dirt, oil, perspiration, and skin debris from the hair and scalp
solute	p. 185	any substance that is dissolved into a solvent to form a solution
solution	p. 185	a stable, uniform mixture of two or more mixable substances made by dissolving a solid, liquid, or gaseous substance in another substance
solvent	p. 185	any substance, usually a liquid, that dissolves the solute to form a solution
sulfate-free shampoo	p. 194	formulated with little to no sulfates so it does not strip natural oils from the hair
surfactant (sur-FAK-tant)	p. 186	a substance that acts as a bridge to allow oil and water to mix or emulsify by reducing surface tension
suspensions (sus-PEN-shunz)	p. 185	formulations in which solid particles are distributed throughout a liquid medium
therapeutic medicated shampoos (thayr-uh-PYOOT-ik MED-ih-kayt-ud sham-POOZ)	p. 194	contain special chemicals or drugs that are very effective in reducing excessive dandruff
treatment or repair conditioners	p. 195	deep, penetrating formulations that help restore moisture and protein in the hair

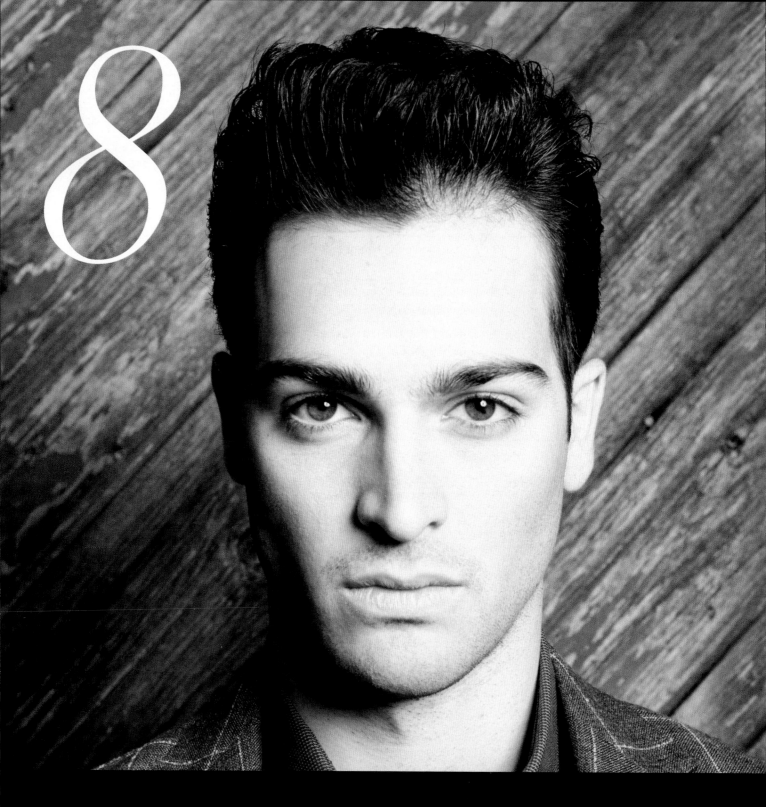

8

BASICS OF

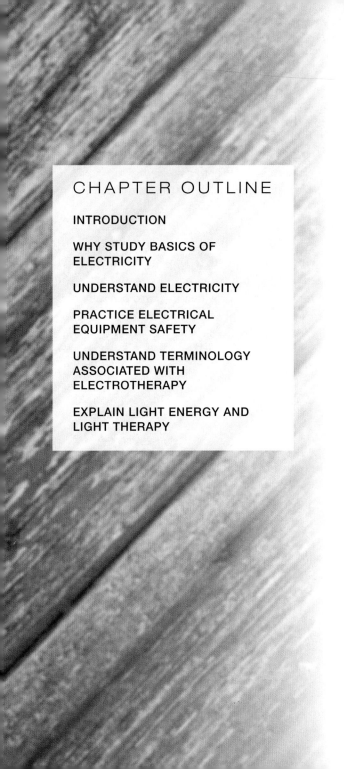

LEARNING OBJECTIVES

After completing this chapter, you will be able to:

LO❶
Define electricity.

LO❷
Define common electrical terms and measurements.

LO❸
Describe electrical safety devices.

LO❹
Examine the modalities a barber might be able to utilize depending on state licensing regulations.

LO❺
Explain the electromagnetic spectrum, visible spectrum of light, and invisible light.

LO❻
Identify devices used in light-therapy treatments.

Introduction

In today's barbershop, haircutting and other services would be very uncomfortable without electricity. It is probably safe to say that most barbers would not like to return to the days of the hand clipper or a lack of air-conditioning. In this chapter, you will learn some important safety precautions regarding the use of electricity in the barbershop. You will also be introduced to different electrical currents used in scalp and facial electrotherapy treatments.

Light-therapy treatments are another service that barbers can offer their clients. Different light rays have different effects on the skin. For this reason, barbers need to know when it is appropriate to apply the thermal and chemical properties associated with light therapy to the skin.

Electricity is a valuable tool for the barber, provided it is used carefully and intelligently. As you study this chapter, think about all the ways electricity and electrical devices will be used in the barbershop.

why study
BASICS OF ELECTRICITY

Barbers should study and have a thorough understanding of the basics of electricity because:

> Barbers use and rely on a variety of electrical appliances and need to know how to use electricity and electrical devices safely.

> Barbers need to understand that special training is required to safely and correctly repair electrical tools and appliances such as clippers, trimmers, and hot towel cabinets. Improperly repaired tools and appliances can result in blown circuit breakers, electric shocks, fires, and personal injury.

> Barbers need to understand the importance of periodic inspections to minimize the risk of fires caused by faulty wiring or overloaded outlets.

Understand Electricity

After reading this section, you will be able to:

LO❶ Define electricity.

LO❷ Define common electrical terms and measurements.

Electricity is not matter because it does not occupy space or have mass; in fact, electricity can move through or across matter and space. Electricity is a form of energy that produces physical, magnetic, chemical, or thermal effects when in motion. This energy is created by the flow of electrons between atoms.

figure 8-1
A complete electric circuit.

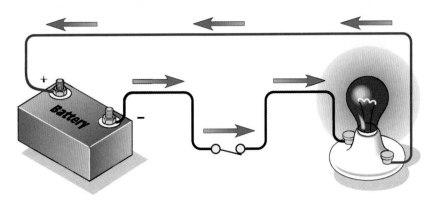

- An **electric current** (ee-LEK-trik KUR-ent) is the flow of electricity along a conductor. All substances can be classified as *conductors* or *insulators*, depending on the ease with which an electric current can be transmitted through them.

- A **conductor** (kahn-DUK-tur) is any substance, material, or medium that conducts electricity. Most metals, carbon, the human body, and watery solutions of acids and salts are good conductors of electricity.

- An **insulator** (IN-suh-layt-ur), or *nonconductor (nahn-kun-DUK-tur)*, is a substance that does not easily transmit electricity. Rubber, silk, dry wood, glass, and cement are good insulators.

- An *electric wire* is composed of fine, twisted metal threads (the conductor), covered with a silk, plastic, or rubber coating (the insulator).

- A **complete electric circuit** (kum-PLEET EE-lec-trick SUR-kit) is the path of an electric current from the generating source through conductors and back to its original source. **Figure 8-1** illustrates the path of a complete direct-current circuit.

> **? DID YOU KNOW?**
> Copper is a highly effective conductor used in electric wiring and electric motors.

TYPES OF ELECTRIC CURRENT

There are two kinds of electric current:

- **Direct current (DC)** (dy-REKT KUR-ent) is a constant, even-flowing current that travels in one direction only and produces a chemical reaction. Battery-operated instruments such as flashlights, cell phones, and cordless tools use DC, as does a car battery.

- **Alternating current (AC)** (AWL-tur-nayt-ing KUR-ent) is a rapid and interrupted current, flowing first in one direction and then in the opposite direction, that produces a mechanical action. Electric clippers, hair dryers, and other tools or appliances that plug directly into a wall outlet use AC.

A **converter** (kun-VUR-tur) is an apparatus that changes DC to AC. A **rectifier** (REK-tih-fy-ur) is an apparatus found within a power supply or adapter that converts AC to DC. Rechargeable cordless clippers and battery chargers use a rectifier to convert the AC from an electrical wall

table 8-1

DIRECT CURRENT (DC) AND ALTERNATING CURRENT (AC)

Direct Current	Alternating Current
Constant, even flow	Rapid and interrupted flow
Travels in one direction	Travels in two directions
Produced by chemical means	Produced by mechanical means

outlet to the DC needed to recharge the batteries. A **rheostat** (REE-oh-stat) is an adjustable resistor that is used for controlling the current in a circuit. Many devices, such as light dimmers, use a rheostat.

Table 8-1 outlines the differences between DC and AC.

Electrical Measurements

An electric current flows through a wire in the same way that water flows through a hose; however, without pressure, neither electricity nor water would flow.

- The **volt (V)** (VOLT) is the unit that measures electrical pressure, which pushes the flow of electrons forward through a conductor, similar to the way water pressure pushes water molecules through a hose. Tools and equipment that depend on electricity to function require different voltages; for example, clippers and blowdryers only require the 120 volts in normal wall sockets, while air conditioners and clothes dryers may require 240 volts. A higher voltage indicates more pressure, more force, and more power. The lower the voltage, the weaker the current (Figure 8-2).

- The **amp (A) (or ampere)** (AM-peer) is the standard unit for measuring the strength or rate of an electric current in a conductor. Just as a water hose must be able to expand as the amount of water flowing through it increases, so an electric wire must expand with an increase in the number of electrons (amps). A cord must be heavy-duty enough to handle the amps put out by the appliance. For example, a hair dryer rated at 10 amps requires a cord that is twice as thick as one rated at 5 amps. If the current, or number of amps, is too strong, the cord can overheat and cause a fire. If the current is not strong enough, the appliance will not operate correctly (Figure 8-3).

- A *milliampere* (mil-ee-AM-peer) is one-thousandth of an ampere. The current for facial and scalp treatments is measured in milliamperes as an ampere current would be much too strong.

- The **ohm (O)** (OHM) is the unit of electrical resistance in an electric current. Unless the force (volts) is stronger than the resistance (ohms), the current will not flow through the wire.

figure 8-2
Volts measure the pressure or force that pushes the electric current forward through a conductor.

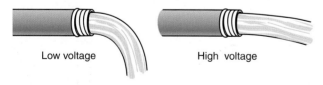

Low voltage   High voltage

figure 8-3
Amps measure the strength of the electric current.

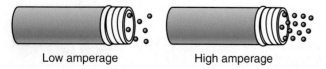

Low amperage   High amperage

- The **watt (W)** (WAHT) is the unit of power (amperes multiplied by volts) and indicates how much electric energy is being used in 1 second. A 40-watt bulb, for example, uses 40 watts of energy per second.

- A kilowatt (kW) is 1,000 watts. The electricity in a house is measured in kilowatt-hours (kWh).

Practice Electrical Equipment Safety

After reading this section, you will be able to:

LO❸ Describe electrical safety devices.

When working with electricity, you must always be concerned with your own safety, as well as the safety of your clients. All electrical equipment should be inspected regularly to determine whether it is in safe working order. Careless electrical connections and overloaded circuits can result in electrical shock, a burn, or even a fire.

SAFETY DEVICES

Safety devices help to prevent serious electrical accidents from happening. You should become familiar with these devices and know where they are located in the shop in the event of an emergency or power outage.

- A **fuse** (FYOOZ) is a safety device that prevents the overheating of electrical wires by preventing excessive current from passing through a circuit. The fuse blows or melts when the wire becomes too hot, which happens when the circuit is overloaded with too much current from too many appliances, or if faulty equipment is used. To reestablish the circuit, the appliance must be unplugged or disconnected and a new fuse inserted in the fuse box. Fuse boxes are often found in older buildings that have not been renovated or modernized (**Figure 8-4**).

- A **circuit breaker** (SUR-kit BRAYK-ar) is a switch that automatically interrupts or shuts off an electric circuit at the first indication of an overload (**Figure 8-5**). When wires become too hot because of overloading or due to a faulty piece of equipment, the breaker will click off and break the circuit. This action prevents the electric wires and the outlet from overheating and causing a fire. In modern electric circuits, circuit breakers have replaced fuses and can be reset. If an electric appliance malfunctions while in operation, disconnect the appliance from the wall socket immediately and check all connections and insulations before resetting.

Grounding

The principle of *grounding* (GROWND-ing) is another important way of promoting electrical safety. All electrical appliances must have at least two electrical connections. One of these connections is neutral and the other is "live" or "hot." When an appliance is plugged into an outlet, it completes the circuit from the live connection to the neutral connection, producing electricity to operate the appliance. The different sizes of the prongs on modern

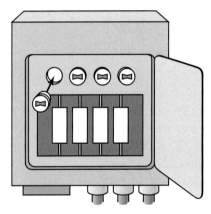

figure 8-4
Fuse box.

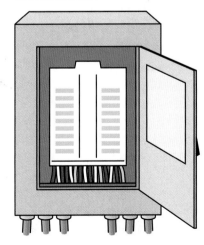

figure 8-5
Circuit breakers.

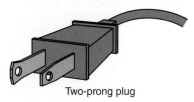

figure 8-6
Two-prong and three-prong plugs.

Two-prong plug

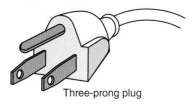

Three-prong plug

figure 8-7
GFI outlet.

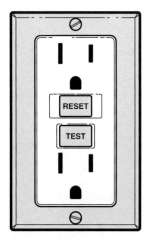

figure 8-8
UL symbol, as it appears
on electrical devices.

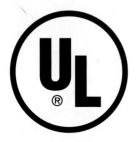

electrical plugs guarantee that the plugs can only be inserted one way. This feature provides protection from electrical shock in the event of a short circuit.

Some appliance plugs have a third circular connection called a *grounding pin* that guarantees a safe path to ground for electricity in the event of a short circuit or faulty wiring. This feature provides the most protection for you and your clients, when the power supply of an appliance is encased in metal. Both two-prong and three-prong plugs are grounded at the circuit breaker (**Figure 8-6**).

Ground Fault Interrupter

A **ground fault interrupter (GFI)** (GROWND FAWLT in-ter-UP-ter) is an outlet that senses imbalances within an electric circuit (**Figure 8-7**). When it "pops" open, it means that it has sensed a ground fault or current leaking to ground. These devices have surge protectors and must be installed properly to operate as intended; otherwise, although the outlet may work, the protection function will be lost. GFIs are required on all outlets located near or around sinks and water sources in the barbershop.

GUIDELINES FOR SAFE USE OF ELECTRICAL EQUIPMENT

Your safety and the safety of your clients should be of primary concern when you are working with electricity. All electrical equipment should be inspected regularly to determine whether it is in safe working order. Careful attention to electrical safety helps to eliminate accidental shocks, fires, and burns. A review of the following reminders will help ensure the safe use of electricity in the barbershop.

- Check that all electrical appliances you use are UL certified (**Figure 8-8**).
- Study the instructions *before* using any electrical equipment.
- Disconnect appliances when not in use.
- Keep all wires, plugs, and equipment in good repair.
- Inspect all electrical equipment frequently.
- Do not overload outlets and power strips (**Figure 8-9**).
- Avoid getting electrical cords wet.
- When using electrical equipment, protect the client at all times.
- Do not touch any metal while using an electrical appliance.
- Do not handle electrical equipment with wet hands.
- Do not allow the client to touch any metal surfaces while being treated with electrical equipment.
- Do not leave the room while a client is connected to an electrical device.

figure 8-9
Use only one plug per outlet on a power strip or on the wall.

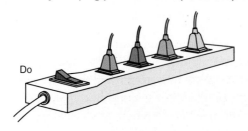

Do

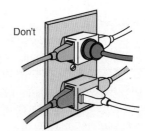

Don't

- Do not attempt to clean around an electric outlet while equipment is plugged in.

- Do not touch two metallic objects at the same time if either is connected to an electric current.

- Do not step on, or set objects on, electrical cords.

- Do not allow electrical cords to become twisted or bent; the fine wires inside the cord will break and the insulation will wear away from the wires.

- Disconnect appliances by pulling on the plug, not on the cord.

- Do not attempt to repair electrical appliances! Send the item to the manufacturer or authorized repair dealer to resolve the problem and to maintain your warranty.

Understand Terminology Associated with Electrotherapy

After reading this section, you will be able to:

LO ❹ Examine the modalities a barber might be able to utilize depending on state licensing regulations.

Electronic facial and scalp treatments are commonly referred to as **electrotherapy** (ee-lek-troh-thair-uh-py). Different types of electric currents are used for facial and scalp treatments. These different types of currents are called **modalities** (MOH-dal-ih-teez) and each modality produces a different effect on the skin. An **electrode** (ee-LEK-trohd) is an applicator used to direct the electric current from the machine to the client's skin. It is usually made of carbon, glass, or metal. Each modality requires two electrodes—one positive and one negative—to conduct the flow of electricity through the body. The only exception to this rule is the Tesla high-frequency current, which is discussed later in this chapter.

DEFINE POLARITY

Polarity (poh-LAYR-ut-ee) indicates the negative or positive pole of an electric current. The electrodes on many electrotherapy devices have one negatively charged pole and one positively charged pole. The positive pole is called the **anode** (AN-ohd), is usually red, and may be marked with a "P" or a plus (+) sign. The negative electrode is called the **cathode** (KATH-ohd). It is usually black and marked with an "N" or a minus (−) sign (**Figure 8-10**). If the electrodes are not marked, contact the manufacturer for more information.

EXPLAIN MODALITIES

Modalities refer to the different types of currents used in electrotherapy treatments. While there are many modalities used in the medical field, this chapter discusses only those modalities that a licensed barber might need. Depending on the rules and regulations in your state, these modalities *may* be galvanic current, microcurrent, and Tesla high-frequency current.

figure 8-10
Anode and cathode.

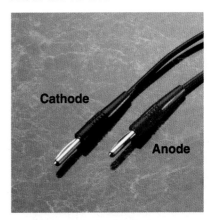

Cathode

Anode

table 8-2

EFFECTS OF GALVANIC CURRENT

Positive Pole (Anode) Cataphoresis	Negative Pole (Cathode) Anaphoresis
• Produces acidic reactions	• Produces alkaline reactions
• Closes the pores	• Opens the pores
• Soothes nerves	• Stimulates and irritates the nerves
• Decreases blood supply	• Increases blood supply
• Contracts blood vessels	• Expands blood vessels
• Hardens and firms tissues	• Softens tissues

figure 8-11
A microcurrent treatment.

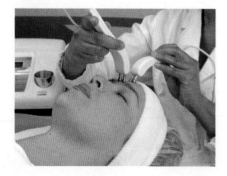

Galvanic Current

Galvanic current (gal-VAN-ik KUR-ent) is a DC, using a negative and positive pole, that is reduced to a safe, low-voltage level. Galvanic current produces chemical changes when passed through body tissues and fluids, and is used to create chemical and ionic reactions in the skin. These reactions depend on the negative or positive polarity of the active electrode that is used on the area being treated. **Table 8-2** shows that the effects produced by the positive pole are the exact opposite of those produced by the negative pole.

- **Desincrustation** (dis-in-krus-TAY-shun) is used to facilitate deep pore cleansing. During this process galvanic current is used to create a chemical reaction that acts to emulsify the sebum and waste in the pores (see Chapter 12).

- **Iontophoresis** (eye-ahn-toh-foh-REE-sus) (meaning "the introduction of ions") is the process of introducing water-soluble products into the skin. Both the positive and negative poles of the galvanic machine are used in the process. Ionic penetration takes place in two ways:

  - **Cataphoresis** (kat-uh-fuh-REE-sus) infuses acidic (positive) substances into the deeper tissues using the galvanic current from the positive pole toward the negative pole
  - **Anaphoresis** (an-uh-for-EES-sus) infuses alkaline (negative) products into the tissues from the negative toward the positive pole.

Microcurrent

Microcurrent is an extremely low level of electricity that mirrors the body's natural electrical impulses. Depending on the machine, one or two probes will be used, although some newer devices have both the negative and positive polarities in one probe. Through the probe(s), microcurrent is directed only to the specific area being treated and does not travel throughout the entire body. Microcurrent can be used for iontophoresis, firming, toning, and soothing the skin, and can help to heal inflamed tissue (**Figure 8-11**). Microcurrents can produce the following effects:

- Improve blood and lymph circulation
- Produce acidic and alkaline reactions

- Open and close hair follicles and pores
- Increase muscle tone
- Restore elasticity
- Reduce redness and inflammation
- Minimize healing time for acne lesions
- Improve the natural protective barrier of the skin
- Increase metabolism
- Produce a firmer, more hydrated appearance to aging skin

Tesla High-Frequency Current

Tesla high-frequency current (TES-luh HY-FREE-quens-ee KUR-ent) is characterized by a high rate of oscillation that produces heat. It is commonly called the *violet ray* and is used for both scalp and facial treatments. Tesla current does not cause muscular contractions; its effects are either stimulating or soothing, depending on the method of application.

The electrodes are made of glass or metal and only one electrode is used to perform a service. The shapes of the electrodes vary depending on the service: the facial electrode is flat and the scalp electrode is rake shaped. As the current passes through the glass electrode, tiny violet sparks are emitted (**Figure 8-12**). All treatments given with high-frequency current should be started with mild current and gradually increased to the required strength. Approximately 5 minutes should be allowed for a general facial or scalp treatment, depending upon the condition being treated. As with all other tools and implements, follow the manufacturer's directions. Tesla high-frequency currents may yield the following benefits:

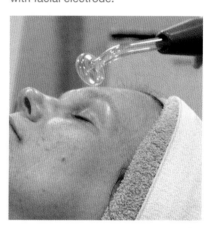

figure 8-12
Applying Tesla high-frequency current with facial electrode.

- Stimulate blood circulation
- Improve glandular activity
- Increase metabolism
- Increase absorption of nutrients and elimination of wastes
- Improve germicidal action
- Relieve skin congestion

Explain Light Energy and Light Therapy

After reading this section, you will be able to:

LO⑤ Explain the electromagnetic spectrum, visible spectrum of light, and invisible light.

LO⑥ Identify devices used in light-therapy treatments.

Electromagnetic spectrum (ee-lek-troh-MAG-ne-tik SPEK-trum), also known as *electromagnetic spectrum of radiation*, refers to all of the forms of energy (or radiation) that exist. These forms of energy are as follows: radio waves

figure 8-13
The electromagnetic spectrum.

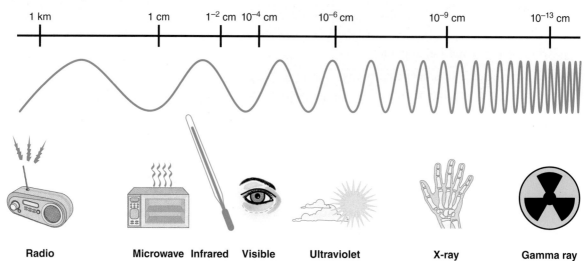

figure 8-14
Waveform patterns of long and
short wavelengths.

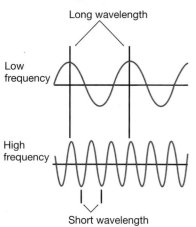

(used by radios and televisions), microwaves (used in microwave ovens), light waves (infrared, visible, and ultraviolet light used for light-therapy services), X-rays (used by physicians and dentists), and gamma rays (used for nuclear power plants) (**Figure 8-13**).

Energy moves through space on waves. Each type of energy has its own **wavelength** (WAYV-length), the distance between successive peaks of electromagnetic waves. A waveform is the measurement of the distance between two wavelengths. Some wavelengths are long and some are short. Long wavelengths have low frequency, meaning the waves pass a point less frequently within a given length of time. Short wavelengths have a higher frequency because the waves pass more frequently within a given length of time. These differences are compared in **Figure 8-14** and **Table 8-3**.

When light passes through a glass prism, it produces the seven colors of the rainbow, arrayed in the following manner: red, orange, yellow, green, blue, indigo, and violet. Within the visible spectrum of light, violet has the shortest wavelength and red has the longest. In the field of barbering, however, we are more concerned with the invisible rays found at the two ends of the visible spectrum: infrared rays, which produce heat, and ultraviolet rays, which produce chemical and germicidal reactions (**Figure 8-15**).

table 8-3

LONG WAVELENGTHS COMPARED WITH SHORT WAVELENGTHS

Long Wavelengths	Short Wavelengths
Low frequency	High frequency
Deeper penetration	Less penetration
Less energy	More energy

figure 8-15
The visible spectrum of light.

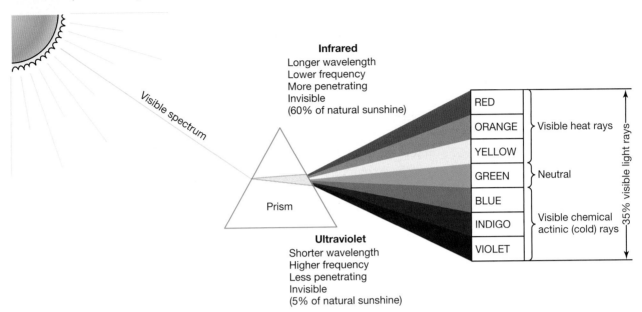

Infrared
Longer wavelength
Lower frequency
More penetrating
Invisible
(60% of natural sunshine)

Ultraviolet
Shorter wavelength
Higher frequency
Less penetrating
Invisible
(5% of natural sunshine)

Visible spectrum

Prism

RED	
ORANGE	> Visible heat rays
YELLOW	
GREEN	> Neutral
BLUE	
INDIGO	Visible chemical
VIOLET	actinic (cold) rays

35% visible light rays

THE VISIBLE SPECTRUM OF LIGHT

The **visible spectrum** (VIZ-uh-buhl SPEK-trum) of light is part of the electromagnetic spectrum. Visible light makes up only 35 percent of natural sunlight. Within the visible spectrum of light, violet is at one end of the spectrum and red is at the other end.

INVISIBLE LIGHT

Invisible light is the light at either end of the visible spectrum of light. Ultraviolet rays and infrared rays are forms of electromagnetic energy that are invisible to the human eye because their wavelengths are beyond the visible spectrum of light. Invisible rays make up 65 percent of natural sunlight at the earth's surface.

- **Ultraviolet light** (ul-truh-VY-uh-let LYT), also known as cold light or actinic light, makes up 5 percent of natural sunlight. It has a short wavelength and is less penetrating than visible light. Ultraviolet (UV) rays can kill microorganisms and cause chemical reactions to happen more quickly than visible light while producing less heat. The three types of UV light are:

  - *UVA* rays are closest to the visible spectrum and are the longest of all the UV rays. These rays are used in tanning booths and penetrate deeply into skin tissue. Overexposure can destroy the elasticity of the skin, causing premature aging, wrinkling, and skin cancer.
  - *UVB* rays are in the middle of the UV range, which produce some effects from both ends of ultraviolet rays. Long exposure to UVB rays will burn the skin and, like UVA rays, can cause skin cancer.
  - *UVC* rays are absorbed by the earth's atmosphere and ozone layer and do not reach the surface. However, UVC light rays are used in ultraviolet germicidal irradiation to inactivate or destroy microorganisms.

- **Infrared light** has a longer wavelength when compared to visible light and penetrates more deeply into the body. It produces more heat than visible light and makes up 60 percent of natural sunlight. Infrared lamps are often used in the barbershop during hair-conditioning treatments to aid product penetration or to accelerate haircolor processing. They are also used in spas to soothe nerves, warm muscles to relieve pain, increase blood circulation, and increase sweat and oil gland production.

LIGHT THERAPY

Light therapy, also known as *phototherapy*, is the application of specific wavelengths of the light spectrum to the skin for the treatment of specific disorders or conditions. In the beauty industry, light-therapy treatments may be accomplished through the use of low-level light therapy or low-level laser therapy, laser (light amplification by stimulated emission of radiation), light-emitting diodes, and therapeutic lamps. There are many light-therapy devices and each one is designed to create specific effects. This is important to know because light changes into electrochemical energy, which creates biochemical reactions in the cells; therefore, different light rays will produce different effects, such as heat, chemical reactions, or germicidal effects in the human body. The most important points to remember are that the equipment to be used is based on the skin type and the condition to be treated and that you will need thorough training in the use of the device.

Depending on the licensing regulations in your state, light therapy may be used to treat a range of skin conditions, from mild eruptions to wrinkles; to treat androgenic alopecia; or to remove unwanted hair. Review the following therapies that you may want to make available to your clients.

LASERS

Lasers (LAY-zurz) are a type of medical device that uses electromagnetic radiation and a medium (solid, liquid, gas, or semiconductor) for hair removal and various skin treatments. Lasers work by *selective photothermolysis* (FOTO-ther-moll-ih-sis), a process that turns the light from a device into heat. Lasers are designed to deliver an intense light beam to a specific depth and to a specific target area without damaging the surrounding tissues. When used in a hair removal treatment the light is converted into heat that is absorbed by the melanin in the follicles, which leads to follicle damage and inhibition of the hair growth. Because most lasers are classified as Level II medical devices or above, an esthetician license and supervision by a qualified physician may be required to operate the laser.

LIGHT-EMITTING DIODE

A **light-emitting diode (LED)** (LYT-EE-mit-ing DYE-ode) is a medical device used to reduce acne, increase skin circulation, and improve collagen content in the skin. The LED works by releasing different colors of light onto the skin to stimulate specific responses at precise depths of the skin tissue. When the colored light reaches a specific depth in the tissue, it triggers a reaction such as stimulating circulation or reducing bacteria. LED treatments should not be performed on anyone who has light sensitivities, has phototoxic reactions, is taking antibiotics, has cancer or epilepsy, is pregnant, or is under a physician's care. Always be certain that your license and state regulations permit the performance of LED treatments.

Depending on the type of equipment used, LEDs use blue, red, yellow, or green light to achieve the following effects:

- Blue light reduces acne and bacteria.

- Red light increases circulation, improves collagen and elastin production in the skin, and stimulates wound healing.

- Yellow light reduces swelling and inflammation, improves lymphatic flow, and detoxifies and increases circulation.

- Green light reduces hyperpigmentation and redness, calms, and soothes.

THERAPEUTIC LAMPS

In the barbershop *therapeutic lamps* may be a more practical solution for delivering light therapies associated with scalp and skin treatments. The lamp usually consists of a dome-shaped reflector mounted on a pedestal with a flexible neck, although several models are available and the bulbs come in various colors for different purposes (**Figure 8-16**). When using therapeutic lamps, the client's eyes must be protected and should be covered with moistened cotton pads or goggles. A general guide for using therapeutic bulbs follows:

- White light relieves pain, relaxes muscles, and produces chemical and germicidal effects.

- Blue light produces little heat, has a tonic effect on bare skin and a soothing effect on nerves, and is used only on clean, dry skin.

- Red light produces heat rays, creates a stimulating effect, and aids the penetration of creams into the skin.

- Ultraviolet light can be used to treat acne, tinea, seborrhea, and dandruff conditions and is applied at a distance of 30 to 36 inches from the skin. Following are guidelines for using ultraviolet light:
  - The skin area to be treated should be clean and dry.
  - Average exposure can produce skin redness; overdoses will cause blistering.
  - To begin with, a short exposure time of 2 to 3 minutes should be used, with the exposure gradually increasing over a period of days to 7 or 8 minutes.

- Infrared light produces heat but does not produce light; therapeutic lamps using infrared light have only a rosy glow when active and should be applied at an average distance of 30 inches from the skin.
  - Skin product ingredients should be checked for contraindications before use.
  - The light path should be frequently broken, by slowly waving your hand through the path during the service, to maintain client's comfort level.
  - Exposure time should not exceed 5 minutes.

Electrotherapy and light-therapy treatments are special client services that new as well as established barbers should consider offering. When the services discussed in this chapter are performed professionally and marketed effectively, the barbershop will benefit from increased revenue, client retention, and new-client referrals.

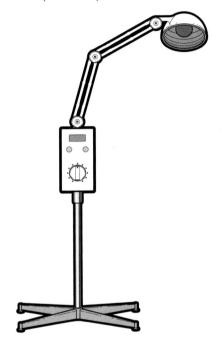

figure 8-16
Therapeutic lamp.

REVIEW QUESTIONS

1. Describe two types of electrical current.

2. Explain the differences between a fuse, circuit breaker, and ground fault interrupter.

3. List and briefly define the three electrical modalities covered in this chapter.

4. What does polarity indicate?

5. Explain the differences between visible and invisible light rays.

6. Explain the differences between ultraviolet and infrared light rays.

7. What conditions can be treated with ultraviolet light rays and what is the recommended range of distance between the lamp and the skin?

8. Explain the effects of infrared light rays on the skin.

9. What is light therapy?

10. List four light-therapy treatments used in the beauty industry.

CHAPTER GLOSSARY

alternating current (AC) (AWL-tur-nayt-ing KUR-ent)	p. 207	rapid and interrupted current, flowing first in one direction and then the opposite direction
ampere (AM-peer) **or amp (A)**	p. 208	standard unit for measuring the strength of an electric current or the rate of flow of charge in a conductor; also called an *amp*
anaphoresis (an-uh-for-EES-sus)	p. 212	process of forcing substances into tissues using galvanic current from the negative toward the positive pole
anode (AN-ohd)	p. 211	positive electrode
cataphoresis (kat-uh-fuh-REE-sus)	p. 212	process of forcing acidic substances into tissues using galvanic current from the positive toward the negative pole
cathode (KATH-ohd)	p. 211	negative electrode
circuit breaker (SUR-kit BRAYK-ar)	p. 209	switch that automatically interrupts or shuts off an electric circuit at the first sign of overload
complete electric circuit (kum-PLEET EE-lec-trick SUR-kit)	p. 207	the path of an electric current from the generating source through the conductor and back to its original source
conductor (kahn-DUK-tur)	p. 207	any substance, medium, or material that conducts electricity
converter (kun-VUR-tur)	p. 207	an apparatus that changes DC to AC
desincrustation (dis-in-krus-TAY-shun)	p. 212	process used to soften and emulsify oil and blackheads in the hair follicles
direct current (DC) (dy-REKT KUR-ent)	p. 207	constant current that travels in one direction only and produces a chemical reaction
electric current (ee-LEK-trik KUR-ent)	p. 207	the flow of electricity along a conductor
electricity	p. 206	a form of energy that produces physical, magnetic, chemical, or thermal effects when in motion
electrode (ee-LEK-trohd)	p. 211	an applicator used to direct electric current from a machine to the skin

electrotherapy (ee-lek-troh-thair-uh-py)	p. 211	electronic scalp and facial treatments
electromagnetic spectrum (ee-lek-troh-MAG-ne-tik SPEK-trum)	p. 213	the range of all forms of electromagnetic radiation
fuse (FYOOZ)	p. 209	device that prevents excessive current from passing through a circuit
galvanic current (gal-VAN-ik KUR-ent)	p. 212	constant and a DC, having a positive and negative pole, that produces chemical changes in tissues and body fluids
ground fault interrupter (GFI) (GROWND FAWLT in-ter-UP-ter)	p. 210	a device that senses imbalances in an electric current
infrared light	p. 215	invisible rays with long wavelengths and deep penetration; produce the most heat of any therapeutic light
insulator (IN-suh-layt-ur)	p. 207	substance that does not easily transfer electricity
iontophoresis (eye-ahn-toh-foh-REE-sus)	p. 212	process of introducing water-soluble products into the skin through the use of electric current
laser (LAY-zur)	p. 216	acronym for light amplification by stimulated emission of radiation
light therapy	p. 216	also known as *phototherapy*, is the application of specific wavelengths of the light spectrum to the skin for the treatment of specific disorders or conditions
light-emitting diode (LED) (LYT-EE-mit-ing DYE-ode)	p. 216	a medical device used to reduce acne, increase skin circulation, and improve collagen content in the skin
modalities (MOH-dal-ih-teez)	p. 211	currents used in electric facial and scalp treatments
ohm (O) (OHM)	p. 208	the unit of electrical resistance to an electric current
polarity (poh-LAYR-ut-ee)	p. 211	negative or positive pole of an electric current
rectifier (REK-tih-fy-ur)	p. 207	apparatus that changes AC to DC
rheostat (REE-oh-stat)	p. 208	an adjustable resistor used for controlling current in a circuit
Tesla high-frequency current (TES-luh HY-FREE-quens-ee KUR-ent)	p. 213	thermal or heat-producing current with a high oscillation rate; also known as the *violet ray*
ultraviolet light (ul-truh-VY-uh-let LYT)	p. 215	invisible rays, with short wavelengths and minimal skin penetration, that produce chemical effects and kill germs; also called *actinic* or *cold rays*
visible spectrum (VIZ-uh-buhl SPEK-trum)	p. 215	electromagnetic spectrum that can be seen by the human eye
volt (V) (VOLT)	p. 208	a unit of electrical pressure that pushes the flow of electrons forward through a conductor
watt (W) (WAHT)	p. 209	the unit of power (amperes multiplied by volts), indicating how much electric energy is being used in 1 second
wavelength (WAYV-length)	p. 214	distance between two successive peaks of electromagnetic waves

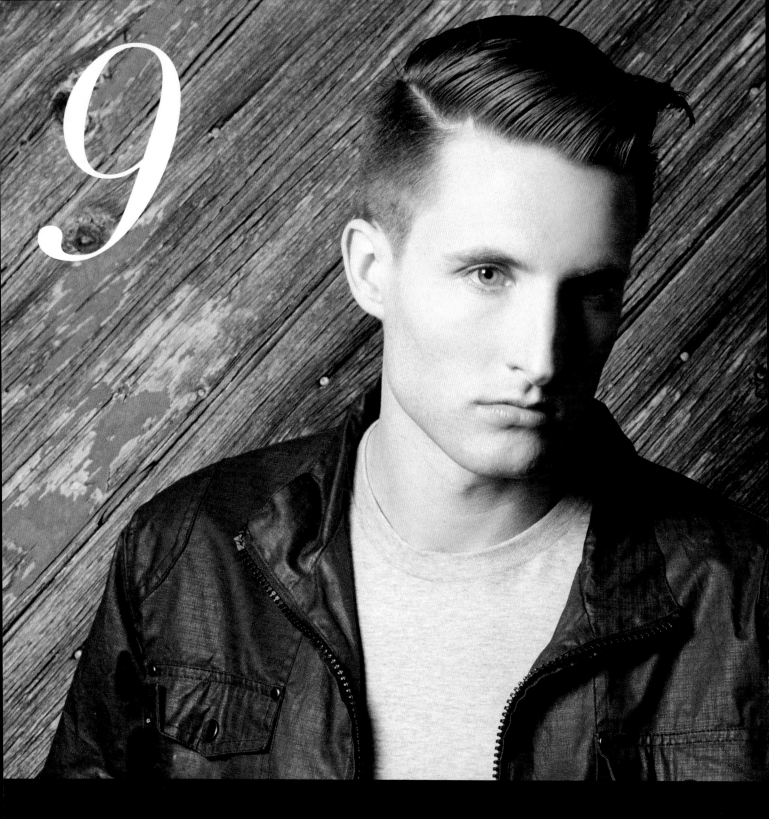

9

THE SKIN—STRUCTURE, DISORDERS, AND DISEASES

LEARNING OBJECTIVES

After reading this chapter, you will be able to:

LO❶
Describe the structure and divisions of the skin.

LO❷
List the functions of the skin.

LO❸
Identify and describe common primary and secondary skin lesions.

LO❹
Describe common skin inflammations and infections.

LO❺
List and describe disorders of the sebaceous and sudoriferous glands.

LO❻
List and describe types of skin pigmentations.

LO❼
Identify common skin hypertrophies.

LO❽
Identify and describe types of skin cancer.

Introduction

As the largest and one of the most important organs of the body, the skin is the body's first line of defense against diseases, protects the organs, and creates a barrier to the environment. **Dermatology** (dur-muh-TAHL-uh-jee) is a branch of medical science that pertains to the study of the skin—its nature, structure, functions, diseases, and treatment. A dermatologist is a physician who specializes in the treatment of the skin, hair, and nails.

why study
THE SKIN—STRUCTURE, DISORDERS, AND DISEASES?

Barbers should study and have a thorough understanding of the skin—structure, disorders, and diseases because:

> Knowing the skin's composition and underlying structures is crucial to performing facials, scalp treatments, and shaving services.

> You will need to recognize and be able to differentiate between normal skin conditions and those that may require medical treatment.

> You will need to recognize abnormal skin conditions that prohibit the performance of certain skin-related services.

Know the Anatomy of the Skin

After reading this section, you will be able to:

LO**1** Describe the structure and divisions of the skin.

LO**2** List the functions of the skin.

Healthy skin is slightly moist, soft, and flexible with a smooth, fine-grained texture. The slightly acidic pH of healthy skin provides a protective barrier against organisms that touch or try to enter it. Ideally, the skin should be free of blemishes and other disorders and have the ability to renew itself.

Skin varies in thickness over different parts of the body. It is thinnest on the eyelids and thickest on the palms of the hands and soles of the feet. Continued pressure over any part of the skin can cause it to thicken and become calloused. A callus is part of the body's natural defense system and should not be removed, as it will generally return thicker and harder. The skin of the scalp is constructed similar to the skin elsewhere on the human body, but the scalp has larger and deeper hair follicles to accommodate the longer hair on the head. The appendages of the skin are hair, nails, sweat glands, and oil glands.

The skin is constructed of two clearly defined divisions: the epidermis and the dermis (**Figure 9-1**).

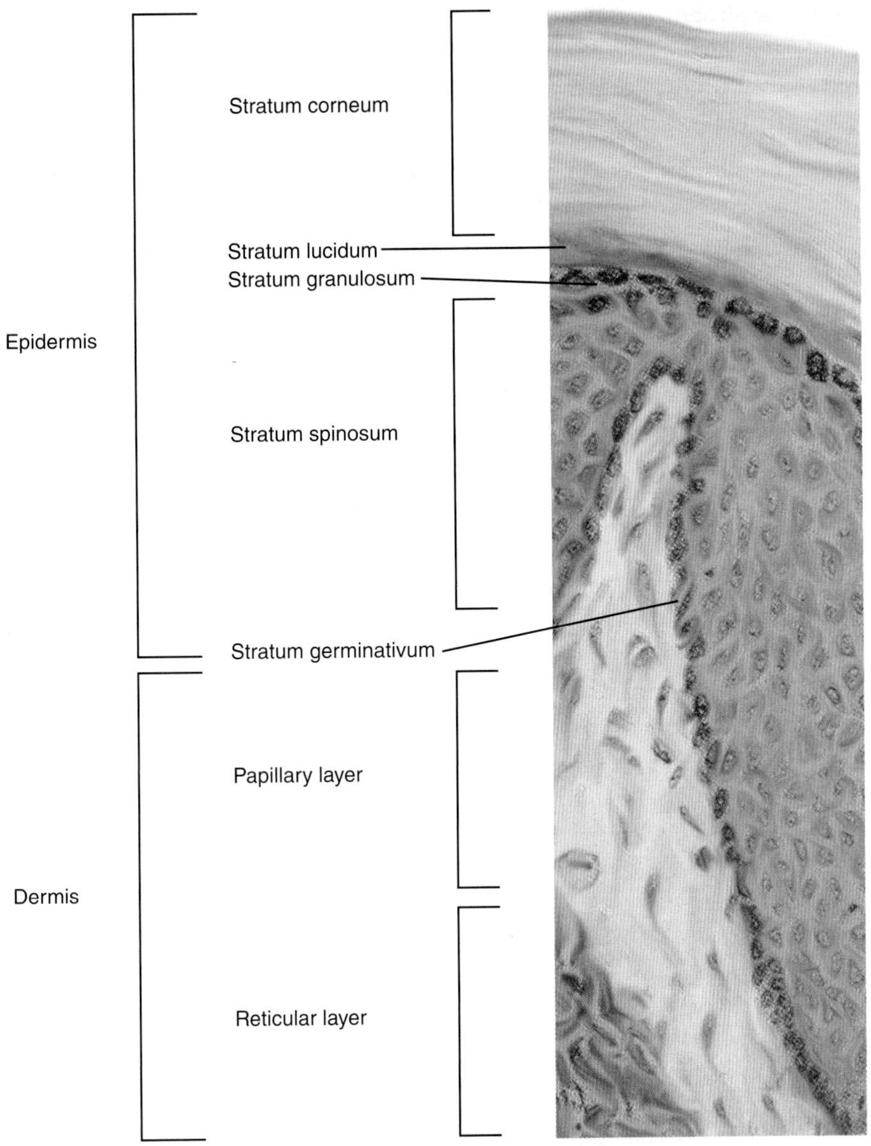

figure 9-1
Layers of the skin.

Epidermis

Stratum corneum

Stratum lucidum

Stratum granulosum

Stratum spinosum

Stratum germinativum

Papillary layer

Dermis

Reticular layer

EPIDERMIS

The **epidermis** (ep-ih-DUR-mus), also known as *cuticle* or *scarf skin*, is the outermost protective layer of the skin and is the thinnest layer of the skin. The epidermis contains no blood vessels, but has many small nerve endings. The layers, or strata, of the epidermis are as follows:

* The **stratum corneum** (STRAT-um KOR-nee-um), or *horny layer*, is the outer layer of the epidermis. This is the layer we see when we look at someone. It consists of tightly packed, scalelike cells that are continually shed and replaced by cells coming to the surface from the underlying layers. These cells are made up of a fibrous protein called *keratin*, which combines with a thin layer of oil (sebum) to help make the stratum corneum a protective, waterproof layer.

* The **stratum lucidum** (STRAT-um LOO-sih-dum), or *clear layer*, lies beneath the stratum corneum and consists of small, transparent cells through which light can pass.

- The **stratum granulosum** (STRAT-um gran-yoo-LOH-sum), or *granular layer*, consists of cells that look like distinct granules and are filled with keratin. These cells are almost dead and are pushed to the surface to replace cells that are shed from the stratum corneum.

- The **stratum spinosum** (STRAT-um spy-NOH-sum), or *spiny layer*, often classified as part of the germinativum, is a sub-layer that lies above the basal strata and beneath the stratum granulosum. The process that causes skin cells to shed begins in this layer.

- The **stratum germinativum** (STRAT-um jur-min-ah-TIV-um), also known as the *malpighian* or *basal cell layer*, is the deepest layer of the epidermis. This layer is responsible for the growth of the epidermis. It also contains melanocytes, which produce a dark pigment called *melanin*, which protects the sensitive cells below from the destructive effects of excessive exposure to ultraviolet light.

DERMIS

The **dermis** (DUR-mis) is the underlying, or inner, layer of the skin. It is also called the **derma** (DURM-uh), *corium, cutis,* or *true skin*. The dermis is about 25 times thicker than the epidermis and consists of a highly sensitive vascular layer of connective tissue. Within its structure are numerous blood vessels, nerves, lymph and oil glands, hair follicles, arrector pili muscles, and papillae. The dermis consists of two layers: the papillary or superficial layer, and the reticular or deeper layer (**Figure 9-2**).

figure 9-2
Structures of the skin.

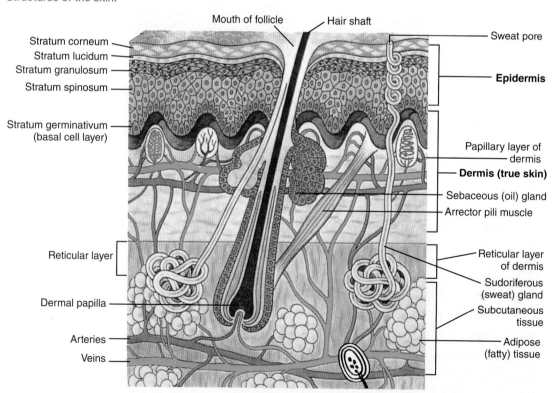

Mouth of follicle — Hair shaft

Stratum corneum
Stratum lucidum
Stratum granulosum
Stratum spinosum

Stratum germinativum (basal cell layer)

Reticular layer

Dermal papilla

Arteries

Veins

Sweat pore

Epidermis

Papillary layer of dermis

Dermis (true skin)

Sebaceous (oil) gland
Arrector pili muscle

Reticular layer of dermis
Sudoriferous (sweat) gland
Subcutaneous tissue
Adipose (fatty) tissue

- The **papillary layer** (PAP-uh-lair-ee LAY-ur) lies directly beneath the stratum germinativum of the epidermis. It contains small, cone-shaped projections of elastic tissue called *papillae* (puh-PIL-eye) that point upward into the epidermis. Some of these papillae contain looped capillaries, which are small blood vessels. Others contain small structures called *tactile corpuscles* with nerve fiber endings that are sensitive to touch and pressure. This layer also contains some melanin (skin pigment). The space at the top of this layer is the epidermal–dermal junction, where the two layers meet.

- The **reticular layer** (ruh-TIK-yuh-lur LAY-ur) is the deeper layer of the dermis, which supplies the skin with oxygen and nutrients. The reticular layer contains the following structures within its network:

  - Fat cells
  - Sweat glands
  - Blood vessels
  - Hair follicles
  - Lymph glands
  - Arrector pili muscles
  - Oil glands

Subcutaneous tissue (sub-kyoo-TAY-nee-us TISH-oo), also known as **adipose tissue** (AD-uh-pohs TISH-oo), is a layer of fatty tissue found below the dermis. Subcutaneous tissue varies in thickness according to age, gender, and general health. It gives smoothness and contour to the body, contains fats for use as energy, and also acts as a protective cushion for the outer skin.

FLUIDS OF THE SKIN

Blood and lymph supply nourishment to the skin in the form of protein, carbohydrates, and fat. From one-half to two-thirds of the body's blood supply is distributed to the skin. As the blood and lymph circulate through the skin, they deliver essential materials for the growth, nourishment, and repair of the skin, hair, and nails. Networks of arteries and lymphatics in the subcutaneous tissue send their smaller branches to hair papillae, hair follicles, and skin glands.

NERVES OF THE SKIN

The skin contains the surface endings of many nerve fibers, which are classified as follows:

- **Motor nerve fibers** (MOH-tur NURV FY-buhrs) are distributed to the arrector pili muscles attached to the hair follicles. These fibers carry impulses from the brain to control muscle movement.

- **Sensory nerve fibers** (SEN-soh-ree NURV FY-buhrs) react to heat, cold, touch, pressure, and pain (**Figure 9-3**). These receptors send messages to the brain.

- **Secretory nerve fibers** (seh-KRUH-toh-ree NURV FY-buhrs) are distributed to the sweat and oil glands of the skin. Secretory nerves regulate the excretion of perspiration from the sweat glands and the flow of sebum from the oil glands to the surface of the skin.

figure 9-3
Sensory nerve endings in the skin.

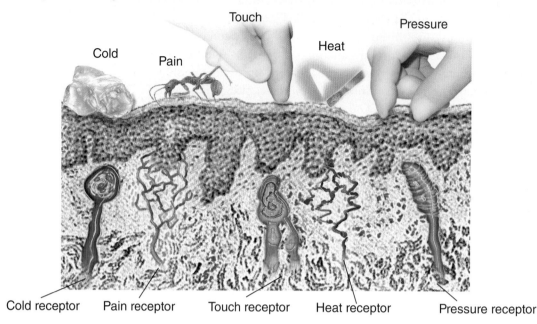

Cold Pain Touch Heat Pressure

Cold receptor · Pain receptor · Touch receptor · Heat receptor · Pressure receptor

Sense of Touch

The papillary layer of the dermis houses the nerve endings that provide the body with the sense of touch. These nerve endings register basic sensations such as touch, pain, heat, cold, pressure, or deep touch. Nerve endings are most abundant in the fingertips. Complex sensations, such as vibrations, seem to depend on the sensitivity of a combination of these nerve endings.

SKIN COLOR

The color of the skin, whether fair or dark, depends on genetics and melanin. Melanin, however, is the primary source of skin color; these grains of pigment are deposited in the stratum germinativum of the epidermis and the papillary layer of the dermis.

Special cells called *melanocytes* produce the pigment granules that are scattered throughout the germinativum and papillary layers. These granules are called *melanosomes* and they produce the complex protein called **melanin** (MEL-uh-nin), a brown-black pigment that gives skin color and serves as the skin's protective screen from the sun's rays. The amount and type of melanin is an inherited trait that varies among races and individuals (**Figure 9-4**). For example, dark skin contains more melanin than light skin.

SKIN ELASTICITY

The skin gets its strength, form, and flexibility from protein fibers within the dermis called *collagen* and *elastin*. **Collagen** (KAHL-uh-jen) fibers make up a large portion of the dermis and help to give support to the many structures found in this layer. When collagen fibers become weakened, wrinkles and sagging of the skin can occur. **Elastin** (ee-LAS-tin) gives the skin its elasticity and flexibility and the ability to regain its shape after stretching. When healthy skin expands, it regains its former shape almost immediately. Conversely, one of the most prominent characteristics of aged skin is its loss of elasticity.

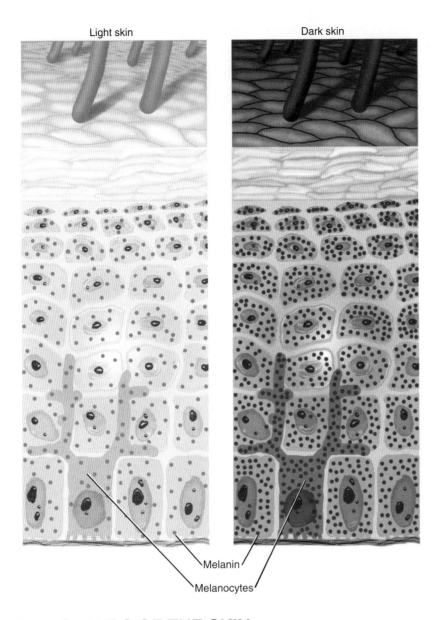

figure 9-4
Melanocytes in the epidermis produce melanin.

Melanin
Melanocytes

THE GLANDS OF THE SKIN

The skin contains two types of duct glands, the *sudoriferous glands*, or *sweat glands*, and the *sebaceous* (sih-BAY-shus) *glands*, or *oil glands*, which extract material from the blood to form new substances (**Figure 9-5**).

Sudoriferous (Sweat) Glands

The **sudoriferous glands** (sood-uh-RIF-uh-rus GLANDZ) consist of a coiled base (called a *fundus*) and a tubelike duct that terminates at the skin surface to form the sweat pore. Practically all parts of the body are supplied with sweat glands, although they are more numerous on the palms, soles, forehead, and armpits.

The nervous system controls the activity of sweat glands, which regulate body temperature and help to eliminate waste products (salt and other chemicals) from the body. Regulation of body temperature occurs when the evaporation of moisture from sweat on the skin cools the body. Heat, exercise, emotion, and certain drugs influence sweat gland activity.

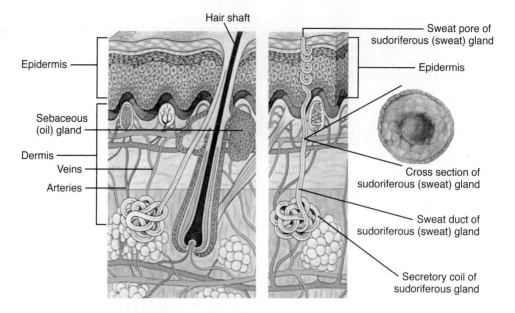

figure 9-5
Sudoriferous glands and the sebaceous gland.

Hair shaft

Epidermis

Sebaceous (oil) gland

Dermis

Veins

Arteries

Sweat pore of sudoriferous (sweat) gland

Epidermis

Cross section of sudoriferous (sweat) gland

Sweat duct of sudoriferous (sweat) gland

Secretory coil of sudoriferous gland

Sebaceous (Oil) Glands

The sebaceous or oil glands of the skin are connected to the hair follicles. These glands consist of little sacs with ducts that open into the hair follicle, where they secrete **sebum** (SEEB-um), which lubricates the skin and preserves the softness of the hair. With the exception of the palms and soles, these glands are found in all parts of the body, particularly the face and scalp.

Sebum is a semifluid, oily substance produced by the oil glands that flows through the oil ducts leading to the mouths of the hair follicles. When the sebum becomes hardened and the duct becomes blocked, a **blackhead** (BLAK-hed) is formed. The primary function of sebum is to act as a shield that prevents moisture from evaporating from the skin surface.

ABSORPTION LEVEL OF THE SKIN

Although the skin serves as a protective barrier against microorganisms and chemical absorption, some topical products and creams are designed to penetrate this barrier for medicinal purposes. Limited absorption occurs through the skin cells, hair follicles, **sebaceous glands** (sih-BAY-shus GLANDZ), and sudoriferous glands and allows for the entry of specialized drugs or chemicals into the body. For example, antiseptics may be used to reduce the risk of skin infections, or vitamin creams used to support skin repair. The amount or level of absorption that takes place is dependent upon the thickness and location of the skin on the body, the concentration of the product, and the frequency of the application.

FUNCTIONS OF THE SKIN

The principal functions of the skin are protection, sensation, heat regulation, absorption, excretion, and secretion.

- **Protection.** The skin protects the body from injury and a multitude of pathogens. The outermost layer of the epidermis is covered with a thin layer of sebum, which renders it waterproof. The skin is resistant to variations in temperature, minor injuries, some chemical substances, and many potential pathogens. The skin also provides protection for internal organs, arteries, veins, and bones.

? DID YOU KNOW?
Many drugs are more effective when the body absorbs them through the skin rather than through the digestive process. Drugs for pain, hormone therapy, and smoking cessation, among others, are safely and effectively delivered through patches that use the absorption properties of the skin to their advantage.

- **Sensation.** The skin responds to heat, cold, touch, pressure, pain, and movement through its sensory nerve endings. Stimulation of a sensory nerve ending sends a message to the brain, which then stimulates a response. When you scratch an itch or pull away from a hot object, you are responding to the stimulation of sensory nerve endings and the message they conveyed to the brain. Some of the sensory nerve endings responsive to touch and pressure lie in close relation to hair follicles.

- **Heat regulation.** Heat regulation is a function of the skin that protects the body from the environment. A healthy body maintains a constant internal temperature of about 98.6 degrees Fahrenheit (37 degrees Celsius). As changes occur in the outside temperature, the blood and sweat glands of the skin make necessary adjustments to facilitate the cooling of the body. Processes such as the evaporation of sweat to cool the body or the closing of pores to retain heat are examples of this adjustment and are regulated by the hypothalamus in the brain.

- **Absorption.** Absorption beyond the top layer of skin is limited, but does occur. Some medications are designed to enter the body through the skin, where they are slowly absorbed and dispersed. Products designed for "skin care" are not intended to be absorbed beyond the top layer of skin.

- **Excretion.** Perspiration is excreted from the skin. Water lost by perspiration carries salt and other chemicals with it. Humans perspire 1 to 2 pints daily; perspiration is made up of made up of water, salt, and chemicals.

- **Secretion.** Sebum is secreted by the sebaceous glands and lubricates the skin and hair, keeping them soft and pliable. Sebum secretion is affected by hormones and emotional stress, which may increase the flow of sebum.

Identify Disorders and Diseases of the Skin

After reading this section, you will be able to:

LO❸ Identify and describe common primary and secondary skin lesions.

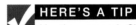

> **HERE'S A TIP**
> Use the mnemonic SHAPES to remember the functions of the skin: sensation, heat regulation, absorption, protection, excretion, and secretion.

Although barbers are not licensed to perform treatments for medical conditions, providing facials and shaves are traditional services well within the barber's scope of expertise. This includes addressing certain skin conditions, such as oily or dry skin, or alleviating minor acne conditions. Before proceeding with services, barbers need to be able to recognize different types of disorders to determine those that might be aggravated by facials or shaving or those that may need medical attention prior to receiving services.

Some skin and scalp disorders may be treated in cooperation with, or under the supervision of a physician or dermatologist. If asked to apply a medicine to the scalp, you must apply the medicine as directed by the physician and the treatment should not extend beyond the number of applications

> **DID YOU KNOW?**
> Barbers are often the first to recognize changes in their client's skin and scalp! Report any changes in a lesion or growth to the client so he or she may pursue diagnosis and treatment.

or date indicated. To protect both the barber and client, the client should provide the barber with a copy of the prescription directions. If a client has a skin or scalp condition you do not recognize, refer the client to a physician.

LESIONS OF THE SKIN

A **lesion** (LEE-zhun) is a mark on the skin that may indicate an injury or damage that changes the structure of tissues or organs. A lesion can be as simple as a freckle or as dangerous as skin cancer. Lesions can indicate skin disorders or diseases and may be symptomatic of other internal diseases. Being familiar with the principal skin lesions will help you to distinguish between conditions that may be compatible with services and those that need to be referred to a physician prior to the provision of services.

PRIMARY LESIONS OF THE SKIN

Primary skin lesions are lesions that are a different color than the color of the skin or lesions that are raised above the surface of the skin. They are often differentiated by size and layers of skin affected. Such lesions may require medical referral. Refer to **Table 9-1** for a description of primary lesions and examples of each.

SECONDARY LESIONS

Secondary skin lesions are characterized by an accumulation of material on the skin surface, such as a crust or scab, or by depressions in the skin surface, such as an ulcer. Refer to **Table 9-2** for a description of secondary lesions and examples of each.

> ⚠️ **CAUTION**
> To safeguard personal and public health, barbers must not perform services on a client who has (or appears to have) an infectious or contagious disorder. This includes parasitic conditions such as pediculosis and scabies. It is also very important that you do not perform services on inflamed skin, whether it is infectious or not. Certain products and services that are applied on inflamed or irritated skin may intensify and worsen the condition. Barbers should be able to recognize such conditions and tactfully suggest that the client seek appropriate medical treatment before receiving services.

table 9-1
PRIMARY LESIONS

Primary Lesion	Image	Graphic	Description	Examples
Bulla (BULL-uh) (plural: bullae [BULL-ay])			Large blister containing a watery fluid; similar to a vesicle. Requires medical referral.	Contact dermatitis, large second degree burns, bullous impetigo, perriphigus.
Cyst (SIST) and **tubercle** (TOO-bur-kul)	© Courtesy DermNet NZ.		Closed, abnormally developed sac that contains pus, semifluid, or morbid matter, above or below the skin. A cyst can be drained of fluid and a tubercle cannot. Requires medical referral.	*Cyst*: Severe acne. *Tubercle*: Lipoma, erythema nodosum.

			Flat spot or discoloration on the skin.	Freckle or "liver" spot.
Macule (MAK-yuhl) (plural: maculae [MAK-yuh-ly])	© wk1003mike/ Shutterstock.com.			
Nodule (NAHD-yul)	© Sue McDonald/Shutterstock.com.		A solid bump larger than 0.4 inches (1 cm) that can be easily felt. Requires medical referral.	Swollen lymph nodes, rheumatoid nodules.
Papule (PAP-yool)	© Ocskay Bence/ Shutterstock.com.		A small elevation on the skin that contains no fluid, but may develop pus.	Acne, warts, elevated nevi.
Pustule (PUS-chool)	© Faiz Zaki/Shutterstock.com.		Raised, inflamed, papule with a white or yellow center containing pus in the top of the lesion.	Acne, impetigo, folliculitis.
Tumor (TOO-mur)	© Courtesy DermNet NZ		Abnormal mass varying in size, shape, and color. Any type of abnormal mass, not always cancer. Requires medical referral.	Cancer.

(Continues)

table 9-1

(*Continued*)

Primary Lesion	Image	Graphic	Description	Examples
Vesicle (VES-ih-kuhl)			Small blister or sac containing clear fluid, lying within or just beneath the epidermis. Requires medical referral if cause is unknown or untreatable with over-the-counter products.	Poison ivy, poison oak.
Wheal (WHEEL)	© Margoe Edwards/ Shutterstock.com.		An itchy, swollen lesion that can be caused by a blow, scratch, bite of an insect, or urticaria (skin allergy), or the sting of a nettle. Typically resolves on its own, but referral to a physician should be considered when the condition lasts more than 3 days.	Hives, mosquito bites.

table 9-2
SECONDARY LESIONS

Secondary Lesion	Image	Graphic	Description	Examples
Crust (KRUST)	© Pan Xunbin/ Shutterstock.com.		Dead cells that form over a wound or blemish while healing; accumulation of sebum and pus, sometimes mixed with epidermal cells.	Scab, sore.
Excoriation (ek-skor-ee-AY-shun)	R. Baran "The Nail in Differential Diagnosis" with permission of Informa (London).		Skin sore or abrasion produced by scratching or scraping.	Nail cuticle damage from nail biting.

			Crack in the skin that penetrates the dermis.	Severely cracked or chapped hands/lips.
Fissure (FISH-ur)	© librakv/Shutterstock.com.			
Keloid (KEE-loyd)			A thick scar resulting from excessive growth of fibrous tissue that will form along any type of scar for people susceptible to these.	
Scale (SKAYL)	© Christine Langer-Pueschel/ Shutterstock.com.		Thin, dry, or oily plate of epidermal flakes.	Excessive dandruff, psoriasis.
Scar (skahr) or **cicatrix** (SIK-uh-triks)	© Geo-grafika/Shutterstock.com.		Slightly raised or depressed mark on the skin formed after an injury or a lesion of the skin has healed.	Postoperative repair.
Ulcer (UL-sur)	© Ilya Andriyanov/ Shutterstock.com.		Open lesion on the skin or mucous membrane of the body, accompanied by loss of skin depth and possibly weeping of fluids or pus. Requires medical referral, particularly for clients with underlying medical conditions, such as diabetes.	Chicken pox, herpes.

Discuss Disorders of the Sebaceous and Sudoriferous Glands

After reading this section, you will be able to:

LO④ Describe common skin inflammations and infections.

LO⑤ List and describe disorders of the sebaceous and sudoriferous glands.

figure 9-6
Comedone.

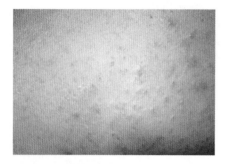

figure 9-7
Milia.

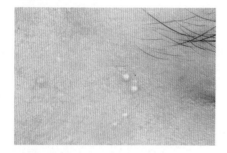

figure 9-8
Acne.

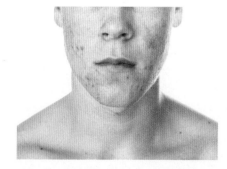

There are several common disorders of the sebaceous (oil) glands that the barber should be able to understand and identify.

An **open comedo**, also known as a *blackhead*, is a hair follicle filled with keratin and sebum. **Comedones** (KAHM-uh-dohnz) appear most frequently on the face, especially in the T-zone, the center of the face (**Figure 9-6**). When the sebum of the comedo is exposed to the environment, it oxidizes and turns black. When the follicle is closed and not exposed to the environment, the sebum remains a white or cream color and is a **closed comedo**, also known as a **whitehead** (WHYT-hed), and appears as a small bump just under the skin surface.

Milia (MIL-ee-uh) are benign, keratin-filled cysts that appear just under the epidermis and have no visible opening. They resemble small sesame seeds and are almost always perfectly round. They are commonly associated with newborn babies but can appear on the skin of people of all ages. They are usually found around the eyes, cheeks, and forehead, and appear as small, whitish masses (**Figure 9-7**).

Acne (AK-nee), also known as *acne vulgaris*, is a skin disorder characterized by chronic inflammation of the sebaceous glands from retained secretions (**Figure 9-8**). Propionibacterium acne occurs when obstructed follicles are deprived of oxygen, which allows acne bacteria to multiply. Fatty acids obtained from sebum in the follicle are the main food source for acne bacteria. The bacteria multiply, causing inflammation and swelling in the follicle and eventually rupture the follicle wall. When the wall ruptures, the immune system causes blood to rush to the ruptured follicle, carrying white blood cells to fight the bacteria. An acne papule is an inflammatory acne lesion resulting from this rupture of the follicle wall and the infusion of blood. A pustule forms from the papule when enough white blood cells accumulate to form pus, which is primarily composed of dead white blood cells. Acne conditions are rated in four grades:

- **Grade I.** Minor breakouts, mostly open comedones, some closed comedones, and a few papules and pustules
- **Grade II.** Many closed comedones, more open comedones, and more papules and pustules
- **Grade III.** Redness and inflammation with many papules and pustules
- **Grade IV.** Cysts with comedones, papules, pustules, and inflammation (cystic acne)

A **sebaceous cyst** is a large, protruding pocket-like lesion filled with sebum. Sebaceous cysts are frequently seen on the scalp and the back and may be surgically removed by a dermatologist.

Seborrheic dermatitis (seb-oh-REE-ick dur-muh-TY-tis) or seborrhea, is a skin condition caused by an inflammation of the sebaceous glands, and is often characterized by redness, dry or oily scaling, crusting, and/or itchiness (Figure 9-9). Excessive oiliness on the skin or scalp may also indicate the presence of seborrhea. The red, flaky skin often appears in the eyebrows and beard, in the scalp and hairline, at the middle of the forehead, and along the sides of the nose. Dandruff and cradle cap are forms of seborrheic dermatitis that are sometimes treated with topical creams.

Rosacea (roh-ZAY-see-uh), previously called *acne rosacea*, is a chronic condition that appears primarily on the cheeks and nose (Figure 9-10). It is characterized by flushing (redness), **telangiectasis** (tel-an-jee-EK-tuh-sus) (distended or dilated surface blood vessels), and, in some cases, the formation of papules and pustules. The cause of rosacea is unknown, but the condition is thought to be genetic. Certain factors are known to aggravate the condition in some individuals. These factors include exposure to heat, sun, and very cold weather; ingestion of spicy foods, caffeine, and alcohol; and stress. Rosacea can be treated and kept under control by using medication prescribed by a physician, using proper skin care products designed for especially sensitive skin, and avoiding the aggravating flare factors listed above.

Asteatosis (as-tee-ah-TOH-sis) is a condition of dry, scaly skin, characterized by the absolute or partial deficiency of sebum. It can be the result of old age, exposure to cold or alkalies, or bodily disorders. **Steatoma** (stee-ah-TOH-muh): a sebaceous cyst or fatty tumor that is filled with sebum. It is a subcutaneous tumor of the sebaceous glands that can range in size from a pea to an orange. A steatoma usually occurs on the scalp, neck, or back and is sometimes called a *wen*.

figure 9-9
Seborrheic dermatitis.

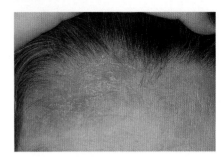

figure 9-10
Rosacea.

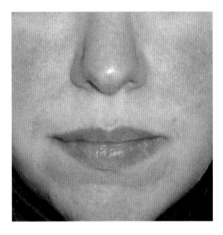

ACNE TREATMENT

Minor forms of acne can be treated without medical referral. Following are the basics of acne treatment:

- Daily use of gentle cleansers, formulated for a specific skin type. The use of harsh cleansers can make skin too dry and sebaceous glands will generate more sebum, creating an even bigger problem. These foamy, rinse-off products remove dirt, debris, and excess oil from the skin. Toners may be helpful for customers with excessively oily skin.

- Follicle exfoliants are leave-on products that help to remove cell buildup from the follicles, allowing oxygen to penetrate the follicles, killing bacteria. Commonly used ingredients in these products are alpha hydroxy acid, salicylic acid, and benzoyl peroxide. Benzoyl peroxide can be especially effective since it helps to shed cellular debris and also kills the acne bacteria. These products are generally not used all over because of their drying properties and are only used as a spot treatment. Clients should be warned about possible allergic reactions to these products and should stop using them if clients experience numbness in the area or swelling of the hands, feet, or mouth.

- Use of a light moisturizer to keep skin balanced and reduce the risk of excess sebum production can be helpful.

IDENTIFY DISORDERS OF THE SUDORIFEROUS GLANDS

There are several disorders of the sudoriferous (sweat) glands that barbers should be able to identify and describe.

- **Anhidrosis** (an-hy-DROH-sis) is a deficiency in perspiration or the inability to sweat, often a result of damage to autonomic nerves. This condition can be life threatening and requires medical attention.

- **Bromhidrosis** (broh-mih-DROH-sis) results in foul-smelling perspiration, usually noticeable in the armpits or on the feet. This condition is generally caused by bacteria; severe cases require medical referral.

- **Hyperhidrosis** (hy-pur-hy-DROH-sis) is characterized by excessive sweating, caused by heat or general body weakness. This condition requires medical referral.

- **Miliaria rubra** (mil-ee-AIR-ee-ah ROOB-rah), also known as *prickly heat*, is an acute inflammatory disorder of the sweat glands, characterized by the eruption of small red vesicles accompanied by burning, itching skin. It is caused by exposure to excessive heat and usually clears in a short time without treatment.

RECOGNIZE COMMON INFLAMMATIONS AND INFECTIONS OF THE SKIN

As a barber, you will need to be able to distinguish between noncontagious and contagious skin inflammations and infections.

- **Dermatitis** (dur-muh-TY-tis) is the general term for an inflammatory condition of the skin. The lesions may appear in various forms, such as vesicles or papules. **Irritant contact dermatitis**, abbreviated ICD, occurs when irritating substances, such as chemicals or tints, temporarily damage the epidermis. Unlike allergic contact dermatitis, irritant contact dermatitis is not usually chronic if precautions are taken, such as wearing gloves when working with chemicals. This condition is also called **dermatitis venenata** (dur-muh-TY-tis VEN-uh-nah-tuh).

- **Eczema** (EG-zuh-muh) is an inflammatory skin disease that may be acute or chronic in nature and present in many forms of dry or moist lesions. Eczema is frequently accompanied by itching or burning and all cases should be referred to a physician for treatment. Eczema is not contagious and its cause is unknown (**Figure 9-11**).

- **Psoriasis** (suh-RY-uh-sis) is a chronic inflammatory skin disease characterized by dry red patches covered with coarse, silvery scales. Psoriasis usually occurs on the scalp, elbows, knees, chest, or lower back, but rarely on the face. If irritated, bleeding points can occur. It is not contagious and its cause is unknown.

- **Herpes simplex I** (HER-peez SIM-pleks ONE) is a recurring viral infection that produces fever blisters or cold sores characterized by a single vesicle

figure 9-11
Eczema.

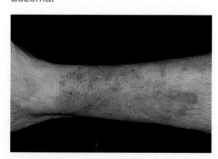

www.dermnet.com

or group of vesicles with red, swollen bases. The blisters usually appear on the lips, nostrils, or other parts of the face, and rarely last more than a week. Herpes simplex II is caused by the same virus and designates occurrences below the waist. Both forms of herpes simplex are contagious and require medical treatment (**Figure 9-12**).

- **Ivy dermatitis** (dur-muh-TY-tis) is a skin inflammation caused by exposure to poison ivy, poison oak, or poison sumac leaves. Blisters and itching develop soon after contact occurs. The condition may spread to other parts of the body by contact with contaminated hands, clothing, objects, or anything that was exposed to the plant itself. If the plant oil, which can be irritating, remains on the skin, it also can be spread from one person to another by direct contact. Serious cases should be referred to a physician.

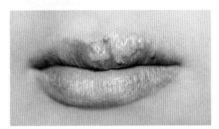

figure 9-12
Herpes simplex I.

Recognize Pigment Disorders and Hypertrophies of the Skin

After reading this section, you will be able to:

LO**6**   List and describe types of skin pigmentations.

LO**7**   Identify common skin hypertrophies.

Barbers are often in the position to notice changes in a client's skin and it is important to be able to differentiate between skin pigmentations and hypertrophies. For example, a flat mole may look like a dark freckle, but if you see a change in the color or growth of the mole, bring it to your client's attention for medical follow up.

IDENTIFY TYPES OF SKIN PIGMENTATIONS

Skin pigment can be affected by internal factors such as heredity or hormonal fluctuations, or by external factors such as prolonged exposure to the sun. Abnormal colorations, known as **dyschromias** (dis-chrome-ee-uhs), accompany skin disorders and are symptoms of many systemic disorders. A change in pigmentation can also be observed when certain medications are being taken, because of photosensitive reactions related to use of certain antibiotics. The following conditions relate to changes in the pigmentation of the skin:

- **Hyperpigmentation** (hy-pur-pig-men-TAY-shun) means darker than normal pigmentation, appearing as dark splotches.

- **Hypopigmentation** (hy-poh-pig-men-TAY-shun) is the absence of pigment, resulting in light or white splotches.

? DID YOU KNOW?

Skin cancer is preventable and early detection is possible, if you know what to look for. Be aware of the following as you service your clients:

- Any unusual lesions on the skin or on the scalp or change in an existing lesion or mole

- Melanomas, irregularly shaped dark spots, sometimes found on the scalp and ears and often first detected by a barber, who can see the back of the head and behind the ears!

- A new lesion or discoloration on the skin or scalp

- A client who complains about sores that do not heal or unexpected skin bleeding

- Recurrent scaly areas that may be rough to the touch, especially in sun-exposed areas such as the face, arms, or hands

Always discuss prevention with every client. If you become aware of any of these conditions, suggest that your client consult a physician.

http://www.dermnet.com.

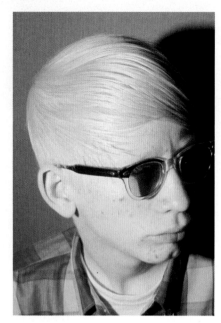

figure 9-13
Albinism.

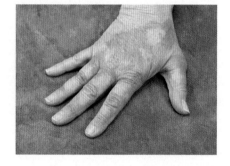

figure 9-14
Port-wine stain.

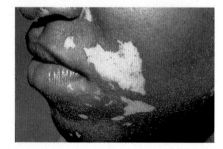

figure 9-15
Vitiligo.

- **Albinism** (AL-bi-niz-em) is congenital hypopigmentation, or absence of melanin pigment in the body, including the skin, hair, and eyes (**Figure 9-13**). Hair is silky white. The skin is pinkish white and will not tan. The eyes are pink, and the skin is sensitive to light and ages early.

- **Chloasma** (kloh-AZ-ma), also known as the *mask of pregnancy*, is a condition characterized by hyperpigmentation on the skin in spots that are not elevated. They are generally caused by cumulative sun exposure and can be helped by exfoliation or treated by a dermatologist.

- **Lentigines** (len-TIJ-e-neez) (singular: lentigo [len-TY-goh]) is the technical term for freckles, small yellow-colored to brown-colored spots on skin exposed to sunlight and air. It is also commonly referred to as *liver spots* in older adults, although there is no relationship to the liver.

- **Leukoderma** (loo-koh-DUR-muh) is a skin disorder characterized by light abnormal patches (hypopigmentation); it is caused by a burn, scar, inflammation, or congenital disease that destroys the pigment-producing cells. Examples are vitiligo and albinism.

- **Nevus** (NEE-vus), also known as a *birthmark*, is a small or large malformation of the skin due to abnormal pigmentation or dilated capillaries.

- **Stain** (STAYN) is an abnormal brown-colored or wine-colored skin discoloration with a circular or irregular shape (**Figure 9-14**). Its permanent color is due to the presence of darker pigment. Stains can be present at birth, or they can appear during aging, after certain diseases, or after the disappearance of moles, freckles, and liver spots. The cause is often unknown.

- **Tan** (TAN) is the change in pigmentation of skin caused by exposure to the sun or ultraviolet light.

- **Vitiligo** (vi-til-EYE-goh) is a hereditary condition that causes hypopigmented spots and splotches on the skin that often appear milky white. Recent research suggests that this disorder is part of an autoimmune disease (**Figure 9-15**). Skin with vitiligo must be protected from overexposure to the sun.

DESCRIBE HYPERTROPHIES OF THE SKIN

As a barber, you can expect to see some common hypertrophies on your clients' face, scalp, or neck during a skin or scalp analysis. An **hypertrophy** (hy-pur-troh-fee) of the skin is an abnormal growth of the skin. Many hypertrophies are benign (harmless) however, if you see any changes occur, be sure to share your observation with your client. Examples of common hypertrophies seen in the barbershop are as follows:

- A **keratoma** (kair-uh-TOH-muh) is an acquired, superficial, thickened patch of epidermis. A callus is a keratoma that is caused by continued, repeated pressure or friction on any part of the skin, especially the hands and feet. If the thickening grows inward, it is called a *corn*.

- A **mole** (MOHL) is a small brownish spot or blemish on the skin, ranging in color from pale tan to brown or bluish black. Some moles are small and flat, resembling freckles; others are raised and darker in color. Large dark hairs often occur in moles. Any change in a mole requires medical attention.

Courtesy Mark Lees Skin Care, Inc.

- A **skin tag** is a small brown-colored or flesh-colored outgrowth of the skin. Skin tags occur most frequently on the neck and chest and can be easily removed by a dermatologist.

- A **verruca** (vuh-ROO-kuh), also known as a **wart**, is an hypertrophy of the papillae and epidermis. It is caused by a virus and is infectious. Verruca can spread from one location to another, particularly along a scratch in the skin. A dermatologist can be helpful in removing and reducing the recurrence of warts.

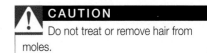

⚠ CAUTION
Do not treat or remove hair from moles.

Understand Skin Cancer

After reading this section, you will be able to:

LO**❽** Identify and describe types of skin cancer.

Skin cancer has become one of the most common cancers. It is also becoming one of the most common causes of cancer-related deaths because of general complacency about prevention and a lack of knowledge about the signs and real risks, particularly in young people. Barbers should recognize the signs of potential skin cancer and always refer clients. In this case, "better safe than sorry" is absolutely true! Do not let someone's young age or general good health stop you from being the one who saves someone's life through early diagnosis and treatment. There are three types of skin cancer (see **Table 9-3**).

table 9-3
TYPES OF SKIN CANCER

Cancer Type	Description	Image
Basal cell carcinoma (BAY-zul SELL kahr-sin-OH-muh)	Most common and least severe skin cancer; characterized by light or pearly nodules and has a 90% survival rate with early diagnosis and treatment.	
Squamous cell carcinoma (SKWAY-mus SELL kahr-sin-OH-muh)	More serious than basal cell carcinoma; characterized by scaly red papules or nodules. It can spread to other parts of the body; survival rates depend on the stage at diagnosis.	
Malignant melanoma (muh-LIG-nent mel-ahn-OH-muh)	Least common of the cancers, but is 100% fatal if left untreated—early detection and treatment can result in a 94% 5-year survival rate, which drops drastically, to 62%, once it reaches local lymph nodes; characterized by black or dark brown patches on the skin that may appear uneven in texture, jagged, or raised.	

Clients should be advised to regularly see a dermatologist for checkups of the skin, especially if any changes in coloration, size, or shape of a mole are detected, if the skin bleeds unexpectedly, or if a lesion or scrape does not heal quickly.

Home self-examinations can also be an effective way to check for signs of potential skin cancer between scheduled doctor visits. You should advise clients to check for—as part of their self-care exam—any changes in existing moles and pay attention to any new visible growths on the skin. Clients should also be advised to ask a spouse, friend, or loved one to check areas they cannot adequately see on a routine basis. These areas would include the back, scalp, and around the ears.

If detected early, anyone with these three forms of skin cancer may be cured. Barbers serve a unique role by being able to recognize the appearance of serious skin disorders and referring the client to a dermatologist for diagnosis and treatment.

Know How to Maintain the Health of Your Skin

Diet and protection are the major factors involved in maintaining the skin's overall health and appearance. Proper and beneficial dietary choices, as well as protecting the skin, help regulate hydration and oil production and optimize the function of cells.

- **Foods.** Eating a well-balanced diet of the three basic food groups of fats, carbohydrates, and proteins is the best way to support the health of the skin.

- **Vitamins and supplements.** Various nutrients aid in healing, softening, and fighting diseases of the skin. Vitamin A supports the overall health of the skin, vitamin C is important to skin and tissue repair, vitamin D promotes healthy and rapid healing of the skin, and vitamin E helps to fight against the harmful effects of the sun's rays. You should always suggest that customers speak to their physician prior to starting any regimen of supplements.

- **Water.** Ingesting plenty of fluid sustains the health of the cells, aids in the elimination of toxins and waste, helps to regulate the body's temperature, and aids in proper digestion.

- **Protection.** Using sunscreen with an SPF30 when being in the sun is necessary, as is avoiding sun exposure when possible, both of which will reduce the risk of cell and tissue damage, which leads to premature aging and possibly cancer. Use moisturizers to assist the surface of the skin to stay soft and supple when in dry environments, such as arid locations, or long-term exposure to water and drying agents.

REVIEW QUESTIONS

1. Briefly describe healthy skin.

2. Name the two main divisions of the skin and describe the layers within each division.

3. Identify the appendages of the skin.

4. How is the skin nourished?

5. Name three types of nerve fibers found in the skin.

6. What determines the color of the skin?

7. Identify two types of glands found in the skin and describe their functions.

8. List the six important functions of the skin.

9. What is a lesion?

10. What are the characteristics of primary skin lesions?

11. Describe the characteristics of secondary skin lesions.

12. List the characteristics of the following: eczema, herpes simplex, psoriasis, irritant contact dermatitis (dermatitis venenata).

13. What are some characteristics of seborrheic dermatitis?

14. Which three disorders of the sudoriferous glands requires medical attention?

15. Define a primary skin lesion and list ten types.

16. Define a secondary skin lesion and list seven types.

17. Name and describe at least five disorders of the sebaceous glands.

18. Name and describe at least five changes in skin pigmentation.

19. Name and describe the three forms of skin cancer.

20. What is the most common type of skin cancer?

CHAPTER GLOSSARY

acne (AK-nee)	p. 234	skin disorder characterized by chronic inflammation of the sebaceous glands from retained secretions
adipose tissue (AD-uh-pohs TISH-oo)	p. 225	a technical term for fat; gives smoothness and contour to the body
albinism (AL-bi-niz-em)	p. 238	congenital leukoderma, or absence of melanin pigment in the body

anhidrosis (an-hy-DROH-sis)	p. 236	a deficiency in perspiration or the inability to sweat, often a result of damage to autonomic nerves
asteatosis (as-tee-ah-TOH-sis)	p. 235	a condition of dry, scaly skin, characterized by the absolute or partial deficiency of sebum
basal cell carcinoma (BAY-zul SELL kahr-sin-OH-muh)	p. 239	most common and least severe type of skin cancer
blackhead (BLAK-hed)	p. 228	an open comedone; consists of an accumulation of excess oil (sebum) that has been oxidized to a dark color
bromhidrosis (bro-mih-DROH-sis)	p. 236	foul-smelling perspiration
bulla (BULL-uh)	p. 230	large blister containing a watery fluid
chloasma (kloh-AZ-ma)	p. 238	non-elevated spots due to increased pigmentation in the skin
closed comedo	p. 234	also known as a *whitehead*; a small bump just under the skin surface with white or cream colored sebum
collagen (KAHL-uh-jen)	p. 226	fibrous protein that gives the skin form and strength
comedone (KAHM-uh-dohn)	p. 234	a mass of hardened sebum and skin cells in a hair follicle that may be open (blackhead) or closed (whitehead)
crust (KRUST)	p. 232	dead cells that have accumulated over a wound while healing
cyst (SIST)	p. 230	a closed, abnormally developed sac containing fluid or morbid matter, above or below the skin
derma (DURM-uh)	p. 224	technical name for skin; also another name for the dermis
dermatitis (dur-muh-TY-tis)	p. 236	an inflammatory condition of the skin
dermatitis venenata (dur-muh-TY-tis VEN-uh-nah-tuh)	p. 236	also known as *irritant contact dermatitis*; an eruptive skin condition due to contact with irritating substances such as tints or chemicals
dermatology (dur-muh-TAHL-uh-jee)	p. 222	a branch of medical science that deals with the study of the skin
dermis (DUR-mis)	p. 224	second or inner layer of the skin; also known as the *derma*, *corium*, *cutis*, or *true skin*
dyschromias (dis-chrome-ee-uhs)	p. 237	abnormal skin colorations
eczema (EG-zuh-muh)	p. 236	inflammatory skin condition characterized by painful itching; dry or moist lesion forms
elastin (ee-LAS-tin)	p. 226	protein base similar to collagen that forms elastic tissue
epidermis (ep-ih-DUR-mus)	p. 223	outermost layer of the skin; also called the *cuticle* or *scarf skin*
excoriation (ek-skor-ee-AY-shun)	p. 232	skin sore or abrasion caused by scratching or scraping
fissure (FISH-ur)	p. 233	a crack in the skin that penetrates to the dermis

herpes simplex I (HER-peez SIM-pleks ONE)	p. 236	fever blister or cold sore; a recurring viral infection
hyperhidrosis (hy-pur-hy-DROH-sis)	p. 236	excessive perspiration or sweating
hyperpigmentation (hy-pur-pig-men-TAY-shun)	p. 237	darker than normal pigmentation, appearing as dark splotches
hypertrophy (hy-pur-troh-fee)	p. 238	abnormal skin growth
hypopigmentation (hy-poh-pig-men-TAY-shun)	p. 237	the absence of pigment, resulting in light or white splotches
irritant contact dermatitis	p. 236	abbreviated ICD; also known as *dermatitis venenata*; occurs when irritating substances temporarily damage the epidermis
ivy dermatitis (EYE-vee dur-muh-TY-tis)	p. 237	a skin inflammation caused by exposure to poison ivy, poison oak, or poison sumac
keloid (KEE-loyd)	p. 233	thick scar resulting from excessive tissue growth
keratoma (kair-uh-TOH-muh)	p. 238	technical name for a callus, caused by pressure or friction
lentigines (len-TIJ-e-neez)	p. 238	technical name for freckles
lesion (LEE-zhun)	p. 230	a structural change in the tissues caused by injury or disease
leukoderma (loo-koh-DUR-muh)	p. 238	skin disorder characterized by abnormal white patches
macule (MAK-yuhl)	p. 231	spot or discoloration of the skin, such as a freckle
malignant melanoma (muh-LIG-nent mel-ahn-OH-muh)	p. 239	most severe form of skin cancer
melanin (MEL-uh-nin)	p. 226	coloring matter or pigment of the skin; found in the stratum germinativum of the epidermis and in the papillary layers of the dermis
milia (MIL-ee-ah)	p. 234	technical name for milk spots; small, benign, whitish bumps that occur when dead skin is trapped in the surface of the skin; commonly seen in infants
miliaria rubra (mil-ee-AIR-ee-ah ROOB-rah)	p. 236	also known as *prickly heat*, is an acute inflammatory disorder of the sweat glands, characterized by the eruption of small red vesicles accompanied by burning, itching skin
mole (MOHL)	p. 238	small brownish spot on the skin
motor nerve fibers (MOH-tur NURV FY-buhrs)	p. 225	nerve fibers distributed to the arrector pili muscles, which are attached to the hair follicles
nevus (NEE-vus)	p. 238	technical name for a birthmark
nodule (NAHD-yul)	p. 231	a solid bump larger than 0.4 inches (1 cm) that can be easily felt
open comedo	p. 234	also known as a *blackhead*; a hair follicle filled with keratin and sebum
papillary layer (PAP-uh-lair-ee LAY-ur)	p. 225	outer layer of the dermis, directly beneath the epidermis

papule (PAP-yool)	p. 231	a small elevation on the skin that contains no fluid, but may develop pus
primary skin lesions	p. 230	lesions that are a different color than the color of the skin or lesions that are raised above the surface of the skin
psoriasis (suh-RY-uh-sis)	p. 236	skin disease characterized by red patches and silvery-white scales
pustule (PUS-chool)	p. 231	raised, inflamed, papule with a white or yellow center containing pus in the top of the lesion
reticular layer (ruh-TIK-yuh-lur LAY-ur)	p. 225	deeper layer of the dermis
rosacea (roh-ZAY-see-uh)	p. 235	chronic congestion of the skin characterized by redness, blood vessel dilation, papules, and pustules
scale (SKAYL)	p. 233	an accumulation of dry or greasy flakes on the skin
scar (skahr) or **cicatrix** (SIK-uh-triks)	p. 233	slightly raised or depressed mark on the skin formed after an injury or a lesion of the skin has healed
sebaceous cyst	p. 234	a large, protruding pocket-like lesion filled with sebum, frequently seen on the scalp and back
sebaceous glands (sih-BAY-shus GLANDZ)	p. 228	oil glands of the skin connected to hair follicles
seborrheic dermatitis (seb-oh-REE-ick dur-muh-TY-tis)	p. 235	is a skin condition caused by an inflammation of the sebaceous glands, and is often characterized by redness, dry or oily scaling, crusting, and/or itchiness
sebum (SEEB-um)	p. 228	an oily substance secreted by the sebaceous glands
secondary skin lesions	p. 230	lesions characterized by an accumulation of material on the skin surface, such as a crust or scab, or by depressions in the skin surface
secretory nerve fibers (seh-KRUH-toh-ree NURV FY-buhrs)	p. 225	nerves regulate the excretion of perspiration from the sweat glands and the flow of sebum from the oil glands
sensory nerve fibers (SEN-soh-ree NURV FY-buhrs)	p. 225	nerves that react to heat, cold, touch, pressure, and pain and send messages to the brain
skin tag	p. 239	a small brown-colored or flesh-colored outgrowth of the skin occurring most frequently on the neck and chest
squamous cell carcinoma (SKWAY-mus SELL kahr-sin-OH-muh)	p. 239	type of skin cancer more serious than basal cell carcinoma, but not as serious as malignant melanoma
stain (STAYN)	p. 238	abnormal brown- or wine-colored skin discoloration
steatoma (stee-ah-TOH-muh)	p. 235	sebaceous cyst or fatty tumor
stratum corneum (STRAT-um KOR-nee-um)	p. 223	outermost layer of the epidermis; the horny layer
stratum germinativum (STRAT-um jur-min-ah-TIV-um)	p. 224	innermost layer of the epidermis, also known as the *basal* or *Malpighian layer*
stratum granulosum (STRAT-um gran-yoo-LOH-sum)	p. 224	granular layer of the epidermis beneath the stratum lucidum; the grainy layer

stratum lucidum (STRAT-um LOO-sih-dum)	p. 223	clear layer of the epidermis, directly beneath the stratum corneum
stratum spinosum (STRAT-um spy-NOH-sum)	p. 224	spiny layer of the epidermis, often considered part of the stratum germinativum
subcutaneous tissue (sub-kyoo-TAY-nee-us TISH-oo)	p. 225	fatty tissue layer that lies beneath the dermis; also called *adipose tissue*
sudoriferous glands (sood-uh-RIF-uh-rus GLANDZ)	p. 227	sweat glands of the skin
tan (TAN)	p. 238	darkening of the skin due to exposure to ultraviolet rays
telangiectasis (tel-an-jee-EK-tuh-sus)	p. 235	distended or dilated surface blood vessels
tubercle (TOO-bur-kul)	p. 230	abnormal solid lump above, within, or below the skin
tumor (TOO-mur)	p. 231	abnormal cell mass resulting from excessive multiplication of cells
ulcer (UL-sur)	p. 233	open skin lesion accompanied by pus and loss of skin depth; a deep erosion; a depression in the skin, normally due to infection or cancer
verruca (vuh-ROO-kuh)	p. 239	technical name for a wart
vesicle (VES-ih-kuhl)	p. 232	small blister or sac containing clear fluid
vitiligo (vih-til-EYE-goh)	p. 238	an acquired leukoderma characterized by milky-white spots
wart	p. 239	also known as *verruca*; an infectious hypertrophy of the papillae and epidermis caused by a virus
wheal (WHEEL)	p. 232	itchy, swollen lesion caused by insect bites or plant irritations, such as nettle
whitehead (WHYT-hed)	p. 234	a closed comedone; consists of accumulated sebum that remains a whitish color because it does not have a follicular opening for exposure to oxygen

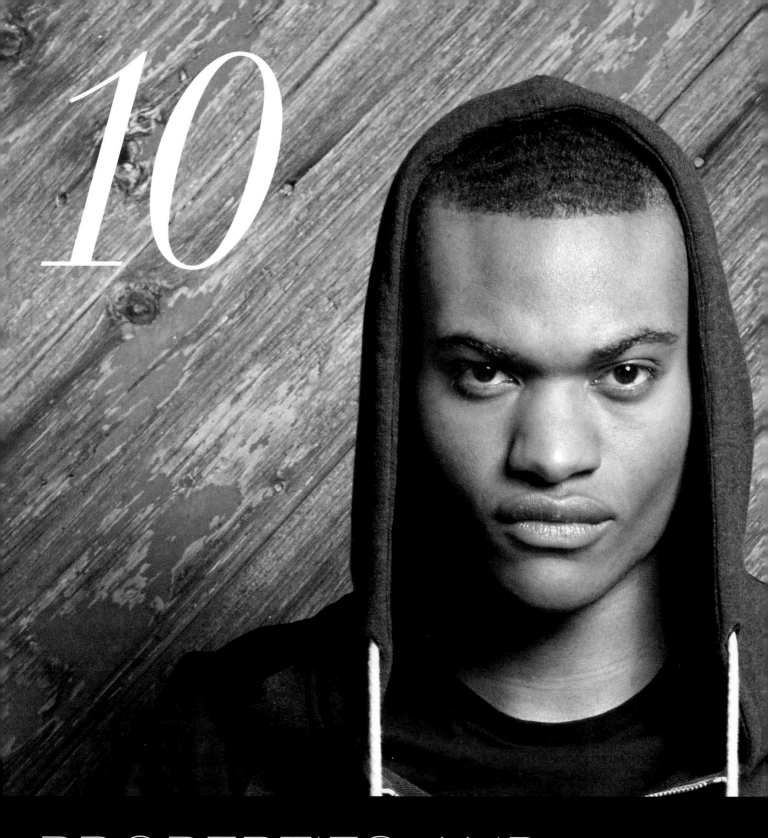

10

PROPERTIES AND DISORDERS OF THE HAIR AND SCALP

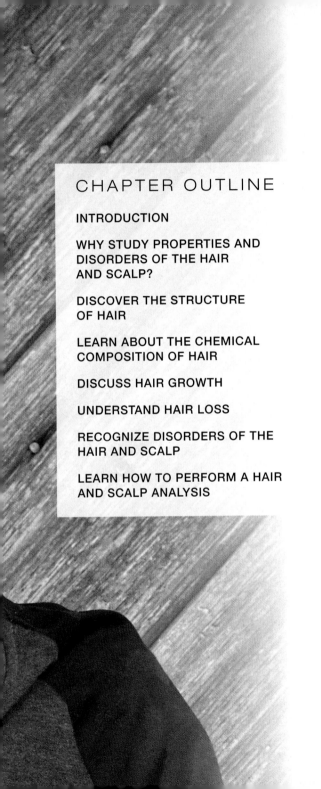

LEARNING OBJECTIVES

After reading this chapter, you will be able to:

LO❶
Identify and distinguish the different structures of the hair root.

LO❷
Identify and distinguish the three layers of the hair shaft.

LO❸
Identify and explain the three types of side bonds of the cortex.

LO❹
Name and describe the three phases of the hair growth cycle.

LO❺
Identify and define seven types of hair loss.

LO❻
Identify and describe two FDA-approved treatments for hair loss.

LO❼
Identify and define common hair disorders.

LO❽
Define common scalp disorders and identify those requiring medical attention.

LO❾
Identify the factors to be observed and considered during a hair and scalp analysis.

Introduction

The scientific study of hair, its disorders, and its care is called **trichology** (trih-KAHL-uh-jee), which comes from the Greek words *trichos* ("hair") and *ology* ("study of"). As you will learn, the hair we see is a part of the integumentary system that protects the head from heat, cold, and injury; it also serves as a source of adornment and an expression of personal style.

why study
PROPERTIES AND DISORDERS OF THE HAIR AND SCALP?

Barbers should study and have a thorough understanding of the properties and disorders of the hair and scalp because:

> Barbers need to know how products and chemicals affect the structure of the hair.

> Barbers need to know how to keep a client's hair and scalp in a healthy condition and how to differentiate between normal and abnormal conditions.

> Barbers need to be able to perform a scalp and hair analysis before performing a service.

Discover the Structure of Hair

After reading this section, you will be able to:

LO Identify and distinguish the different structures of the hair root.

LO Identify and distinguish the three layers of the hair shaft.

figure 10-1
Structures of the hair.

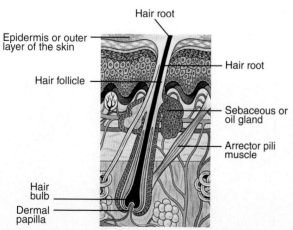

Epidermis or outer layer of the skin

Hair follicle

Hair bulb

Dermal papilla

Hair root

Hair root

Sebaceous or oil gland

Arrector pili muscle

Hair is an appendage of the skin, in the form of a slender, threadlike outgrowth of the skin and scalp. It is composed chiefly of a fibrous protein called **keratin** (KAIR-uht-in), which is present in all horny growths such as nails, claws, and hoofs. Full-grown human hair is divided into two parts: the hair root and the hair shaft. The **hair root** (HAYR ROOT) is that portion of the hair enclosed within the follicle beneath the skin surface. The **hair shaft** (HAYR SHAFT) is the portion of the hair we see extending above the skin surface.

STRUCTURES OF THE HAIR ROOT

The main structures of the hair root are the follicle, bulb, dermal papilla, sebaceous glands, and arrector pili muscle (**Figure 10-1**).

The hair **follicle** (FAWL-ih-kul) is the tubelike depression or pocket in the skin or scalp that contains the hair root. Hair follicles are distributed all over the body, with the exception of the palms of the hands and the soles of the feet. The follicle extends downward from the epidermis into the dermis, where it surrounds the dermal papilla. Follicles vary in depth, depending on the thickness and location of the skin. Sometimes, more than one hair will grow from a single follicle. The funnel-shaped mouths of hair follicles make this area breeding places for germs and the accumulation of sebum and dirt. Proper shampooing and rinsing procedures help to minimize the occurrence of scalp and hair disorders caused by the germs and dirt.

The **hair bulb** (HAYR BULB) is club-shaped structure that forms the lower part of the hair root and is the lowest part of the hair strand. The lower part of the hair bulb is hollow and fits over and covers the dermal papilla.

The **dermal papilla** (DUR-mul puh-PIL-uh) is a small, cone-shaped elevation at the base of the hair follicle that fits into the hair bulb. The dermal papilla contains the blood and nerve supply that provides the nutrients needed for hair growth, because of that some people refer to the dermal papilla as the *mother* of the hair.

The sebaceous glands consist of small, saclike structures with ducts that are attached to each hair follicle. They secrete an oily substance called *sebum* that lubricates the skin. Some of the factors that influence sebum production are subject to personal control. These factors are diet, blood circulation, emotional disturbance, stimulation of the endocrine glands, and certain drugs.

- *Diet* influences the general health of the hair. Overindulgence in sweet, starchy, and fatty foods may cause the sebaceous glands to become overactive and to secrete too much sebum, which can cause an oily scalp condition.

- *Blood circulation* is a factor because the hair and scalp derive their nourishment from the blood supplied to them; in turn, proper blood supply depends upon the nutrients derived from the foods eaten.

- *Emotional disturbances* are linked to the health of the hair through the nervous system. The hair's condition is affected by stress.

- *Endocrine glands* are ductless glands. Their secretions go directly into the bloodstream, which in turn influences the welfare of the entire body. The condition of the endocrine glands influences their secretion. During adolescence, endocrine glands are very active; after middle age, their activity usually decreases. Endocrine gland disturbances influence the hair as well as other aspects of health.

- *Medication*, such as hormones, may adversely affect the hair.

The **arrector pili** (ah-REK-tohr PY-leh) is a minute, involuntary muscle fiber in the skin attached to the base of the hair follicle. Strong emotions or cold causes it to contract, which makes the hair stand up straight, resulting in *goose bumps*.

STRUCTURES OF THE HAIR SHAFT

The three main layers of the hair shaft are the cuticle, cortex, and medulla (**Figure 10-2**). The hair **cuticle** (KYOO-tih-kul) is the outermost layer of the hair. It consists of a single overlapping layer of transparent, scalelike cells that look like shingles on a roof.

figure 10-2
Cross section of hair cuticle.

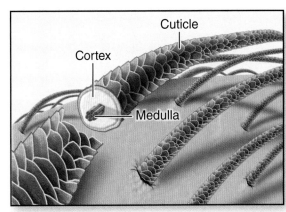

figure 10-3
Hair cuticle layer.

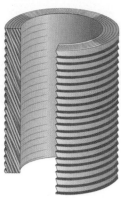

figure 10-4
Hair shaft with part of the hair cuticle stripped off, exposing the cortex.

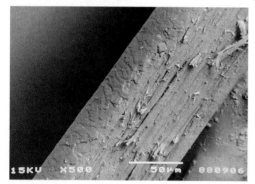

The cuticle layer provides a barrier that protects the inner structure of the hair as it lies tightly against the cortex. These scales can be felt by holding a strand of hair between the thumb and forefinger of one hand while moving the thumb and fingers of the other hand down the hair strand from its end to the scalp. The hair feels rough when you move from its end to the scalp because you are going against the cuticle layer. A healthy, compact cuticle layer is the hair's primary defense against damage and protects the inner structure of the hair; it is also responsible for the shine and silkiness of the hair. Conversely, heat and certain chemical solutions can raise the scales of the cuticle layer to allow for penetration and absorption of substances into the cortex.

A cross section of hair shows that although the cuticle scales overlap, each individual cuticle scale is attached to the cortex, thereby creating only one cuticle layer (Figure 10-3). Swelling the hair with high-pH products, such as oxidation tints, permanent waving solutions, or chemical hair relaxers, raises the cuticle layer and opens the spaces between the scales, allowing liquids to penetrate into the cortex.

The **cortex** (KOR-teks) is the middle layer of the hair. It is a fibrous protein core formed by elongated cells that contain melanin pigment. About 90 percent of the total weight of the hair comes from the cortex. Its unique protein structure provides strength, elasticity, and natural color to the hair. The changes that take place in the hair during chemical services occur within the cortex (Figure 10-4).

The **medulla** (muh-DUL-uh) is the innermost layer of the hair and is composed of round cells. Although mature male beard hair contains a medulla, this layer of the hair may be absent in very fine and naturally blond hair.

Photography: Courtesy of P&G Beauty, from the World of Hair by John Gray.

Learn about the Chemical Composition of Hair

After reading this section, you will be able to:

LO**3**   Identify and explain the three types of side bonds of the cortex.

Hair is composed of protein that grows from cells that originate within the hair follicle. This is where the hair shaft begins. When these living cells form, they begin a journey upward through the follicle, where they mature through a process called **keratinization** (kair-uh-ti-ni-ZAY-shun). As the newly formed cells mature, they fill up with a fibrous protein called *keratin*, move upward, lose their nuclei, and die. By the time the hair shaft emerges from the scalp, the cells are completely keratinized and no longer living. The hair shaft that we see is a nonliving fiber composed of keratinized protein.

Human hair is approximately 90 percent protein. Protein is made of chemical units called **amino acids** (uh-MEE-noh AS-udz) and amino acids are made of elements. The essential elements in the human hair are carbon, oxygen, hydrogen, nitrogen, and sulfur, often referred to as the *COHNS elements* (KOH-nz EL-uh-mentz). These elements are also found in skin and nails. Table 10-1 shows the percentage of each element in a typical strand of hair; this chemical composition, however, varies with color.

table 10-1
THE COHNS ELEMENTS

Element	Percentage in Normal Hair
Carbon	51
Oxygen	21
Hydrogen	6
Nitrogen	17
Sulfur	5

Proteins are made of long chains of amino acids. These amino acids are joined end to end in a definite order by chemical bonds known as **peptide bonds** (PEP-tyd BAHNDZ) or **end bonds** (END BAHNDZ). A long chain of amino acids linked by peptide bonds is called a **polypeptide chain** (pahl-ee-PEP-tyd CHAYN). **Proteins** (PROH-teenz) are long, coiled complex polypeptides made of amino acids. The spiral shape of a coiled protein is called a **helix** (HEE-licks), which is created when the polypeptide chains intertwine with each other (Figure 10-5).

SIDE BONDS OF THE HAIR CORTEX

Within the hair cortex, a more complex structure is formed when millions of polypeptide chains are cross-linked by **side bonds** (SYD BAHNDZ) (formerly known as *cross-bonds*), to form a ladderlike structure (Figure 10-6). Side bonds are of three types, consisting of hydrogen, salt, and disulfide bonds, which account for the strength and elasticity of human hair. These bonds play a critical role in the blowdrying, wet setting, thermal styling, and chemical processes. Table 10-2 summarizes the properties of the types of bonds found within the protein structure of hair.

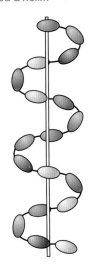

figure 10-5
Polypeptide chains intertwine in a spiral shape called a *helix*.

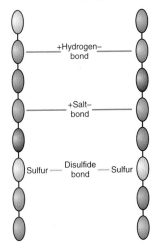

figure 10-6
Side bonds between polypeptide chains.

+Hydrogen–bond
+Salt–bond
Sulfur — Disulfide bond — Sulfur

table 10-2
BONDS OF THE HAIR

Bond	Type	Strength	Broken By	Re-formed By
Hydrogen	Side bond	Weak, physical	Water or heat	Drying or cooling
Salt	Side bond	Weak, physical	Changes in pH	Normalizing pH
Disulfide	Side bond	Strong, chemical	Thio perms and thio relaxers	Oxidation with neutralizer
			Hydroxide relaxers	Cannot be re-formed; water converts broken disulfide bonds to lanthionine bonds
			Extreme heat	Cannot be re-formed; water converts broken disulfide bonds to lanthionine bonds
Peptide	End bond	Strong, chemical	Chemical depilatories or cutting	Cannot be re-formed; hair dissolves

A **hydrogen bond** (HY-druh-jun BAHND) is a weak, physical, cross-link side bond that is easily broken by water or heat. Although individual hydrogen bonds are weak, they are so numerous in the hair that they account for about one-third of the hair's overall strength. Hydrogen bonds are broken when hair gets wet (**Figure 10-7**), which allows the hair to be stretched. The hydrogen bonds re-form when the hair dries, which explains how blowdrying techniques work when the barber works with a comb or brush to style the hair into place while drying.

A **salt bond** (SAWLT BAHND) is a weak, physical side bond, which cross-links the polypeptide chains, but reacts to changes in pH. Salt bonds depend on pH and are easily broken by strong acidic or alkaline solutions (**Figure 10-8**). Although weak, salt bonds are numerous and account for another one-third of the hair's total strength.

A **disulfide bond** (dy-SUL-fyed BAHND), also known as a *sulfur bond*, is a strong covalent bond that is different from the physical side bond of hydrogen or salt bonds. Disulfide bonds join the sulfur atoms of two neighboring **cysteine** (SIS-tuh-een) amino acids to create one *cystine* (SIS-teen). The cystine joins together two polypeptide strands. Although there are fewer disulfide bonds in the hair, they are stronger than hydrogen or salt bonds and account for the final third of the hair's total strength. Unlike hydrogen and salt bonds, disulfide bonds are not broken by heat or water—they are broken by permanent waves and chemical relaxers that alter the shape of hair. Normal amounts of heat, such as those used for normal thermal styling, do not break disulfide bonds. However, extremely high heat, such as that from a very hot flat iron, can break the disulfide bond. Thioglycolate permanent waves break disulfide bonds, which are then

figure 10-7
Changes in hair cortex during wet setting.

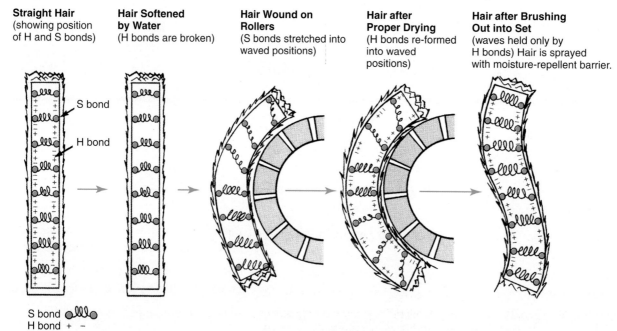

Straight Hair
(showing position of H and S bonds)

Hair Softened by Water
(H bonds are broken)

Hair Wound on Rollers
(S bonds stretched into waved positions)

Hair after Proper Drying
(H bonds re-formed into waved positions)

Hair after Brushing Out into Set
(waves held only by H bonds) Hair is sprayed with moisture-repellent barrier.

S bond
H bond + −

figure 10-8
Changes in hair cortex during permanent waving.

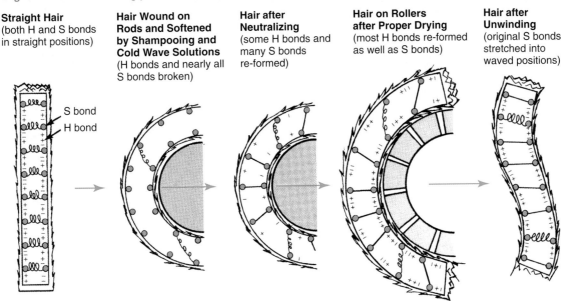

| **Straight Hair** (both H and S bonds in straight positions) | **Hair Wound on Rods and Softened by Shampooing and Cold Wave Solutions** (H bonds and nearly all S bonds broken) | **Hair after Neutralizing** (some H bonds and many S bonds re-formed) | **Hair on Rollers after Proper Drying** (most H bonds re-formed as well as S bonds) | **Hair after Unwinding** (original S bonds stretched into waved positions) |

re-formed with neutralizers. Hydroxide chemical hair relaxers also break disulfide bonds, which are then converted to lanthionine bonds when the relaxer is rinsed from the hair. Disulfide bonds broken by hydroxide relaxers are permanently broken and cannot be re-formed. The more disulfide bonds in the hair, the more resistant it will be to chemical processes.

HAIR PIGMENT

Natural hair color is the result of the melanin pigment found within the cortex. **Melanin** are the tiny grains of pigment in the cortex that give natural color to the hair. There are two types of melanin:

* **Eumelanin** (yoo-MEL-uh-nin) provides brown and black color to hair.

* **Pheomelanin** (fee-oh-MEL-uh-nin) provides natural hair colors that range from red and ginger to yellow and light blond tones.

All natural color is dependent on the ratio of eumelanin to pheomelanin, along with the total number and size of the pigment granules. Gray hair contains only a few scattered melanin granules and white hair contains no melanin.

WAVE PATTERN

The **wave pattern** (WAYV PAT-URN) of hair refers to the shape of the hair strand and is described as straight, wavy, curly, and extremely curly (Figure 10-9).

Natural wave patterns are the result of genetics. Although there are many exceptions, as a general rule, Asians and Native Americans tend to have extremely straight hair, Caucasians tend to have straight, wavy, or curly hair, and African Americans tend to have extremely curly hair.

figure 10-9
Straight, wavy, curly, and extremely curly hair strands.

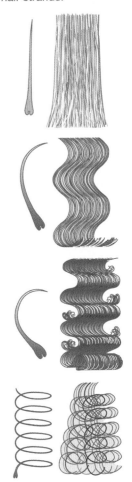

Basis of Hair Color and Texture

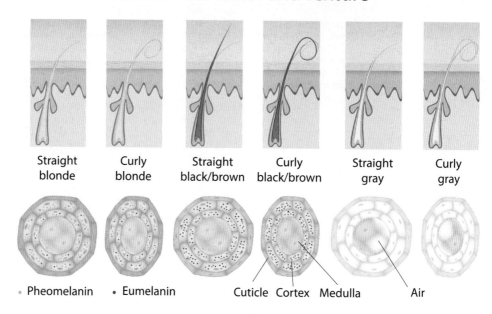

figure 10-10
Individuals with curly hair often have straighter hair in the crown and tighter curls in other areas.

Straight blonde   Curly blonde   Straight black/brown   Curly black/brown   Straight gray   Curly gray

• Pheomelanin   • Eumelanin   Cuticle   Cortex   Medulla   Air

© Alia Medical Media/Shutterstock.com.

But straight, wavy, curly, and extremely curly hairs occur in all races—anyone of any race, or mixed race, can have hair with varying degrees of curl from straight to extremely curly. The wave pattern may also vary from strand to strand on the same person's head. It is not uncommon for an individual to have different amounts of curl in different areas of the head. Individuals with curly hair often have straighter hair in the crown and tighter curls in other areas (**Figure 10-10**).

Several theories attempt to explain the cause of natural curly hair, but there is no single, definite answer that explains why some hair grows straight and other hair grows curly. The most popular theory claims that the shape of the hair's cross section determines the amount of curl. This theory claims that hair with a round cross section is straight, hair with an oval-to-flattened oval cross section is wavy or curly, and hair with a flattened-to-flattened oval cross section is extremely curly (**Table 10-3**).

table 10-3
WAVE PATTERN AND CROSS SECTIONS

	Wave Pattern	Shape of Cross Section
⬤	Straight Hair	Round cross section
⬤	Wavy or Curly Hair	Oval to round cross section
⬤	Extremely Curly Hair	Elliptical cross section

EXTREMELY CURLY HAIR

Extremely curly hair grows in long twisted spirals. Cross sections appear flattened and vary in shape and thickness along their length. Compared to straight or wavy hair, which tends to possess a fairly regular and uniform diameter along a single strand, extremely curly hair is of fairly irregular thickness, showing varying diameters along a single strand. Some extremely curly hair have a natural tendency to form a coil like a telephone cord. Coiled hair usually has a fine texture, with many individual strands winding together to form the coiled locks. Extremely curly hair often has low elasticity, breaks easily, and has a tendency to knot, especially on the ends. Gentle scalp manipulations, conditioning shampoo, and a detangling rinse help minimize tangles.

Discuss Hair Growth

After reading this section, you will be able to:

LO❹ Name and describe the three phases of the hair growth cycle.

The two main types of hair are vellus hair and terminal hair (Figure 10-11).

- **Vellus hair** (VEL-us HAYR), or **lanugo** (luh-NOO-goh) hair, is the short, fine, unpigmented, downy hair. It almost never has a medulla or melanin and helps in the efficient evaporation of perspiration. In adults, vellus hair is found in places normally considered hairless (forehead, eyelids, and bald scalp).

- **Terminal hair** (TUR-mih-nul HAYR) is the long, coarse hair found on the scalp, legs, arms, and bodies of males and females. Hormonal changes during puberty cause some areas of fine vellus hair to be replaced with thicker terminal hair. All hair follicles are capable of producing either vellus or terminal hair, depending on genetics, age, and hormones. In occurrences of male pattern baldness, the follicles stop making terminal hair and revert back to producing the vellus type.

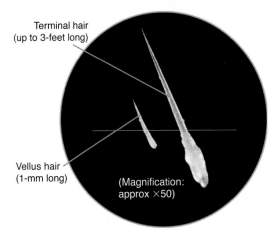

figure 10-11
Vellus hair and terminal hair.

Terminal hair
(up to 3-feet long)

Vellus hair
(1-mm long)

(Magnification:
approx ×50)

Pfizer Inc.

GROWTH CYCLES OF HAIR

The average growth rate of healthy hair on the scalp is about ½ (0.5) inch per month. The rate of growth will differ over specific parts of the body, between sexes, among races, and with age. The growth of scalp hair occurs more rapidly between the ages of 15 and 30 and declines sharply between 50 and 60. Hair growth is also influenced by such factors as the seasons of the year, nutrition, and hormonal changes within the body.

In normal, healthy hair, hair growth occurs in cycles. Each complete cycle has three phases that are repeated over and over throughout life. These three phases are known as the *anagen, catagen,* and *telogen phases.*

Anagen: The Growth Phase

During the **anagen phase** (AN-uh-jen FAYZ), or *growth phase*, new hair is produced. New cells are manufactured in the hair follicle. During this phase, hair cells are produced faster than any other normal cell in the body. About 90 percent of scalp hair is in the anagen phase—that is, growing—at any given time. The anagen phase generally lasts from 3 to 5 years, but can last as long as 10 years. The anagen phase determines how long the hair will grow before shedding; therefore, the longer the anagen phase is, the longer the hair can grow. This explains why some people can grow their hair to extremely long lengths and others cannot.

Catagen: The Transition Phase

The **catagen phase** (KAT-uh-jen FAYZ) is a transition period between the growth and resting phases of a hair strand. During the catagen phase the follicle shrinks, the hair bulb disappears, and the shrunken root end forms a rounded club. The catagen phase lasts from 1 to 2 weeks. Less than 1 percent of the hair is in the catagen phase at any given time.

Telogen: The Resting Phase

The **telogen phase** (TEL-uh-jen FAYZ), or *resting phase*, is the final phase of the hair growth cycle. The hair either sheds during this phase or remains in place until it is pushed out by the growth of a new hair in the next anagen phase. Less than 10 percent of scalp hair is in the telogen phase at any given time. The telogen phase lasts for approximately 3 to 6 months or until the hair is shed. As soon as the telogen phase ends, new hair in the anagen phase begins the cycle again. On average, the entire growth process repeats itself once every 4 or 5 years.

Hair growth is not increased by shaving, trimming, cutting, singeing, or the application of ointments or oils. Hair growth is also not stimulated by scalp massage, although it does increase blood flow and relax the nerves of the scalp. Minoxidil and finasteride are the only treatments that have been scientifically proven to increase hair growth and are approved for that purpose by the Food and Drug Administration (FDA). Products that claim to increase hair growth are regulated as drugs and are not cosmetics.

NORMAL HAIR SHEDDING

It is normal to lose an average of 75 to 100 hairs per day. This shedding process makes room for new hair that is in the process of growing. Hair loss beyond this estimated average indicates some problem. Eyebrow hairs and eyelashes are replaced every 4 to 5 months.

GROWTH PATTERNS

It is important when cutting and styling hair to consider the hair's natural growth patterns. Doing so will produce a more natural-looking haircut and a style that the client will have less trouble duplicating for everyday wear. Growth patterns that result in creating hair streams, whorls, and cowlicks are determined by the angle at which the hair emerges from the hair follicle.

- A **hair stream** (HAYR STREEM) is hair that flows in the same direction. It is the result of follicles being arranged and sloping in a uniform manner. When two such streams slope in opposite directions, they form a natural part in the hair.
- A **whorl** (WHORL) is hair that grows in a circular or swirl pattern. Whorls are most often seen at the crown.
- A **cowlick** (KOW-lik) is a tuft of hair that stands straight up. Cowlicks are usually more noticeable at the front hairline, but they may be located anywhere on the scalp. Styles should be chosen to minimize the upright effects of cowlicks.

MYTHS AND FACTS ABOUT HAIR GROWTH

As a barber, you may hear opinions about hair growth from your clients or from other professionals. Here are some myths and facts about hair growth:

Myth. Shaving, clipping, and cutting the hair on the head makes it grow back faster, darker, and coarser.

Fact. Although it may *seem* to grow back faster, darker, and coarser, shaving or cutting the hair on the head has no effect on hair growth. When hair is blunt cut to the same length, it may grow back more evenly.

Myth. Scalp massage increases hair growth.

Fact. Scalp massages are very stimulating to the scalp and can increase blood circulation, relax the nerves in the scalp, and tighten the scalp muscles. However, it has not been scientifically proven that any type of stimulation or scalp massage increases hair growth.

Myth. Gray hair is coarser and more resistant than pigmented hair.

Fact. Other than the lack of pigment, gray hair is exactly the same as pigmented hair. Although gray hair may be resistant, it is not resistant simply because it is gray. Pigmented hair on the same person's head is just as resistant as the gray hair. Gray hair is simply more noticeable than pigmented hair.

Myth. The amount of natural curl is always determined by racial background.

Fact. Anyone of any race, or mixed race, can have hair from straight to extremely curly. It is also true that within races, individuals have hair with varying degrees of curl in different areas of the head.

Understand Hair Loss

After reading this section, you will be able to:

LO **5** Identify and define seven types of hair loss.

LO **6** Identify and describe two FDA-approved treatments for hair loss.

We all lose some hair every day as a result of the normal shedding that takes place during the hair's natural growth and replacement cycle. A hair that is shed in the telogen phase is replaced by a new hair, in that same follicle, in the next anagen phase. This natural shedding of hair accounts for normal daily hair loss, which averages 75 to 100 hairs per day.

THE EMOTIONAL IMPACT OF HAIR LOSS

Although the medical community does not always recognize hair loss as a medical condition, the anguish felt by those who suffer abnormal hair loss is very real and often overlooked. Results from a study that investigated perceptions of bald and balding men showed that compared to men with hair, bald men were perceived as

- less physically attractive (by both sexes);
- less assertive;
- less successful;
- less personally likeable;
- older than their actual age (average 5 years).

Over 63 million men and women in the United States suffer from abnormal hair loss. As a professional barber, it is likely that you will be the first person that a hair loss sufferer confides in, so it is important that you have a basic understanding of the different types of hair loss and the services that are available.

IDENTIFY TYPES OF ABNORMAL HAIR LOSS

Abnormal hair loss is called **alopecia** (al-oh-PEE-shah). Understandably, hair loss for either sex can be a traumatic experience, so conversations about it should be handled tactfully. Alopecia may appear in different forms as a result of a variety of abnormal conditions. These forms include androgenic alopecia, alopecia prematura, alopecia areata, alopecia totalis, alopecia universalis, alopecia senilis, and alopecia syphilitica.

Androgenic alopecia (an-druh-JEN-ik al-oh-PEE-shah) is hair loss that occurs as a result of genetics, age, and hormonal changes that cause the miniaturization of terminal hair, converting it to vellus hair (**Figure 10-12**).

Androgenic alopecia can begin as early as in the teens (**alopecia prematura** ([al-oh-PEE-shah pree-muh-TOO-ruh]) and is frequently seen by the age of 40. Almost 40 percent of men and women show some degree of hair loss by age 35. In men, androgenic alopecia is known as *male pattern baldness* and usually progresses to the familiar horseshoe-shaped fringe of hair (Figure 10-13).

Alopecia areata (al-oh-PEE-shah ay-reh-AH-tuh) is an autoimmune disorder that causes the affected hair follicles to be mistakenly attacked by the person's own immune system, which stops hair growth at the anagen phase. It is characterized by the sudden falling out of hair in round patches, which creates bald spots, and can progress to total scalp hair loss,

figure 10-12
Miniaturization of the hair follicle.

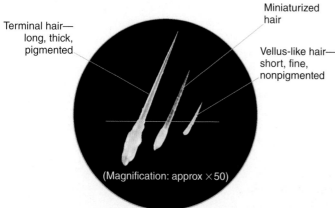

Terminal hair— long, thick, pigmented

Miniaturized hair

Vellus-like hair— short, fine, nonpigmented

(Magnification: approx ×50)

Pfizer Inc.

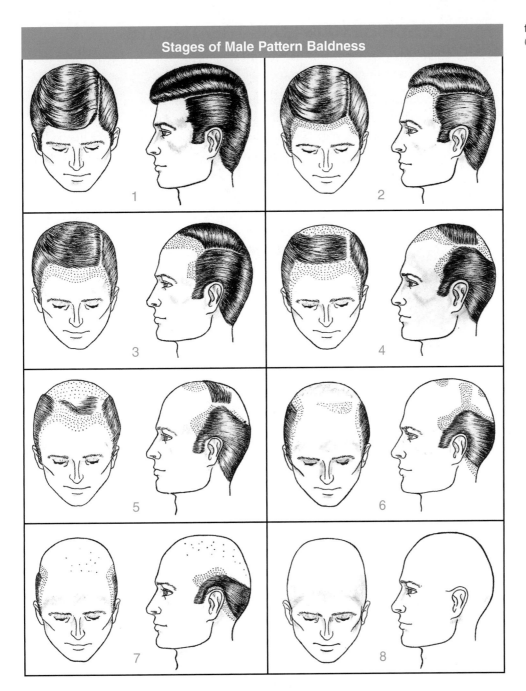

Stages of Male Pattern Baldness

Gradual balding process.

known as **alopecia totalis** (al-oh-PEE-shah toe-TAL-is), or complete body hair loss, called **alopecia universalis** (al-oh-PEE-shah yoo-nih-vur-SAA-lis). It is a highly unpredictable skin disease that may occur on the scalp and elsewhere on the body. Clients who exhibit symptoms of alopecia areata should be referred to a physician. **Alopecia senilis** (al-oh-PEE-shah seh-NIL-is) is the normal loss of scalp hair occurring in old age and is permanent. **Alopecia syphilitica** (al-oh-PEE-shah sif-il-IT-ih-kuh) is caused by syphilis. The non-inflamed bald areas look molted or moth-eaten, and the disease may also affect the beard and eyebrow areas. The hair usually grows back once the disease is cured.

DESCRIBE HAIR LOSS TREATMENTS

The only FDA-approved hair loss treatments, which have been proven to stimulate hair growth, are minoxidil and finasteride.

- *Minoxidil* is a topical treatment that has been proven to stimulate hair growth. Applied to the scalp twice a day, it is sold over the counter as a nonprescription drug under the brand names Rogaine and Theroxidil. Minoxidil is available for both men and women. It is available in two strengths: 2 percent (regular) and 5 percent (extra strength). It is not known to have any negative side effects.

- *Finasteride* is an oral prescription medication for men, sold under the brand name Propecia, and is for use only by men. This drug is extremely effective in slowing the rate of hair loss and can even grow new hair; however, once you stop using the drug all the hair loss returns. Although finasteride is considered more effective and convenient than minoxidil, side effects are possible, which include weight gain and loss of sexual function.

In addition to the medicinal treatments described above, there are also several surgical options available. A hair transplant is the most common *permanent* hair replacement technique. The process consists of removing small sections of hair that include the follicle, papilla, and bulb from areas of thick hair growth and transplanting them into the bald area. Only licensed surgeons may perform this procedure and several surgeries are usually necessary to achieve the desired results. The cost of each surgery ranges from about $8,000 to over $20,000.

With proper training, barbers can offer several nonmedical options to camouflage hair loss. These include hair replacement systems, wigs, hair weaves, and hair extensions (see Chapter 15).

Recognize Disorders of the Hair and Scalp

After reading this section, you will be able to:

LO**7** Identify and define common hair disorders.

LO**8** Define common scalp disorders and identify those requiring medical attention.

RECOGNIZE DISORDERS OF THE HAIR

Hair disorders are noncontagious conditions that include disorders such as canities, hypertrichosis, trichoptilosis, trichorrhexis nodosa, monilethrix, and fragilitas crinium.

- **Canities** (kah-NISH-ee-eez) is the technical term for gray hair. Congenital canities exists at or before birth and generally is part of a disorder known as *albinism* (albino) that affects all pigment throughout the body. Acquired canities develops with age and is the result of genetics.

- Ringed hair is a variation of canities, characterized by alternating bands of gray and pigmented hair throughout the length of the hair strand.

- **Hypertrichosis** (hy-pur-trih-KOH-sis), also known as *hirsuties* (hur-SOO-teez) is a condition of abnormal growth of hair. It is characterized by the growth of terminal hair on areas of the body that are normally covered with only vellus hair.

- **Trichoptilosis** (trih-kahp-tih-LOH-sus) is the technical term for split ends. Hair conditioning and oils will smooth split ends, but the only way to remove them is to cut them.

- **Trichorrhexis nodosa** (trik-uh-REK-sis nuh-DOH-suh) is the technical term for knotted hair. It is characterized by brittleness and nodular swellings along the hair shaft. Treatments include softening the hair with conditioners and moisturizers.

- **Monilethrix** (mah-NIL-ee-thriks) is the technical term for beaded hair. The hair breaks easily between the beads or nodes. Treatments include hair and scalp conditioning.

- **Fragilitas crinium** (fruh-JIL-ih-tus KRY-nee-um) is the technical term for brittle hair. The hairs may split at any point along their length. Treatments include hair and scalp conditioning and haircutting above the split to prevent further damage.

IDENTIFY DISORDERS OF THE SCALP

The skin of the scalp is constantly renewing itself, just as skin does on all parts of the body. Problems with the skin of the scalp can range from irritating and embarrassing to painful and dangerous.

RECOGNIZE TYPES OF DANDRUFF

Pityriasis (pit-ih-RY-uh-sus) is the technical term for dandruff, which is characterized by the excessive production and accumulation of skin cells. Instead of the normal, one-at-a-time shedding of tiny individual skin cells, dandruff is the shedding of an accumulation of large, visible clumps of skin cells. It can be easily mistaken for dry scalp because the symptoms of both conditions are a flaky, itchy, irritated scalp, but a dry scalp does not have the oily scalp that is common to dandruff. An unhealthy scalp—due to poor blood circulation, infection, injury, improper diet, or poor personal hygiene—can contribute to this accumulation, as can the use of strong shampoos and/or insufficient rinsing of the hair. Although the cause of dandruff has been debated for over 150 years, current research confirms that dandruff is the result of a fungus called **malassezia** (mal-uh-SEEZ-ee-uh), formerly named pityrosporum. Malassezia is a naturally occurring fungus that is present on all human skin, but develops the symptoms of dandruff when it grows out of control. Factors including stress, age, hormones, and hygiene can cause the fungus to multiply and dandruff symptoms to worsen. Antidandruff shampoos containing antifungal ingredients such as pyrithione zinc, selenium sulfide, or ketoconazole help control dandruff by suppressing the growth of malassezia.

figure 10-14
Pityriasis capitis simplex, commonly known as dandruff.

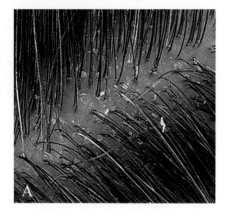

figure 10-15
Pityriasis steatoides.

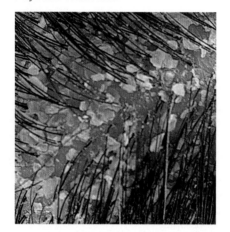

figure 10-16
Tinea capitis.

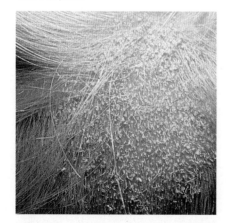

The two principal types of dandruff are pityriasis capitis simplex and pityriasis steatoides.

- **Pityriasis capitis simplex** (pit-ih-RY-uh-sus KAP-ih-tus SIM-pleks) is the technical term for classic dandruff, characterized by scalp irritation, large flakes, and an itchy scalp (**Figure 10-14**). The scales may be attached to the scalp in masses or scattered loosely throughout the hair. Topical treatments for controlling dandruff include the use of antidandruff shampoos, scalp massage and treatments, and medicated scalp ointments.

- **Pityriasis steatoides** (pit-ih-RY-uh-sus stee-uh-TOY-deez) is a more severe form of dandruff that is characterized by an accumulation of greasy or waxy scales mixed with sebum (**Figure 10-15**). This excessive shedding mixed with sebum causes the scales to adhere to the scalp in patches, where they can cause itching and irritation. When this condition is accompanied by redness and inflammation, it is called *seborrheic dermatitis*, which can also be found on the eyebrows and beard. You should not perform a service on anyone who has dandruff, as the scalp is irritated and itchy. Antidandruff shampoos can be recommended to a client with mild conditions, but severe cases should be referred to a physician.

At one time, dandruff was thought to be contagious; however, current research has determined that it is not. Regardless of whether or not dandruff is contagious, barbers are prohibited by state barber board rules to use their tools and implements on more than one client without first disinfecting the items. Barbers must always practice approved cleaning and disinfection procedures in the barbershop before and after each client service. It is also advisable to wear gloves when shampooing a client with a dandruff condition.

IDENTIFY FUNGAL INFECTIONS: TINEA

Tinea (TIN-ee-uh) is the medical term for ringworm. Ringworm is caused by fungal organisms and is characterized by itching, scales, and, sometimes, painful circular lesions. It usually starts with a small, reddened patch of little blisters that spreads outward and then heals in the middle, with a scalelike appearance. If the ringworm has spread, several patches may be present at one time.

All forms of tinea are highly contagious. Infected skin scales or hair containing the fungi are known to spread the disease; public showers, swimming pools, and unclean personal articles (such as brushes) are also sources of transmission. Practicing approved cleaning and disinfection procedures will help prevent the spread of ringworm in the barbershop. Clients with suspected or confirmed tinea should be referred to a physician for medical treatment and must not receive services in the barbershop until the condition has cleared.

- **Tinea capitis** (TIN-ee-uh KAP-ih-tus) is commonly known as *ringworm* of the scalp (**Figure 10-16**). It is characterized by red papules or spots at the openings of the hair follicles. As the patches spread, the hair becomes brittle and lifeless and breaks off, leaving a stump, or falls from the enlarged, open follicles.

- **Tinea barbae** (TIN-ee-uh BAR-bee) is a superficial fungal infection caused by dermatophytes occurring chiefly over the bearded area of the face (**Figure 10-17**). Beginning as small, round, slightly scaly, inflamed patches, the areas enlarge, clearing up somewhat at the center with elevation at the borders. As the parasites invade the hairs and follicles, hard, lumpy swellings develop. In severe cases, pustules form around the hair follicles and rupture, forming crusts. In the later stage, the hairs become dry, break off, and fall out or are readily extracted. Tinea barbea is highly contagious and medical treatment is required.

- **Tinea favosa** (TIN-ee-uh fah-VOH-suh) is also known as *tinea favus* (TIN-ee-uh FAY-vus) or *honeycomb ringworm*. It is characterized by dry, sulfur-yellow, cuplike crusts on the scalp having a peculiar, musty odor—these are called **scutula** (SKUT-yoo-lah). Scars from favus are bald patches that are pink or white and shiny. Tinea favosa is very contagious and should be referred to a physician.

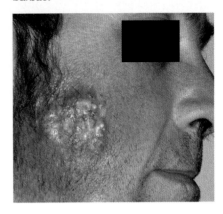

figure 10-17
Folliculitis barbae or tinea (ringworm) barbae.

RECOGNIZE PARASITIC INFESTATIONS

The two most common parasitic infestations barbers may see in the barbershop are pediculosis capitis and scabies.

- **Pediculosis capitis** (puh-dik-yuh-LOH-sis KAP-ih-tus) is the infestation of the hair and scalp with head lice (**Figure 10-18**). The parasites feed on the scalp and cause severe itching. You can distinguish head lice from dandruff or other conditions by looking at the scalp and hair closely—with a magnifying glass if necessary. The scalp usually appears reddened from scratching, and you should be able to see mature lice moving through the hair. The nits, or eggs, attach to individual hair strands and are difficult to remove without a special comb made for that purpose. The nits can also withstand some products used to treat the infestation, so repeat applications of the preparation is usually required. Commercially prepared products for the treatment of head lice are sold over the counter and are readily available at most drug stores.

    The head louse is transmitted from one person to another by contact with infested hats, combs, brushes, and other personal items; so following proper cleaning and disinfection procedures is extremely important.

    Head lice are tenacious creatures that can live away from the human body for up to 48 hours, so it is equally important to disinfect all household and personal items to avoid reinfestation. Occurrences of head lice must not be treated in the barbershop, and the client should be referred to a physician or pharmacist.

- *Scabies* is a highly contagious skin disease caused by mites that burrow under the skin. Vesicles and pustules usually form from the irritation caused by the parasites or from scratching the affected areas (**Figure 10-19**). Excessive itching is a characteristic of scabies and can lead to infections of the affected area. A client with this condition should be referred to a physician. As with all disorders and diseases, the practice of approved cleaning and disinfection procedures will help to limit the spread of scabies.

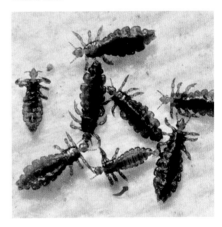

figure 10-18
Head lice.

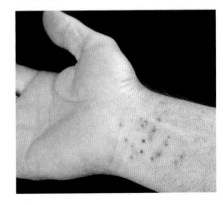

figure 10-19
Scabies.

www.dermnet.com.

Courtesy of the National Pediculosis Association,® Inc.

RECOGNIZE BACTERIAL INFECTIONS

Barbers may also encounter bacterial staphylococci infections in the barbershop in the form of different types of folliculitis. Folliculitis can occur anywhere on the body as a result of bacterial or viral infection and is characterized by the inflammation or infection of one or more hair follicles. Some of its more common forms are folliculitis barbae, pseudofolliculitis barbae, sycosis vulgaris, furuncles, and carbuncles.

Folliculitis barbae and *pseudofolliculitis barbae* are inflammations of the follicle caused by bacterial or viral infection, irritation, or ingrown hairs. The cause of the inflammation is what differentiates the two conditions, but both can be triggered from damaged follicles caused by friction, blockages, or improper shaving methods, for example, close shaving, too much pressure, dull blades, dirty blades, or shaving against the grain.

Folliculitis barbae (fah-lik-yuh-LY-tis BAR-bee), or barber's itch, is an infection of the hair follicles characterized by inflamed pustules in the bearded areas of the face and neck that may have hairs growing through the pustule.

- Staphylococcus bacteria most often cause the infection; however, a herpes simplex virus can spread to other hair follicles during shaving, resulting in similar pustule formation and infection.

- Treatments include topical or oral antibiotics as prescribed by a physician.

Pseudofolliculitis barbae (SUE-doe-fah-lik-yuh-LY-tis BAR-bee), also referred to as *razor bumps*, is a chronic inflammatory condition that resembles folliculitis in terms of papules and pustules, but is generally accepted to be caused by ingrown hair. The disorder is most often seen in men and women of Mediterranean, African, Hispanic, and Jewish ethnicity, but can occur to anyone with any type of hair texture.

- Pseudofolliculitis barbae can be caused by improper shaving or by broken hair below the skin surface that grows into the side of the follicle, causing irritation and swelling that cuts off oxygen to the bottom of the follicle. Bacteria then have a perfect environment for growth, which can lead to the development of pus and, if left untreated, folliculitis.

- Nonmedical treatments for pseudofolliculitis barbae include the use of proper shaving techniques, antibiotic or antifungal preparations, and the use of electric razors or razors designed to cut hair above the skin to minimize outbreaks and irritation. Clients should also be instructed to change razor blades frequently as dull, dirty blades also increase all types of folliculitis. Warm compresses and clear gel masks that soothe and heal may help to relieve symptoms.

With an understanding of folliculitis and pseudofolliculitis, barbers can help clients to determine if the condition is caused by chemical or mechanical means. Preparations that contain salicylic acid to break up impactions and kill bacteria are available for the prevention of ingrown hairs. Physicians may prescribe topical and oral antibiotics for more serious conditions. When mechanical causes, such as improper shaving, are the source of the condition, the barber can offer the client some instructions in proper shaving techniques.

Sycosis vulgaris (sy-KOH-sis vul-GAYR-is), also known as *sycosis barbae*, is a chronic bacterial infection involving the areas surrounding the follicles of the beard and mustache areas. It may be contracted through the use of contaminated towels or implements or by contact with public resting areas. The condition can be worsened by irritation caused by shaving or continual nasal discharge. The main lesions are papules and pustules pierced by hairs and crusts that form after eruption. The surrounding skin is tender, reddened, swollen, and itchy. Medical treatment is required and a client with this condition should be referred to a physician. This infection should not be confused with **tinea sycosis** (TIN-ee-uh sy-KOH-sis), which is due to ringworm fungus.

A **furuncle** (FYOO-rung-kul), or boil, is an acute bacterial infection of a hair follicle, producing constant pain. A furuncle is the result of an active inflammatory process limited to a definite area that subsequently produces a pustule perforated by a hair (**Figure 10-20**). A client with this condition should be referred to a physician.

A **carbuncle** (KAHR-bung-kul) is the result of an acute, deep-seated bacterial infection in the subcutaneous tissue. It appears similar to a furuncle, but is larger and should also be referred to a physician.

figure 10-20
Furuncle (boil).

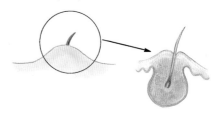

Learn How to Perform a Hair and Scalp Analysis

After reading this section, you will be able to:

LO**9** Identify the factors to be observed and considered during a hair and scalp analysis.

Barbering services include a variety of applications that benefit from a barber's ability to analyze the condition of a client's scalp and hair. In addition to wave and growth patterns, barbers should be able to analyze the hair's texture, density, porosity, and elasticity.

Knowledge and skill in performing a hair analysis can be acquired by observation and practice using the senses of sight, hearing, smell, and touch.

- **Sight.** Observation will impart some knowledge immediately, such as whether the hair looks dry or oily. Sight alone, however, will not provide an accurate judgment of the hair's quality.

- **Hearing.** Some clients will volunteer information about their hair, health problems, or experiences with products and medications. Since all of these factors are important when deciding how to treat the hair, it is advisable to listen carefully.

- **Smell.** Certain scalp disorders will create an odor. If the client is in general good health and the scalp is clean, the hair should be odor free.

- **Touch.** The sense of touch is key to analyzing hair condition and texture. This sense needs to be developed to its fullest capacity for the barber to provide truly professional services.

PERFORM A SCALP ANALYSIS

Always begin the analysis with checking the scalp first since any disorders or conditions found there could prohibit a service from being performed.

When analyzing the scalp, comb through the hair gently while parting it to check for hypertrophies, abrasions, and parasites; do not scrape the scalp.

- Do not begin any service if parasites are present.

- Do not proceed with chemical services if there are signs of irritation or abrasions.

- Hypertrophies, such as moles or warts, require extreme care when combing through the hair to avoid catching the comb on these abnormal skin growths. If you see changes in a hypertrophy from one client visit to another, suggest that your client see a physician. Barbers play a significant role in the early detection of many skin cancers, so any unusual-looking pigmentation or growth on the scalp should be referred to a physician.

PERFORM A HAIR ANALYSIS

Observe and consider hair texture, density, porosity, and elasticity when performing a hair analysis.

Hair texture (HAYR TEKS-chur) refers to the degree of coarseness or fineness of individual hair strands, which may vary on different parts of the head. Hair texture is measured by the diameter of the hair strand and is classified as coarse, medium, or fine.

- Coarse hair has the largest diameter and tends to be stronger than fine hair. It also has a stronger structure, which may require more processing or stronger products during chemical services than medium or fine hair. Generally, it is more difficult for hair lighteners, haircolors, waving solutions, and relaxing creams to penetrate coarse hair (Figure 10-21).

- Medium hair texture is the most common and is the standard to which other hair is compared. Medium hair is the hair texture that is considered normal and does not usually pose any special problems or concerns during a haircut (Figure 10-22).

- Fine hair has the smallest diameter and is generally more fragile, easier to process, and more susceptible to damage from chemical services than coarse or medium hair. Some fine or very fine hair does not possess a medulla, which helps to account for the smaller diameter of the strand (Figure 10-23).

figure 10-21
Coarse hair.

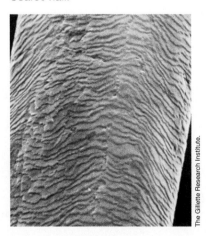

The Gillette Research Institute.

figure 10-22
Medium hair.

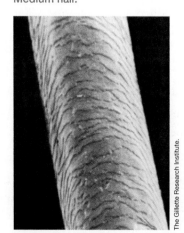

The Gillette Research Institute.

figure 10-23
Fine hair.

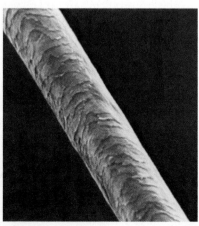

The Gillette Research Institute.

- Wiry hair, whether coarse, medium, or fine, has a hard, glassy finish because the cuticle scales lie flat against the hair shaft. It usually takes longer to give this type of hair a chemical service.

Testing for Hair Texture

Hair texture can be determined by feeling a single strand of dry hair between the fingers. Hold the strand securely with one hand while rolling it between the thumb and forefinger of the other hand. With practice, you will be able to feel the difference between coarse, medium, and fine hair textures (Figure 10-24).

HAIR DENSITY

Hair density (HAYR DEN-sih-tee) refers to the number of individual hair strands per square inch of scalp area and is classified as thick, average, or thin or as high, medium, or low density.

- Hair density is different from hair texture in that individuals with the same hair texture can have different densities or different amounts of hair per square inch. For example, one person may have thick, fine hair while another has thin, fine hair.

- The average hair density is approximately 2,200 strands per square inch, with the average head containing about 100,000 individual strands.

- The number of hairs on the head varies with the color of the hair—blonds usually have the highest density and redheads the least density per square inch (Table 10-4).

HAIR POROSITY

Hair porosity (HAYR puh-RAHS-ut-ee) is the ability of the hair to absorb moisture. The degree of porosity is directly related to the condition of the cuticle layer of the hair. A compact cuticle layer is naturally more resistant to penetration, whereas porous hair has a raised cuticle layer that easily absorbs water. The porosity level of hair can be classified as low porosity, average porosity, and high porosity or as resistant, normal, and overly porous.

- Hair that has moderate or average porosity is considered normal (Figure 10-25). This hair type presents no special problems and chemical applications usually process as expected.

- Hair that is classified as having low porosity is considered resistant (Figure 10-26). This hair type absorbs the least amount of moisture and may require a more alkaline solution than other hair types.

- Hair with a high porosity level is considered overly porous and is usually the result of previous overprocessing (Figure 10-27). Hair in this condition is dry, damaged, fragile, and brittle. Although overly porous hair may absorb liquids quickly, the damaged and open cuticle scales may make it difficult for the hair to retain haircoloring pigments or to react favorably to chemical texture services. Reconditioning treatments, the use of low-pH products, and strands tests are recommended prior to performing chemical services on hair in this condition.

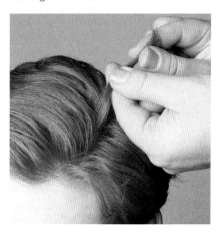
figure 10-24
Testing hair texture.

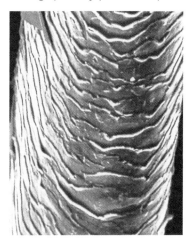
figure 10-25
Average porosity (normal hair).

table 10-4

AVERAGE NUMBER OF HAIRS ON THE HEAD BY HAIR COLOR

Hair Color	Average Number of Hairs on Head
Blond	140,000
Brown	110,000
Black	108,000
Red	80,000

figure 10-26
Low porosity (resistant hair).

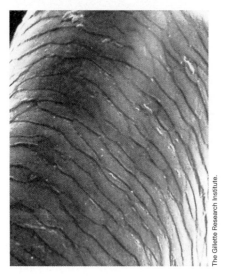

figure 10-27
High porosity (overly porous hair).

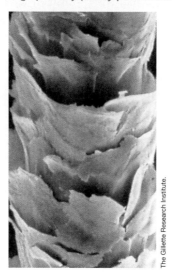

figure 10-28
Testing for hair porosity.

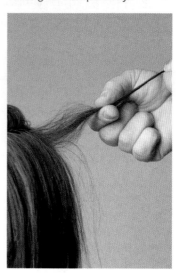

Testing for Hair Porosity

The porosity of the hair can be checked by holding multiple strands of dry hair between the fingers while sliding the thumb and forefinger of the other hand down toward the scalp (**Figure 10-28**). If the hair feels smooth and the cuticle is compact, it is considered resistant. If you can feel a slight roughness or the imbrications of the cuticle scales, the hair is porous. Should the hair break or feel very rough, the hair is probably over-porous.

HAIR ELASTICITY

Hair elasticity (HAYR ee-las-TIS-ut-ee) is the ability of the hair to stretch and return to its original length without breaking and is an indication of the strength of the side bonds in the hair. Hair with normal elasticity tends to hold the curl from sets and permanent waves without excessive relaxing of the curl. Hair with low or poor elasticity is brittle and breaks easily. Hair in this condition may have been overprocessed during previous chemical applications or may be the result of poor nutrition or internal disorders.

Testing for Hair Elasticity

Gently tug a few strands of clean, wet hair as shown in **Figure 10-29**.

- Hair with normal elasticity will stretch and return to its original length without breaking.

- Curly or wavy hair may stretch up to 50 percent of its original length and return to that length without breaking.

- Hair that breaks easily or fails to return to its normal length has low elasticity.

figure 10-29
Testing for hair elasticity.

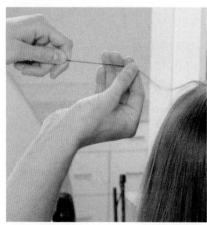

REVIEW QUESTIONS

1. Why is the study of the properties and disorders of the hair and scalp important to barbers?

2. Name the five main structures of the hair root

3. List the three layers of the hair shaft.

4. Describe the process of keratinization.

5. Describe polypeptide chains.

6. List and describe the three types of side bonds.

7. Name and describe the two types of melanin responsible for natural hair color.

8. Define and describe the two types of body hair and where they are found on the body.

9. List and describe the steps in the hair growth cycle.

10. Define and describe androgenic alopecia, alopecia areata, and alopecia totalis.

11. Name two FDA-approved treatments for hair loss.

12. Identify the hair and scalp disorders that must be referred to a physician for treatment.

13. Explain the similarities and differences associated with folliculitis barbae and pseudofolliculitis barbae.

14. Describe the factors to be observed and considered in a hair and scalp analysis.

CHAPTER GLOSSARY

alopecia (al-oh-PEE-shah)	p. 258	abnormal hair loss
alopecia areata (al-oh-PEE-shah ay-reh-AH-tuh)	p. 258	the sudden falling out of hair in patches or spots—autoimmune disorder
alopecia prematura (al-oh-PEE-shah pree-muh-TOO-ruh)	p. 258	hair loss that occurs before middle age
alopecia senilis (al-oh-PEE-shah seh-NIL-is)	p. 259	hair loss occurring in old age
alopecia syphilitica (al-oh-PEE-shah sif-il-IT-ih-kuh)	p. 258	hair loss as a result of syphilis
alopecia totalis (al-oh-PEE-shah toe-TAL-is)	p. 259	total loss of scalp hair
alopecia universalis (al-oh-PEE-shah yoo-nih-vur-SAA-lis)	p. 259	complete loss of body hair
amino acids (uh-MEE-noh AS-udz)	p. 250	the building blocks or units of structure in protein
anagen phase (AN-uh-jen FAYZ)	p. 256	growth phase in the hair cycle
androgenic alopecia (an-druh-JEN-ik al-oh-PEE-shah)	p. 258	hair loss that occurs as a result of genetics, age, and hormonal changes; male pattern baldness
arrector pili (ah-REK-tohr PY-leh)	p. 249	involuntary muscle fiber attached to the base of the hair follicle
canities (kah-NISH-ee-eez)	p. 260	technical term for gray hair
carbuncle (KAHR-bung-kul)	p. 265	the result of an acute, deep-seated bacterial infection in the subcutaneous tissue
catagen phase (KAT-uh-jen FAYZ)	p. 256	transition phase of the hair growth cycle that signals the end of the growth phase

cortex (KOR-teks)	p. 250	middle layer of the hair shaft
cowlick (KOW-lik)	p. 257	tuft of hair that stands straight up
cuticle (KYOO-tih-kul)	p. 249	outermost layer of the hair shaft
cysteine (SIS-tuh-een)	p. 252	an amino acid with a sulfur atom that joins together two peptide chains
dermal papilla (DUR-mul puh-PIL-uh)	p. 249	small, cone-shaped elevation located at the base of the hair follicle that fits into the hair bulb
disulfide bond (dy-SUL-fyed BAHND)	p. 252	also known as a *sulfur bond*; a type of chemical cross bond found in the hair cortex
end bonds (END BAHNDZ)	p. 251	also known as *peptide bonds*; chemical bonds that join amino acids end to end
eumelanin (yoo-MEL-uh-nin)	p. 253	melanin that gives brown and black color to hair
follicle (FAWL-ih-kul)	p. 248	tubelike depression in the skin that contains the hair root
folliculitis barbae (fah-lik-yuh-LY-tis BAR-bee)	p. 264	also known as *barber's itch*; a bacterial infection of the hair follicles with inflamed pustules in the bearded areas of the face and neck; may have hairs growing through the pustule
fragilitas crinium (fruh-JIL-ih-tus KRY-nee-um)	p. 261	technical term for brittle hair
furuncle (FYOO-rung-kul)	p. 265	an acute bacterial infection of a hair follicle, producing constant pain; also known as a *boil*
hair bulb (HAYR BULB)	p. 249	club-shaped structure that forms the lower part of the hair root
hair density (HAYR DEN-sih-tee)	p. 267	the amount of hair per square inch of scalp
hair elasticity (HAYR ee-las-TIS-ut-ee)	p. 268	the ability of the hair to stretch and return to its original length
hair porosity (HAYR puh-RAHS-ut-ee)	p. 267	the ability of the hair to absorb moisture
hair root (HAYR ROOT)	p. 248	the part of the hair that is encased in the hair follicle
hair shaft (HAYR SHAFT)	p. 248	the part of the hair that extends beyond the skin
hair stream (HAYR STREEM)	p. 257	hair that flows in the same direction
hair texture (HAYR TEKS-chur)	p. 266	measures the diameter of a hair strand: coarse, medium, fine
helix (HEE-licks)	p. 251	the spiral shape of a coiled protein created when polypeptide chains intertwine
hydrogen bond (HY-druh-jun BAHND)	p. 252	weak, physical, cross-link side bond that is easily broken by water or heat
hypertrichosis (hy-pur-trih-KOH-sis)	p. 261	a condition of abnormal hair growth
keratin (KAIR-uht-in)	p. 248	the protein of which hair is made
keratinization (kair-uh-ti-ni-ZAY-shun)	p. 250	process by which protein cells mature within the follicle to form hair
lanugo (luh-NOO-goh)	p. 255	vellus hair
malassezia (mal-uh-SEEZ-ee-uh)	p. 261	fungus that causes dandruff
medulla (muh-DUL-uh)	p. 250	innermost or center layer of the hair shaft

melanin	p. 253	tiny grains of pigment in the cortex that give natural color to the hair
monilethrix (mah-NIL-ee-thriks)	p. 261	technical term for beaded hair
pediculosis capitis (puh-dik-yuh-LOH-sis KAP-ih-tus)	p. 263	the infection of the hair and scalp with head lice
peptide bonds (PEP-tyd BAHNDZ)	p. 251	end bonds; chemical bonds that join amino acids end to end
pheomelanin (fee-oh-MEL-uh-nin)	p. 253	melanin that gives red to blond colors to hair
pityriasis (pit-ih-RY-uh-sus)	p. 261	technical term for dandruff
pityriasis capitis simplex (pit-ih-RY-uh-sus KAP-ih-tus SIM-pleks)	p. 262	dry dandruff
pityriasis steatoides (pit-ih-RY-uh-sus stee-uh-TOY-deez)	p. 262	waxy or greasy dandruff
polypeptide chain (pahl-ee-PEP-tyd CHAYN)	p. 251	long chain of amino acids linked by peptide bonds
proteins (PROH-teenz)	p. 251	are made of chemical units called amino acids
pseudofolliculitis barbae (SUE-doe-fah-lik-yuh-LY-tis BAR-bee)	p. 264	a chronic inflammatory form of folliculitis known as *razor bumps* resembling folliculitis papules and pustules; generally accepted to be caused by ingrown hair
salt bond (SAWLT BAHNDZ)	p. 252	a physical side bond within the hair cortex
scutula (SKUT-yoo-lah)	p. 263	dry, sulfur-yellow, cuplike crusts on the scalp seen in tinea favosa
side bonds (SYD BAHNDZ)	p. 251	also known as *cross bonds*; hydrogen, salt, and sulfur bonds in the hair cortex
sycosis vulgaris (sy-KOH-sis vul-GAYR-is)	p. 264	chronic bacterial infection of the bearded areas of the face
telogen phase (TEL-uh-jen FAYZ)	p. 256	resting phase of the hair growth cycle
terminal hair (TUR-mih-nul HAYR)	p. 255	long hair found on the scalp, beard, chest, back, and legs
tinea (TIN-ee-uh)	p. 262	technical name for ringworm
tinea barbae (TIN-ee-uh BAR-bee)	p. 263	also known as barber's itch, a superficial fungal infection that commonly affects the skin; it is primarily limited to the bearded areas of the face and neck or around the scalp
tinea capitis (TIN-ee-uh KAP-ih-tus)	p. 262	a fungal infection of the scalp characterized by red papules, or spots, at the opening of the hair follicles
tinea favosa (TIN-ee-uh fah-VOH-suh)	p. 263	ringworm characterized by dry, sulfur-yellow crusts on the scalp
tinea sycosis (TIN-ee-uh sy-KOH-sis)	p. 265	ringworm of the bearded areas on the face
trichology (trih-KAHL-uh-jee)	p. 248	the science dealing with the hair, its diseases, and its care
trichoptilosis (trih-kahp-tih-LOH-sus)	p. 261	the technical term for split ends; hair conditioning and oils will smooth split ends, but the only way to remove them is to cut them
trichorrhexis nodosa (trik-uh-REK-sis nuh-DOH-suh)	p. 261	technical term for knotted hair
vellus hair (VEL-us HAYR)	p. 255	soft, downy hair that appears on the body
wave pattern (WAYV PAT-URN)	p. 253	amount of movement in the hair strand; straight, wavy, curly, and coiled
whorl (WHORL)	p. 257	hair that grows in a circular pattern

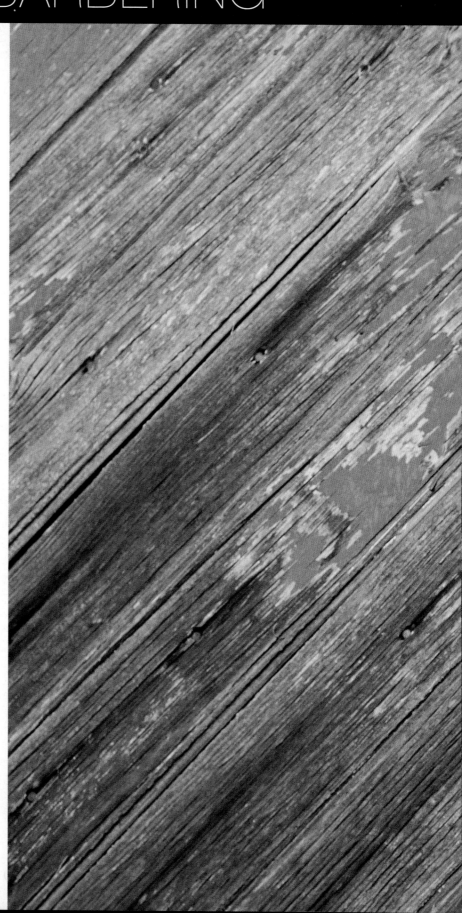

PART 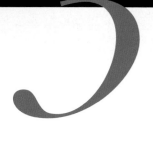 THE PRACTICE OF BARBERING

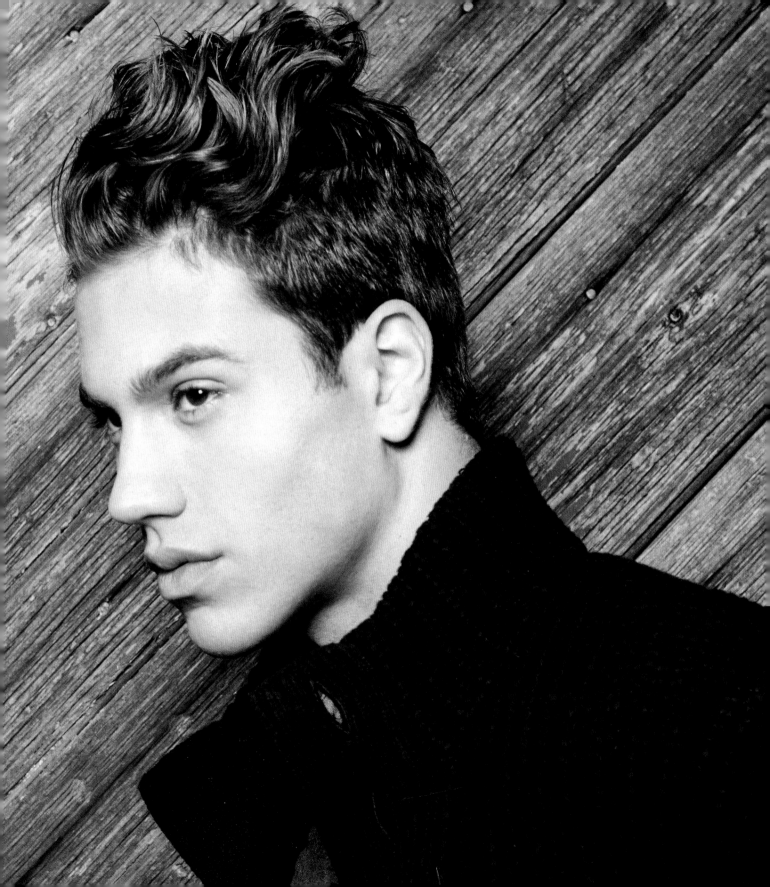

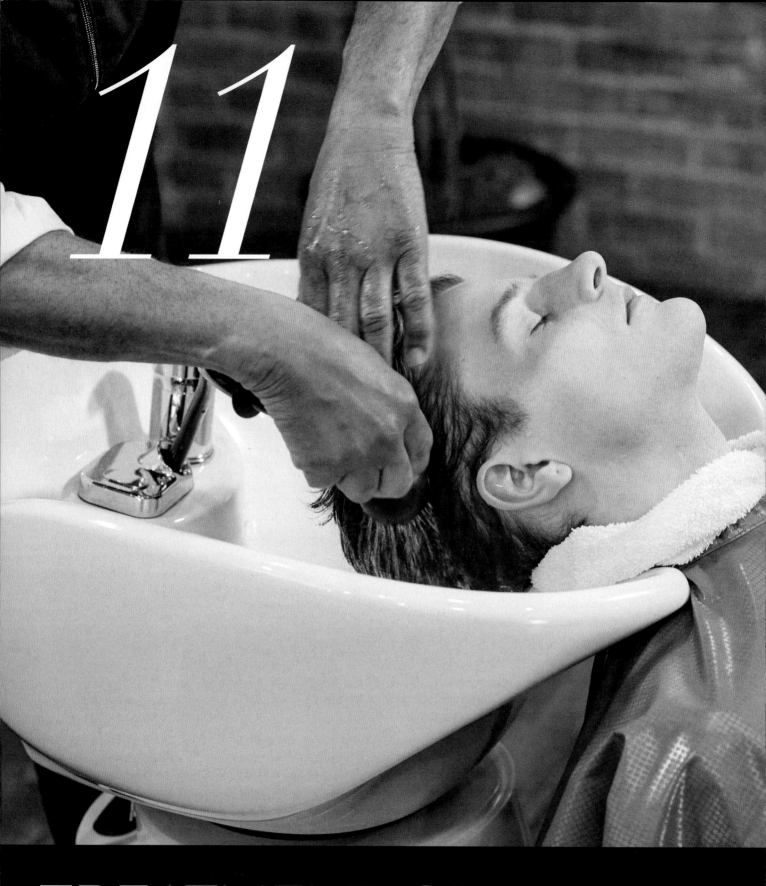

11

TREATMENT OF THE HAIR AND SCALP

LEARNING OBJECTIVES

After completing this chapter, you will be able to:

LO❶
Discuss the benefits of a shampoo service.

LO❷
Select products for different hair types and textures.

LO❸
Describe proper draping procedures for various services.

LO❹
Identify basic considerations for performing a shampoo service.

LO❺
Describe two shampooing methods.

LO❻
Discuss reasons why a client may find fault with a shampoo service.

LO❼
Describe scalp massage manipulations and techniques.

LO❽
Explain services that may be included in a hair or scalp treatment.

Introduction

The treatment of the hair and scalp includes shampooing, scalp massage, conditioning, and special treatments for hair and scalp conditions. When performed correctly, these services are relaxing and effective in helping to ensure the health of clients' hair and scalp. Providing such professional services can also increase client retention and referrals and helps to promote a positive reputation for the barber and barbershop.

why study
TREATMENT OF THE HAIR AND SCALP?

Barbers should study and have a thorough understanding of treatments for the hair and scalp because:

> Analyzing the client's hair and scalp helps to identify conditions that may prohibit services.

> Professionally delivered scalp massage during shampooing and treatments provides hygienic, circulatory, and relaxation benefits to the client.

> Special services, such as electrotherapy or light therapy treatments, require advanced knowledge and skills to perform correctly and safely.

Discuss the Shampoo Service

After reading this section, you will be able to:

LO**❶** Discuss the benefits of a shampoo service.

LO**❷** Select products for different hair types and textures.

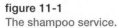
figure 11-1
The shampoo service.

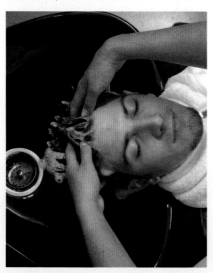

Shampooing the hair before cutting ensures that you are working with clean hair that is free from oils or products that can interfere with cutting tools and haircut results. Follow-up conditioning treatments after the shampooing help to keep hair in a healthy and manageable condition for the client and the barber (**Figure 11-1**). It is your responsibility to know how shampoos and conditioners affect the hair and scalp so that you can select or recommend the right products for your clients. As a professional barber, you need to take the time to read the specific information found on product labels or manufacturers' websites. **Table 11-1** shows a general guideline for selecting shampoos and conditioners for different hair types and textures.

REVIEW SHAMPOOS AND CONDITIONERS

The purpose of a shampoo product and service is to cleanse the scalp and hair. This may seem obvious, but some barbers still encounter clients who use bar soap or other detergent products, which can leave the hair dry or coated with soap residues. As you may know from your study of chemistry,

table 11-1

MATCHING PRODUCTS TO HAIR TYPES

Hair Type	Hair Texture		
	Fine	Medium	Coarse
Straight	Volumizing shampoo Detangler, if necessary Protein treatments Fine-hair shampoo	pH-balanced shampoo Finishing rinse Protein treatments	Moisturizing shampoo Leave-in conditioner Moisturizing treatments
Wavy, curly, extremely curly	Light leave-in conditioner Protein treatments Spray-on thermal protectors	pH-balanced shampoo Leave-in conditioner Moisturizing treatment	Leave-in conditioner Protein and moisturizing treatments
Dry and damaged (perms, color-treated, relaxers, blowdrying, sun, hot irons)	Gentle cleansing shampoo Light leave-in conditioner Protein and moisturizing repair treatments Spray-on thermal protection	Shampoo for chemically treated hair Moisturizing conditioner Protein and moisturizing repair treatments	Deep-moisturizing shampoo for damaged hair Leave-in conditioner Deep-conditioning treatments and hair masks

shampoos (sham-POOz) are oil-in-water emulsions with a pH range of 4.5 to 7.5. Since these products do not contain the harsh alkalis found in soaps and detergents, they leave the hair in a more manageable condition.

Conditioners can refer to either hair conditioners or scalp conditioners.

- Generally, **hair conditioners** (HAYR kun-DIH-shun-urz) moisturize the hair and help to restore some of the oils and/or proteins. Hair conditioners typically range from 3.0 to 5.5 on the pH scale.

- **Scalp conditioners** (SKALP kun-DIH-shun-urz), usually in cream or ointment form, are available for overall scalp maintenance or to treat conditions requiring a medicinal product.

> **⏱ REMINDER**
> Display and use the shop's retail products at the workstation or shampoo sink to promote product sales and your endorsement of the products.

Know How to Drape

After reading this section, you will be able to:

LO❸ Describe proper draping procedures for various services.

Before any barbering service can begin, the client needs to be appropriately draped for the service. **Draping** is the term used to describe the covering of the client's skin and clothing with a cape and a barrier at the neckband for their protection. Proper draping for the service being performed is required to maintain compliance with state barber laws and infection control standards in the barbershop.

Depending on the procedure to be performed, you will drape a client for either a wet service or a dry service. Wet services, such as shampooing

figure 11-2
Draped shampoo cape.

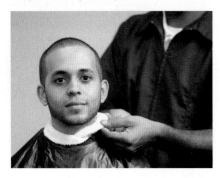

figure 11-3
Draped haircutting cape.

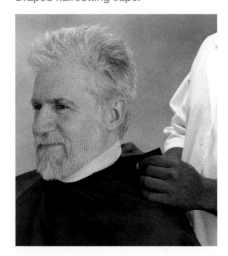

REMINDER

If a shampoo service precedes the haircut, replace the vinyl cape and towel with a nylon cape and neck strip.

? DID YOU KNOW?

Paper towels designed for barbering services are available and preferred by some barbers. They typically measure 12 × 24 inches and can be used

- in place of a neck strip;
- as a wiping towel for lather during razor work;
- as a towel wrap over the hand to remove hair clippings or to apply products.

---

and chemical applications, require protection from liquids. Dry services, such as a haircut or beard trim, do not require this type of protection, so it is important to use the appropriate drape for the service.

The two main types of drapes used are shampoo capes (or wet capes) and haircutting capes (also known as *chair cloths*).

- *Shampoo capes* are waterproof drapes made of vinyl that are used to protect the client's skin and clothing from water, liquids, and chemical processes (see **Figure 11-2**).

- *Haircutting capes* are made of nylon or other synthetic materials. These draping fabrics are usually more comfortable for the client because they do not hold in as much body heat as vinyl capes. From the barber's standpoint, these fabrics are also more effective for shedding wet and dry hair. Wet hair has a tendency to stick to vinyl capes, making it more difficult to shake loose hairs off the drape (**Figure 11-3**).

LEARN DRAPING METHODS

The method of draping to be used depends on the service to be performed. There are several draping methods used in the barbershop and all require the use of a barrier (towel or neck strip) between the client's neck and the neckband of the cape. The barriers used are listed below; review Procedures 11-1 and 11-2 for guidelines on draping for wet, chemical, and haircutting services.

- **Shampoo service.** A cloth towel is positioned under the cape and folded over the neckband once the cape is secured. Another option for the shampoo service is to place a second towel over the cape neckline, secured with a clip, to use for blotting the hair after the shampoo procedure.

- **Chemical service.** A chemical service always requires a cloth towel under the cape and folded over the neckband once the cape is secured, followed by a cloth towel over the cape neckline and secured with a clip to provide protection from solution or chemical drips.

- **Haircut service.** For a haircut service, draping includes the use of a neck strip under and then folded over the neckband of the cape.

- **Mustache/beard trim service.** This service requires either a neck strip or a cloth towel placed under and then folded over the neckband of the cape. Some barbers prefer to use a terry cloth towel for beard trims because the cloth fibers are more effective in trapping hair clippings than a neck strip.

- **Shave service.** The shave service requires a special draping method to ensure that a barrier between the client's skin and the drape remain in place during the procedure. This method is described in detail in Chapter 13.

ⓟ 11-1 **Draping for Wet and Chemical Services** *pages 286–287*

ⓟ 11-2 **Draping for Haircutting Services** *pages 288–289*

Although several draping methods are presented in this text, your instructor's methods would be correct as well, as long as there is a barrier between the client's neck and the neckband of the cape.

Consider Important Guidelines for Draping

Important guidelines that apply to all draping methods are as follows:

- Prepare materials and supplies for the service.
- Wash your hands.
- Ask the client to remove jewelry if any and store it in a safe place.
- Turn the client's collar to the inside if applicable (**Figure 11-4**).
- Proceed with the appropriate draping method.

Understand the Shampoo Service

After reading this section, you will be able to:

LO④ Identify basic considerations for performing a shampoo service.

LO⑤ Describe two shampooing methods.

LO⑥ Discuss reasons why a client may find fault with a shampoo service.

The basic considerations for performing a shampoo service include proper draping and positioning of the client, scalp manipulations to facilitate the shampoo procedure, and proper body positioning of the barber. Most barber-shops are equipped with shampoo bowls either within a working booth area or placed in a separate section of the shop. Typically, the barber stands beside the client and shampoo bowl while performing the shampoo. Some shops, however, are equipped with the European-style shampoo bowl, which is a freestanding unit that allows the barber to stand in back of the client's head.

DESCRIBE TWO METHODS OF SHAMPOOING AND RINSING

The two methods used for shampooing and rinsing are the reclined and inclined methods.

- The *reclined method* of shampooing is the most commonly used method. The hydraulic or shampoo chair is reclined and the client's head positioned in the neck rest of the shampoo bowl (**Figure 11-5**). This method is favored because it is more comfortable for the client and permits greater speed and efficiency by the barber.

- The *inclined method* can be used when a standard shampoo bowl is not available or when the client cannot use the reclined method. This method requires the client to bend his head forward over the shampoo bowl or sink (**Figure 11-6**). The client may also sit on a stool or chair positioned close to the sink.

SHAMPOOING CLIENTS WITH SPECIAL NEEDS

If a client is disabled or wheelchair bound, ask the client how he would like to be shampooed. Some wheelchairs can be positioned comfortably at the shampoo bowl while others may require the client to use the inclined method. Always make the client's comfort and safety a priority.

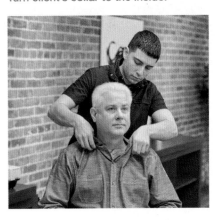

figure 11-4
Turn client's collar to the inside.

> **? DID YOU KNOW?**
> The purpose of the towel or neck strip in draping procedures is to prevent the cape from having direct contact with the client's skin and to maintain compliance with state barber laws and infection control standards. This barrier is a requirement of every state's barber rules and regulations.

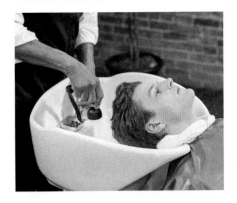

figure 11-5
Reclined method.

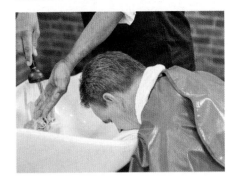

figure 11-6
Inclined method.

The Barber's Physical Presentation

To prevent muscle aches, back strain, and fatigue, it is important that you maintain good posture at the shampoo bowl. Review the following suggestions to maintain a good posture while shampooing.

- Stand as close as possible to the back of the client's head.
- Flex the knees slightly and position your body directly over your feet to maintain good balance.
- Try to keep your chin parallel to the floor to avoid neck strain. Your head should be raised, with the chest up, abdomen flat, and shoulders relaxed.
- Do not bend or twist sideways from the waist or lean too far forward.

Perform a Superior Shampoo Service

An excellent shampoo service requires you to give individual attention to each client's needs. The effectiveness of the shampoo service will depend on the manner in which you apply and rinse the shampoo, the quality of the scalp massage, the temperature of the water used, and the use of the shampoo best suited to the condition of the client's scalp and hair.

Some of the more common reasons that a client may find fault with the shampoo service include

- improper shampoo selection;
- insufficient scalp massage;
- extreme water temperatures: either too hot or too cold;
- shampoo or water that runs onto the client's face, ears, or eyes;
- wetting or soiling the client's clothing;
- scraping or scratching the client's scalp with fingernails;
- improper hair blotting;
- insufficient cleansing and rinsing.

An excellent shampoo service therefore requires preparation and set-up, product selection, water temperature testing, shampoo application, and shampoo massage manipulations.

Preparation and Setup

Following consultation with the client, preparation is the first step in performing a shampoo service. Assemble all necessary supplies or have them stored in an area convenient to the shampoo bowl. Supplies include cleansing and conditioning products, waterproof drapes, and terry cloth towels.

Analysis and Product Selection

It is essential that you be knowledgeable about the products you use on your clients. Always read product labels and follow the manufacturer's directions. To determine which product to use, you must first perform a scalp and hair analysis (Figure 11-7). Six characteristics of the scalp and hair that should be considered before choosing products are:

- **Condition of the scalp.** Dry, oily, normal, and/or the presence of abrasions or disorders such as tinea or pediculosis capitis (if abrasions or disorders are present, do not proceed with the service)

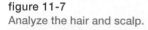

figure 11-7
Analyze the hair and scalp.

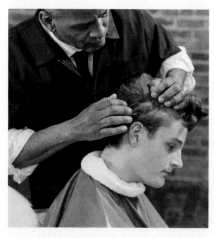

- **Condition of the hair.** Dry, brittle, fragile, oily, normal, or chemically treated

- **Hair density.** Thin, medium, thick

- **Hair texture.** Fine, average, coarse

- **Hair porosity.** Low (resistant), average (normal), high (overly porous)

- **Hair elasticity.** Low (breaks easily), average (normal)

With practice and experience, you will learn the effects of different products on the hair and scalp. For example, moisturizing shampoos are not alkaline enough to cleanse an oily scalp and hair condition; heavy, cuticle-coating conditioners can weigh down fine hair, leaving it flat or oily; and dry, coarse hair may require a humectant-rich moisturizing conditioner to increase manageability.

Water Temperature

The water should be comfortably warm for the client. Cold water, in addition to causing discomfort, tends to reduce lathering. Hot water, in addition to burning the client, can cause the scalp to flake or become dry. Warm water is more comfortable and relaxing for the client and reacts favorably during the foaming process. Always test the water temperature before applying it to your client's head (**Figure 11-8**).

Shampoo Application

Applying the shampoo product is not difficult but some basic guidelines can help you perform this step more efficiently and effectively. Refer to Procedure 11-3 to review the following guidelines:

- Dampen the client's hair thoroughly.

- Dispense shampoo product onto your hand and distribute it over both palms to facilitate spreading it throughout the client's hair.

- Spread sections of the hair apart with the thumbs and fingers to distribute the shampoo onto the scalp and hair.

- Gradually add warm water to work up a rich, creamy lather.

- Avoid getting shampoo lather on the client's face.

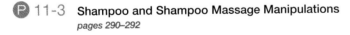 11-3   Shampoo and Shampoo Massage Manipulations
pages 290–292

Other Shampoo Applications

Occasionally, you may be called upon to visit a client who is bedridden or in a condition where a wet shampoo service may not be feasible. In such a case, liquid-dry or powder shampoo applications can be used to freshen the client's hair and scalp (refer to Procedure 11-4).

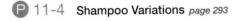 11-4   Shampoo Variations page 293

Most state boards require out-of-shop services of this nature to be recorded in the appointment book, with the name, times, and destination clearly documented.

figure 11-8
Test water temperature before applying to client's head.

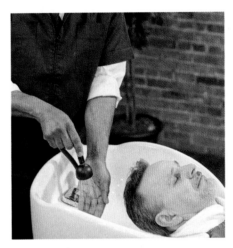

Learn about Scalp and Hair Treatments

After reading this section, you will be able to:

LO❼ Describe scalp massage manipulations and techniques.

LO❽ Explain services that may be included in a hair or scalp treatment.

EXPLAIN SCALP MASSAGE MANIPULATIONS

Massage manipulations performed during a shampoo or scalp treatment start at the hairline and should be performed with even pressure and continuous synchronized movements to achieve the following effects:

- Increased blood and lymph flow
- Soothed nerves
- Stimulated scalp muscles and glands
- A more flexible scalp

The shampoo massage is usually performed using a combination of rotary or circular movements and back and forth scrubbing-type movements. A scalp massage as part of a scalp treatment most often includes rotary and sliding massage movements.

These massage manipulations are performed as follows:

- A *rotary movement* uses the thumbs and/or fingertips to produce overlapping circular movements with moderate to firm pressure throughout the scalp area (**Figure 11-9**).

- A *sliding movement* uses the thumbs and fingertips to produce sliding strokes with moderate to firm pressure and often overlap as the hands meet over a section of the head (**Figure 11-10**).

- A *back and forth movement* uses the thumbs and/or fingertips to produce a brisk back and forth movement with moderate to firm pressure (**Figure 11-11**).

figure 11-9
Rotary movement.

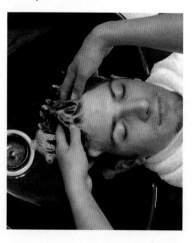

figure 11-10
Sliding movement.

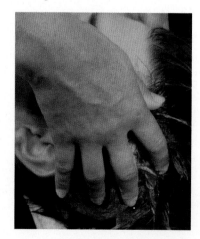

figure 11-11
Back and forth movement.

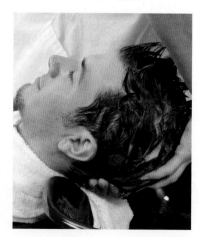

Guidelines for performing a scalp massage are as follows:

- Apply firm pressure on the upward strokes.
- Firm rotary movements loosen the scalp tissues and help to improve the health of hair and scalp by increasing blood circulation to the scalp and hair papillae.
- Massage manipulations should be slow and rhythmic.
- Avoid pulling the hair in any way.
- With each movement, the hands are placed under the hair with the fingertips resting on the scalp. The length of the fingers, the balls of the fingertips, and the cushions of the palms all help to stimulate muscles, nerves, and blood vessels in the scalp area. Table 11-2 shows the influence of massage movements on the scalp.

DESCRIBE SCALP AND HAIR TREATMENTS

The purpose of scalp and hair treatments is to preserve the health and appearance of the hair and scalp. These treatments also help to prevent or combat disorders such as dandruff, dry hair or scalp, and oily hair or scalp.

Cleanliness and stimulation are essential requirements for healthy hair and scalp; because the scalp and hair are so interrelated, many scalp disorders need correction to maintain the health of the hair. A healthy scalp will help to maintain healthy hair. Some common scalp and hair disorders you are likely to encounter in the barbershop are described below:

- *Dry scalp and hair* may be caused by the inactivity of the oil glands, poor blood circulation to the scalp, or the excessive removal of natural oil by products that strip hair oils. Select scalp preparations that contain moisturizing agents. Avoid the use of strong soaps, greasy preparations, and lotions with high alcohol content.

table 11-2

MASSAGE AND ITS INFLUENCE ON THE SCALP

Section of the Head	Service	Movement	Muscles	Nerves
Sides to top of head	Scalp treatment Shampoo	Sliding Rotary	Auricularis superior, temporalis, frontalis	Fifth and seventh cranial nerves
Behind ears and neck-to-crown	Scalp treatment Shampoo	Rotary and sliding Rotary/back and forth	Auricularis posterior, sternocleidomastoideus, occipital, aponeurosis, trapezius	Eleventh cranial and spinal nerves
Forehead-to-crown	Scalp treatment Shampoo	Sliding Rotary/back and forth	Frontalis, aponeurosis, temporalis	Fifth and seventh cranial and spinal nerves
Front hairline	Scalp treatment Shampoo	Rotary Rotary	Frontalis	Fifth cranial nerves

- *Oily scalp and hair* is most often caused by overactive sebaceous glands; however, an improper diet or lack of hygienic practices can be contributing factors as well. Manipulating the scalp will increase circulation and help to release hardened sebum from the follicles; regular shampooing can minimize oil buildup.

- *Dandruff*, caused by the fungus malassezia, is indicated by white scales on the hair and scalp and may be accompanied by itching. Conditions vary from dry flakes and scales to greasy, waxy scales that build up on the scalp. If a client has a prescribed topical medication from his physician, do not apply it without the prescription directions and be sure to save a copy with the client's record card.

- *Alopecia* is the term used to describe abnormal hair loss. The chief causes of alopecia are heredity; poor blood circulation; lack of proper stimulation; improper nourishment; certain infectious skin diseases, such as ringworm; and constitutional disorders. Conditions of alopecia may benefit from stimulation of the blood supply to the germinal papilla through scalp treatments.

- A *corrective hair treatment* deals with the hair shaft rather than the scalp. Dry and damaged hair can be greatly improved by reconditioning treatments that contain proteins, humectants, and other ingredients that help to strengthen the hair while making it soft and pliable.

Scalp treatments may be given separately or combined with hair treatments. In many cases, a product that is good for the scalp is also good for the hair. In other cases, separate products may need to be used. Conditions caused by neglect, such as a tight scalp, overactive or underactive oil glands, or tense nerves may be corrected by proper scalp treatments. Depending on the client's needs, hair and scalp treatment services may include

- cleansing with a suitable shampoo;

- steaming the scalp;

- massage with the hands or an electrical appliance;

- use of infrared and/or ultraviolet lamps, or high-frequency current;

- the application of cosmetic preparations such as hair tonics, astringents, antiseptics, or ointments.

Scalp Steam

A **scalp steam** (SKALP STEEM) is effective in preparing the scalp for scalp massage manipulations and treatments. Steam relaxes the pores, softens the scalp and hair, and increases blood circulation.

- A scalp steamer assures a constant and controlled source of steam; steam towels can also be used effectively.

    - To use a scalp steamer, fill the container with water, fit the hood over the client's head, and turn on the current.

    - Some hood models have openings on the side so the barber's hands can be inserted to perform a scalp massage during the scalp steam.

- Hot towels can be used in the absence of a scalp steamer (Figure 11-12).

  - Towels can be prepared in advance and stored in a hot-towel cabinet or prepared one at a time by soaking in hot water; wring out the excess water before applying towel to client's head.

  - As one towel cools, apply another in its place; two or three towel applications are usually sufficient.

Scalp massage should be performed as a series of treatments, once a week for normal scalp and more frequently for scalp disorders under the direction of a dermatologist. Review Procedures 11-5 and 11-6 for the steps involved in scalp steam and scalp massage treatments.

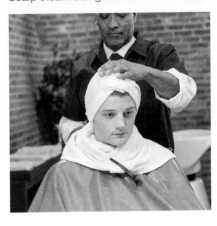

figure 11-12
Scalp steam using hot towels.

Ⓟ 11-5   **Scalp Steam** *page 294*

Ⓟ 11-6   **Scalp Massage Treatment** *pages 295–296*

Scalp Treatment with an Electric Massager

As you learned in Chapter 5, an electric massager, sometimes called a *vibrator* or *hand massager*, is an electrical device that is used to perform a stimulating scalp massage. The vibrations are transmitted through the cushions of the fingertips of the barber's hand. The same movements are followed as for a regular hand scalp massage. Following are guidelines for use:

figure 11-13
Handheld electric massager.

  - Before using an electric massager, adjust the device on the back of the hand, leaving the thumb and fingers free; then turn on the current.

  - When using the electric massager on the scalp, be careful to regulate the intensity and duration of the vibrations, as well as the pressure applied (Figure 11-13).

  - Scalp massage is most effective when given in a series of treatments and may be advised for general scalp maintenance, to promote hair growth, or to correct a scalp condition.

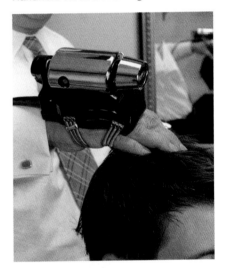

Refer to Procedure 11-7 for detailed descriptions of many variations in scalp treatment.

Ⓟ 11-7   **Scalp Treatment Variations** *pages 297–300*

Hair Tonic Treatments

Scalp steamers, steam towels, vibrators, and scalp manipulations may all be used with hair tonics.

The steps for a hair tonic treatment are as follows:

- Apply the hair tonic.

- Massage the scalp.

- Apply scalp steam.

- Massage again with hands or a vibrator.

- Comb the hair into the desired style.

> ⚠ **CAUTION**
> Barbers are prohibited from treating scalp disorders caused by parasitic infestations or staphylococcus infections. Clients with abnormal scalp conditions should be referred to a physician.

DRAPING FOR WET AND CHEMICAL SERVICES

MATERIALS, IMPLEMENTS, AND EQUIPMENT

☐ Clip
☐ Terry cloth towels
☐ Waterproof cape

PREPARATION

1 Assemble supplies.

2 Seat the client in a comfortable and relaxed position.

3 Wash your hands.

PROCEDURE

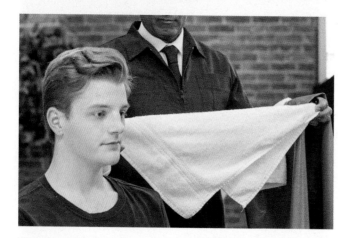

1 Hold the towel lengthwise in front of you. Grasp the towel by opposite diagonal corners and fold on the diagonal to maximize the length.

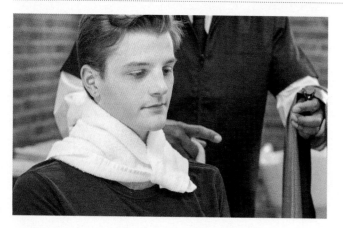

2 Place the towel lengthwise around the client's neck and shoulders, crossing the ends beneath the chin.

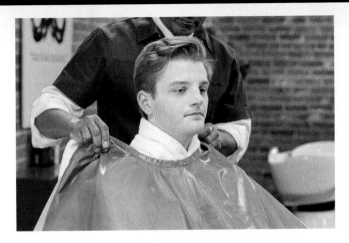

3 Drape a waterproof cape over the towel and fasten it at the back so that the cape does not touch the client's skin.

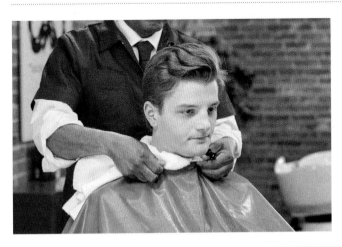

4 Position and flatten the top edge of the towel down over the neckline of the cape.

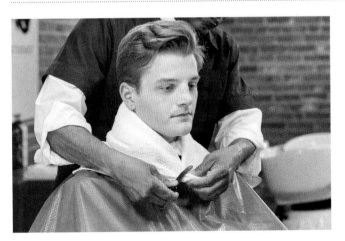

5 Options: Place another towel over the cape and secure it in front with a chair cloth clip; or fold the second towel in thirds and place it in the neck rest of the shampoo bowl to create a barrier between the client and the sink.

DRAPING FOR HAIRCUTTING SERVICES

MATERIALS, IMPLEMENTS, AND EQUIPMENT

☐ Haircutting cape

☐ Neck strips

PREPARATION

1. Assemble supplies.

2. Seat the client in a comfortable and relaxed position.

3. Wash your hands.

PROCEDURE

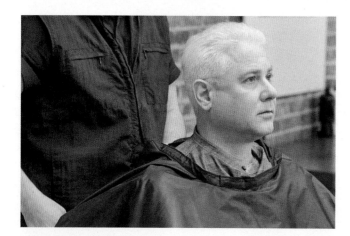

1. Drape the nylon cape loosely across the client's chest and shoulders.

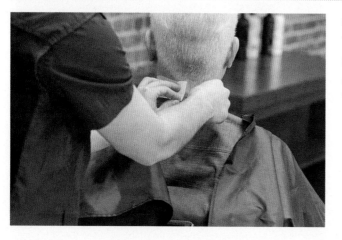

2. Place the neck strip around the client's neck from front to back.

3. Hold one end of the neck strip against the client's skin at the back or side of the neck while wrapping the rest of the strip.

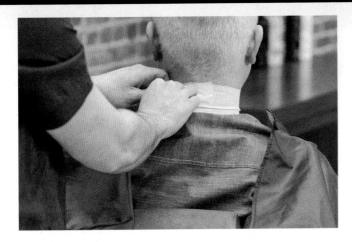

4 Secure the second end of the neck strip by tucking it neatly into the band of the neck strip.

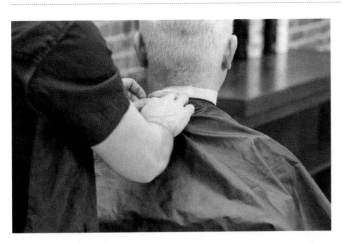

5 Lift the cape from across the client's shoulders, slide it into place around the neck, and fasten it at the back of the neck.

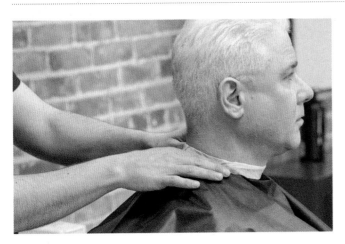

6 Fold and flatten the top edge of the neck strip over the neckline of the cape to prevent the client's skin from touching the drape.

SHAMPOO AND SHAMPOO MASSAGE MANIPULATIONS

MATERIALS, IMPLEMENTS, AND EQUIPMENT

☐ Comb

☐ Shampoo and conditioner

☐ Shampoo bowl

☐ Terry cloth towels

☐ Waterproof cape

PREPARATION

1. Assemble supplies.

2. Seat the client in a comfortable and relaxed position.

3. Wash your hands.

PROCEDURE

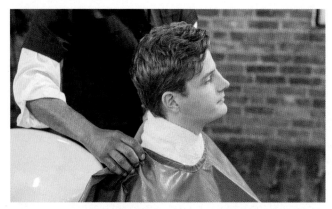

1. Drape the client for the shampoo service.

2. Consult with the client about products, hair and scalp problems, or any questions the client has about his or her hair or scalp.

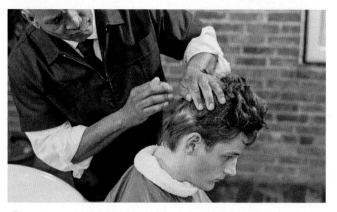

3. Examine the condition of the client's hair and scalp. Use back and forth movement to lightly massage the scalp to loosen epidermal scales, debris, and scalp tissues.

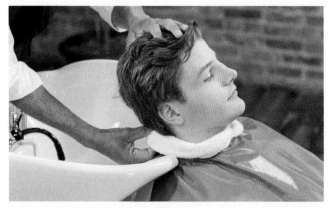

4. Position the client for the shampoo service. Recline the client while draping the back of the cape over the back of the chair.

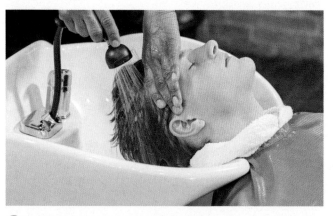

5. Saturate the hair with warm water, protecting the face and ears against splashes. Support the head while saturating the nape and back sections.

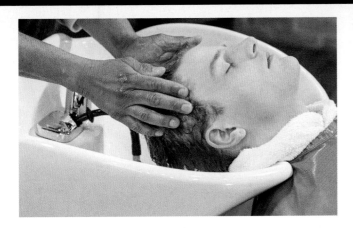

6 Apply shampoo to all parts of the scalp.

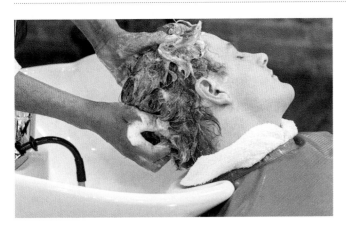

7 Starting at the front hairline, work along the sides toward the back and nape areas to massage and produce a lather. Use rotary movements over the entire head area to massage the scalp for several minutes. Repeat these movements over the top, side, and back sections several times.

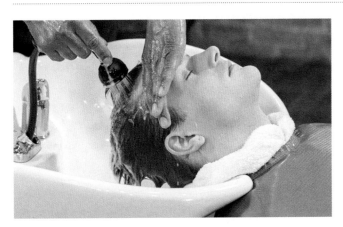

8 Remove excess lather with a sweep of the palm from the front of the head to the back; rinse hair thoroughly with warm water using a moderate to strong spray. Repeat lathering step if necessary and rinse.

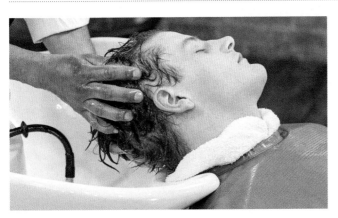

9 Apply conditioner, massage through hair, and rinse thoroughly.

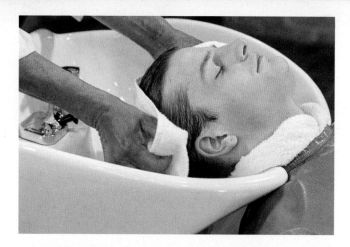

10 Blot the hair.

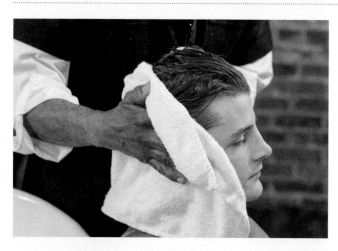

11 Raise the client to a sitting position and lightly towel-dry the hair; wipe the face and ears if necessary.

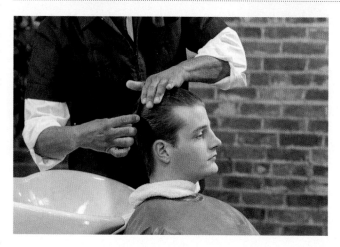

12 Comb the hair into position for cutting.

CLEAN-UP AND DISINFECTION

☐ Clean and disinfect the tools and implements used.

☐ Clean and disinfect the work area.

☐ Dispose of single-use items. Place all used linens, towels, and capes in the laundry.

☐ Wash your hands.

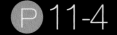
SHAMPOO VARIATIONS

MATERIALS, IMPLEMENTS, AND EQUIPMENT

☐ Brush

☐ Comb

☐ Cotton pledget or cotton-tipped applicator

☐ Liquid-dry shampoo, dry or powder shampoo

☐ Terry cloth towels

☐ Waterproof cape

PREPARATION

1. Assemble supplies.

2. Seat or recline the client in a comfortable and relaxed position.

3. Wash your hands.

A. LIQUID-DRY SHAMPOO APPLICATION

PROCEDURE

1. Drape the client for shampoo service.

2. Perform hair and scalp analysis.

3. Brush the hair thoroughly and comb it lightly.

4. Part the hair into small sections.

5. Saturate a piece of cotton with the liquid-dry shampoo and squeeze out excess or use a cotton-tipped applicator to apply to the scalp along each part line. Follow by swiftly rubbing the scalp with a towel along the same area. Repeat this procedure over the entire head.

6. Saturate more cotton with the product and apply down the length of the hair strands.

7. Rub the hair strands with a towel to remove the soil.

8. Remoisten the hair lightly with liquid and comb it into the desired style.

B. DRY OR POWDER SHAMPOO APPLICATION

PROCEDURE

1. Drape the client for a shampoo service.

2. Perform hair and scalp analysis.

3. Sprinkle the product into the hair, working it in one section at a time.

4. Brush hair thoroughly to remove the powder.

CLEAN-UP AND DISINFECTION

☐ Clean and disinfect the tools and implements used.

☐ Clean and disinfect the work area.

☐ Dispose of single-use items. Place all used linens, towels, and capes in the laundry.

☐ Wash your hands.

SCALP STEAM

MATERIALS, IMPLEMENTS, AND EQUIPMENT

☐ Comb
☐ Shampoo bowl
☐ Terry cloth towels
☐ Waterproof cape

PREPARATION

1. Assemble supplies.
2. Seat the client in a comfortable and relaxed position.
3. Wash your hands.

PROCEDURE

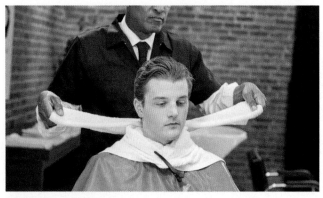

1. Drape the client for a shampoo service.
2. Perform hair and scalp analysis.

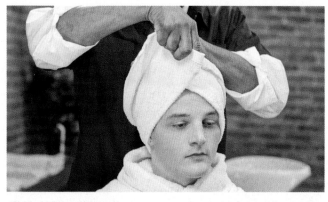

3. Wrap prepared steam towel around head.

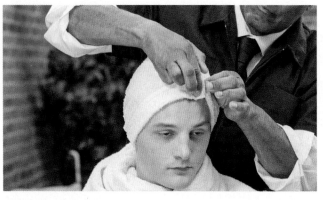

4. Tuck in edge to secure.

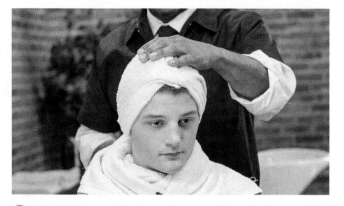

5. Mold the towel to client's head.
6. Repeat process two or three times.

CLEAN-UP AND DISINFECTION

☐ Clean and disinfect the tools and implements used.
☐ Clean and disinfect the work area.

☐ Dispose of single-use items. Place all used linens, towels, and capes in the laundry.
☐ Wash your hands.

SCALP MASSAGE TREATMENT

Note: The following is one method of performing a scalp massage treatment. Your instructor may have developed a different procedure, which would be equally correct.

MATERIALS, IMPLEMENTS, AND EQUIPMENT

☐ Scalp cream or hair tonic if desired by the client

☐ Towel or neck strip

☐ Waterproof cape

PREPARATION

1. Assemble supplies.
2. Seat the client in a comfortable and relaxed position.
3. Wash your hands.

PROCEDURE

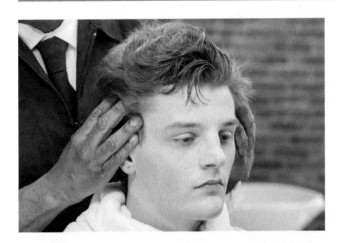

1. Drape the client as for a shampoo service.
2. Perform hair and scalp analysis.
3. Stand behind the client to start manipulations.
4. Place the fingertips of each hand at the hairline on each side of the client's head, hands pointing upward. Firmly slide the fingers upward, spreading the fingertips. Continue until the fingers meet at the center or top of the scalp. Repeat three or four times.

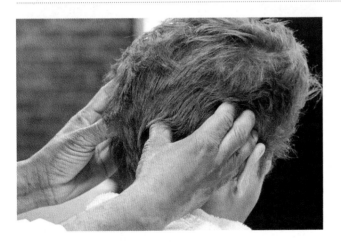

5. Place the fingers of each hand on the sides of the client's head, behind the ears. Use a rotary movement and the thumbs to massage from behind the ears toward the crown. Repeat four or five times. Move the fingers until both thumbs meet at the hairline at the back of the neck. Rotate the thumbs upward toward the crown.

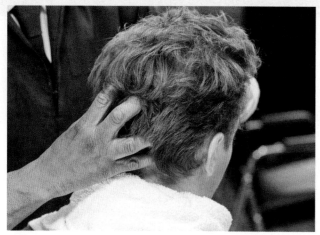

6 Move to the side of the client. Place one hand at the back of the head. Place the thumb and fingers of the other hand against and over the forehead, just above the eyebrows. With the cushion tips of the thumb and fingers of the right hand, use a sliding movement to massage slowly and firmly across the top of the head toward the crown while keeping the left hand at the back of the head in a fixed position. Repeat four or five times.

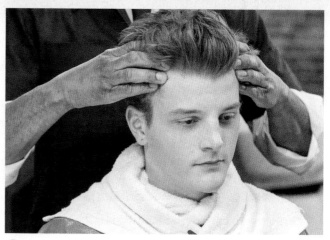

7 Move behind the client. Place the hands on each side of the head at the front hairline. Rotate the fingertips three times. On the fourth rotation, apply a quick, upward twisting motion, firm enough to move the scalp. Continue this movement on the sides and top of the scalp. Repeat three or four times.

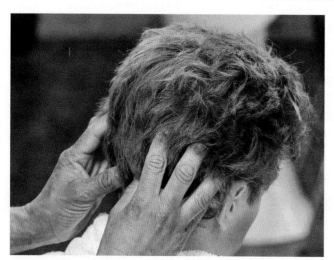

8 Place the fingers of each hand below the back of each ear. Rotate the fingers upward from behind the ears to the crown. Repeat three or four times. Move the fingers toward the back of the head and repeat the movement with both hands. Apply rotary movements in an upward direction toward the crown.

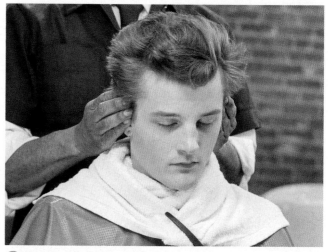

9 Place one hand at either side of the head. Keep fingers close together and position at the hairline above the ears. Firmly move the hands directly upward to the top of the head in a sliding movement. Repeat four times. Move the hands to above the ears and repeat the movement. Move the hands to back of the ears and repeat the movement.

10 Follow scalp massage with a shampoo service.

CLEAN-UP AND DISINFECTION

☐ Clean and disinfect the tools and implements used.

☐ Clean and disinfect the work area.

☐ Dispose of single-use items. Place all used linens, towels, and capes in the laundry.

☐ Wash your hands.

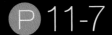
SCALP TREATMENT VARIATIONS

MATERIALS, IMPLEMENTS, AND EQUIPMENT FOR ALL TREATMENTS

- ☐ Brush
- ☐ Comb
- ☐ Cotton or cotton-tipped swabs
- ☐ Eye protectors for client
- ☐ Gloves

- ☐ High-frequency current appliance with assorted electrodes
- ☐ Infrared lamp
- ☐ Safety goggles
- ☐ Scalp conditioners or ointments
- ☐ Scalp lotions or tonics

- ☐ Scalp steamer (optional)
- ☐ Shampoo bowl
- ☐ Shampoos and conditioners
- ☐ Terry cloth towels
- ☐ Waterproof cape

PREPARATION FOR ALL TREATMENTS

The preparation for a variety of scalp treatments is as follows:

1. Assemble supplies.
2. Seat the client in a comfortable and relaxed position.
3. Wash your hands.
4. Drape the client for a shampoo service.
5. Perform hair and scalp analysis.

A. TREATMENT FOR HEALTHY SCALP AND HAIR

The purpose of a general scalp treatment is to keep the scalp and hair clean and healthy. Regular scalp treatments can also help to prevent baldness.

PRODUCTS

- ☐ Scalp conditioner or ointment, if desired
- ☐ Scalp lotion or tonic, if desired
- ☐ Shampoo and conditioner for normal hair and scalp

PROCEDURE

1. Brush the hair for a few minutes to loosen dead skin cells.
2. Part the hair and apply a scalp conditioner or ointment directly to the scalp with cotton or cotton swab.
3. Apply an infrared lamp for 3 to 5 minutes.

    1. Massage the scalp for 10 minutes.

    2. Shampoo the hair and towel-dry.

    3. Optional: Stimulate the scalp with high-frequency current for 2 to 3 minutes.

    4. If desired, apply a suitable scalp lotion or tonic and work it into the scalp; comb and style the hair.

B. TREATMENT FOR DRY SCALP AND HAIR

PRODUCTS

☐ Mild shampoo and moisturizing conditioner for dry hair

☐ Scalp conditioning cream for dry hair and scalp

PROCEDURE

1. Brush the client's hair.

2. Massage and stimulate the scalp for 3 to 5 minutes.

3. Apply a scalp preparation for this condition.

4. Steam the scalp with hot towels or scalp steamer for 7 to 10 minutes.

5. Shampoo the hair using a mild shampoo suitable for dry scalp and hair.

6. Towel-dry the hair, making sure the scalp is thoroughly dried.

7. Apply scalp cream sparingly with a rotary, frictional motion.

8. Apply an infrared lamp over the scalp for 3 to 5 minutes.

9. Stimulate the scalp with direct high-frequency current, using a glass rake electrode, for about 5 minutes.

10. Rinse the hair thoroughly.

11. Comb the hair into the desired style.

> **⚠ CAUTION**
> Never use a scalp or hair treatment product that contains alcohol *before* applying high-frequency current. Products with alcohol can only be safely applied *after* the high-frequency treatment.

C. TREATMENT FOR OILY SCALP AND HAIR

PRODUCTS

☐ Balancing shampoo and conditioner for oily hair and scalp

☐ Medicated scalp astringent

☐ Medicated scalp lotion

PROCEDURE

1. Brush the hair gently.

2. Apply a medicated scalp lotion to the scalp only.

3. Apply an infrared lamp or scalp steamer for 3 to 5 minutes.

4. Massage the scalp.

5. Shampoo with a product suitable for oily scalp and hair and towel-dry the hair.

6. Apply direct high-frequency current for 3 to 5 minutes.

7. Apply a medicated lotion or astringent to the scalp only.

8. Comb the hair into the desired style.

D. TREATMENT FOR A DANDRUFF CONDITION

PRODUCTS

☐ Antidandruff shampoo and conditioner

☐ Antiseptic lotion, cream, or ointment

☐ Prescribed cream or ointment, if applicable

PROCEDURE

1. Seat the client in a comfortable and relaxed position.

2. Drape the client.

3. Apply gloves and perform hair and scalp analysis.

4. Shampoo with antidandruff shampoo according to the type of dandruff and towel-dry.

5. Apply antiseptic product to the scalp.

6. Apply steam towels or scalp steamer for 3 to 5 minutes.

7. Massage the scalp.

8. Shampoo and condition with antidandruff products.

9. Both the barber and the client should put on tinted safety goggles.

10. Expose the scalp to ultraviolet rays (for its germicidal effects) for 5 to 8 minutes, parting the hair every half inch.

11. Apply a leave-in antiseptic or prescribed medication to the scalp.

12. Expose the scalp to an infrared lamp for 5 to 8 minutes at a distance of 30 inches to help penetration of the product. Slowly wave your hand through the path of the lamp to avoid burning the client's scalp.

Alternate Step 12: High-frequency currents may be applied for 3 to 5 minutes but only if the antiseptic or prescribed medication *does not* contain alcohol.

13. Comb the hair into desired style.

E. SCALP TREATMENT FOR ALOPECIA

PRODUCTS

☐ Prescribed medicated scalp ointment, if applicable (check for alcohol content)

☐ Shampoo for normal, dry, or oily hair and scalp

PROCEDURE

1. Apply regular scalp manipulations.

2. Shampoo the hair and scalp with an appropriate product.

3. Dry the scalp thoroughly.

4. Both the barber and the client should put on tinted safety goggles.

5. Expose the scalp to ultraviolet rays for about 5 minutes at a distance of 30 to 36 inches.

6. Apply a non-alcohol-based medicated scalp ointment as directed by client's physician.

7. Apply indirect high-frequency current (with the client holding the wire glass electrode between both hands) for about 5 minutes.

8. Comb the hair into the desired style.

F. TREATMENT FOR DRY OR DAMAGED HAIR

PRODUCTS

☐ Leave-in conditioner

☐ Protein and moisturizing repair treatments

☐ Shampoo appropriate for hair texture

PROCEDURE

1 Massage and stimulate the scalp for 3 to 5 minutes.

2 Apply a mild shampoo and rinse thoroughly.

3 Blot hair with a towel.

4 Apply a deep-conditioning agent according to the manufacturer's directions.

5 Apply a plastic cap; set the client under a dryer and apply heat for 10 minutes.

6 Rinse the conditioner thoroughly; comb hair into the desired style.

CLEAN-UP AND DISINFECTION FOR ALL TREATMENTS

☐ Clean and disinfect the tools and implements used.

☐ Clean and disinfect the work area.

☐ Dispose of single-use items. Place all used linens, towels, and capes in the laundry.

☐ Wash your hands.

REVIEW QUESTIONS

1. What services are associated with the treatment of the hair and scalp?

2. Why is performing a shampoo before a haircut a good idea?

3. Why is proper draping required?

4. Explain the purpose of the towel or neck strip in draping.

5. Describe the type of cape that should be used for wet and chemical services and why.

6. Describe the type of cape that should be used for haircutting services and why.

7. Where are massage manipulations started from relative to the client's head and how should they be performed?

8. Compare the massage manipulations used in a shampoo service to the manipulations used in a scalp massage.

9. Review the Procedures section and list the scalp treatments that include the application of ultraviolet rays and/or infrared rays in the treatment.

10. Identify three important cautions associated with scalp treatments.

CHAPTER GLOSSARY

draping	p. 277	the term used to describe the covering of the client's clothing with a cape for their protection
hair conditioners (HAYR kun-DIH-shun-urz)	p. 277	products designed to moisturize the hair or restore some of the hair's oils or proteins
scalp conditioners (SKALP kun-DISH-un-urz)	p. 277	cream-based products and ointments used to soften and improve the health of the scalp
scalp steam (SKALP STEEM)	p. 284	process of using steam towels or a steaming unit to soften and open scalp pores
shampoos (sham-POOz)	p. 277	hair and scalp cleansing products

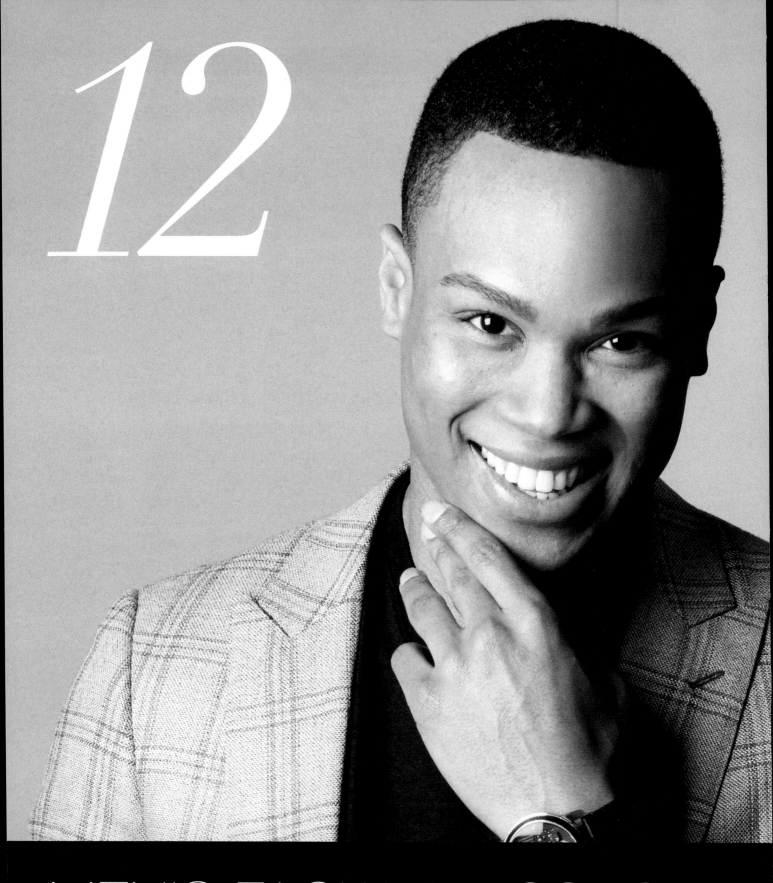

12

MEN'S FACIAL MASSAGE AND TREATMENTS

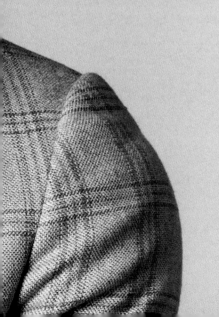

LEARNING OBJECTIVES

After completing this chapter, you will be able to:

LO❶
List the modalities that affect muscle action.

LO❷
Know the muscles of the scalp, face, and neck.

LO❸
List the modalities that affect nerve responses.

LO❹
Know the main cranial nerve branches of the scalp, face, and neck.

LO❺
Identify arteries and veins affected by facial massage.

LO❻
Describe the physiological effects of massage.

LO❼
Name and describe massage manipulations.

LO❽
Explain the use of facial and electrotherapy equipment.

LO❾
Identify skin types, facial treatments, and products.

Introduction

Providing for men's skin care needs is an important and lucrative service in today's personal appearance market. Male clients represent about 20 percent of the skin care clientele in spas and salons, and this percentage is expected to grow. The data, which follows the trend of spas and salons specifically, indicates a market base that may not have been well served in the past few decades by the very branch of the industry that once catered to the male market—barbers and barbershops! Historically, hot towels and rolling cream facials were standard customer services performed by the barber. Although products and technological options have changed over the years, the concept of providing psychologically and physiologically rewarding services has not. Facial massage and skin care treatments are services that you should master and promote to build your clientele.

In this chapter, you will review anatomical features of the face and neck as they relate to massage manipulations and facial treatments. You will also learn how to analyze skin types so that you can recommend appropriate products and treatments to your clients.

why study
MEN'S FACIAL MASSAGE AND TREATMENTS?

Barbers should study and have a thorough understanding of men's facial massage and treatments because:

> Barbers need to be competent in all of the services for which they are licensed to perform.

> The current trend among men is that they wish to experience the benefits of facial massage and treatments.

> Regularly scheduled facials can produce noticeable improvement in the client's skin tone, texture, and appearance, and this outcome can lead to repeat clients and referrals.

> Barbers need to know how to perform the aspects of a facial that are part of the finishing steps after a shave.

Review Subdermal Systems

After reading this section, you will be able to:

LO**1** List the modalities that affect muscle action.

LO**2** Know the muscles of the scalp, face, and neck.

LO**3** List the modalities that affect nerve responses.

LO④ Know the main cranial nerve branches of the scalp, face, and neck.

LO⑤ Identify arteries and veins affected by facial massage.

The muscles, nerves, and arteries of the head, face, and neck are three of the subdermal systems associated with the performance of facial treatments. As you learned in Chapter 6,

- *muscles* are fibrous tissues that have the ability to stretch and contract to produce all body movements;

- *nerves* are long, white, fibrous cords that act as message carriers from the brain and spinal column to and from all parts of the body;

- *arteries* are elastic, muscular, thick-walled blood vessels that transport blood under high pressure;

- *veins* are thin-walled vessels that contain valves that keep the blood flowing to the heart and prevent it from flowing backward.

Since massage manipulations and facial treatments can affect all of these systems it is important to have a good understanding of their location and functions so you can perform facial services safely and effectively.

DESCRIBE THE MODALITIES THAT AFFECT MUSCLE ACTION

The effect of a facial service on a muscle can be calming or stimulating, depending on the modality used. These modalities are

- massage (hand massage and electric massager);

- electric currents (high frequency, galvanic, and microcurrent);

- light rays (infrared and ultraviolet, low-level light therapy or low-level laser therapy [LLLT], and light-emitting diodes [LED]);

- heat (heat lamps, heating caps, infrared devices, lasers);

- moist heat (steamers and hot towels);

- nerve impulses (through the nervous system and motor points);

- chemicals (certain acids, salts, and microdermabrasion).

DISCUSS THE MUSCLES AFFECTED BY FACIAL MASSAGE

When performing a facial massage, you will be concerned with the voluntary muscles of the head, face, and neck. Study **Figures 12-1** and **12-2** and **Table 12-1** to review the location of these muscles and what they control so you can apply skillful massage manipulations.

figure 12-1
Muscles of the head, face, and neck.

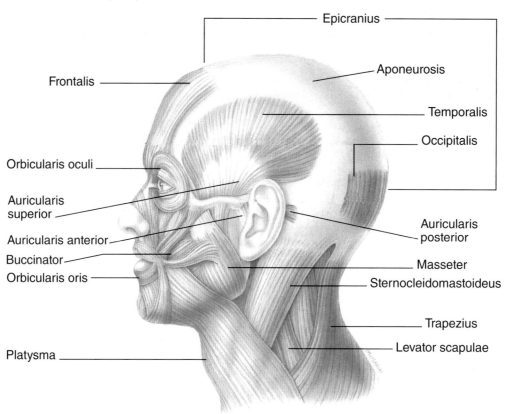

figure 12-2
Muscles of the face.

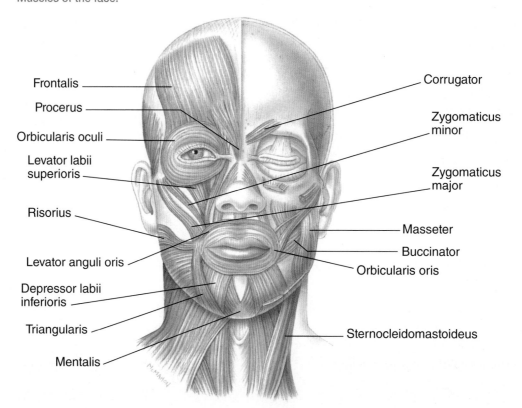

table 12-1

MUSCLES OF THE SCALP, FACE, AND NECK

Muscle	Location	Description and Function
Epicranius (occipitofrontalis)	Scalp	Broad muscle that covers the top of the skull
Frontalis	Scalp	Muscle at the front portion of the epicranius that draws scalp forward and causes wrinkles across the forehead
Occipitalis	Scalp	Muscle at the back part of the epicranius that draws the scalp backward
Epicranial aponeurosis	Scalp	Tendon that connects the occipitalis and frontalis
Orbicularis oculi	Eyebrows	Muscle that surrounds the eye socket and closes the eyelid
Corrugator	Eyebrows	Muscle beneath the frontalis and orbicularis oculi that draws the eyebrows down and in and wrinkles the forehead vertically
Procerus	Nose	Muscle that covers the top of the nose, depresses the eyebrow, and causes wrinkles across the bridge of nose; other nasal muscles contract and expand the openings of the nostrils
Levator labii superioris (quadratus labii superioris)	Mouth	Muscle surrounding the upper lip that elevates the upper lip and dilates the nostrils, for example, when expressing distaste
Depressor labii inferioris (quadratus labii inferioris)	Mouth	Muscle that surrounds the lower part of the lip, depresses the lower lip, and draws it to one side, for example, when expressing sarcasm
Buccinator	Mouth	Thin, flat muscle between the upper and lower jaws; compresses the cheeks and expels air between the lips
Levator anguli oris (caninus)	Mouth	Muscle that raises angle of mouth and draws it inward
Mentalis	Mouth	Muscle at the tip of the chin that elevates the lower lip and raises and wrinkles the skin of the chin
Orbicularis oris	Mouth	Flat band of muscle around the upper and lower lips that compresses, contracts, puckers, and wrinkles the lips
Risorius	Mouth	Muscle that extends from the masseter muscle to the angle of the mouth that draws the corner of the mouth out and back, for example, when grinning
Zygomaticus major	Mouth	Muscle on both sides of the face that extends from the zygomatic bone to the angle of the mouth that pulls the mouth upward and backward, for example, when laughing or smiling
Zygomaticus minor	Mouth	Muscle on both sides of the face that extends from the zygomatic bone to the upper lip and that pulls the mouth upward, inward, and backward, for example, when smiling
Triangularis	Mouth	Muscle that extends along the side of the chin that draws the corner of the mouth down
Masseter and the temporalis	Mastication muscles	Muscles that coordinate opening and closing mouth; chewing muscles
Auricularis superior	Ears	Muscle above the ear that draws the ear upward

(continues)

table 12-1

(Continued)

Muscle	Location	Description and Function
Auricularis posterior	Ears	Muscle behind the ear that draws the ear backward
Auricularis anterior	Ears	Muscle in front of the ear that draws the ear forward
Platysma	Neck	Broad muscle extending from the chest and shoulder muscles to the side of the chin; responsible for depressing the lower jaw and lip
Sternocleidomastoideus	Neck	Muscle that extends from the collar and chest bones to the temporal bone in back of the ear that bends and rotates the head
Trapezius	Neck	Muscle that covers the back of the neck allowing movement of the shoulders

DISCUSS THE MODALITIES THAT AFFECT NERVE RESPONSES

Nerve stimulation causes muscles to expand and contract. Heat and moist heat on the skin cause relaxation and cold causes contraction. Nerve stimulation may be accomplished by any of the following means:

- Chemicals (certain acids, salts, and microdermabrasion)
- Massage (hand massage and electric massager)
- Electrical current (high frequency and microcurrent)
- Light rays (infrared, LLT, and LED)
- Heat (heat lamps, heating caps, infrared devices, lasers)
- Moist heat (steamers and hot towels)

DISCUSS THE MAIN CRANIAL NERVES AFFECTED BY FACIAL MASSAGE

There are 12 pairs of cranial nerves and all are connected to a part of the brain surface. When performing facials and scalp treatments, the cranial nerves of most interest are the fifth, seventh, and eleventh cranial nerves. Refer to Chapter 6 to review the nerves of the scalp, face, and neck in greater detail.

- **Fifth cranial nerve (also known as trifacial or trigeminal nerve).** The chief sensory nerve of the face that also serves as the motor nerve that controls chewing
- **Seventh cranial nerve (facial nerve).** The sensory-motor nerve that controls motions of the face, scalp, and neck and sections of the palate and tongue
- **Eleventh cranial nerve (accessory nerve).** The motor nerve that controls motions of the neck muscles

Spinal (cervical) nerves can also be affected by facial massage. The cervical nerves originate at the spinal cord and their branches supply the muscles and scalp at the back of the head and neck.

DISCUSS ARTERIES AND VEINS AFFECTED BY FACIAL MASSAGE

Arteries are vessels that transport *oxygenated* blood from the heart to all parts of the body. The primary arteries affected by facial massage are as follows:

- **Common carotids.** The main sources of blood supply to the head, face, and neck; located at the sides of the neck
- **External maxillary (facial artery).** Supplies the lower region of the face, mouth, and nose
- **Superficial temporal.** A continuation of external carotid; supplies muscles, skin, and scalp on the front, side, and top of the head
- **Occipital.** Supplies the scalp and back of the head up to the crown
- **Posterior auricular.** Supplies the scalp behind and above the ear

Veins transport *deoxygenated* blood from various parts of the body to the heart. The deoxygenated blood from the head, face, and neck returns to the heart through the internal jugular and external jugular veins located on each side of the neck. Refer to Chapter 6 to review the arteries and veins of the scalp, face, and neck in greater detail.

Understand the Theory of Massage

After reading this section, you will be able to:

LO**6** Describe the physiological effects of massage.

LO**7** Name and describe massage manipulations.

Most clients enjoy a properly administered facial treatment for its stimulating or relaxing effects. Facial massage involves the manual or mechanical external manipulation of the face and neck and requires a skillful touch when using the hands or an electric massager. Each massage movement is performed to obtain a specific result and the benefits to be gained will depend on the

- type of massage movement used;
- amount of pressure used;
- direction of the movement;
- duration of the massage manipulation.

DISCUSS THE PHYSIOLOGICAL EFFECTS OF MASSAGE

Skillfully applied massage influences the structures and functions of the body, either directly or indirectly. The immediate effect of massage is first noticed on the skin. The part being massaged reacts with an increase in its functional activities, such as more active circulation, secretion, nutrition, or excretion. There is scarcely an organ of the body that is not affected favorably by scientific massage. Following are some beneficial results that may be obtained by proper massage:

- The skin and all its structures are nourished.
- Muscle fiber is stimulated and strengthened.
- The nerves are soothed and rested.
- Fat cells are reduced.
- Circulation of blood is increased.
- The activity of the skin and scalp glands is stimulated.
- The skin is rendered soft and pliable.
- Pain is sometimes relieved.

KNOW ABOUT MASSAGE MANIPULATIONS

A **motor point** (MOH-tur POYNT) is a point on the skin where nerves that control the underlying muscle are located. When electrical stimulation is applied to the nerve through electrodes, the muscle responds by contracting. Every muscle has a motor point. This is important to know because in order to obtain the maximum benefit from electrotherapy treatments, you must consider the motor points that affect the underlying muscles of the face and neck. The location of a motor point, however, varies among individuals due to differences in body structure. **Figure 12-3** illustrates the areas where motor points are generally found.

figure 12-3
Motor points of the face.

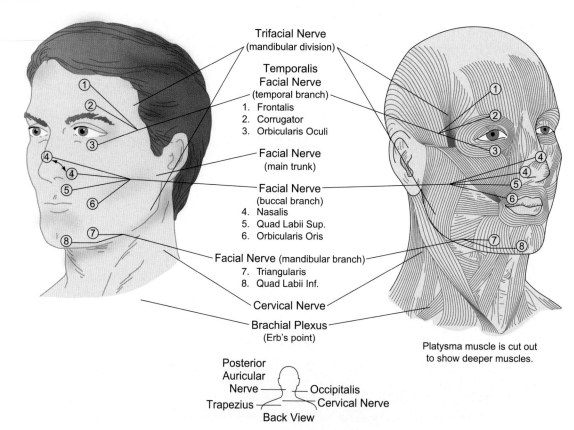

Trifacial Nerve (mandibular division)

Temporalis
Facial Nerve (temporal branch)
1. Frontalis
2. Corrugator
3. Orbicularis Oculi

Facial Nerve (main trunk)

Facial Nerve (buccal branch)
4. Nasalis
5. Quad Labii Sup.
6. Orbicularis Oris

Facial Nerve (mandibular branch)
7. Triangularis
8. Quad Labii Inf.

Cervical Nerve

Brachial Plexus (Erb's point)

Platysma muscle is cut out to show deeper muscles.

Posterior Auricular Nerve — Occipitalis
Trapezius — Cervical Nerve
Back View

A **trigger point** is a tender area in a muscle caused by a localized knot or spasm in the muscle fiber that can radiate pain to other locations in the body. A trigger point exhibits hypersensitivity to electrical stimulation and pressure, which makes it more responsive to electrotherapy or massage. When used in facial massage, gentle but direct pressure can be applied to a trigger point for about 30 seconds, followed by stroking movements to help relieve painful areas.

Review the position of motor points and trigger points in **Figure 12-3**.

Massage Manipulations

Effleurage (EF-loo-rahzh) is a stroking movement. It is a light, continuous movement that should be applied in a slow and rhythmic manner over the skin, with no pressure (**Figure 12-4**). The palms are used over large surfaces and the fingertips work the small surfaces, such as those around the eyes. Effleurage is frequently used on the forehead, face, and scalp for its soothing and relaxing effects and to apply lotions or creams.

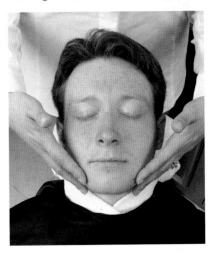

figure 12-4
Stroking movement with the fingertips.

- To correctly position the fingers for the stroking movement, slightly curve the fingers with just the cushions of the fingertips touching the skin. Do not use the ends of the fingertips for these massage movements since they are pointier than the cushions and the fingernails may scratch the client's skin.

- When using the palms for the stroking movement, keep your hands loose and your wrists and fingers flexible. Curve your fingers and palms to conform to the shape of the area being massaged.

Pétrissage (PEH-treh-sahzh) is a kneading movement that is performed with light, firm pressure.

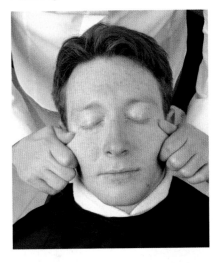

figure 12-5
Pétrissage.

- In this movement, the skin and flesh are grasped between the thumb and fingers. As the tissues are lifted from their underlying structures, they are gently squeezed, rolled, or pinched with a light, firm pressure.

- Pétrissage exerts an invigorating effect on the area being massaged. These kneading movements provide deeper stimulation to the muscles, nerves, and skin glands and also help to improve circulation.

- Although kneading movements are usually used on large surfaces such as the shoulders and back, the fingertips can be used to gently knead the cheeks with light pinching movements (**Figure 12-5**).

Friction (FRIK-shun) is a deep rubbing movement in which pressure is applied on the skin with the fingers or palms while moving over an underlying structure. Friction has been proven to be beneficial to the circulation and glandular activity of the skin (**Figure 12-6**).

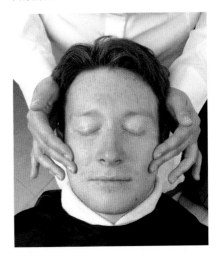

figure 12-6
Friction.

- Light circular friction is used on the face and neck.

- Circular friction movements with more pressure can be used during scalp massages.

Percussion (pur-KUSH-un) or **tapotement** (tah-POT-ment) consists of short, quick tapping, slapping, or hacking movements. Percussion movements

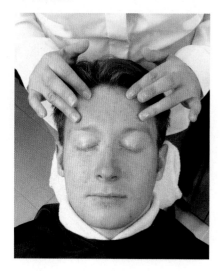

figure 12-7
Percussion.

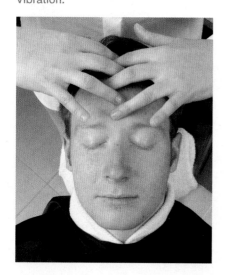

figure 12-8
Vibration.

stimulate the nerves to tone the muscles and impart a healthy glow to the part being massaged. Since percussion is the most stimulating form of massage, it needs to be performed with care and discretion.

- Tapping movements are the gentlest form of tapotement and can be used in facial massage by bringing the fingertips down against the skin in rapid succession with even force (Figure 12-7).

- In slapping movements, the lower points to midpoints of the fingers are used to strike the skin lightly and rapidly. One hand follows the other and should lift the skin slightly with each slapping stroke.

- Hacking, or chopping movements, employs the outer edges of the hands to strike against the skin in alternate succession. Hacking should only be used on the back and shoulders.

Vibration (vy-BRAY-shun) is a rapid shaking movement over the skin section with the fingertips or an electric massager or vibrator. Both methods are used to transmit a trembling movement to the skin and its underlying structures.

- Vibration should be used sparingly and not exceed a few seconds' duration on any one area to avoid overstimulation (Figure 12-8).

- Deep vibration with a mechanical vibrator or massager can stimulate blood circulation and increase muscle tone.

Guidelines for Performing Facial Massage Manipulations

When massaging areas of the head, face, or neck, any pressure employed should be applied in an upward direction to avoid loss of skin resiliency. This rule should be followed in all massage manipulations, whether they are intended to stimulate, relax, or soothe the skin. When applying rotary manipulations, any pressure used should be applied on the upward swing of the circular movement. Review Procedure 12-1 to know about facial massage manipulations.

- A thorough client consultation and accurate skin analysis is crucial to determining the method and duration of massage manipulations to be used.

- Be sure that the direction of massage movements is from the insertion of the muscle toward its origin. The insertion of a muscle is the attachment point to a movable bone and the origin of a muscle is the attachment point to an immovable bone.

- Perform massage manipulations systematically and rhythmically.

- Curve the fingertips or palms slightly to conform to the area being massaged.

- Gradually reduce the pressure when removing your hands from the client's face to gently feather-off from the skin surface.

- When facial hair is present, direct massage movements in the direction of the beard growth. Massage manipulations that go against or across the grain may cause discomfort to the client.

- The frequency of facial or scalp massages depends on the condition of the skin, age of the client, and the condition being treated. Generally speaking, a normal skin or scalp can be kept in good condition with weekly treatments and proper home care.

- Massage should always be performed in moderation and based on good judgment.

- Massage should never be recommended or employed when any of the following conditions are present:

  - Acute inflammation of the skin

  - Severe skin lesions

  - Pus-containing pimples

  - High blood pressure

  - Skin infections

 12-1 **Facial Massage Manipulations** *pages 326–328*

REMINDER

Massage manipulations on the face are usually performed with upward movements; however, the presence of facial hair may require a different approach. Direct massage movements in the direction of beard growth. Massage manipulations that go against or across the grain may cause discomfort to the client.

Know the Purpose of Facial Equipment

After reading this section, you will be able to:

LO **8** Explain the use of facial and electrotherapy equipment.

In addition to employing hands for massages, appliances, electrical currents, microdermabrasion, and light rays can be used to enhance a facial treatment service. However, thorough training in the application of any of these modalities and licensure compliance is required before using them on a client.

The following section provides an overview of some appliances and modalities that may be used in facial services.

IDENTIFY FACIAL APPLIANCES

The **electric massager** (ee-LEK-trik muh-SAJH-ur), most often used in barbershops, is a handheld unit that transmits vibrations through the barber's hand and fingertips to the client's skin and muscles. This type of massager is typically used over heavy muscle tissue such as the scalp and shoulders to produce a succession of stimulating impulses. It has an invigorating effect on muscle tissue, increases the blood supply to the parts treated, is soothing to the nerves, increases glandular activity, and stimulates the skin and scalp. When used correctly with a light and gentle touch, electric massagers can also be used to perform vibratory facials. Following are some rules for using an electric massager:

- Do not use a massager when the client has a known weakness of the heart or on a client with fever, abscesses, or skin inflammations.

HERE'S A TIP

Some hand massager appliances are heavy and cumbersome for smaller hands. Always try one on for size before purchasing.

- Regulate the number of vibrations to avoid overstimulation; do not use the massager for too long in any one spot.

- Vary the amount of pressure in accordance with the results desired.

- Do not apply vibrations over the upper lip as it may cause discomfort.

- For soothing and relaxing effects, use slow, light vibrations; for stimulating effects, use light vibrations of moderate speed and duration; to reduce fatty tissues, use moderately timed, fast vibrations with firm pressure.

A **brush machine** is an electrical appliance with interchangeable brushes that attach to the rotating head of the unit. Brushing is a form of mechanical exfoliation that helps to stimulate, cleanse, and remove dead cells from the skin surface. Many models are available from a variety of manufacturers. Typically, these units have two or three brush attachments of various bristle textures that can be attached and rotated at different speeds, depending on the features of the unit (**Figure 12-9**). Following are guidelines for use (see also Procedure 12-2):

- Apply a moisturizing cleansing cream or lotion to the face before using the brush machine.

- Use the softer brush attachments on facial skin.

- Always thoroughly clean and disinfect brushes between clients.

- Do not apply pressure; allow the brush and rotating head to do the work with the bristles remaining straight.

- Remoisten the brush as needed during the process. Drier skin requires a slow, steady rotation. Thicker, oily skins may tolerate a higher speed.

Ⓟ 12-2 **Using the Brush Machine** *page 329*

A *hot-towel cabinet* ensures a ready supply of warm towels for facial services. To prepare towels, fold the towel lengthwise and then in half. Run hot water over the towel, wring out the excess water, and place the towel in the cabinet. Towels can also be prepared for a witch hazel steam by soaking dampened towels in a hot water witch hazel bath prior to wringing.

A **facial steamer** is an electrical appliance that produces and projects moist, uniform steam that can be positioned over sections of the head or face for softening and cleansing purposes (**Figure 12-10**). The steam warms the skin, stimulates circulation, induces the flow of sebum and sweat, and has an antiseptic effect on problematic skin. Steam also helps to soften follicle accumulations such as comedones, making them easier to extract.

Professional steamers are available in various sizes and models, from tabletop units to facial machine components. Most units have a heating coil that boils the water and a pipe through which the steam flows so it can be directed toward the skin area. Following are two guidelines for use:

- Use only distilled or filtered water to avoid mineral and calcium deposits, which can damage the unit.

- In general, administer steam at the beginning of the facial treatment.

figure 12-9
The brush machine helps cleanse and lightly exfoliate the skin.

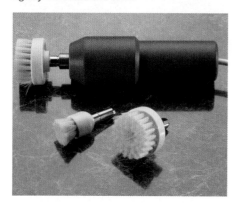

> ⚠ **CAUTION**
> Brushing should never be performed on skin that has been treated with Retin-A® or other drugs that thin or exfoliate the skin.

> 🕐 **REMINDER**
> Brushing machines must always be thoroughly cleaned and disinfected between clients. Position brushes so they will not lose their shape while drying and then store in a clean, closed container.

figure 12-10
The steamer provides many benefits during the facial treatment.

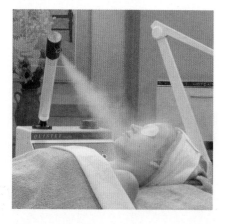

Steamers may also be used in place of hot towels for scalp treatments. When positioned over the scalp, the steam softens the skin, increases perspiration, and softens accumulations in the follicles for more thorough cleansing during the shampoo. Refer to Procedure 12-3 for guidelines for using a facial steamer.

(P) 12-3 **Using a Facial Steamer** *page 330*

IDENTIFY ELECTROTHERAPY EQUIPMENT

Facial treatments performed with facial machines that produce electrical currents are a form of electrotherapy. The two modalities most often used in facial treatments are high-frequency current and galvanic current. Other currents, such as faradic or sinusoidal current, should only be performed by a licensed physician.

Electrodes

Each modality requires an *electrode* to apply and direct the current to the client's skin. The high-frequency appliance requires only one electrode (Figure 12-11). Galvanic machines have two electrodes, one positive and one negative, to conduct the flow of electricity through the body. A positive electrode (anode) is red with a plus sign (+) and a negative electrode (cathode) is black with a minus sign (–) (Figure 12-12).

High-Frequency Machine

High-frequency current (also known as *tesla current*) is characterized by a high rate of oscillation that is used for both scalp and facial treatments. Although it is sometimes called the violet ray because of its color, there are no ultraviolet rays in high-frequency current.

The primary actions of high-frequency current are thermal and antiseptic. Its rapid vibrations do not produce muscular contractions or chemical changes, so the physiological effects are either stimulating or soothing, depending on the method of application.

The electrodes for high-frequency machines are made of glass or metal. Their shapes vary from the flat facial electrode to the rake-shaped scalp electrode. As the current passes through the glass electrode, tiny violet sparks are emitted. All high-frequency treatments should be started with a mild current that is gradually increased to the required strength. The length of the treatment depends upon the condition to be treated. For general facial or scalp treatments, no more than 5 minutes should be allowed.

The high-frequency machine is a versatile tool that can benefit the client's skin in the following ways:

- Stimulates blood circulation
- Helps to oxygenate the skin
- Increases glandular activity
- Aids in elimination and absorption
- Increases cell metabolism
- Promotes antiseptic and germicidal action
- Generates a warm feeling that has a relaxing effect on the skin

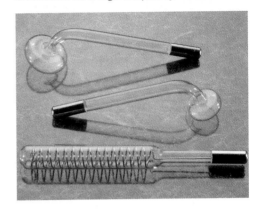

figure 12-11
Electrodes for a high-frequency machine.

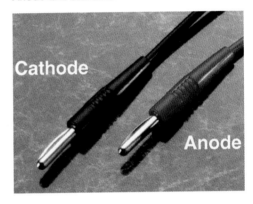

figure 12-12
Anode and cathode.

⚠ **CAUTION**
When performing electrotherapy treatments, the barber and the client must avoid contact with metals or water.

figure 12-13
The high-frequency machine produces a heat effect that stimulates circulation and has an antiseptic effect on the skin.

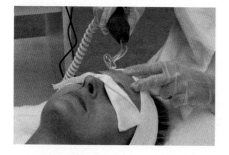

figure 12-14
Indirect application method using high frequency.

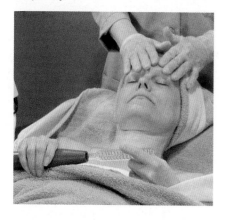

Following are guidelines for cleaning and disinfecting high-frequency electrodes.

1. Wipe the glass electrode with a soap and water solution. Do not immerse the electrode directly in water.

2. Place only the end of the electrode into a disinfectant solution, for 20 minutes.

3. Rinse with cool water, but do not let the metal parts get wet.

4. Dry with a clean towel and store in a clean, covered container.

High-Frequency Application Methods

Always follow the manufacturer's directions for the proper use of high-frequency current. The two primary methods are direct surface application and indirect application. Direct surface application is the method most conducive for use in the barbershop.

Direct surface application is performed with the mushroom or rake-shaped electrode for its calming and germicidal effect on the skin (Figure 12-13).

- The heat that is generated has a sedative effect, and oily or acne-prone skin can benefit from its germicidal action.

- Germicidal benefits of high-frequency current are produced only with the direct application method.

- Direct surface application can be used on clean, dry skin, over facial creams, or over gauze for a sparking effect.

Indirect application is performed with the client holding the wire glass electrode between both hands (Figure 12-14).

- To prevent shock, the power is turned on *after* the client holds the electrode firmly and turned off before the electrode is removed from the client's hand. At no time is the electrode held by the barber or stylist.

- Indirect application of the current produces both a toning and stimulating effect on the skin and is ideal for aging or sallow skin.

Galvanic Machine

The galvanic machine converts the alternating current received from an outlet into a direct current. The electrons then flow continuously in the same direction. This produces a relaxation response that can be regulated to target-specific nerve endings in the epidermis. Galvanic current is used to produce chemical (desincrustation) and ionic (iontophoresis) reactions in the skin. This treatment is beneficial for oily skin problems and acne.

The galvanic machine has two poles, negative (−) and positive (+). Both are used for different effects. Several types of electrodes are available for the galvanic machine. The most popular are the desincrustrator and the ionizing roller.

Galvanic Current Applications

Galvanic current accomplishes two basic tasks: desincrustation and iontophoresis.

Galvanic Current Reactions

Desincrustation is used to facilitate deep pore cleansing. To ensure proper contact, each electrode is wrapped in wet cotton and the active electrode is applied to the oily areas of the face for 3 to 5 minutes. The inactive electrode is held by the client in the right hand or is attached to a pad placed in contact with the client's right shoulder. To perform desincrustation, an acid-based solution is applied to the skin's surface. During the process, a chemical reaction takes place that helps to emulsify or liquefy sebum and waste that can be easily extracted with gentle pressure.

Iontophoresis (eye-ahn-toh-foh-REE-sus) is the process of using galvanic current to enable ion-containing water-soluble solutions to penetrate the skin. Negative current applied to the skin allows products with negative ions to penetrate the skin; conversely, positive current applied to the skin allows products with positive ions to penetrate (**Figure 12-15**). Products suitable for iontophoresis applications will be labeled as such by the manufacturers.

The process of ionic penetration takes place in two forms: cataphoresis and anaphoresis.

Cataphoresis (kat-uh-foh-REE-sus) is the use of the positive pole (anode) to introduce an acid-pH product, such as an astringent solution, into the skin. Products that have a slightly acidic pH are considered positive. The positive pole may also be used to close the follicles or pores after the treatment; decrease redness, as in mild acne; prevent inflammation after comedone and blemish treatment (by decreasing blood supply); soothe nerves; and harden tissues.

Anaphoresis (an-uh-foh-REE-sus) is the use of the negative pole (cathode) to force an alkaline-pH product, such as a desincrustation lotion, into the skin. Products with an alkaline pH are considered to be negative. The negative pole may be used to stimulate the circulation of blood to dry skin, stimulate nerves, and soften tissues. The procedure for ionization is the same as that used in the desincrustation process.

Microcurrent

Microcurrent (MI-kroh-CUR-ent) is a type of galvanic treatment that uses a very low level of electrical current for many applications in skin care. It is best known for toning the skin and producing a lifting effect on aging skin, which lacks elasticity.

Microdermabrasion

Microdermabrasion (MI-kroh-DERMA-bray-shun) is a form of mechanical exfoliation that involves spraying aluminum oxide or other microcrystals across the skin's surface to exfoliate dead cells. These exfoliated cells are then vacuumed off by means of suction. Microdermabrasion produces fast, visible results and can be used to treat surface wrinkles and aging skin. Although the machine and service are not standard features of most barbershops, they may be found in some high-end men's spas or grooming parlors.

Light Therapy

Light therapy is the process of using light exposure to treat certain conditions of the skin and scalp. Ultraviolet rays, infrared rays, and more currently, LEDs are used to produce different therapeutic effects on the skin.

figure 12-15
Multifunctional machine.

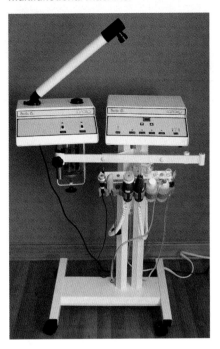

> ⚠ **CAUTION**
> It is critically important to be fully trained in the use of electrotherapy equipment, products, and treatments prior to performing a service. Be guided by your instructor or research manufacturers and suppliers that offer education and training in this modality.

> ⚠ **CAUTION**
> Always check with your state regulatory agency to determine which skin and scalp treatments are allowed to be performed under your barber license and the electrotherapy machines approved for use in your state.

Ultraviolet-Ray Lamps

Ultraviolet rays are at the shorter-wavelength end of the visible spectrum and create different effects depending on the type of ultraviolet bulb used as follows:

- UVA rays—tonic rays
- UVB rays—therapeutic rays
- UVC rays—germicidal rays

Generally speaking, ultraviolet lamps may be used to treat acne, tinea, seborrhea, or dandruff conditions and may produce the following effects:

- Increase the elimination of waste products
- Improve the flow of blood and lymph
- Assist the body in producing vitamin D
- Increase melanin production that produces a tan

Following are guidelines for use of ultraviolet applications:

- Position the lamp 30 to 36 inches from the skin.
- Apply light rays to clean, dry skin.
- Start with a 2- or 3-minute exposure and gradually increase exposure time to 7 or 8 minutes.
- Average exposure may produce skin redness; overdoses can cause blistering.
- Protect the client's eyes with opaque eye protectors.
- Protect your eyes with tinted safety goggles or sunglasses.

Infrared-Ray Lamps

Infrared rays generally produce a soothing and beneficial type of heat that extends for some distance into the tissues of the body. Listed below are some effects of infrared rays on the exposed skin area:

- Heats and relaxes the skin without increasing overall body temperature
- Soothes nerves, dilates blood vessels, and increases circulation
- Increases metabolism and chemical changes within skin tissues
- Increases production of perspiration and oil on the skin
- Relieves pain in sore muscles

Following are guidelines for application of infrared-ray lamps:

- Position lamp at a distance of 30 inches from the skin.
- Protect the client's eyes with opaque eye protectors.
- Do not allow rays to remain on a skin area for more than a few seconds; move your hand back and forth through the light path to break constant exposure.
- Total exposure time should not exceed 5 minutes.

> **⚠ CAUTION**
> Do not permit infrared rays to remain on the body tissues for more than a few seconds at a time. Move your hand back and forth across the rays' path to break constant exposure on the client's skin. The total exposure time should not exceed 5 minutes.

> **⚠ CAUTION**
> Overexposure to ultraviolet rays can destroy skin tissue. Start with a 2- or 3-minute exposure time and gradually increase exposure time to 7 or 8 minutes.

Contraindications for Electrotherapy

A **contraindication** (kahn-trah-in-dih-KAY-shun) is any product, procedure, or treatment that should be avoided because it may cause undesirable side effects or be harmful to the individual. Electrotherapy should never be performed on clients with any of the following conditions:

- Seizures or epilepsy
- Heart conditions
- Nerve disorders
- Fever or any infection
- Asthma
- Pregnancy
- High blood pressure
- Open or broken skin, including pustular acne
- Sinus blockages or conditions
- Pacemakers
- Metal implants

If in doubt, request that clients get approval from their physician before receiving an electrotherapy treatment.

Review Safety Precautions for Using Electrical Equipment

It is especially important to handle electrical equipment safely when applying a device to a client's skin or scalp. Adhere to the following safety precautions when using any electrical item in the barbershop:

- Disconnect any appliances when they are not being used.
- Study instructions before using any electrical equipment.
- Keep all wires, plugs, and equipment in a safe condition.
- Inspect all electrical equipment frequently.
- Avoid getting electrical cords wet.
- Clean and disinfect all electrodes properly.
- Protect the client at all times.
- Do not touch any metal while using electrical appliances.
- Do not handle electrical equipment with wet hands.
- Do not allow the client to touch metal surfaces when electrical treatments are being performed.
- Do not leave the room when the client is attached to any electrical device.
- Do not attempt to clean around an electric outlet when equipment is plugged in.
- Do not touch two metallic objects at the same time while connected to an electric current.
- Do not use any electrical equipment without first obtaining full instruction in its care and use.

The protection and safety of the client should be your primary concern as carelessness can result in shocks or burns. Barbers who practice safety precautions help to eliminate accidents, assuring greater comfort and satisfaction for their clients.

Learn about Facial Treatments

After reading this section, you will be able to:

LO❾ Identify skin types, facial treatments, and products.

Barbers do not treat skin diseases; however, they should be able to recognize various skin disorders that need to be referred to a physician. Facials performed in the barbershop are considered to be either preservative or corrective treatments.

- *Preservative treatments* help maintain the health of facial skin through correct cleansing, toning, and massage.

- *Corrective treatments* correct skin conditions such as dryness, oiliness, blackheads, aging lines, and minor acne.

As with other forms of massage, facial treatments help to increase circulation and metabolism, relax the nerves, activate skin glands, maintain muscle tone, and improve skin texture and complexion.

DESCRIBE SKIN TYPES

There are four basic skin types that the barber will need to be able to recognize before the appropriate products can be chosen for a facial treatment. Skin type is primarily based on the amount of oil that is produced in the follicles from the sebaceous glands and the amount of lipids found between the cells. Dry, normal, combination, and oily are the four basic skin types. Any of these skin types can be sensitive to products, irritation, or the environment.

- *Dry skin*, also known as alipidic (a-la-pid-ic or a-li-pid-ic) skin, does not produce enough sebum to prevent the evaporation of cell moisture. This leaves the skin in a dehydrated state. When analyzed using a magnifying lamp, dry skin may be flaky or dry looking with small fine lines and wrinkles. The objective of a facial treatment for dry skin is to stimulate oil production for protection of the skin surface. Hydrating the skin with moisturizers and humectants, in addition to drinking plenty of water, can help minimize the negative effects of dryness and dehydration (Figure 12-16).

- *Normal skin* has a good water–oil balance. The follicle pores are a normal size and the skin is free of blemishes. Maintenance and preservative care is the goal for this type of skin (Figure 12-17).

- *Oily skin* is characterized by excess sebum production and may appear shiny or greasy. The follicle size is larger and contains more oil. Oily skin requires more cleansing and exfoliation than other skin types, yet over-cleansing can strip and irritate the skin. If the skin is overdried, it is not balanced and the body will try to produce additional oil to compensate for the dryness on the surface.

figure 12-16
Dry skin.

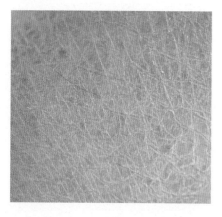

figure 12-17
Normal skin.

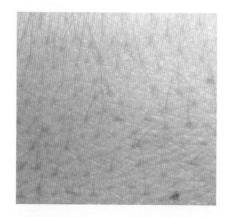

Proper exfoliation and a water-based hydrator help keep oily skin clean and balanced (Figure 12-18).

- *Combination skin* can be both oily and dry in different areas of the face. The T-zone is the section of the face that incorporates the forehead, nose, and chin area (Figure 12-19). These areas tend to have more sebaceous glands and larger pores. The cheek and outer areas of the face tend to be dry. Water-based products work best for combination skin types.

- *Wrinkles* are depressions in the skin that have developed from repetitious muscle action moving in the same direction (Figure 12-20). Other factors that influence the formation of wrinkles include

  - loosening of the elastic skin fibers due to abnormal tension or relaxation of the facial muscles;

  - shrinking of the skin tissue as a result of aging;

  - excessive dryness of the skin;

  - improper facial care.

Skin Analysis

It is preferable to analyze the skin with a magnifying lamp or light (Figure 12-21), but if one is not available, a close inspection of the skin will suffice. When analyzing the skin, it is important to note the client's skin type and condition and the skin's visible appearance and texture.

Guidelines for performing a skin analysis and client consultation include the following:

1. Observe client's skin type, condition, and appearance; feel the texture.

2. Ask the client questions relating to the skin's appearance and home care routine.

3. Discuss the facial procedure and/or treatment plans as well as the products that will be used and why.

4. Encourage the client to ask questions and then determine a course of action together.

5. Record information for the client's next visit.

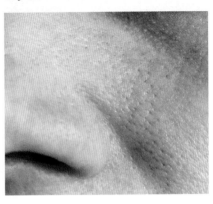

figure 12-18
Oily skin.

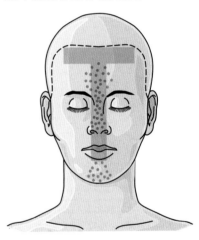

figure 12-19
The T-zone area of the face.

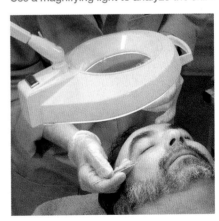

figure 12-21
Use a magnifying light to analyze the skin.

figure 12-20
Wrinkles.

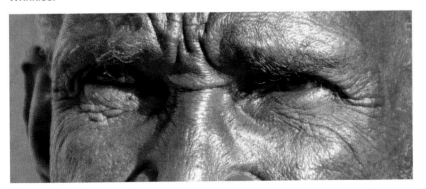

REMINDER

All products should be removed from their containers with a disinfected or disposable spatula to prevent contamination of the product. Do not dip your fingers into containers!

Skin Care Products

There are many types of skin care products available for use in the barbershop or for the client's home use. These products are usually designed for specific skin types or conditions and can be categorized as cleansers, exfoliants, skin tonics, masks, and moisturizers. Products such as toners, massage creams, and moisturizers will also be used following a shave service. *Cleansing* products should be mild and easy to rinse from the skin. They are available as face washes, lotions, and creams for different types of skin and skin conditions.

* Face washes are usually water-based products with a neutral or slightly acidic pH effective on oily and combination skin types.

* Cleansing lotions are water-based emulsions for normal and combination skin that contain emollients or oils to soften the skin.

* Cleansing creams are heavier oil-based emulsions that are used primarily to dissolve dirt and makeup.

Skin tonics, which include **fresheners**, **toners**, and **astringents** (uh-STRIN-jentz), help to rebalance the pH of the skin and remove product residue after cleansing. Skin tonics have a temporary tightening effect on the skin and vary in strength and alcohol content.

* *Fresheners* usually have the lowest alcohol content (0 to 4 percent) and are suitable for dry, mature, and sensitive skin.

* *Toners* are designed to tone or tighten the skin and may be used on normal and combination skin types. The alcohol content range of toners is usually 4 to 15 percent.

* *Astringents* may contain up to 35 percent alcohol and may be used for oily and acne-prone skin.

Moisturizers are formulated to add moisture to the skin surface. They contain moisture-attracting humectants and emollients that prevent moisture from evaporating from the skin. Moisturizing creams and lotions are available with varying humectant-to-emollient ingredient ratios for dry, normal, and oily skin types. As a barber, you will use moisturizers as one of the final steps in facial and shave services.

Mechanical exfoliants are products that help to physically remove dead cells from the skin surface and to clear clogged pores. Granular scrubs are available in cream, lotion, and gel forms for a variety of skin types. **Rolling cream** (ROHL-ing KREEM) is a thick, smooth, *nongranular* exfoliating cream, usually pink in color, which has been used in barbershops for decades. It is applied in a thin layer over the skin and then rolled off with firm, stroking motions. As the rolling takes place, dead-cell buildup and trapped impurities are lifted from the skin surface. The skin is left soft and smooth with increased circulation to the surface.

Rolling cream should only be used on clients with normal, oily, or thick skin; it is not recommended on dry, acne-prone, sensitive, or thin-textured skin.

Chemical exfoliants, such as alpha hydroxy acids or enzyme peels, loosen or dissolve dead-cell buildup on the skin surface. The use of chemical exfoliants requires advanced training and in some cases, certification, to meet compliance standards.

Masks help to draw impurities out of pores; depending on the ingredients, they can tighten, tone, hydrate, soothe, and nourish the skin. They are available

DID YOU KNOW?

Witch hazel works as an astringent and can be used as a toning tonic in facial treatments and shave services.

in cream, gel, or clay forms and should be used according to skin type. These products differ in their composition and application, as discussed below.

A mask is usually a setting product, which means that it dries after application, providing complete closure to the environment on top of the skin. Masks are most often applied directly to the skin and are known for their tightening and sebum-absorbing effects.

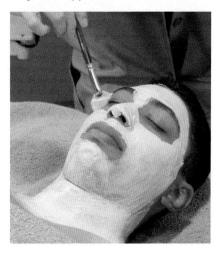

figure 12-22
Clay mask application.

- Clay masks are used to stimulate circulation and temporarily contract the skin pores. They absorb sebum and are used on oily and combination skin types. Applied with a mask brush, they are allowed to set until dry, usually about 10 minutes (**Figure 12-22**).

- Cream masks often contain humectants and emollients and have a strong moisturizing effect; consequently, they do not dry hard like clay masks do and are often used on dry skin types.

- Gel masks use hydrators and soothing ingredients to add moisture to sensitive or dehydrated skin for a more supple appearance.

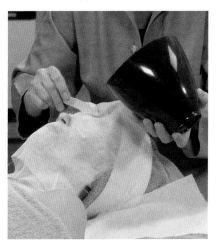

figure 12-23
Paraffin wax application.

- Paraffin wax masks employ the pack application method. Specially prepared paraffin is melted at a temperature that is slightly higher than body temperature before application. The client's skin is prepared by cleansing, followed by the application of a treatment cream. Eye pads are used and the paraffin is applied over gauze to prevent the facial hair from sticking to the wax (**Figure 12-23**).

Gauze is often used to hold cream or gel masks in place over the skin or to prevent paraffin wax from sticking to the skin or facial hair.

High-quality masks and packs should feel comfortable while producing slight tingling and tightening sensations. Always follow the manufacturer's directions for preparation, application, and removal of the product from the skin.

Massage creams are creams, lotions, or oils that provide slip during a massage while also softening and moisturizing the skin.

A general outline of the order in which skin care products will be used during a basic facial treatment in this text is as follows:

1. Cleansing cream or lotion

2. Exfoliant (scrub or rolling cream)

3. Massage cream

4. Cleansing cream or lotion

5. Freshener (low alcohol content)

6. Mask or pack

7. Toner or astringent

8. Moisturizer

However, your instructor's recommended order of product application would be equally correct.

A Note about Men's Skin Care Products

There are many product lines that have been developed specifically with males in mind and each year more men are experiencing the benefits of using skin care products on a regular basis.

When choosing men's skin care products for use in the barbershop, it is important to think about the specific characteristics of a product that might appeal to men. For example, some men do not like highly fragranced or multistep products. Creams should be simple, non-fragranced, and absorbent, with a matte finish rather than greasy or oily. Men also seem to prefer simpler routines and multipurpose products. For example, a skin tonic that also serves as an aftershave may be chosen over the purchase and use of two separate products.

Although the quality of the product must be the first consideration in choosing products, packaging also needs to be taken into consideration. Typically, tube packaging is preferred over jars, and size can be a factor for the client who travels often. One option is to stock retail shelves with larger containers for clients' home use and smaller, more convenient sizes for travel. Smaller packaged goods can also be used for shop promotions and marketing strategies. As a general rule, any products sold in the barbershop should also be visible on backbars and stations and used during client services.

IDENTIFY DIFFERENT FACIAL TREATMENTS

As a professional barber, you should be able to provide different facial treatments and products for different skin conditions. Review the following sections to become familiar with the types of facial treatments you should be able to offer your clients.

Basic Facial

The *basic facial*, sometimes known as the *scientific rest facial*, is the foundation for all other facial treatments covered in this chapter. A basic facial includes cleansing, exfoliating, massage manipulations, toning, a mask or pack, and moisturizing. These actions help to stimulate the functions of the skin while exercising or relaxing facial muscles. Refer to Procedure 12-4 to learn how to perform a basic facial at the barber's chair. This procedure may be changed to conform to your instructor's method, different equipment, or new procedures in the industry.

 12-4 **Basic Facial Procedure** *page 331–333*

Vibratory Facial

A *vibratory facial* is often performed using a combination of hand massage and an electric massager. To avoid heavy contact or pressure that can be uncomfortable for the client, you will need to learn how to apply the electric massager to the client's skin directly and indirectly.

- *Direct application* is performed by attaching the massager to your dominant hand and allowing the vibrations to travel through your fingertips or palms to the client's skin. This method is appropriate for less sensitive facial areas such as the jaw or forehead.

- *Indirect application* requires that you place your nondominant palm or fingertips on the client's skin with the hand holding the massager on top of your hand. In this way, the vibrations will flow through your nondominant hand before reaching the client's skin, making the vibrations more suitable for delicate areas, such as those around the nose and upper cheek.

> ⚠ **CAUTION**
> Do not use a massager when the client has a known weakness of the heart or on a client with fever, abscesses, or skin inflammations.

Facial for Dry Skin

Dry skin is caused by an insufficient flow of sebum from the sebaceous glands. The objective of a facial for dry skin is to help moisturize it. Dry skin facials can be supplemented with infrared rays, galvanic current, or high-frequency current to help stimulate sebum production.

Facial for Oily Skin

Oily skin and/or blackheads (comedones) are caused by hardened masses of sebum formed inside a follicle. The sebaceous material in the follicle darkens when it is exposed to oxygen and forms a blackhead.

Acne is a disorder of the sebaceous glands; clients with a serious condition require medical attention. If the client is under medical care, the barber *may* be able to perform facial treatments prescribed by a client's physician as indicated on the prescription depending on state rules and regulations. If in doubt, contact the physician and your state barber board directly. Because acne contains infectious matter, you will need to wear gloves and use only effleurage movements to apply gentle massage or products to avoid spreading infectious matter to other areas of the client's skin.

With a physician-prescribed treatment plan, barbers are limited to performing the following related procedures:

- Reduction of oil on the skin through topical applications
- Removal of blackheads using proper procedures
- Application of medicated or prescribed preparations

Guidelines for Facial Treatments

To ensure successful facial treatments that can result in repeat bookings and referrals, follow the guidelines below:

- Help the client relax by speaking in a quiet and professional manner.
- Explain the benefits of the service and products during the consultation.
- Provide a quiet atmosphere.
- Work efficiently.
- Maintain clean conditions and arrange supplies neatly.
- Analyze the skin and follow a systematic procedure for performing the facial.
- Protect the client's eyes when applying products.
- Keep your nails smooth and short to avoid scratching the client's skin.
- Keep your hands smooth; warm cold hands before applying to client's skin.
- Always test hot towels before applying them to the client's skin.
- Avoid excessive or rough massage manipulations.
- Avoid leaving excess product on the skin.
- Avoid excessive conversations that do not facilitate client relaxation.

REMINDER

Some clients are sensitive to latex. Use latex-free gloves, sponges, applicators, and so on to avoid causing a negative reaction.

FACIAL MASSAGE MANIPULATIONS

MATERIALS, IMPLEMENTS, AND EQUIPMENT

- ☐ Barber chair with headrest
- ☐ Container for paper and cotton products
- ☐ Container for soiled towels
- ☐ Cotton pads or pledgets
- ☐ Drape
- ☐ Electric massager

- ☐ Headrest covering (paper or cloth towels)
- ☐ Hot-towel cabinet
- ☐ Massage cream
- ☐ Sink
- ☐ Spatula
- ☐ Terry cloth towels

PREPARATION

1. Assemble supplies.
2. Wash your hands.
3. Perform client consultation.
4. Drape the client, recline the chair, and cover the client's hair with towel or plastic cap.
5. Analyze the client's skin.

PROCEDURE

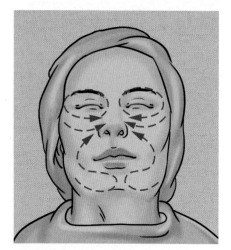

1. Remove the massage cream from container with a clean spatula. Disperse the product over your hands and apply the cream lightly over the client's face with stroking, spreading, and circulatory movements.

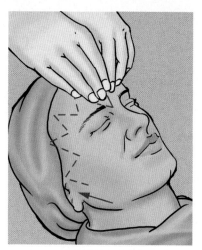

2. Stroke your fingers across the client's forehead with up and down movements.

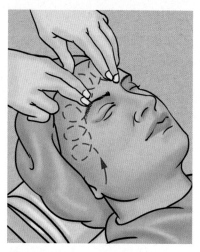

3. Manipulate fingers across the forehead using circular movements.

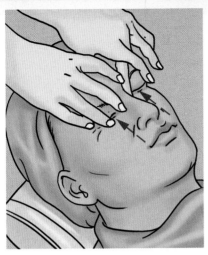

4 Stroke fingers upward along the sides of the nose.

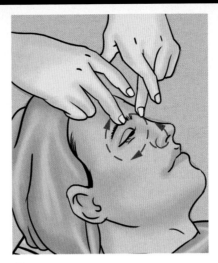

5 Work the circular movements up using a light stroking movement between and around the eyes.

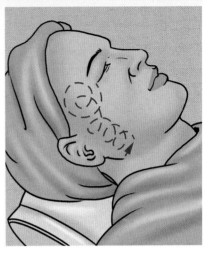

6 Manipulate the temples and then the front and back of the ears with larger circular movements.

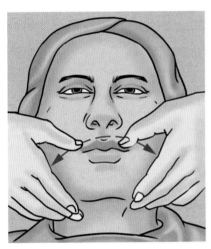

7 Gently stroke both thumbs across the upper lip from center to corners.

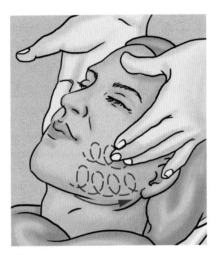

8 Manipulate fingers from the corners of the mouth to the cheeks and temples with a circular movement; start next set of rotations from the tip of the chin through jaw area to the ear using same technique.

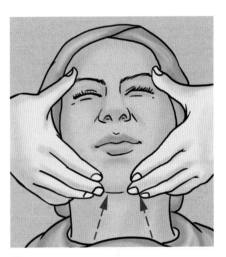

9 Manipulate fingers from under the chin and neck to the back of the ears and up to the temples.

10 Remove massage cream with a warm towel and pat dry.

11 Proceed with the appropriate facial treatment.

CLEAN-UP AND DISINFECTION

☐ Clean and disinfect all tools and implements.

☐ Store products and soiled towels appropriately.

☐ Dispose of single-use items. Place all used linens, towels, and capes in the laundry.

☐ Clean and disinfect the work area.

☐ Wash your hands.

Facial Massage Variation: Electric Massager

1. After completing the above preparation steps 1 to 5, perform the following massage movements with an electric massager.

2. Remove the massage cream from the container with a clean spatula. Disperse the product over your hands and apply the cream lightly over the face with stroking, spreading, and circulatory movements.

3. Adjust the massager on your dominant hand and place the fingertips of your other hand on the client's left nostril. Place the fingers of the vibrating hand over the fingers of the opposite hand to deliver vibrations to the skin.

4. Vibrate the skin with a few light up-and-down movements on the left side of the nose.

5. Gently slide your fingers along the upper cheek area and direct them toward the center of the forehead.

6. Place the vibrating hand onto the skin and perform rotary movements toward the left temple. Pause for a moment.

7. Continue the rotary movements down along the jawline toward the tip of the chin.

8. Massage from the chin back toward the cheek, using wider, firmer movements.

9. Continue with a slow, light stroke at the temple, around the left ear, over the jawbone, toward the center of the neck, and then below the chin.

10. Vibrate rotary movements over the neck, behind the ear, up to the temple, and then toward the center of the forehead.

11. Repeat steps 2 through 9 on the right side of the face.

12. Remove massage cream with a warm towel and pat dry.

13. Proceed with the appropriate facial treatment.

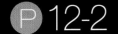

USING THE BRUSH MACHINE

MATERIALS, IMPLEMENTS, AND EQUIPMENT

- ☐ Barber chair with headrest
- ☐ Brush machine with attachments
- ☐ Cleansing cream
- ☐ Container for paper and cotton products
- ☐ Container for soiled towels
- ☐ Cotton pads or pledgets

- ☐ Drape
- ☐ Headrest covering (paper or cloth towels)
- ☐ Hot-towel cabinet
- ☐ Sink
- ☐ Spatula
- ☐ Terry cloth towels

PREPARATION

1. Assemble supplies.
2. Wash your hands.
3. Perform client consultation.
4. Drape the client, recline the chair, and cover the client's hair with towel or plastic cap.
5. Analyze the client's skin.

PROCEDURE

1. Perform a light cleansing on the skin.
2. Insert the appropriate size brush for the face into the handheld device.
3. Apply more cleansing cream to the skin.
4. Dip the bristles into water and begin the rotation movement at the forehead.
5. Continue rotating down the cheeks, nose, upper lip, chin, jaw, and neck areas.
6. Remoisten the brush as needed during the process.
7. Remove cleansing cream with a warm towel and pat dry.
8. Proceed with the appropriate facial treatment.

CLEAN-UP AND DISINFECTION

- ☐ Clean and disinfect all tools and implements.
- ☐ Store products and soiled towels appropriately.
- ☐ Dispose of single-use items. Place all used linens, towels, and capes in the laundry.
- ☐ Clean and disinfect the work area.
- ☐ Wash your hands.

USING A FACIAL STEAMER

MATERIALS, IMPLEMENTS, AND EQUIPMENT

- □ Barber chair with headrest or facial bed
- □ Cleansing cream
- □ Container for paper and cotton products
- □ Container for soiled towels
- □ Cotton pads or pledgets
- □ Drape
- □ Draping sheet or large towel

- □ Facial steamer
- □ Headrest covering (paper or cloth towels)
- □ Hot-towel cabinet
- □ Sink
- □ Spatula
- □ Terry cloth towels

PREPARATION

1. Assemble supplies.
2. Pour distilled water into the steamer and allow the unit to preheat.
3. Wash your hands.
4. Perform client consultation.
5. Drape the client so the neck and shoulders are protected from steam or dripping water.
6. Recline the chair and cover the client's hair with towel or plastic cap.
7. Analyze the client's skin.

PROCEDURE

1. Position the steamer arm to the correct angle and height for the client's position.
2. Turn the machine away from the client and flip the switch on. Do not turn on the vaporizer switch until steam is visible.
3. When the water boils and steam is visible, flip on the vaporizer switch and slowly adjust the steamer arm to a position about 15 inches from the client's face. Move the steamer farther away if the steam becomes too hot or uncomfortable for the client.
4. Upon completion of the steam treatment, turn off the vaporizer switch first and then the on-off switch.
5. Proceed with the appropriate facial treatment.

> ⚠ **CAUTION**
> Placing steam too close to the skin can cause overheating, burning, and irritation.

CLEAN-UP AND DISINFECTION

- □ Clean and disinfect all tools and implements.
- □ Store products and soiled towels appropriately.
- □ Clean and disinfect the work area.

- □ Wash your hands.
- □ Dispose of single-use items. Place all used linens, towels, and capes in the laundry.

BASIC FACIAL PROCEDURE

MATERIALS, IMPLEMENTS, AND EQUIPMENT

- ☐ Barber chair with headrest
- ☐ Cleansing cream
- ☐ Container for paper and cotton products
- ☐ Container for soiled towels
- ☐ Cotton pads or pledgets
- ☐ Exfoliating scrub
- ☐ Head covering
- ☐ Headrest covering (paper or cloth towels)
- ☐ Hot-towel cabinet
- ☐ Mask or pack

- ☐ Massage cream
- ☐ Moisturizer
- ☐ Nylon or vinyl drape
- ☐ Rolling cream
- ☐ Sink
- ☐ Spatulas
- ☐ Talc
- ☐ Terry cloth towels
- ☐ Tonics (toners, fresheners, astringents)

PREPARATION

1. Assemble supplies.
2. Wash your hands.
3. Perform client consultation.
4. Drape the client, recline the chair, and cover the client's hair with towel or plastic cap.
5. Analyze the client's skin.

PROCEDURE

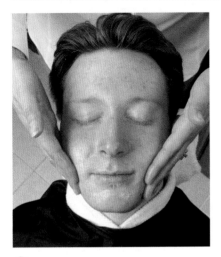

1. Apply cleansing cream over the client's face, using stroking and rotary movements.

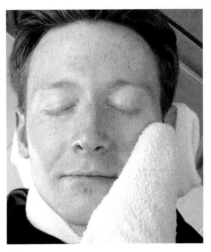

2. Remove the cleansing cream with a warm, damp towel.

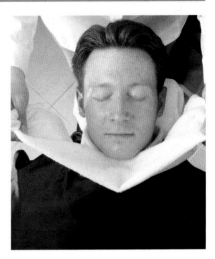

3. Apply two or three steam towels to open pores and loosen imbedded dirt and oils.

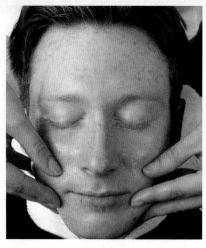

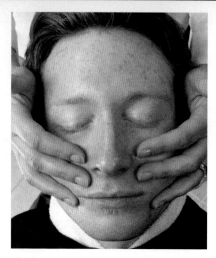

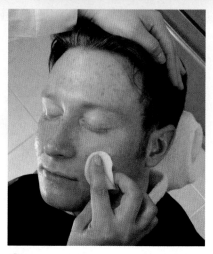

4 Reapply cleansing cream to the skin with your fingertips.

5 Gently massage the face with your hands or a brush machine, using continuous and rhythmic movements.

6 Wipe off excess cleansing cream with a warm towel.

7 Apply an exfoliating product and lightly massage over the skin.

8 Wipe off excess product with a warm towel until the skin is free of exfoliating residue.

9 Apply massage cream and perform effleurage, pétrissage, and tapotement manipulations.

10 Remove excess massage cream with a warm towel and gently wipe selected tonic over the face and pat dry.

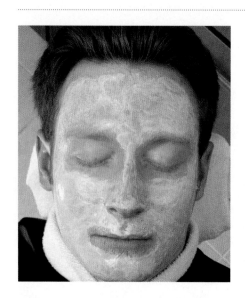

11 Apply the mask or pack and allow to dry.

12 Apply a tepid-to-warm towel to moisten mask or pack. Wipe off product until free of residue.

13 Again, gently wipe a toner or astringent over the face and pat dry.

14 Apply a light coat of moisturizer using the effleurage movement.

15 Apply a light dusting of talc if the client desires it. Remove any excess.

16 Slowly raise the hydraulic chair and assist the client to a sitting position.

☐ Dispose of single-use items. Place all used linens, towels, and capes in the laundry.

☐ Wipe containers and close tightly. Store in an appropriate place.

☐ Clean and then disinfect all non-disposable implements and tools.

☐ Clean and then disinfect work area.

☐ Wash your hands.

Basic Facial Variation: Rolling Cream Facial

1. Perform basic facial steps 1 to 5.

2. Step 6: Apply a rolling cream instead of exfoliating scrub.

3. Apply thin dabs of the rolling cream product to the client's chin, cheeks, and forehead.

4. Dampen the fingertips of both your hands with water and spread the cream evenly over the face and neck with smooth, stroking movements.

5. Massage the face and neck with uniform rotary, stroking, and rubbing movements with the cushion tips of the fingers in an upward direction until most of the cream has dried and rolled off.

6. Apply a small amount of cleansing cream to the face and neck, using lighter manipulations to remove residue.

7. Continue with basic facial from step 7 to finish.

REVIEW QUESTIONS

1. Identify three characteristics of the skin that may benefit from regularly scheduled facial services.

2. List the ways muscles can be stimulated or calmed.

3. Explain what stimulation of the nerves achieves.

4. List the ways in which nerves may be stimulated.

5. Identify three cranial nerves that are important in massaging the head, face, and neck.

6. Identify the main arteries that supply blood to the entire head, face, and neck.

7. Identify the principal veins by which blood from the head, face, and neck is returned to the heart.

8. List and describe five basic massage movements and their effects on the skin.

9. List the benefits of facial massage.

10. List and describe the basic skin types.

11. List 11 caution elements presented in this chapter.

CHAPTER GLOSSARY

anaphoresis (an-uh-foh-REE-sus)	p. 317	process of forcing substances into tissues using galvanic current from the negative toward the positive pole
astringents (uh-STRIN-jentz)	p. 322	tonic lotions with an alcohol content of up to 35 percent; used to remove oil accumulation on oily and acne-prone skin
brush machine	p. 314	an electrical appliance with interchangeable brushes that is used to mechanically cleanse, stimulate, and exfoliate the skin surface
cataphoresis (kat-uh-foh-REE-sus)	p. 317	process of forcing acidic substances into tissues using galvanic current from the positive toward the negative pole
contraindication (kahn-trah-in-dih-KAY-shun)	p. 319	any product, procedure, or treatment that should be avoided because it may cause undesirable side effects or be harmful to the individual
desincrustation	p. 317	the process of deep pore cleansing using an electrode and acid-based solution to create a chemical reaction that helps to emulsify or liquefy sebum and waste from the skin
direct surface application	p. 316	high-frequency current performed with the mushroom- or rake-shaped electrodes for its calming and germicidal effect on the skin
effleurage (EF-loo-rahzh)	p. 311	light, continuous stroking movement applied with the fingers (digital) or the palms (palmar) in a slow, rhythmic manner
electric massager (ee-LEK-trik muh-SAJH-ur)	p. 313	massaging unit that attaches to the barber's hand to impart vibrating massage movements to the skin surface
facial steamer	p. 314	an electrical appliance that produces and projects moist, uniform steam for softening and cleansing purposes

fresheners	p. 322	skin tonics with the lowest alcohol content of 0 to 4 percent; usually designed for dry, mature, and sensitive skin types
friction (FRIK-shun)	p. 311	deep rubbing movement requiring pressure on the skin with the fingers or palm while moving the hand over an underlying structure
indirect application	p. 316	high-frequency current administered with the client holding the wire glass electrode between both hands
iontophoresis (eye-ahn-toh-foh-REE-sus)	p. 317	the process of using galvanic current to enable ion-containing water-soluble solutions to penetrate the skin
microcurrent (MI-kroh-CUR-ent)	p. 317	a type of galvanic treatment that uses a very low level of electrical current for different applications in skin care
microdermabrasion (MI-kroh-DERMA-bray-shun)	p. 317	a form of mechanical exfoliation that involves spraying aluminum oxide or other microcrystals across the skin's surface to exfoliate dead cells
motor point (MOH-tur POYNT)	p. 310	a point on the skin, over a muscle, where pressure or stimulation will cause contraction of that muscle
percussion (pur-KUSH-un)	p. 311	another name for tapotement
pétrissage (PEH-treh-sahzh)	p. 311	kneading movement performed by lifting, squeezing, and pressing the tissue with a light, firm pressure
rolling cream (ROHL-ing KREEM)	p. 322	cleansing and exfoliating product used in facials to lift dead skin cells and dirt from the skin surface
skin tonics	p. 322	toners, fresheners, and astringents; products used to help rebalance skin pH, remove product residue, and create a temporary tightening effect on the skin
tapotement (tah-POT-ment)	p. 311	most stimulating massage movement, consisting of short, quick tapping, slapping, and hacking movements
toners	p. 322	skin tonics with an alcohol content of 4 to 15 percent; most are designed for use on normal and combination skin types
trigger point	p. 311	a tender area in a muscle caused by a localized knot or spasm in the muscle fiber that can radiate pain to other locations in the body
vibration (vy-BRAY-shun)	p. 312	in massage, the rapid shaking of the body part while the fingertips are pressed firmly on the point of application

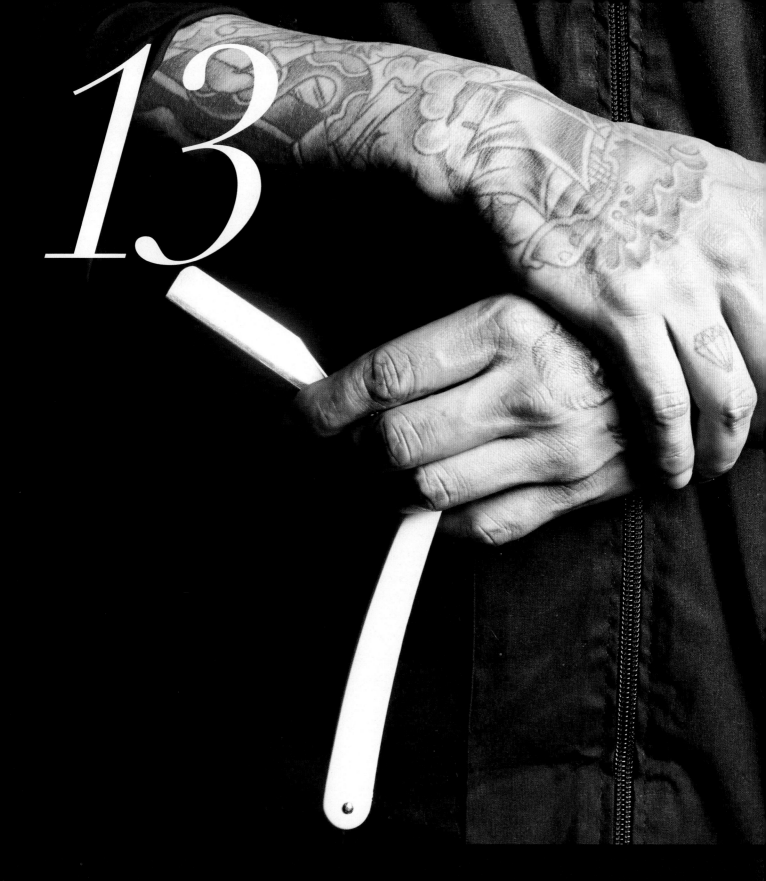

13

SHAVING AND
FACIAL-HAIR DESIGN

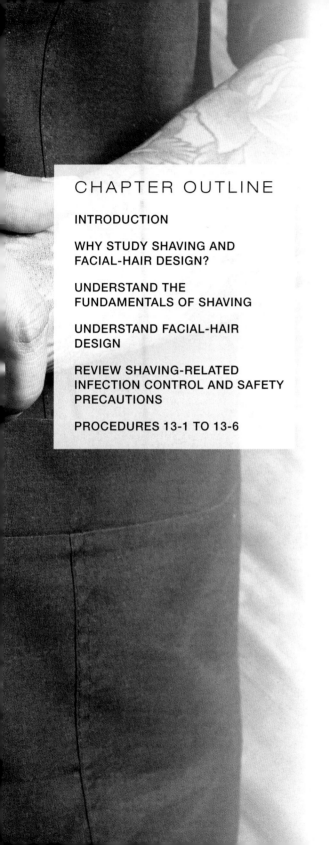

LEARNING OBJECTIVES

After completing this chapter, you should be able to:

LO❶
List basic guidelines for shaving a client.

LO❷
Identify the 14 shaving areas of the face.

LO❸
Explain what you need to know about razor positions and strokes to perform a shave safely and effectively.

LO❹
Describe the differences between various facial-hair designs.

LO❺
Discuss Infection Control and safety precautions associated with shaving.

LO❻
Demonstrate how to handle a straight razor safely.

LO❼
Demonstrate the freehand, backhand, reverse-freehand and reverse-backhand positions and strokes.

LO❽
Demonstrate a shave service.

LO❾
Demonstrate a neck shave.

LO❿
Demonstrate a mustache trim.

LO⓫
Demonstrate cutting in beard designs.

Introduction

When performed correctly, a full facial shave, complete with hot towels, lotions, and massage, is one of the most relaxing, yet rejuvenating, services men can enjoy in the barbershop. And although safety and electric razors may have made it more convenient for men to shave at home, this self-service approach does not provide the preparation, relaxation, and finishing elements of a well-executed barbershop shave.

Your client can also benefit from mustache and beard trims being performed in the barbershop, since the barber is better positioned and trained to create a more balanced and even facial-hair design.

why study
SHAVING AND FACIAL-HAIR DESIGN?

Barbers should study and have a thorough understanding of shaving and facial-hair design because:

> It is important to understand that shaving requires careful attention, skill, and practice to perfect.

> Shaving and facial-hair designs require knowledge about bone structure and facial features.

> Shaving is a traditional skill that separates barbering from other professions and helps to ensure the longevity of the profession.

> **⚠ CAUTION**
>
> It is critical that student barbers read and study the entire shaving section of this chapter before practicing a facial shave.

Understand the Fundamentals of Shaving

After reading this section, you will be able to:

LO❶ List basic guidelines for shaving a client.

LO❷ Identify the 14 shaving areas of the face.

LO❸ Explain what you need to know about razor positions and strokes to perform a shave safely and effectively.

Shaving is one of the basic services performed in the barbershop; its primary objective is to remove the visible part of facial and neck hair without causing irritation to the skin. A changeable-blade or conventional straight razor, hot towels, and warm lather are used in a professional shave.

Although there are general shaving principles that apply to all men, there are also exceptions that will require consideration. For example, the application of hot towels is a standard procedure in preparing the beard for shaving. However, some clients may not be able to tolerate a hot towel on their skin. Other individual characteristics such as hair texture, growth pattern, and product sensitivity are variables that barbers must consider and make educated judgments about before proceeding with the shave service.

CONSIDER BASIC GUIDELINES FOR SHAVING A CLIENT

There are some basic guidelines that you need to be aware of before shaving any client. These include some general dos and don'ts, characteristics of facial hair that need to be considered, and customer service concerns. Consider these important guidelines related to performing a shave service.

DOS AND DON'TS

- The client's skin must be analyzed before beginning the shave. Do not proceed with the service if the client has a skin infection or pustules. Doing so could spread the infection to other parts of the client's face or to you.

- The client's hair growth pattern must be analyzed before beginning the shave to identify grain changes and growth patterns in the beard.

- Do not use hot towels on skin that is chapped, blistered, thin, or sensitive.

- Do not perform a deep cleansing facial immediately after a shave as it may irritate or damage the skin.

- Be careful when shaving sensitive areas beneath the lower lip, on the lower part of the neck, and around the Adam's apple to avoid irritation or injury.

- Use pH-balanced fresheners or toners when stronger astringents are too harsh for sensitive skin.

- Heavy beard growth may require more thorough lathering and more hot-towel applications to prepare it for the shave.

- When a client wears a mustache, trim and shape it prior to the shave service to prepare it for finish work with the razor during the shave.

Hair Type Considerations

Curly facial hair requires special care because it grows in a looped direction as it grows out of the follicle; if not shaved correctly, it can bend back into the skin surface where it may cause ingrown hairs (pseudofolliculitis). Ingrown hairs are often the result of improper hair removal by a razor, tweezers, or trimmer. Improper hair removal includes excessively close shaving, shaving in the wrong direction, and/or excessive pressure with clippers, trimmers, or razors. Any of these methods can cause new hair to be trapped or pushed under the skin and if left untreated may result in infected bumps both on and under the skin surface (folliculitis). Sometimes, it may even initiate a keloid condition.

Hair Growth Considerations

You will need to analyze the direction and pattern of hair growth before beginning the shave to identify where the grain changes occur and to observe growth patterns that may influence the procedure.

- As hair emerges from the skin surface it flows in a particular direction. This direction of hair growth creates the *grain* of the hair. A *grain change* occurs when hair growing in one direction meets hair that is growing in a different or an opposite direction.

- Hair growth patterns are visible indicators of the direction of the hair as it emerges from the skin surface. Growth patterns determine hairline shapes and whether the hair lies down as it emerges from the skin or results in a whorl, cowlick, or other growth feature.

- The direction of hair growth determines the razor positions and strokes that need to be used to shave *with the grain* of the hair during the service.

While men's facial hair usually grows in the same direction in each of the 14 shaving areas, there are always exceptions. Occasionally, a section of the beard or neck hair will grow in a whorl pattern and may require the barber to use a different razor stroke than the stroke generally used in that particular shaving area. This is a perfectly acceptable practice when the growth pattern warrants the use of a different razor position or stroke.

Customer Satisfaction

While there are many reasons why a client may find fault with a shave procedure, the most common include

- dull or rough razors;
- unclean hands, towels, or drape;
- cold fingers;
- heavy touch;
- poorly heated towels (either too hot or too cold);
- poorly heated lather (either too hot or too cold);
- glaring overhead lights;
- unshaven hair patches;
- scraping the skin and close shaving;
- offensive body odor or foul breath of the barber.

IDENTIFY THE SHAVING AREAS OF THE FACE

There are 14 shaving areas of the face to be shaved during the *first-time-over* part of the service. These areas are shaved systematically and sequentially from one section to another using a specific razor position to shave *with the grain* in each area.

Refer to **Figures 13-1** through **13-6** and **Table 13-1** to review the 14 shaving areas of the face.

Shaving Areas for the Right-Handed Barber

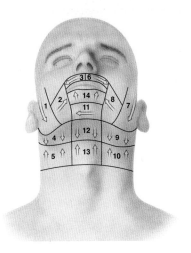

figure 13-1
Areas of the face for right-handed shaving: front.

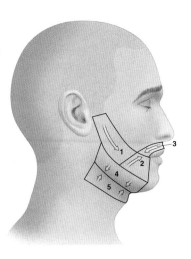

figure 13-2
Areas of the face for right-handed shaving: right side.

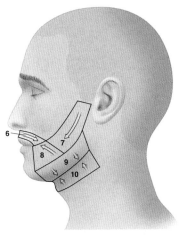

figure 13-3
Areas of the face for right-handed shaving: left side.

Shaving Areas for the Left-Handed Barber

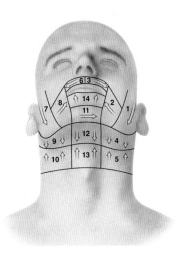

figure 13-4
Areas of the face for left-handed shaving: front.

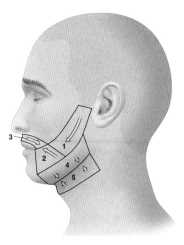

figure 13-5
Areas of the face for left-handed shaving: left side.

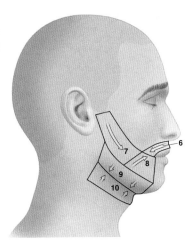

figure 13-6
Areas of the face for left-handed shaving: right side.

table 13-1

SHAVING MOVEMENTS FOR LEFT-HANDED AND RIGHT-HANDED BARBERS

Shaving Area	Area of Face for Left-Handed Barber	Position and Stroke	Direction of Stroke	Area of Face for Right-Handed Barber
1	From left sideburn toward jawbone and angle of mouth	Freehand	Down	From right sideburn toward jawbone and angle of mouth
2	From angle of mouth toward point of chin	Backhand	Down	From angle of mouth toward point of chin
3	From center of upper lip to corner of mouth on left side	Freehand	Down	From center of upper lip to corner of mouth on right side
4	From left jawbone to grain change	Freehand	Down	From right jawbone to grain change
5	Left side of neck to grain change	Reverse freehand	Up	Right side of neck up to grain change
6	From center of lip to corner of right side of mouth	Backhand	Down	From center of lip to corner of left side of mouth
7	From right sideburn toward jawbone and angle of mouth	Backhand	Down	From left sideburn toward jawbone and angle of mouth
8	From angle of mouth toward point of chin	Freehand	Down	From angle of mouth toward point of chin
9	From right jawbone to grain change	Backhand	Down	From left jawbone to grain change
10	Right side of neck to grain change	Reverse freehand	Up	Left side of neck to grain change
11	Across chin from right to left	Freehand	Across	Across chin from left to right
12	Under chin to grain change	Freehand or backhand	Down	Under chin to grain change
13	Center of neck to grain change	Reverse freehand	Up	Center of neck to grain change
14	Beneath lower lip	Reverse freehand	Up	Beneath lower lip

UNDERSTAND RAZOR POSITIONS AND STROKES

The term used to describe the correct angle of cutting with a razor is called the **cutting stroke** (KUT-ing STROHK). To achieve a proper cutting stroke, the razor is positioned at a slight angle to the skin surface and stroked with the point leading (**Figure 13-7**). This should be a light-handed forward gliding motion that is most often positioned to shave with the grain of the hair, not against it.

The four razor positions used in the practice of barbering are **freehand** (FREE-HAND), **backhand** (BAK-HAND), **reverse freehand** (ree-VURS FREE-HAND), and **reverse backhand** (ree-VURS BAK-HAND). The three positions and strokes used in facial shaving are freehand, backhand, and reverse freehand (see **Figures 13-8 to 13-10**).

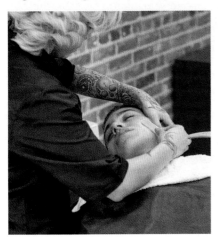

figure 13-7
Angle of cutting stroke (on skin).

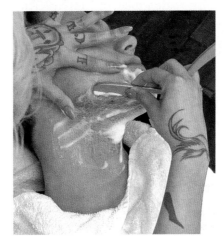

figure 13-8
Freehand position.

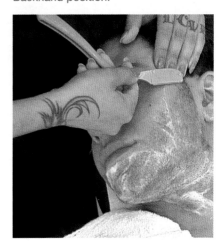

figure 13-9
Backhand position.

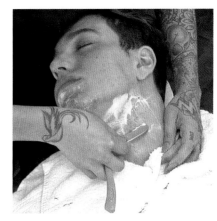

figure 13-10
Reverse-freehand position.

Position refers to the way the razor is held in the barber's hand to perform a stroke movement. For example, your instructor may direct you to "hold the razor in the freehand position" or "position the razor at about a 30-degree angle." The stroke is the actual movement of the razor as it is held in one of the four positions, for example, "a freehand stroke is used to shave area 1" or "use a gliding stroke toward you."

You will need to know and practice the following skills for each of the 14 shaving areas (refer to Procedures 13-1 and 13-2):

Ⓟ 13-1   **Handling a Straight Razor** *pages 353–354*

Ⓟ 13-2   **Razor Position and Strokes Practice** *pages 355–357*

- Where to use a particular razor position and stroke
- How to hold the razor for each position and stroke to
  - position the fingers, wrist, and elbow of the dominant hand in relation to the razor
  - position the opposite hand on the client's skin in relation to the razor
  - position your body in relation to the client to facilitate a razor position and stroke
- How to hold or stretch the skin to
  - find the balance between stretching the skin too much or too little
  - use the cushions of the fingertips to stretch the skin with the proper amount of pressure
  - use the thumb and second finger as the primary digits for stretching the skin
  - stretch different areas of the skin in the opposite direction that the razor will travel
- How to position and stroke the razor on the surface of the skin to
  - angle the razor about 30 degrees relative to the skin surface
  - use a forward gliding movement that leads with the point of the razor

- use the proper stroke length on different areas of the face
- use strokes of 1 inch to 3 inches to avoid shaving too far from the stretching point
- use shorter strokes around the mouth, over the ears, and in other tight areas
- develop a medium stroke speed to avoid very fast or very slow movements
- adjust the rate of speed of the stroke according to the area being shaved
- use smooth strokes that carry through once started without stopping and starting

- How to recognize growth patterns and the grain of the hair in different areas of the face to
  - identify areas where the direction of hair growth changes
  - use the appropriate razor position and stroke for the area to be shaved
  - adjust stroke speed and pressure to accommodate the texture or density of the hair
  - recognize use of the terms *with the grain*, *against the grain*, and *across the grain*

- How to work efficiently and effectively to
  - perform strokes so little to no lather is left behind
  - keep the nondominant thumb and fingertips dry for stretching purposes
  - start strokes from a clean skin surface into the lathered surface
  - wipe residual lather and hair from the razor in a safe and clean manner
  - check your work for rough or missed patches

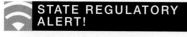

STATE REGULATORY ALERT!

Some states prohibit the use of conventional straight razors and allow only changeable-blade razors. Be guided by your state barber board rules and regulations.

FREEHAND POSITION AND STROKE

How to hold the razor

The position of the right hand is as follows (refer to Procedure 13-1):

- Take the razor in the right hand. The handle of the razor should rest between the third and fourth fingers, with the tip of the little finger resting on the tip of the tang of the razor. The thumb should sit securely on the side of the shank near the shoulder of the blade. The third finger should lie at the pivot of the shank and the handle with the first and second fingers in front of it on the back of the shank.
- Turn the hand slightly outward from the wrist with the elbow at a comfortable level.

The position of the left hand is as follows:

- Keep the fingers of the left hand dry in order to prevent them from slipping on the face.
- Use the left hand to stretch the skin in the opposite direction of the stroke under the razor.

How to perform the freehand stroke

- Use a gliding stroke toward you.

- Lead with the point of the razor in a forward, gliding movement.

Where to use the freehand stroke

- The freehand position and stroke is used in 6 of the 14 shaving areas. See Shaving Areas 1, 3, 4, 8, 11, and 12 in **Figures 13-1** through **13-6**.

BACKHAND POSITION AND STROKE

How to hold the razor

The position of the right hand is as follows:

- The shank of the razor should be held firmly between the thumb and first two fingers at the pivot with the razor held in a relatively straight position.

- The underside of the handle rests on the third and fourth fingers.

- An alternative method is to bend the handle slightly so the third finger barely rests at the end of the tang and the fourth finger is bent into the palm.

- Turn the back of the hand away from you and bend the wrist slightly downward. Then raise the elbow so that you can move the arm freely. This is the position used for the backhand stroke with the arm movement. Some practitioners prefer to use a wrist movement, in which case the arm is not held as high.

The position of the left hand is as follows:

- Keep the fingers of the left hand dry in order to prevent them from slipping.

- Stretch the skin under the razor in the opposite direction of the stroke.

How to perform the backhand stroke

- Use a gliding stroke away from you.

- Direct the stroke with the point of the razor leading in a forward, gliding movement.

Where to use the backhand stroke

The backhand stroke is used in 4 of the 14 shaving areas and if preferred, in area 12. See Shaving Areas 2, 6, 7, and 9 in **Figures 13-1** through **13-6**.

REVERSE-FREEHAND POSITION AND STROKE

The hand and razor position in the reverse-freehand stroke is similar to that of the freehand stroke, but the stroke is performed in an upward rather than a downward direction, usually with the barber standing behind the client's shoulder or head.

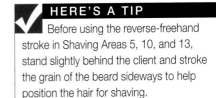

HERE'S A TIP

Before using the reverse-freehand stroke in Shaving Areas 5, 10, and 13, stand slightly behind the client and stroke the grain of the beard sideways to help position the hair for shaving.

How to hold the razor

The position of the right hand is as follows:

- Hold the razor firmly in a freehand position.
- Turn the hand slightly toward you so that the razor edge is turned upward

The position of the left hand is as follows:

- Keep the hand dry and use it to pull the skin taut under the razor.
- Position the fingers below or in back of the razor opposite the blade edge and direction of the stroke.

How to perform the reverse-freehand stroke

- Use an upward, semi-arced stroke toward you with the point leading in a gliding movement.
- The movement is from the elbow to the hand with a slight twist of the wrist.

Where to use the reverse-freehand stroke

The reverse-freehand stroke is used in 4 of the 14 shaving areas. See Shaving Areas 5, 10, 13, and 14 in Figures 13-1 through 13-6.

REVERSE-BACKHAND POSITION AND STROKE

figure 13-11
Reverse-backhand stroke.

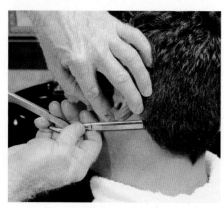

The reverse-backhand position and stroke require diligent practice to master. The holding position of the razor for the reverse-backhand stroke is the same as that for the backhand stroke, except that the elbow is positioned downward (closer to the barber's body) and the forearm is held upward. When using this stroke, employ a downward gliding stroke that follows along the natural hairline along the side of the neck (see Figure 13-11).

How to hold the razor

The position of the right hand is as follows:

- Hold the razor firmly in the backhand position.
- Turn the wrist to the right so that the palm of the hand faces upward.
- Drop the elbow close to the side.

The position of the left hand is as follows:

- Position the left hand so as to be able to draw the skin taut under the razor.
- Position your hand above the razor.

How to perform the reverse-backhand stroke

- Use a smooth, gliding stroke, directed downward, that leads with the point of the razor.
- Proceed with short cutting strokes directed downward and slightly outward.

Where to use the reverse-backhand stroke

The reverse-backhand stroke is only used during a neck shave with the client sitting in an upright position. Typically, the right-handed barber uses a reverse-backhand stroke when shaving the client's left sideburn outline and behind the left ear along the side of the neck. The left-handed barber uses a reverse-backhand stroke to shave these areas on the client's right side.

The cutting strokes described in this section illustrate the holding and stroking positions that should be employed by the right-handed barber. Right-handed barbers start the shave on the client's right side; left-handed barbers start on the client's left side (see **Table 13-1**).

UNDERSTAND BODY POSITIONING

The shave procedure begins with the barber standing at the client's side; right-handed barbers stand at client's right side; left-handed barbers stand at client's left side.

- Gently turn the client's head to the position needed to accommodate the stroke.

- Take half steps or shift your body weight from one foot to the other to change position to perform the shaving strokes; following are four common body positions with corresponding shaving areas for the right-handed barber:

  - Stand slightly at front of client's right side (**Figure 13-12**): Shaving Areas 1, 4, and 12 (if using freehand)

  - Stand centered at client's right side (**Figure 13-13**): Shaving Areas 2, 3, 6, 8, 11, and 12 (if using backhand)

  - Stand at client's right shoulder (**Figure 13-14**): Shaving Areas 7 and 9

  - Stand behind client's right shoulder (**Figure 13-15**): Shaving Areas 5, 10, 13, and 14

figure 13-12
Stand slightly at front of client's right side.

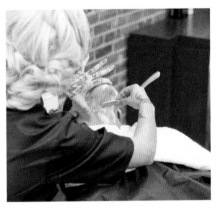

figure 13-13
Stand centered at client's right side.

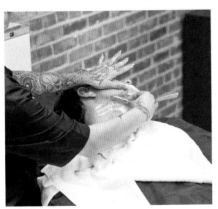

figure 13-14
Stand at client's right shoulder.

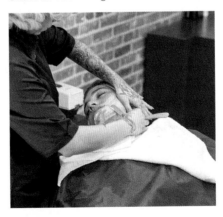

figure 13-15
Stand behind client's right shoulder.

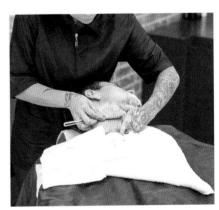

DESCRIBE THE PROFESSIONAL SHAVE

The three main steps of a standard professional shave are preparation, shaving, and finishing (refer to Procedure 13-3). Preparation includes draping the client for the shave, preparing hot towels, and preparing the client's face for the shave.

- Draping (refer to Procedure 13-3: Preparation)

- Preparing hot towels

- Preparing the face for shaving involves steaming and lathering the face.
  - Steaming helps to soften the hair cuticle, provides lubrication by stimulating oil glands, and relaxes the client.
  - Lathering with a shaving cream or gel cleanses the skin, softens the hair, helps to hold the hair in an upright position for shaving, and creates a smooth surface for the razor. Use an electric latherizer to prepare warm shaving lather.

Shaving involves safely removing the hair in the 14 shaving areas without causing irritation or injury to the skin, and completing the finishing steps of the service.

- Razor strokes should be correct and systematic. Proper coordination of both hands is necessary.

- While the right hand holds and strokes the razor, the fingers of the left hand gently stretch the skin area being shaved. Taut skin allows the beard hair to be cut more easily.

- Loose skin tends to push out in front of the razor and can result in cuts or nicks. Stretching the skin too tightly, however, will cause irritation. The skin must be held firmly, neither too loosely nor too tightly, to create the correct shaving surface for the razor.

- To prevent slipping and to see the area to be shaved, remove excess lather with the thumb. If needed, dry the skin area where you will place your fingers for stretching.

- Keep the fingers of the nondominant hand dry at all times.

Finishing includes massaging moisturizer into the skin, toning to remove residual cream product, and a light powder dusting to leave a matte finish, if desired. Traditionally, a neck shave is also offered at this time.

KNOW THE TYPES OF SHAVES

There are several terms that both barbers and clients may use to describe either a type of shave or the different steps performed in a standard shave service. These terms have remained consistent for decades, so it is important that you become familiar with the terminology.

The First-Time-Over Shave

The **first-time-over shave** (FIRST-TYM-OH-ver SHAYV) is actually the primary shave in a standard shave service that is performed on lathered facial hair. The objective is to remove the beard growth without causing irritation and to leave a smooth skin surface. The *first-time-over* shave is followed by the **second-time-over shave** (SEK-und-TYM-OH-ver SHAYV) to remove any rough or uneven spots.

The Second-Time-Over Shave

The second-time-over shave is performed for one of two reasons, either as a step that follows the first-time-over shave or as part of a close shave as described in a later section (see The Close Shave). Following the first-time-over shave, the barber checks the client's skin for any rough or uneven spots. The client's skin is moistened with a warm towel or water and a freehand stroke is used to shave *with* or *across the grain* to remove any remaining hair.

The Once-Over Shave

The **once-over shave** (WONCE-OH-ver SHAYV) requires less time for a complete shave service and was popular when men patronized barbershops daily for their shave. This shave should result in a smooth face without being a close shave. To perform a once-over shave, use a few more strokes while shaving *across the grain* in each shaving area. This practice should ensure a complete and even shave with a single lathering. Remember to use a light hand to avoid causing irritation.

The Close Shave

Close shaving (KLOHS SHAYV-ing) is the practice of shaving the beard *against the grain* during the second-time-over phase of the shave. This practice is undesirable because it may irritate the skin and lead to infection or ingrown hairs; therefore, barbers do not traditionally employ close-shaving methods. That said, if a client's beard growth warrants it and he has requested a close shave, the barber should be able to perform the service.

The Neck Shave and the Outline Shave

A **neck shave** (NEK SHAYV) traditionally accompanies a facial shave and involves shaving the neckline on both sides of the neck behind the ears and across the nape if desired or necessary (refer to Procedure 13-4). Conversely, a complete *outline shave* includes the sideburn, around the ear, behind the ear areas, and sometimes the front hairline, and typically follows a haircut (refer to Chapter 14).

> **⏱ REMINDER**
> Be sure to check the hairline and neck areas for moles, warts, or other hypertrophies before beginning the neck shave; follow the natural hairline for best results.

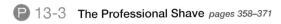 P 13-3 **The Professional Shave** *pages 358–371*

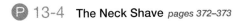 P 13-4 **The Neck Shave** *pages 372–373*

Understand Facial-Hair Design

LO❹ Describe the differences between various facial-hair designs.

In addition to cutting and styling hair, you should be able to offer your clients a full range of services for grooming facial hair. Because today's style is one of individuality, barbers should become proficient, or even specialize, in the design and trimming of men's facial hair. The client who wears a mustache and/or beard will frequent a shop that can provide both haircutting and facial-hair design services.

figure 13-16
Thicker mustache design for heavier facial features.

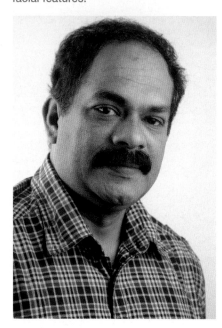

figure 13-17
Thinner mustache design for finer facial features.

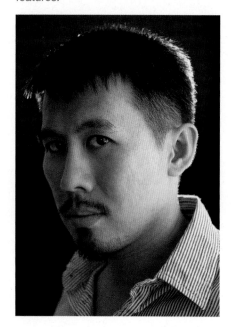

TRIMMING THE MUSTACHE

A mustache is most often worn for personal adornment and men are usually very particular about how it is designed and maintained. Care, artistry, and sensitivity to the client's preferences are required for this service. Corrective shaping or redesign of the mustache can help clients with their daily maintenance and trimming until their next visit to the barbershop.

In addition to knowing how to trim and shape mustaches, barbers should be able to understand and apply certain principles of mustache design.

Mustache Design

Factors to consider when consulting with a client about suitable mustache designs are his facial features, hair growth and texture, and personal taste. Consider the following factors when discussing mustache design options with your client:

- The size of the mustache should correspond to the size of the client's features, for example, larger, thicker designs for heavier facial features and smaller, thinner designs for finer features (**Figures 13-16** and **13-17**).

- Following are important facial characteristics that influence mustache design:

  - Width of the mouth

  - Size of the nose

  - Shape of upper lip area

  - Width of the cheeks, jaw, and chin

  - Density and texture of hair growth

- As a general rule, be guided by the client's hair growth pattern and avoid cutting too deeply into natural hairlines. This approach will help to minimize daily maintenance as new growth occurs.

- Following are guidelines for mustache design and proportion:

  - *Large, coarse facial features:* heavier-looking mustache

  - *Prominent nose:* medium to large mustache

  - *Long, narrow face:* narrow to medium mustache

  - *Extra-large mouth:* pyramid-shaped mustache

  - *Extra-small mouth:* medium, short mustache

  - *Smallish, regular features:* smaller, triangular mustache

  - *Wide mouth with prominent upper lip:* heavier handlebar or large divided mustache

  - *Round face with regular features:* semisquare mustache

  - *Square with prominent features:* heavier, linear mustache with ends slightly curving downward

- Additional services that may be offered with a mustache trim include:

  - waxing mustache ends;

  - penciling with temporary color;

  - coloring for evenness or compatibility with scalp hair color.

DESIGNING THE BEARD

Like mustaches, beards can be used to balance the appearance of facial features. As with their mustaches, men are usually very particular about the design of their beards. Again, a careful approach, artistry, and sensitivity to the client's preferences are required for this service.

If the client is getting a haircut along with his beard trim, the decision must be made as to which service will be performed first. This is completely a matter of choice for the barber; you will have your own reasons for performing one service before or after the other. For example, many barbers cut and style the hair before the beard trim so they can balance the length and fullness of the beard with the finished haircut more effectively.

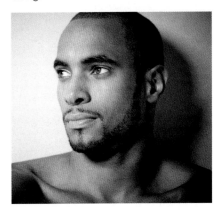

figure 13-18
A balanced and proportioned beard design.

Beard Design

The correct shaping or design of the beard can emphasize pleasant facial features, minimize less desirable ones, and camouflage flaws. As with other hair design, it is important to develop a good eye for balance and proportion (Figure 13-18). Since very few individuals have perfectly symmetrical face shapes, it may be challenging to create the illusion of symmetry and balance in design. Following are some important practical tips for beard design:

- Analyze the density and distribution of the hair to identify uneven growth areas; cutting the hair too short in the area surrounding these sections will result in emphasizing the *bald spot* with no way to provide coverage of the uneven area.

- Work with the natural hairline in the sideburn, cheek, and mustache areas to guide the design and to minimize daily maintenance.

- Consider where hair growth under the chin and jaw changes direction to help determine design options for outlines in this area.

- Leave the facial hair slightly longer than the desired end result during the first trimming to avoid cutting the hair too closely. Remember, you can always cut more off. This is also a good time to face the client to the mirror so he can check the progress of the trim and to clarify or ask anything you need to know to finish the service.

- Beard trimming and design is usually performed with a combination of the shears, comb, outliner and/or clippers, and razor.

- Even-all-over clipper-cutting is most successful on beards with even density and texture. This is important to note because sometimes cutting the beard at all the same length will leave whorls or patches, especially in wavy hair.

  - When creating a uniform length throughout the beard, start with a blade size close to the length of the client's beard. If more than a light trim is required, select the next size blade that will cut the hair to a shorter length. Repeat as necessary until the desired length is achieved.

  - Follow up clipper work with shears, outliner, and/or razor for final trimming and detail work.

Perfecting your mustache and beard design skills will help you meet the service needs of your clients while providing an outlet for creative design and an additional income source (refer to Procedures 13-5 and 13-6).

P 13-5   **Mustache Trim** *pages 374*

P 13-6   **Beard Designs** *pages 375–380*

Review Shaving-Related Infection Control and Safety Precautions

After reading the next section, you will be able to:

LO⑤   Discuss infection control and safety precautions associated with shaving.

Use **Table 13-2** as a guide for complying with infection control and safety precautions associated with shaving as you perform the procedures in this chapter.

table 13-2
INFECTION CONTROL AND SAFETY PRECAUTIONS

- Clean and disinfect razors and blades before use.
- Discard used blades in a sharps container.
- Wash your hands before servicing a client.
- Use clean linens, capes, and paper products.
- Provide a clean cloth or paper barrier between the client's head and the headrest.
- Treat small cuts or nicks using standard precautions and exposure incident procedures.
- Lock the chair once the client is properly draped and in position for the shave.
- Prepare facial hair for the shave with warm or hot towels and lather.
- Use a light touch and a forward gliding motion that leads with the point of the blade.
- Observe the hair growth pattern and shave with it, not against it.
- Lather against the grain *gently* to place the hair in a position to be shaved.
- Keep your fingers dry to stretch or hold the skin firmly during the shave.
- Use the cushions of the fingertips to stretch skin in the opposite direction of the razor stroke.
- Keep the fingers and thumb of the nondominant hand away from the path of the razor.
- Apply lather neatly to the areas to be shaved and replace as necessary.
- Keep the skin moist while shaving.
- Follow through with shaving strokes from one shaving area to another; do not stop short or shave over an area repeatedly.

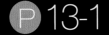

HANDLING A STRAIGHT RAZOR

After practicing this procedure, you should be able to:

LO**6** Demonstrate how to handle a straight razor safely.

Note: The first step in learning how to shave is to master the fundamentals of handling the razor. Review the parts of the razor to become familiar with terms associated with this tool.

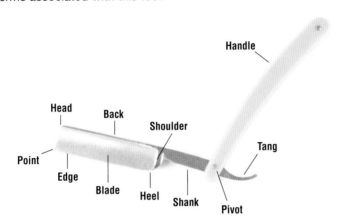

MATERIALS, IMPLEMENTS, AND EQUIPMENT	PREPARATION
□ Straight razor with blade	1 Assemble supplies.
	2 Wash your hands.

PROCEDURE

1 To open the razor, grasp the back of the blade between the thumb and index finger of the dominant hand while holding the handle with the opposite thumb and index finger.

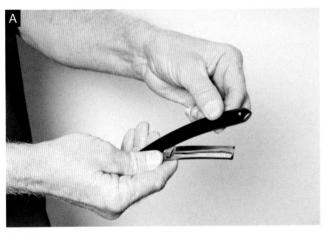

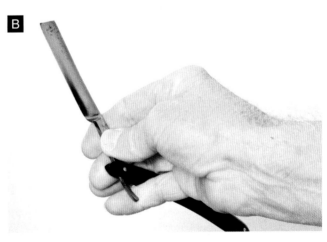

2 As the blade and handle separate by way of the pivot, reposition the little finger of the dominant hand to rest on the tang as the handle is placed in an upward position.

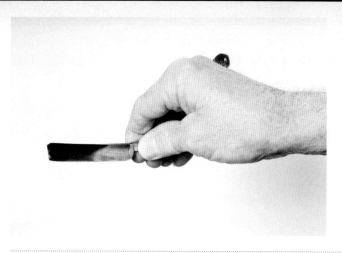

③ Hold the razor between the thumb and index finger on the sides of the shank near the shoulder of the blade and rest across the second and third fingers, with the little finger bracing the razor.

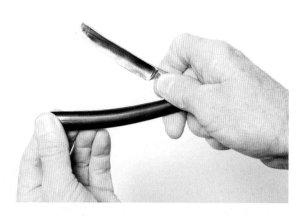

④ When closing the razor, release the little finger and bring the handle to the blade. Be careful the cutting edge does not strike the handle.

CLEAN-UP AND DISINFECTION

☐ Clean and disinfect the tools and implements.

☐ Clean and then disinfect the work area.

☐ Deposit used blades in a sharps container.

☐ Dispose of single-use items. Place all used linens, towels, and capes in the laundry.

☐ Wash your hands.

> ⚠ **CAUTION**
> Always handle razors with extreme care. Warped or loose handles may cause the blade to pass through to the fingers when closing the razor.

RAZOR POSITION AND STROKES PRACTICE

After practicing this procedure, you should be able to:

LO ❼ Demonstrate the freehand, backhand, reverse-freehand, and reverse-backhand positions and strokes.

Note: After mastering this procedure, repeat the steps using a bladed straight razor on a live model (or as directed by your instructor) before advancing to Procedure 13-3.

MATERIALS, IMPLEMENTS, AND EQUIPMENT

☐ Beardless male mannequin and stand

☐ Straight razor (without a blade)

PREPARATION

❶ Assemble supplies.

❷ Wash your hands.

PROCEDURE

A. FREEHAND POSITION AND STROKE

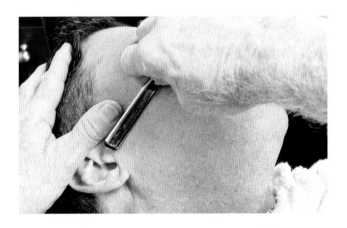

❶ Hold the razor in the right hand. The handle should rest between the third and fourth fingers, with the tip of the little finger resting on the tip of the tang. The thumb should sit securely on the side of the shank near the shoulder of the blade. The third finger should lie at the pivot with the first and second fingers in front of it on the back of the shank.

❷ Turn the hand slightly outward from the wrist with the elbow at a comfortable level.

❸ Keep the fingers of the left hand dry to prevent slipping.

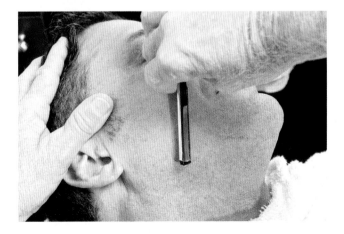

❹ Use the left hand to stretch the skin in the opposite direction of the stroke.

❺ Use a gliding stroke toward you.

❻ Lead with the point of the razor in a forward, gliding movement.

Note: The freehand position and stroke is used in 6 of the 14 shaving areas. See Shaving Areas 1, 3, 4, 8, 11, and 12 in Figures 13-1 through 13-6.

B. BACKHAND POSITION AND STROKE

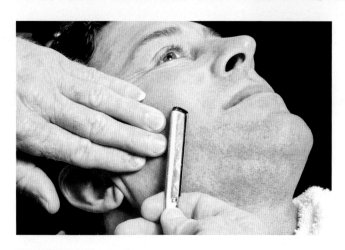

7 The shank of the razor should be held firmly between the thumb and first two fingers at the pivot with the razor held in a relatively straight position.

8 The underside of the handle rests on the third and fourth fingers.

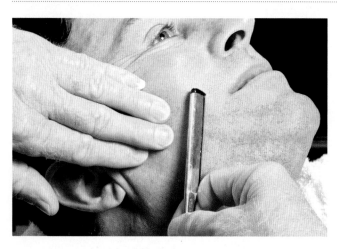

9 An alternative method is to bend the handle slightly so the third finger barely rests at the end of the tang and the fourth finger is bent into the palm.

10 Turn the back of the hand away from you and bend the wrist slightly downward. Then raise the elbow so that you can move the arm freely. This is the position used for the backhand stroke with the arm movement. Some practitioners prefer to use a wrist movement, in which case the arm is not held as high.

11 Keep the fingers of the left hand dry in order to prevent them from slipping.

12 Stretch the skin under the razor in the opposite direction of the stroke.

13 Use a gliding stroke away from you.

14 Direct the stroke with the point of the razor leading in a forward, gliding movement.

Note: The backhand stroke is used in 4 of the 14 shaving areas and if preferred, in area 12. See Shaving Areas 2, 6, 7, and 9 in Figures 13-1 through 13-6.

C. REVERSE-FREEHAND POSITION AND STROKE

The hand and razor position of the reverse-freehand stroke is similar to that of the freehand stroke, but the stroke is performed in an upward rather than a downward direction, usually with the barber standing at the client's shoulder or behind the client's head.

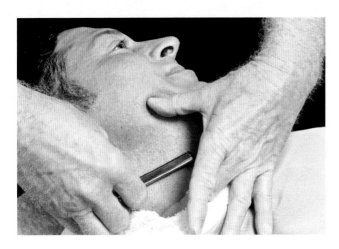

15 Hold the razor firmly in a freehand position.

16 Turn the hand slightly toward you so that the razor edge is turned upward.

17 Keep the hand dry and use it to pull the skin taut under the razor.

18 Position the fingers below or at the back of the razor opposite to the blade edge and direction of the stroke.

19 Use an upward, semi-arced stroke toward you in a gliding movement.

20 The movement is from the elbow to the hand with a slight twist of the wrist.

Note: The reverse-freehand stroke is used in 4 of the 14 shaving areas. See Shaving Areas 5, 10, 13, and 14 in Figures 13-1 through 13-6.

D. REVERSE-BACKHAND POSITION AND STROKE

The holding position of the razor for the reverse-backhand stroke is the same as the backhand stroke except that the elbow is positioned downward (closer to the barber's body) and the forearm in held upward. When using this stroke, employ a downward gliding stroke that follows along the natural hairline along the side of the neck.

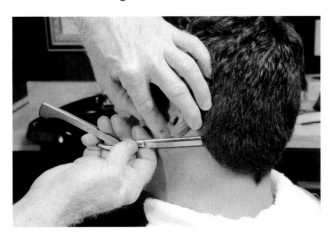

21 Hold the razor firmly in the backhand position.

22 Turn the wrist so that the palm faces upward.

23 Drop the elbow close to the side.

24 Position the left hand so as to be able to draw the skin taut under the razor.

25 Position your hand above the razor.

26 Use a smooth, gliding stroke.

27 Direct the stroke downward along the side of the neck.

Note: The reverse-backhand stroke is used for shaving the left side behind the ear along the side of the neck by the right-handed barber and on the right side along the side of the neck by the left-handed barber.

CLEAN-UP AND DISINFECTION

☐ Clean and disinfect the tools and implements.

☐ Clean and then disinfect the work area.

☐ Deposit used blades in a sharps container.

☐ Dispose of single-use items. Place all used linens, towels, and capes in the laundry.

☐ Wash your hands.

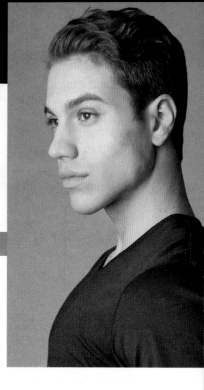

THE PROFESSIONAL SHAVE

After practicing this procedure, you should be able to:

LO⑧ Demonstrate a shave service.

REMINDERS

☐ Analyze the client's skin and hair growth patterns.

☐ Keep client's skin moist.

☐ Keep your fingers dry.

☐ Position the client's head as needed.

☐ Remove excess lather with thumb before beginning stroke.

☐ Right-handed barbers stand at the client's right side; left-handed barbers stand at the client's left side.

☐ Shift your body position as needed.

☐ Stretch the skin of the area to be shaved.

☐ Use gliding strokes with the point leading.

MATERIALS, IMPLEMENTS, AND EQUIPMENT

☐ Barber chair with headrest

☐ Barber's paper towels

☐ Comb and brush

☐ Cotton pledgets or tissues

☐ Covered container for soiled towels

☐ Covered trash can

☐ Electric latherizer

☐ Haircutting cape

☐ Headrest cover

☐ Hot-towel cabinet

☐ Moisturizing cream

☐ Sharps container

☐ Shaving cream or gel

☐ Sink

☐ Straight razor and blades

☐ Terry cloth towels

☐ Toner or astringent

PREPARATION

① Assemble supplies.

② Wash your hands.

PROCEDURE

A. PREPARE CLIENT FOR THE SHAVE

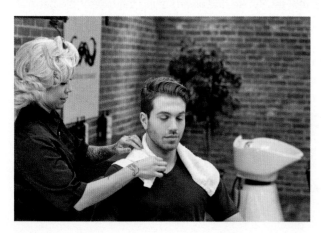

① Seat the client comfortably in the chair.

② If applicable, ask the client to loosen his collar; turn collar to inside. Position a terry cloth towel from back to front.

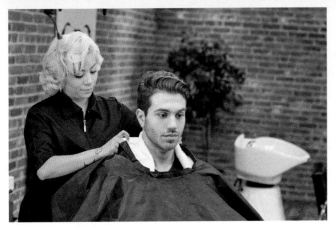

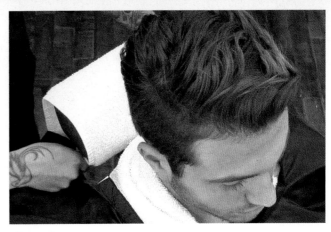

3 Lay the cape loosely over the client's shoulders from the front without it coming into contact with the client's neck.

4 Apply a fresh headrest cover and adjust the headrest to the proper height.

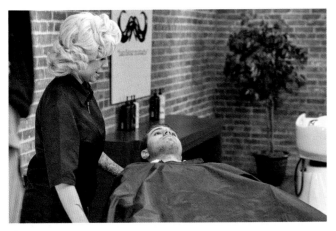

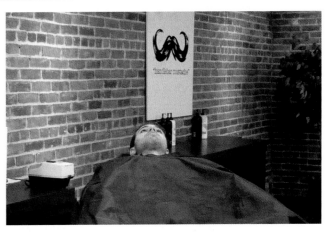

5 Recline the chair to a comfortable working angle for you and the client.

6 Adjust and lock the chair to the proper height.

7 Wash your hands with soap and warm water, and dry them thoroughly.

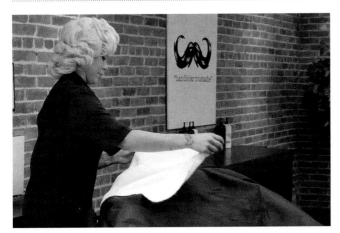

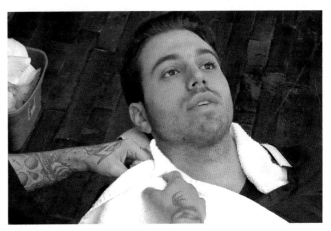

8 Unfold a clean terry cloth towel, and lay it diagonally across the client's chest.

9 Tuck one corner of the towel along the right side of the client's neck. Secure the tucked edge by sliding a finger inside the neckband.

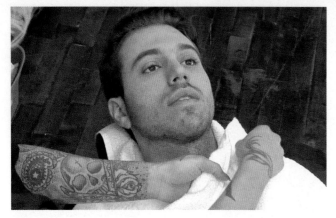

10 Cross the lower end of the towel to the other side of the client's neck and tuck under the neckband using the same sliding motion.

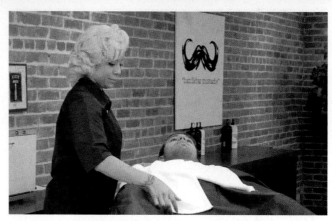

11 Tuck a paper strip or paper towel into the neckband and lay it across the client's chest. Use for wiping the razor clean during the shave.

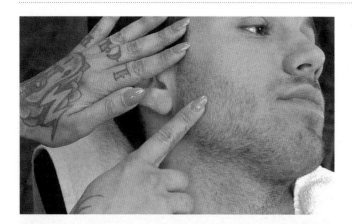

12 Analyze client's skin, hair texture, and hair growth patterns.

B. PREPARE CLIENT'S FACE FOR SHAVING

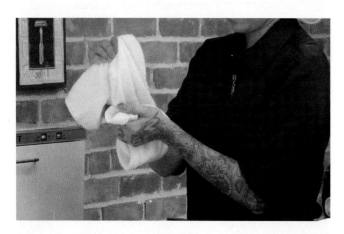

13 Retrieve a pre-warmed towel from the hot-towel cabinet.

14 Test the temperature of the towel on your wrist. If it is too hot, hold the towel by the top corners and gently fan it back and forth for a few seconds. Test the towel again before applying it to the client's face.

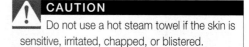

⚠ CAUTION
Do not use a hot steam towel if the skin is sensitive, irritated, chapped, or blistered.

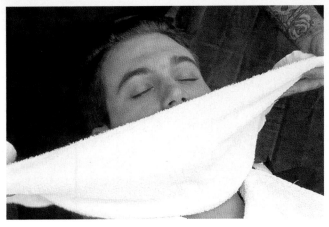 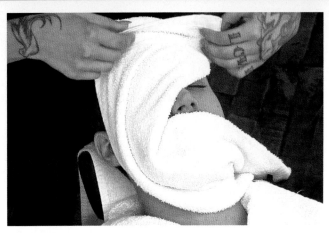

15 Standing behind the client's head, position the hot towel under and in front of the client's chin. Fold the towel over the client's mouth and upper lip area to just under his nose.

16 Cross the right-hand section of the towel over to the client's right temple area.

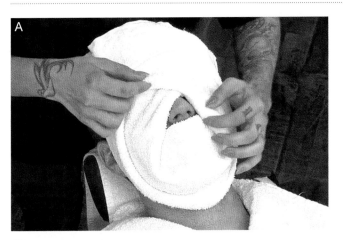 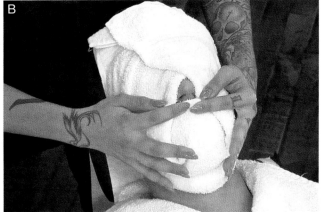

17 Bring the left-hand section of the towel over toward the client's left side and smooth the fold. Mold towel to client's face.

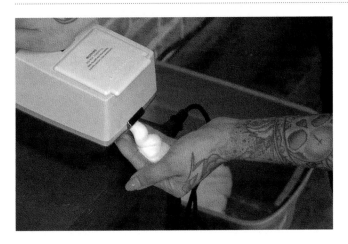

18 Transfer a quantity of warm shaving lather from the electric latherizer into your hand.

19 Remove the hot towel, and spread lather evenly over the bearded areas to be shaved.

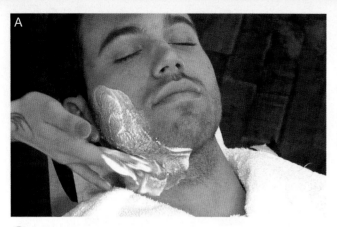

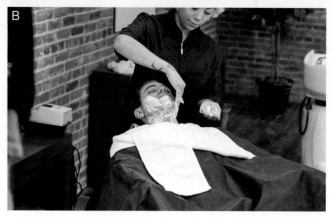

20 Starting at the neck and working up the right side of the face, use brisk, rotary movements with the cushions of the fingertips to work the shaving cream into a lather in the bearded areas of the face. Repeat on the left side of the neck and face until all areas to be shaved are covered. Rub for 1 to 2 minutes depending on the stiffness and density of the beard.

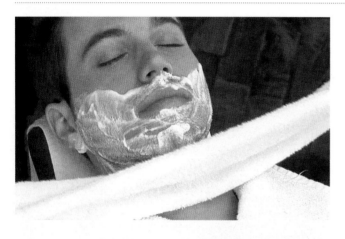

21 Test the temperature of the second hot towel and apply it over the lather. Mold or pat towel to conform to client's face. Repeat the steaming process if the beard is extremely coarse or dense.

22 Prepare the razor while the hot towel is on the client's face.

   a. When using a conventional straight razor, strop the razor, immerse it in a disinfectant solution, rinse, and wipe dry.

   b. When using a changeable-blade razor, disinfect the razor and new blade, rinse, wipe dry, and assemble.

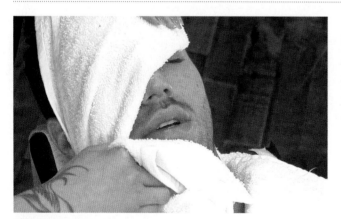

23 Remove hot towel and wipe the lather off in one smooth operation.

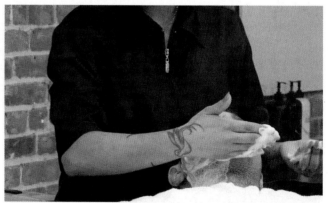

24 Re-lather the beard and wipe the lather from your hands.

C. THE FACIAL SHAVE

First-Time-Over Shave

Shaving Area No. 1—Freehand stroke

25 Stand at the right side of chair and shift weight to right foot; gently turn the client's face to the left. Remove the lather from the hairline with the thumb of the left hand. Hold the razor in a freehand position.

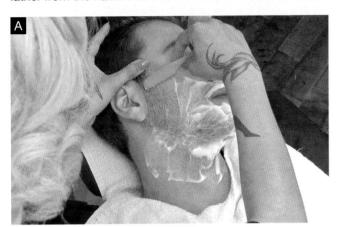
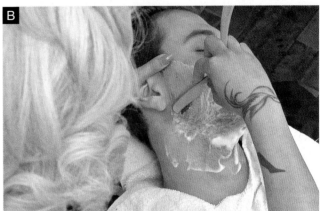

26 Stretch the skin and begin at the hairline of the right sideburn. Use a gliding diagonal stroke that leads with the point of the razor; shave downward toward the corner of the mouth and jawbone.

27 Wipe razor clean.

Shaving Area No. 2—Backhand stroke

28 Shift your weight to the left foot; hold razor in backhand position.

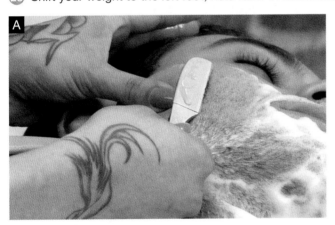
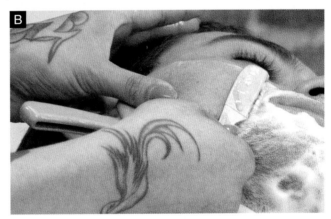

29 Stretch the skin and use a diagonal stroke from point to heel to shave the right side from the angle of the mouth to the point of the chin.

30 Wipe razor clean.

Shaving Area No. 3—Freehand stroke

31 Maintain the same body position; hold razor in freehand position.

32 To shave beneath the nostril, slightly lift the tip of the nose, taking care not to interfere with the client's breathing. Stretch the upper lip by placing the fingers of the left hand against the nose while holding the thumb below the lower corner of the lip.

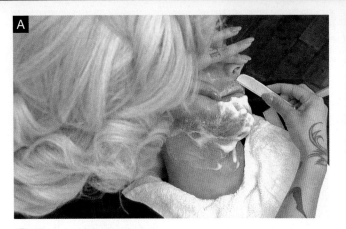

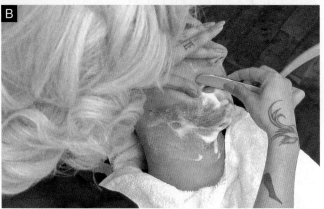

33 Shave beneath the nostrils and over the right side of the upper lip; use fingers of left hand to stretch the underlying skin. If the client wears a mustache, shave the outline with the razor at this time.

34 Wipe razor clean.

> **REMINDER**
> Shaving strokes on the upper lip are performed on a slight diagonal to follow the curves of the face; however, remember to shave *with the grain* in this area.

Shaving Area No. 4—Freehand stroke

35 Shift your body position to face the front of the right side of the client's face.

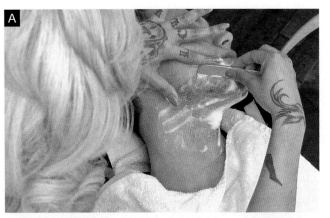

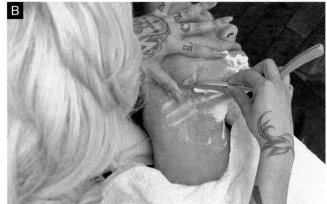

36 Starting at chin level, stretch the skin, and shave that portion of the neck below the jawbone down to the change in the grain of the beard. Be sure to hold the skin taut between the thumb and fingers of left hand.

37 Wipe razor clean.

Shaving Area No. 5—Reverse-freehand stroke

38 Move behind the chair; hold the razor for the reverse-freehand stroke.

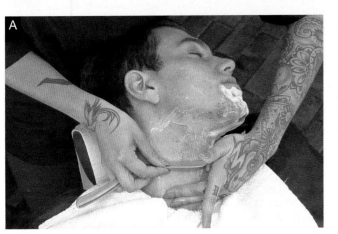
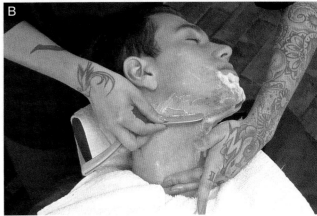

39 Stretch the skin from the bottom of Shaving Area No. 5 and shave upward with the grain. Do not expect to complete this shaving area in one stroke.

40 After completing the first stroke, reposition the razor just right of the previously shaved section until the entire area is shaved. This movement completes shaving of the right side of the face the first time over.

41 Wipe razor clean.

> **REMINDER**
> The beard should be shaved with the grain of the hair; therefore, you must determine when the reverse hand positions and strokes are the correct procedure for shaving the client's beard. For example, when the hair in Shaving Area No. 5 grows downward, the freehand stroke may be a better choice than the reverse-freehand stroke.

Shaving Area No. 6—Backhand stroke

42 Stand to the right side of the client; turn the client's face to access left upper lip. Re-lather if necessary. Hold the razor in the backhand position.

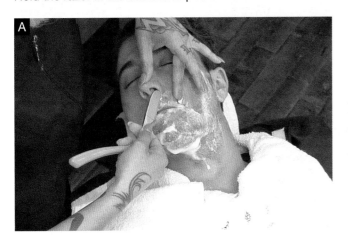
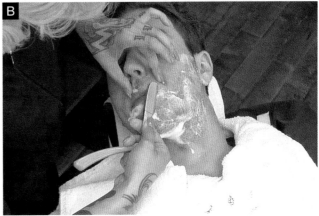

43 While gently pushing the tip of the nose to the right with the thumb and fingers of the left hand, stretch the skin and shave left side of upper lip.

44 Wipe razor clean.

Shaving Area No. 7—Backhand stroke

45 Move toward client's right shoulder and gently turn his face to the right. Re-lather the left side of the face.

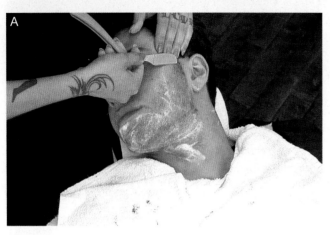

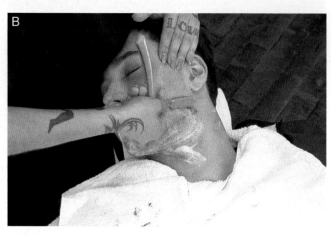

46 Using the thumb, wipe lather from the hairline. Stretch the skin taut and shave downward and slightly forward toward the corner of the mouth and jawbone.

47 Wipe razor clean.

Shaving Area No. 8—Freehand stroke

48 Stand at client's right and position his head to access this shaving area.

49 Hold razor in a freehand position.

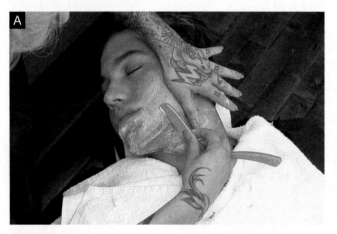

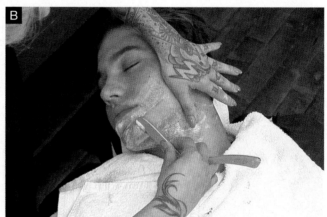

50 Stretch the skin and shave downward on the left side from the angle of the mouth to the point of the chin.

51 Wipe razor clean.

Shaving Area No. 9—Backhand stroke

52 Shift body position to access Shaving Area No. 9; hold razor for backhand stroke.

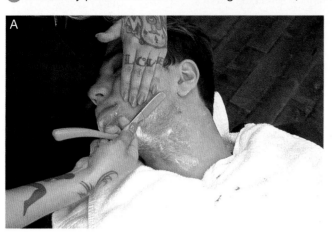
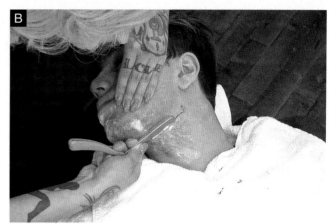

53 With the fingers of the left hand stretching the skin, shave downward from the point of the chin to where the grain of the beard changes on the neck.

54 Wipe razor clean.

Shaving Area No. 10—Reverse-freehand stroke

55 Stand behind client; hold razor in reverse-freehand position.

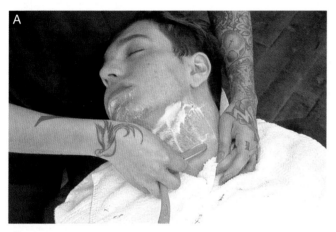
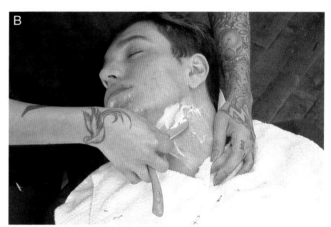

56 Stretch skin from the bottom of Shaving Area No. 10 with the left hand; shave left side of lower neck area upward to where the grain changes.

57 Similar to Shaving Area No. 5, after completing the first stroke, reposition the razor just left of the previously shaved section until the entire area is shaved. This completes the shaving of the left side of the face.

58 Wipe razor clean.

Shaving Area No. 11—Freehand stroke

59 Stand at the client's side; reposition his face to access Shaving Area No. 11.

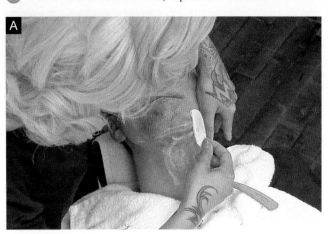

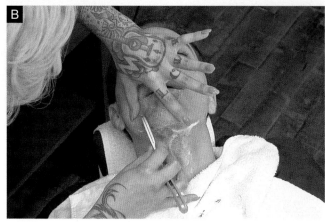

60 Hold the razor in a freehand position and stretch the skin; shave across the chin. Continue shaving until the entire chin area has been shaved to a point just below the jawbone.

61 Wipe razor clean.

> **? DID YOU KNOW?**
> In Shaving Area Nos. 11 and 14, the client can help to stretch the skin if he rolls his bottom lip slightly over his bottom teeth. This is sometimes called *balling-the-chin*.

Shaving Area No. 12—Freehand or backhand stroke

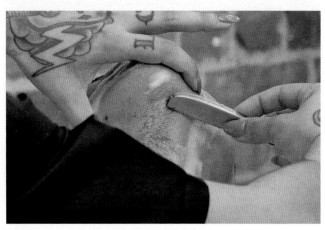

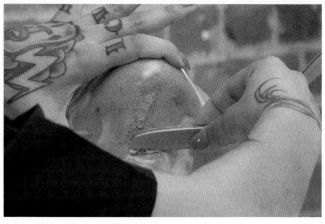

62 Using the freehand stroke, stretch the skin with the left hand and position the razor to arc downward just below the chin.

63 Continue this stroke until the grain of the beard changes.

64 Wipe razor clean.

65 Alternate method: Some barbers prefer to use the backhand stroke in Shaving Area No. 12.

Shaving Area No. 13—Reverse-freehand stroke

66 Stand behind the chair; hold razor for reverse-freehand stroke.

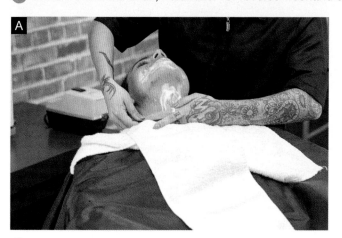
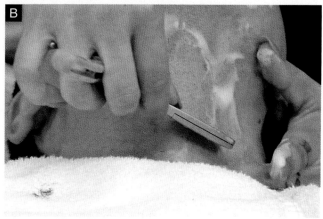

67 Stretch the skin from below Shaving Area No. 13 under the chin; shave upward on the lower part of the neck. Stretch the skin away from the Adam's apple and shave on a slight diagonal to prevent nicks.

68 Wipe razor clean.

Shaving Area No. 14—Reverse-freehand stroke

69 Remain behind the chair. Cup the client's chin and stretch the skin.

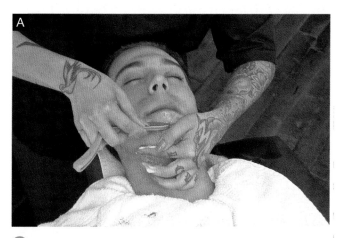
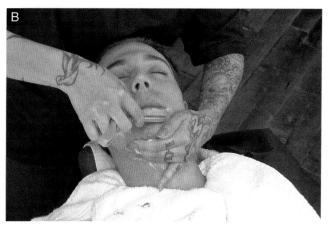

70 Using the reverse-freehand stroke, use a few short scooping strokes to shave upward from the top of the chin toward the lower lip. You may also ask the client to ball his chin for this step.

71 Wipe the razor clean and discard the towel or paper strip. This completes the first-time-over shave procedure.

Second-Time-Over Shave

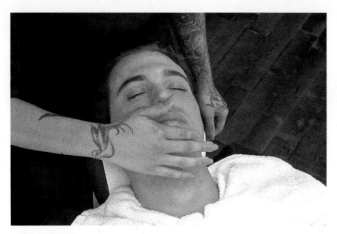

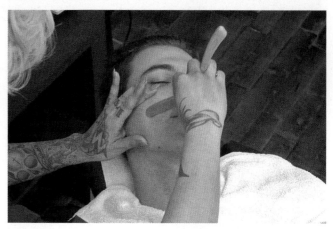

72 Dampen the client's face with water, checking for rough or uneven spots as you moisten the skin.

73 Stretch the skin and use freehand strokes with a light touch to shave with or across the grain to remove any residual facial hair.

74 Remove and dispose of wiping towel or paper. Lay a clean towel across client's chest.

D. FINISHING STEPS OF THE SHAVE

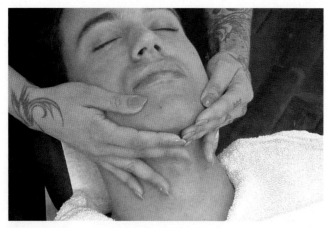

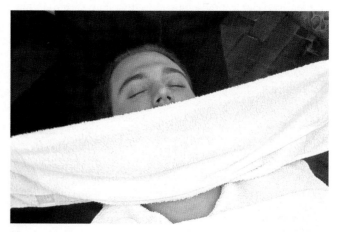

75 Apply light facial cream or moisturizing lotion with an effleurage massage movement. Massage the cream into the skin using pétrissage massage movements.

76 Apply a moderately warm towel over client's face.

77 Remove the towel and wipe off excess product in one operation.

> ⚠ **CAUTION**
> Avoid hot towels as the skin may be sensitive after the shave service.

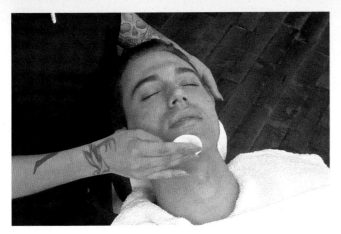

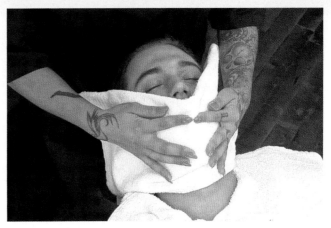

78 Apply a skin toner or other mild astringent using cotton pledgets or a soft tissue to remove residual cream product. Pat gently; do not wipe or scrape against the skin.

79 Remove the towel from the client's chest and position yourself behind the chair. Spread the towel over the client's face. Pat dry the lower part of the face; then the upper part. Remove the towel and fan the face dry.

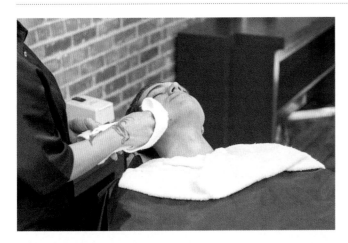

80 Move to the side of the chair and wrap a clean dry towel around your hand. Sprinkle a small amount of talcum powder on the towel and apply evenly to the face, if desired by client.

81 Slowly return the client to a sitting position.

82 Offer to perform a neck shave.

83 Comb the hair neatly as desired.

84 Wipe off loose hair, lather, or powder from the client's face, neck, and clothing. Proceed with mustache trim, if not performed before shave service, or neck shave, as desired. Remove draping.

CLEAN-UP AND DISINFECTION

☐ Clean and disinfect the tools and implements.

☐ Clean and then disinfect the work area.

☐ Sweep up hair and deposit in a closed receptacle.

☐ Deposit used blades in a sharps container.

☐ Dispose of single-use items. Place all used linens, towels, and capes in the laundry.

☐ Wash your hands.

THE NECK SHAVE

After practicing this procedure, you should be able to:

LO❾ Demonstrate a neck shave.

MATERIALS, IMPLEMENTS, AND EQUIPMENT

- ☐ Barber chair
- ☐ Barber's paper towels
- ☐ Comb and brush
- ☐ Covered container for soiled towels
- ☐ Covered trash can
- ☐ Electric latherizer
- ☐ Haircutting cape

- ☐ Sharps container
- ☐ Shaving cream or gel
- ☐ Sink
- ☐ Straight razor and blades
- ☐ Terry cloth towels
- ☐ Witch hazel or antiseptic

PREPARATION

1. Assemble supplies.
2. Following the facial shave, raise the chair slowly to an upright position.
3. Wash your hands.
4. Tuck a towel around the back of the neck, leaving the cape and towel loose enough to access the sides and bottom of the neckline.

PROCEDURE

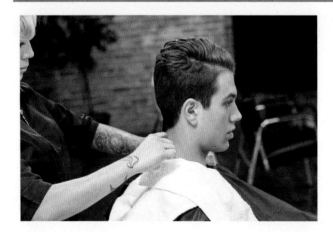

1. Tuck neck strip or paper towel into the neckline of drape for wiping the razor. Check the neckline and behind-the-ear areas for moles, blemishes, or other conditions.

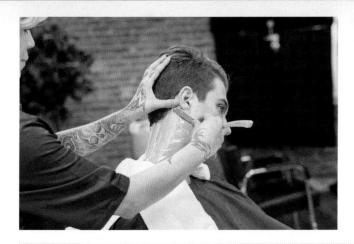

2 Apply lather. Stretch the skin behind the right ear with the thumb and shave along the natural hairline down the side of the neck using a freehand stroke.

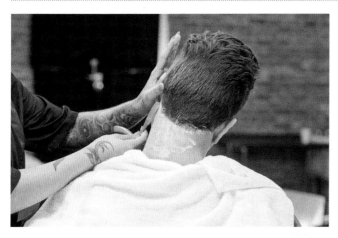

3 Repeat on left side using a reverse-backhand stroke.

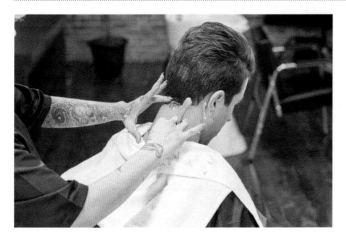

4 Use a freehand stroke to shave the nape area. Clean the shaven part of the neckline with a towel or neck strip moistened with witch hazel, antiseptic, or warm water. Remove the towel from around the neck and dry thoroughly.

5 Stand behind the chair, place a clean dry towel around the client's neck, and comb or style the hair as desired by the client.

6 Take the towel from the back of the neck and fold it around the right hand. Remove all traces of powder and any loose hair.

7 Discard the towel and remove the chair cloth from the client.

CLEAN-UP AND DISINFECTION

☐ Clean and disinfect the tools and implements.

☐ Clean and then disinfect the work area.

☐ Sweep up hair and deposit in a closed receptacle.

☐ Deposit used blades in a sharps container.

☐ Dispose of single-use items. Place all used linens, towels, and capes in the laundry.

☐ Wash your hands.

MUSTACHE TRIM

After practicing this procedure, you should be able to:

LO**10** Demonstrate a mustache trim.

MATERIALS, IMPLEMENTS, AND EQUIPMENT

- ☐ Barber chair with headrest
- ☐ Barber's paper towels
- ☐ Comb and brush
- ☐ Covered container for soiled towels
- ☐ Covered trash can

- ☐ Electric latherizer
- ☐ Haircutting cape
- ☐ Haircutting shears
- ☐ Headrest cover
- ☐ Outliner or trimmer

- ☐ Sharps container
- ☐ Shaving cream or gel
- ☐ Sink
- ☐ Straight razor and blades
- ☐ Terry cloth towels

PREPARATION

1 Assemble supplies.

2 Wash your hands.

3 Drape the client as for a haircut service.

4 Consult with the client regarding mustache shape preferences.

PROCEDURE

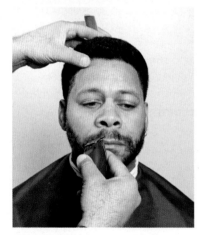

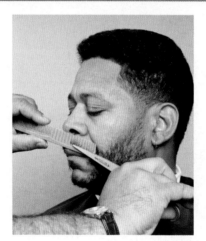

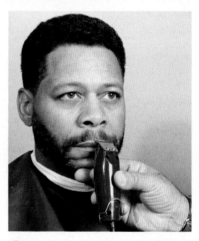

1 Trim the mustache to desired length with an outliner. Check for evenness of length at the corners of the mouth.

2 For safety, remove bulk from the mustache using the shear-over-comb or outliner-over-comb technique.

3 Shape and detail mustache with an outliner or razor. If using a razor, apply shaving cream or gel, wipe off excess product with thumb or finger, and proceed with razor outlining.

CLEAN-UP AND DISINFECTION

- ☐ Clean and disinfect the tools and implements.
- ☐ Clean and then disinfect the work area.
- ☐ Sweep up hair and deposit in a closed receptacle.
- ☐ Deposit used blades in a sharps container.

- ☐ Dispose of single-use items. Place all used linens, towels, and capes in the laundry.
- ☐ Wash your hands.

BEARD DESIGNS

After practicing this procedure, you should be able to:

LO⓫ Demonstrate cutting in beard designs.

MATERIALS, IMPLEMENTS, AND EQUIPMENT

☐ Barber chair with headrest

☐ Barber's paper towels

☐ Clippers

☐ Comb and brush

☐ Covered container for soiled towels

☐ Covered trash can

☐ Electric latherizer

☐ Haircutting cape

☐ Haircutting shears

☐ Headrest cover

☐ Outliner or trimmer

☐ Sharps container

☐ Shaving cream or gel

☐ Sink

☐ Straight razor and blades

☐ Terry cloth towels

PREPARATION

1 Assemble supplies.

2 Wash your hands.

3 Drape the client as for a haircut service.

4 Consult with the client as to his desired design of the beard. Determine any preferences regarding length, density (thickness), and shape.

> **✓ HERE'S A TIP**
> A cloth towel is a good alternative to a neck strip, especially if the client has a lot of hair growth on his neck.

PROCEDURE

A. BEARD TRIM ON MEDIUM-TEXTURED FACIAL HAIR

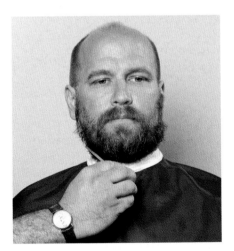

1 Gently comb through the beard and check for hidden moles or growths.

2 Apply a fresh headrest cover. Adjust the headrest so the client's neck is supported while leaning his head back. The chair back may also be reclined at a slight angle, depending on your preference for reaching areas under the chin. Place a towel underneath the chin to protect the client's neck from stray hairs (optional).

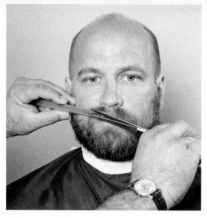

3 Trim excess mustache hair using the shear-over-comb or clipper-over-comb technique.

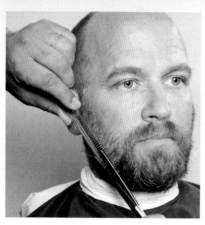

4 Trim excess hair in cheek areas.

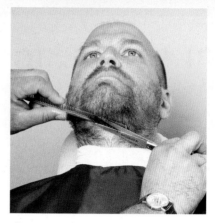

5 Trim excess hair under chin.

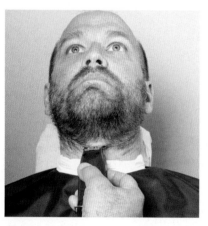

6 Start in the center directly under the chin and establish a guide with the outliner.

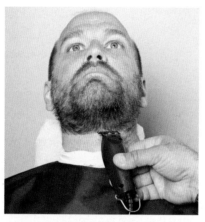

7 Work left and right of center to establish design line to back of the jaws.

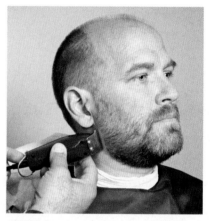

8 Move to the client's right side and cut in the design from the sideburn down to the guide at the back of the jaw. Repeat on the left side.

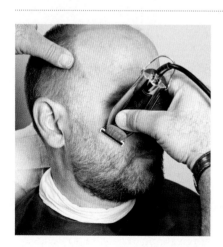

9 Use trimmer to outline the cheek and upper areas of the beard, blending with the sideburn area.

10 Using the shear-over-comb or clipper-over-comb technique, taper and blend the beard from the outlined areas up to just under the bottom lip, mustache, and cheek areas.

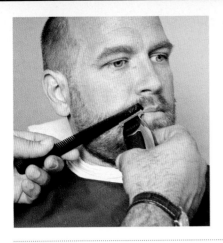

11 Trim and blend the mustache into the beard using the shear-, clipper-, or outliner-over-comb technique.

12 Recline client, apply steam towel, lather areas to be shaved, shave carefully at the outline, and wipe clean. Apply aftershave or tonic lotion.

13 Return client to sitting position.

14 Remember to check the proportion and shape of the beard in the mirror when the client is returned to a sitting position. Retouch the beard design with shears or outliner wherever necessary.

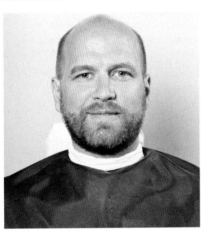

15 Style or cut the hair as needed for a finished look.

B. BEARD REDESIGN ON MEDIUM-TEXTURED FACIAL HAIR

The following steps show the procedure for creating a new mustache and beard design starting from the trim just performed.

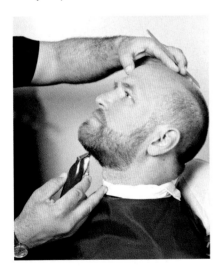

16 Use outliner to create a new guide starting in the center under the chin.

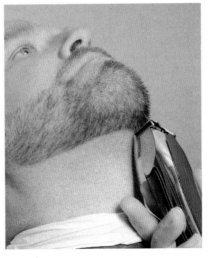

17 Cut right and left of center to establish new design line.

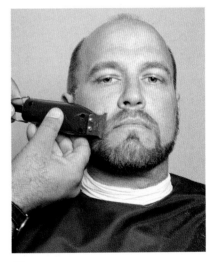

18 Reshape mustache and chin areas.

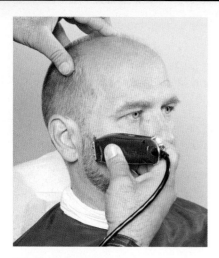

19 Cut in a new design line in the cheek areas. Make sure design line connects with the corners of the mustache outline.

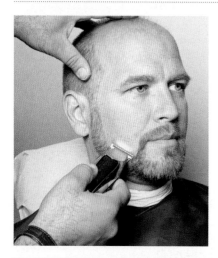

20 With outliner blades facing up, remove excess hair in cheek areas.

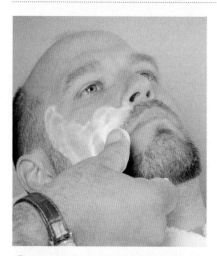

21 Recline client and apply shaving cream along new outlines.

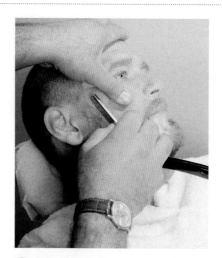

22 Shave sideburn outline.

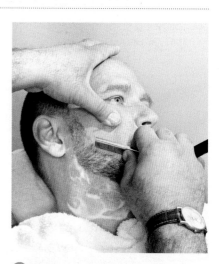

23 Shave cheek outline.

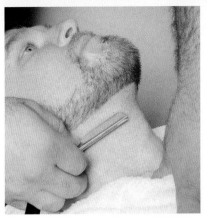

24 Shave neck areas 5 and 10.

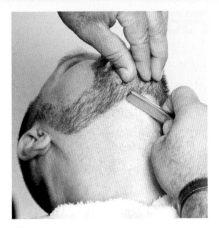

25 Shave neck areas 12 and 13.

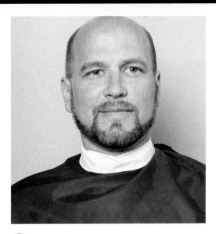

26 Finish design.

C. BEARD TRIM ON CURLY-TEXTURED FACIAL HAIR

Note: This procedure shows the progression of three designs from a full beard to a patch and goatee.

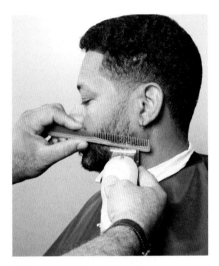

27 Trim excess hair using the clipper-over-comb technique.

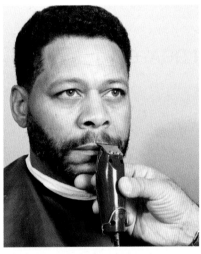

28 Trim and shape mustache.

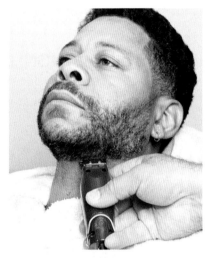

29 Establish design line under chin.

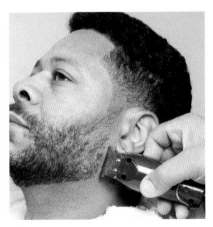

30 Establish design line at jaw and sideburn areas.

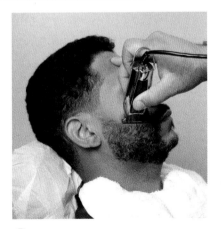

31 Establish design line in cheek areas.

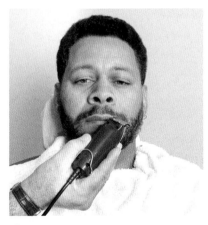

32 Contour under mustache above top lip. This completes design no. 1.

D. BEARD REDESIGN: FULL GOATEE

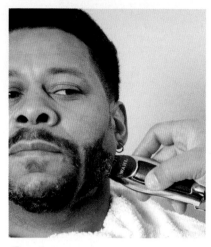

33 Remove cheek and side hair to create a full goatee.

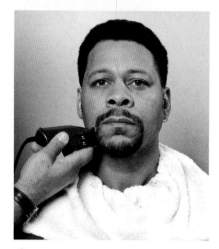

34 Contour full goatee design line. This completes design no. 2.

E. BEARD REDESIGN: CHIN GOATEE

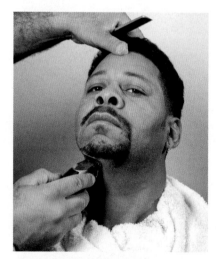

35 Remove excess hair under chin to create a chin goatee; shape the patch.

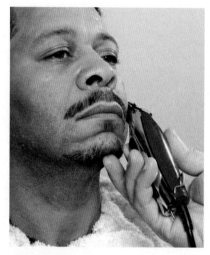

36 Establish length of mustache at corners.

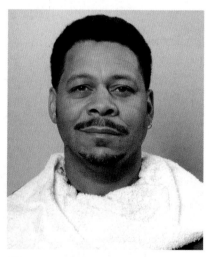

37 This completes design no. 3.

CLEAN-UP AND DISINFECTION

☐ Clean and disinfect the tools and implements.

☐ Clean and then disinfect the work area.

☐ Sweep up hair and deposit in a closed receptacle.

☐ Deposit used blades in a sharps container.

☐ Dispose of single-use items. Place all used linens, towels, and capes in the laundry.

☐ Wash your hands.

REVIEW QUESTIONS

1. Identify three client characteristics that barbers should be aware of before beginning the shave service.

2. List the steps to prepare the client for a shave.

3. What effect does shaving cream have on facial hair?

4. Describe how to work shaving cream into a lather.

5. What effect do hot towels have on facial hair?

6. Identify several skin conditions that may prohibit the application of hot steam towels.

7. Identify the four razor-holding positions or strokes.

8. What three razor strokes are used in facial shaving?

9. Shaving strokes should be performed in what relation to the grain of the hair?

10. Identify the number of shaving areas of the face.

11. What two types of shaves are performed in a standard shave service?

12. Explain the difference between the first-time-over shave and the once-over shave.

13. List the finishing steps of a facial shave.

14. Explain how a close shave differs from a standard shave and why it may be undesirable.

15. List the important characteristics used to determine a mustache design.

16. Explain why some barbers prefer to cut and style the hair before performing a beard trim service.

CHAPTER GLOSSARY

backhand (BAK-HAND)	p. 342	razor position and stroke used in 4 of the 14 basic shaving areas: nos. 2, 6, 7, and 9; optional position for area 12
close shaving (KLOHS SHAYV-ing)	p. 349	the procedure of shaving facial hair against the grain during the second-time-over shave
cutting stroke (KUT-ing STROHK)	p. 342	the correct angle of cutting the beard with a straight razor
first-time-over shave (FIRST-TYM-OH-ver SHAYV)	p. 348	first part of the standard shave consisting of shaving the 14 areas of the face; followed by the second-time-over shave to remove residual missed or rough spots
freehand (FREE-HAND)	p. 342	razor position and stroke used in 6 of the 14 shaving areas: nos. 1, 3, 4, 8, 11, and 12
neck shave (NEK SHAYV)	p. 349	shaving the areas behind the ears down the sides of the neck, and at the back neckline
once-over shave (WONCE-OH-ver SHAYV)	p. 349	single-lather shave in which the shaving strokes are made across the grain of the hair
reverse backhand (ree-VURS BAK-HAND)	p. 342	razor position and stroke used by right-handed barbers for shaving the left side of the neck behind the ear and used by left-handed barbers behind the right ear
reverse freehand (ree-VURS FREE-HAND)	p. 342	razor position and stroke used in 4 of the 14 basic shaving areas: nos. 5, 10, 13, and 14
second-time-over shave (SEK-und-TYM-OH-ver SHAYV)	p. 348	follows a regular shave to remove any rough or uneven spots using water instead of lather; may be considered a form of close shaving
styptic powder (STIP-tik POW-dur)	p. 352	alum powder or liquid used to stop bleeding of nicks and cuts

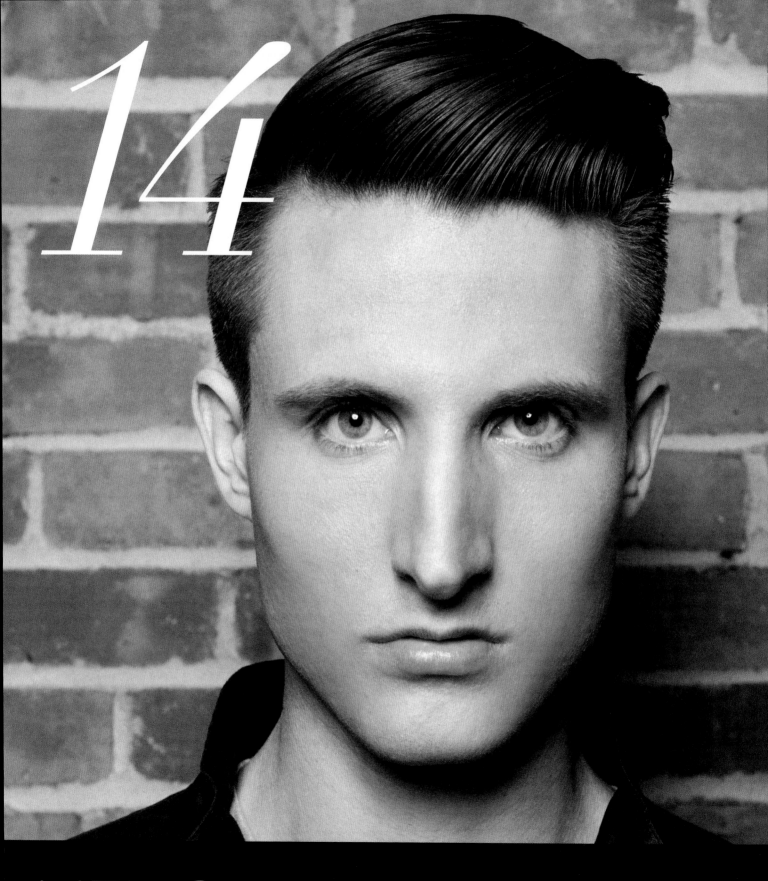

14

MEN'S HAIRCUTTING
AND STYLING

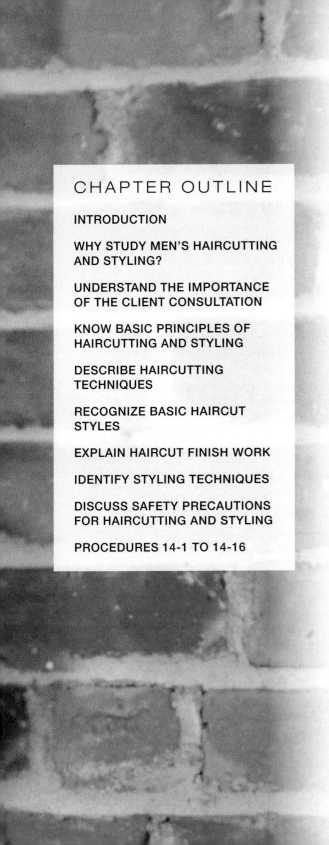

LEARNING OBJECTIVES

After completing this chapter, you will be able to:

LO❶
Explain the importance of the client consultation and consider questions that help you envision the client's desired outcome.

LO❷
Describe anatomical features that influence haircutting and styling.

LO❸
Identify the sections of the head as applied to haircutting.

LO❹
Identify tapering and blending areas.

LO❺
Define design elements used in haircutting and styling.

LO❻
Define basic terms used in haircutting and styling.

LO❼
Explain basic cutting techniques using shears, clippers, and razors.

LO❽
Describe basic haircut styles.

LO❾
Describe haircut finish work.

LO❿
Describe basic styling techniques.

LO⓫
Discuss haircutting and styling safety precautions.

LO⓬
Demonstrate basic haircuts and styling techniques.

Introduction

The art of haircutting involves the precise designing, cutting, and shaping of the client's hair. Mastering this art requires the competent use of a variety of tools, implements, and techniques. The same general techniques are used in men's and women's haircutting. The differences between the two are usually evident in the overall design line, the contour or shape, and the finished style.

A good haircut is the foundation of a good hairstyle. The importance of this simple truth cannot be overstated. To perform a good haircut, you need to be able to cut, blend, and taper the hair using clippers, shears, and razors. Diligent practice and application of these skills will help form the foundation for your future success; however, the learning doesn't stop with your barber license. When working in the barbershop, there will be occasions when a client requests a haircut that you might not feel confident about performing or that requires you to step out of your comfort zone. This is to be expected, so do not panic. If you've learned the basics while in school, you should be able to create a plan of action that utilizes the skills you've mastered so that you can perform the haircut with confidence.

Hairstyling has been defined as the art of arranging the hair in a particular style that is appropriately suited to the cut and that best fits the client's physical characteristics and personality. In men's haircutting, very often the finished cut *is* the style; when we use the term *styling*, we usually refer to combing, brushing, blowdrying, or other methods used to redirect or place the hair into its finished look. Both the haircut and style should accentuate the client's best features and minimize the weakest ones. This rule requires that the barber consider the client's head shape, facial features, neck length, hairline, and hair texture. The barber also needs to be guided by the client's preferences, personality, and lifestyle so the client can manage the style in between shop visits.

why study
MEN'S HAIRCUTTING AND STYLING?

Barbers should study and have a thorough understanding of men's haircutting and styling because:

> Haircutting is a basic skill that provides the foundation for hair design and styling.

> Practicing skills and techniques is critical to being able to perform balanced and proportionate haircuts and styles for clients.

> The more practice and experience barbers have, the better able they will be to meet their clients' needs.

> Meeting clients' haircutting and styling needs results in satisfied customers and the opportunity to build repeat business.

Understand the Importance of the Client Consultation

After reading this section, you will be able to:

LO❶ Explain the importance of the client consultation and consider questions that help you envision the client's desired outcome.

The client consultation is a conversation between you and the client about the client's desires and expectations of the service you will perform. It also facilitates the hair and scalp analysis step so that you can determine what can or cannot be done with the client's hair and helps to eliminate any guesswork about the haircut or style to be performed. During the consultation you should be able to:

- determine what the client wants his hair to look like or to be able to do with his hair;
- discuss the client's lifestyle as it relates to his daily hair maintenance routine;
- identify hair conditions, such as density, texture, or length, that may limit or enhance cutting and styling options;
- discover scalp conditions that may prohibit moving forward with the service;
- identify hair conditions that require special treatment;
- offer your professional advice or alternative suggestions;
- agree with the client on the type of haircut and finishing services to be performed.

With this information you can make a more informed judgment about what can or cannot be done to meet the client's expectations (Figure 14-1).

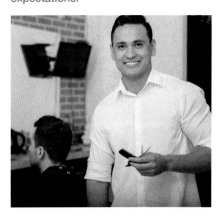

figure 14-1
Know if you can meet your client's expectations.

© antoniodiaz/Shutterstock.com.

DISCUSS COMMON QUESTIONS ASKED DURING A CONSULTATION

After draping the client and facing him toward the mirror you can begin the consultation with a few basic questions:

- *How long has it been since your last haircut?*

  Knowing that on average hair grows at the rate of about ½ inch per month, you should be able to envision the preferred length of the hair before it grew out and needed to be cut again.

- *Do you prefer a similar style or are you looking for something new?*

  The answer to this question can lead you directly to the cutting stage or to further discussion with the client about appropriate styles and options.

- *What is your usual morning routine (shampoo, blowdry, etc.)?*

  This answer will indicate how much time the client is willing to spend on his hair care every day.

- *Did you have any particular problems with your previous cut or style?*

  This question provides the client an opportunity to open dialogue about specific hair-related issues such as problem areas, length, fullness, growth and wave patterns, hair texture, density, and color.

Next, you will need more details to visualize what the finished cut and style should look like. While analyzing the client's hair and scalp (**Figure 14-2**), ask specific questions about the style the client expects and then clarify the answers; "a little off the top," "just a trim," and "over the ears" are some commonly heard phrases in the barbershop; but what do these phrases actually tell you about the haircut? Would you feel confident about cutting the client's hair without finding out just what the client means? Consider some of the reasons why these phrases do not provide enough information for you to proceed with the haircut; as you may note, they do not confirm what the client means:

- How is "a little" measured? Is it ¼ inch, 1 inch, or somewhere in between?

- What does the client consider a "trim"? Clean up the hairline, take ½ inch off all over, or something else?

- To the client, does "over the ears" mean covering the ears or cutting around the ears?

These are just a few examples of misinterpretations that can occur during a consultation and why it is so important that you listen and understand what the client is telling you. Before beginning the haircut, explain or summarize what you will be doing based on what the client has told you. Use the mirror to show him how you have interpreted what he has said (**Figure 14-3**). When in doubt, ask more questions for clarity. This will benefit you, your client, and the final result. With practice and experience, you will develop your own questions to gain the information you need to perform the haircut with confidence and a clear plan of execution. Asking these questions helps you **envisioning** (EN-vijg-ohn-ing) the haircut before beginning the actual procedure.

A Word about Trims

When a client uses the term *trim*, what he usually means is that he doesn't want his hair cut too close or wants to retain some length. If the client makes this request, you will need to understand what his concept of a *trim* is during the consultation.

The term *trim* may also mean that the client just wants his outline cleaned up in-between haircuts; a little outliner work and he is all set until his next appointment. A *tape-up* also fits into this category of trims and should consist of no more than an outline cleanup because, once you start *taping up* or cutting above the hairline, you will have to keep blending into the interior sections, which makes the service a haircut.

In still other cases, clients may ask for a trim with the idea that the price of the service will be adjusted down because less hair is cut off.

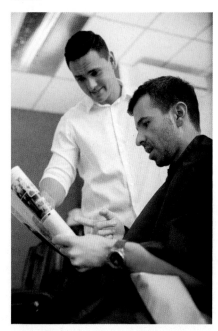

figure 14-2
Communicate specifics with your client.

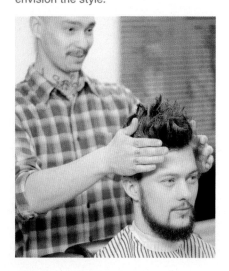

figure 14-3
Use the mirror to help your client envision the style.

© antoniodiaz/Shutterstock.com.

© Dmytro Zinkevych/Shutterstock.com.

In reality, there really isn't any such thing as a trim when used in this context because regardless of the *amount* of hair cut off, you will still have to perform a series of steps to cut the various hair sections and the service should be priced accordingly.

The best way to avoid any confusion or pricing issues for any of these interpretations of a trim is to clearly define the services on the price menu and to educate your clients about the difference in the services being offered.

Know Basic Principles of Haircutting and Styling

After reading this section, you will be able to:

LO② Describe anatomical features that influence haircutting and styling.

LO③ Identify the sections of the head as applied to haircutting.

LO④ Identify tapering and blending areas.

LO⑤ Define design elements used in haircutting and styling.

LO⑥ Define basic terms used in haircutting and styling.

Every haircut is a representation and advertisement of the barber's work. Pay attention to details such as client comfort, sideburn lengths, outlines, balance, and proportion and always remember that the haircut is the foundation of the hairstyle. In order to provide services that will make your clients' barbershop experience an exceptional one, you need to have a good understanding of the anatomical features, terminology, and techniques that relate to haircutting and styling.

RECOGNIZE ANATOMICAL FEATURES

As a barber, the anatomical features that will most influence the haircut and style design options for your client are his facial shape, head shape, profile, neck length, and the size and placement of his ears.

Facial Shapes

The consultation should provide sufficient information about the client's lifestyle and personality to suggest a suitable style, but a study of facial shapes will assist you in determining the best style for a client's features. The **facial shape** (FAY-shul SHAYP) of each individual is determined by the position and prominence of the facial bones. The seven general facial shapes are oval, round, inverted triangular, square, pear-shaped, oblong, and diamond. In order to recognize each facial shape for the purpose of offering correct advice, you will need to be acquainted with the characteristics of each type. With this information, you can suggest a haircut and style that complements the facial shape, similar to the way that certain clothes flatter the body.

figure 14-4
Determine facial shapes.

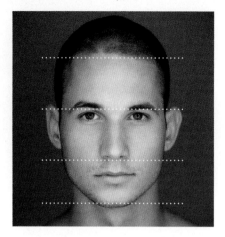

To determine a facial shape, divide the face into three zones: forehead to eyebrows, eyebrows to end of nose, and end of nose to chin (Figure 14-4). Envision these divisions while reviewing the following facial shapes.

Oval. The oval-shaped face is generally recognized as the ideal shape.

- Any hairstyle that maintains the oval shape is usually suitable.
- Change the part or redirect the hair to experiment with different looks (**Figure 14-5**).

Round. The aim here is to slim the face.

- Hair that is too short will emphasize the fullness of the face.
- Create some height on the top to lengthen the look of the face.
- An off-center part and some waves at eye level will also help lessen the full appearance of the face.
- Beards should be styled to make the face appear more oval (**Figure 14-6**).

Inverted triangular. This facial shape has over-wide cheekbones and a narrow jawline.

- Keep the hair close at the crown and temples and longer in back.
- Try changing the part and the direction of the hair.
- A full beard helps to fill out the narrow jaw (**Figure 14-7**).

Square. This shape has angular features at the forehead and jaw.

- Use wavy bangs that blend into the temples to an asymmetrical line.
- Minimize the square look by directing more hair to the temple areas.
- Beards should be styled to slenderize the face (**Figure 14-8**).

Pear-shaped. This shape is narrow at the top and wide on the bottom.

- Create width and fullness at the top, temples, and sides to produce balance.
- Short, full styles are best, ending just above the jawline where it joins the ear area.

figure 14-5
Oval face shape.

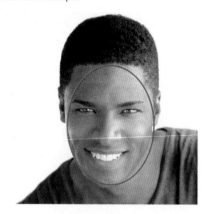

figure 14-6
Round.

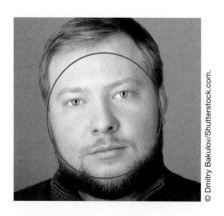

figure 14-7
Inverted triangular.

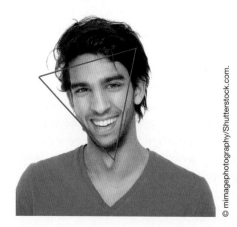

figure 14-8
Square.

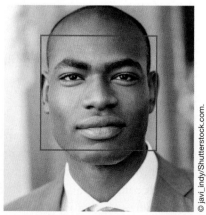

figure 14-9
Pear.

figure 14-10
Oblong.

figure 14-11
Diamond.

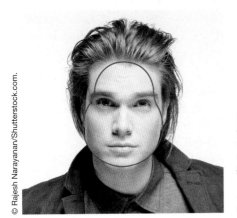

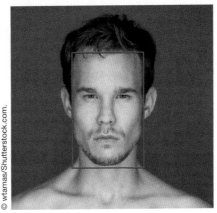

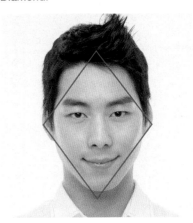

- A body wave or medium-size curl perm is another way to achieve width at the top.
- Beards should be styled to slenderize the lower jaw area (**Figure 14-9**).

Oblong. The long face needs to be visually shortened and its angularity softened.

- Layered bangs brushed to the sides over the temples can camouflage the front hairline, giving the illusion of a shorter facial shape.
- Wearing a mustache also helps to shorten the look of a longer face shape (**Figure 14-10**).

Diamond. This face shape is narrow at the temples and chin.

- Create a style with width or fullness at the temples.
- Keep hair close to the head at the widest points of the face.
- Direct bangs off the face and into the sides to broaden the appearance of the forehead.
- A full, square, or rounded beard is also appropriate (**Figure 14-11**).

Head Shapes

Generally speaking, the basic shape of the head consists of rounded portions, such as the crown, parietal, and occipital areas; concave curved areas as found below the occipital to the nape; and portions of flat areas in the top and side sections. However, not every client's head shape conforms to this general description and that can create particular haircutting and styling challenges for the barber. For example, a head shape that is more pointed at the apex may require longer hair lengths between the temporal and top areas to create the illusion of roundness and evenness through that section. In other cases, the client might have one or more ridges of scalp through the occipital area, rather than a smooth curve to the nape area; leaving the hair slightly longer in this area can help camouflage the ridges while close cutting only makes them more visible. As a barber, you will see many variations of head shapes and these variations will influence the cutting techniques you use and the styles you recommend.

figure 14-12
Straight.

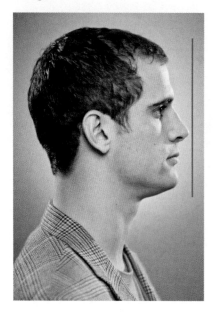

Profiles

You should be aware of your client's profile since it can influence the appropriateness of the haircut or style he wears. You will need to study the position, shape, and size of the forehead, nose, and chin from both side (profile) and full-face views to determine the best look for your client.

Straight profiles tend to be the most balanced and proportioned because the forehead and chin align with only a slight curvature; a variety of hairstyles are appropriate for this profile type (**Figure 14-12**).

Concave profiles have a prominent forehead and chin. Use a close hair arrangement at the forehead to minimize the bulge of the forehead (**Figure 14-13**).

Convex profiles recede at the forehead and chin. This profile can appear straighter by creating the appearance of balance from the forehead to the chin. Experiment with arranging the hair at the front hairline to add volume and suggest the client wear a beard or goatee; this will help to balance out the projection of the nose by adding bulk to the features that recede (**Figure 14-14**).

Angular profiles have a receding forehead, but the chin tends to jut forward. This profile can appear more balanced by arranging the hair over the forehead and by adding a mustache and a close-cut beard to minimize the look of the protruding chin (**Figure 14-15**).

Prominent nose shapes include a hooked nose, large nose, or pointed nose. Style the hair forward at the forehead and back on the sides to minimize the prominence of the nose; beards and mustaches can also be used to balance the features (**Figure 14-16**).

Small to average nose shapes usually require shorter haircut styles because the size or heavy features associated with prominent nose shapes are not an issue. Experiment with different part lines or by combing the hair in different directions on the sides (**Figure 14-17**).

Neck Lengths

The length of the client's neck is also a factor in determining the overall shape of the haircut and style. In most cases, it is advisable to follow the

figure 14-13
Concave.

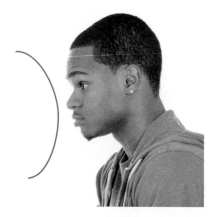

figure 14-14
Convex.

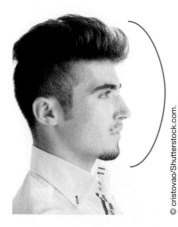

figure 14-15
Angular.

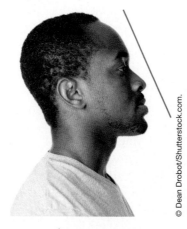

figure 14-16
Prominent nose.

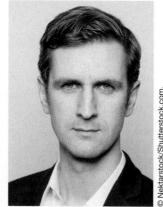

figure 14-17
Smaller nose.

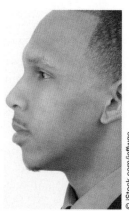

client's natural hairline; however, sometimes an overly long or very short neck limits the options. You will have to consider the length of the hairline and the growth pattern and density of the hair at the nape to determine the most suitable design for your client. Review the following guidelines for working with different neck lengths:

- A long neck can appear shorter if the hair is left fuller or longer at the nape. Avoid cutting into or above the natural hairline as this will only make the neck appear longer (**Figure 14-18**).

- A short neck can appear longer if the hair does not extend below the natural hairline at the nape. Tapering this area and fine blending at the natural hairline will also help create the illusion of a longer neck (**Figure 14-19**).

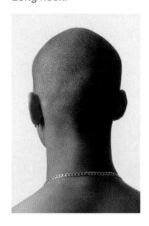

© Simon Wilkinson/The Image Bank/Getty Images.

figure 14-18
Long neck.

Ear Size and Placement

The size and placement of the client's ears is important to a haircut design because these characteristics help to determine the most appropriate length or thickness for the hair at the sides of the client's head and for the length of his sideburns. For example, a client whose ears have a tendency to stick out might prefer a style that leaves the hair fuller on the sides or a style that covers the top of the ear. Either option will create the illusion of less distance between the client's ears and his head. The size and placement of the client's ears also influences his options for the length, thickness, and shape of his sideburns, as explained in the following section.

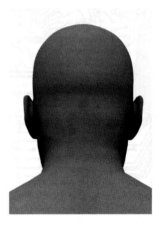

© VICTOR HABBICK VISIONS/Science Photo Library/Getty Images.

figure 14-19
Short neck.

Sideburn Lengths and Designs

To determine the most suitable length and shape for the client's sideburns, you will need to consider his hairstyle, facial structure and features, natural hair growth, and the size and placement of his ears. Consider the relationships of these factors to sideburn designs, as discussed below.

The sideburns will look short, medium, or long relative to client's facial features and structure. For example, a 1-inch-long sideburn may appear short to medium on a client with a larger, longer facial structure or too long on a client with smaller or shorter facial features.

The client's natural hair growth is a consideration because it determines his natural hairline and the density and texture of his hair. These characteristics affect the amount of hair there is to work within the sideburn areas and the design options you will have to create a balanced and proportioned look. For example, if the client has light, thin sideburn hair, very close cutting can result in creating patches or exposing the underlying skin. Conversely, dark, thick sideburn hair may require very close cutting and tapering to reduce the appearance of weight and to create balance with the haircut.

Like his facial structure, the size and placement of the client's ears will determine if the sideburns are considered short, medium, or long relative to his particular features. For example, a short sideburn for a client with small features might be ½-inch long and a short sideburn for a client with larger features might be ¾-inch long.

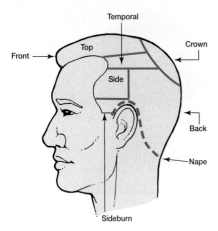

figure 14-20
Sections of the head: side view.

Some guidelines for designing sideburns are as follows:

- The length, shape, and density of the sideburns influence the look of the haircut and the client's facial features overall. Be aware of balance, color, and proportion when cutting in the sideburns.

- Sideburns should *appear* even in length and thickness when viewed from the front, preferably in a mirror.

- The density of the sideburns should blend gradually from the hairline into the side sections.

- Anatomical features, such as the facial bones, may be used as a general guide for trimming sideburns but it must be remembered that few people have truly symmetrical features. Therefore, a ½-inch-long sideburn on the right side might need to be slightly shorter or longer on the left side to appear even when viewing the client from the front.

- Sideburns should complement the facial shape and hairstyle.

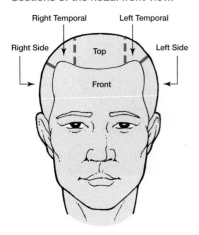

figure 14-21
Sections of the head: front view.

LEARN THE SECTIONS OF THE HEAD FORM

To create consistent and successful results in haircutting, it is necessary to understand the shape of the head. Hair responds differently in different areas of the head because of the curves and changes from one section to the next. Visualizing the sections of the head form as presented in this textbook will help you to:

- Know where to start a haircut

- Develop patterns or steps for cutting specific styles

- Eliminate technical mistakes when blending from one section to another

- Reduce confusion when cutting because you will know where you are in the cut

- Facilitate easier checking of the final result

The sections of the head form as depicted in **Figures 14-20** through **14-22** include the

- Front

- Top (apex)

- Temporal (crest, parietal ridge, hatband, horseshoe)

- Crown (tonsure area)

- Sides

- Sideburns

- Back

- Nape

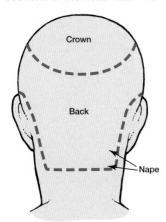

figure 14-22
Sections of the head: back view.

Reference points (REF-err-ence POYNTZ) are points on the head that mark areas where the surface of the head changes or the behavior of the hair changes as a result of the surface changes. These points are used to establish proportionate design lines and contours.

The **parietal ridge** (puh-RY-ate-uhl RIJ) is also known as the **crest** (KREST), *temporal*, *horseshoe*, or *hatband* area of the head. It is the widest section of the head, starting at the temples and ending just below the crown. When a comb is placed flat against the head at the sides, the parietal ridge begins where the head starts to curve away from the comb (**Figure 14-23**). The parietal ridge is one of the most important sections of the head when cutting hair because it serves as a transition area from the top to the front, sides, and back sections.

The occipital bone protrudes at the base of the skull. When a comb is placed flat against the nape area, the occipital begins where the head curves away from the comb (**Figure 14-24**). The apex is the highest point on the top of the head (**Figure 14-25**). The four corners are located by crossing two diagonal lines at the apex (**Figure 14-26**). The lines will point to the front and back corners of the head.

Tapering and Blending Areas

Taper (TAYP-uhr) or tapering is the action of gradually increasing the length of the hair from one point on the head to another without any lines of demarcation such as gaps or steps. The primary tapering areas of a cut are determined by the style. For example, in a standard taper cut, gradual tapering occurs from the hairline through the back and side sections up to the top; in the case of a bald fade, most of the tapering takes place around the parietal ridge. Tapering and blending areas refer to the sections or levels within the haircut where transitions between hair lengths occur.

Clients often describe their desired style in terms of length using such words as *long*, *medium*, *short*, *close* or *extra-short*, or *faded*. Tapering and

figure 14-23
The parietal ridge.

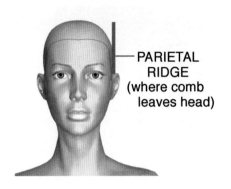

PARIETAL RIDGE
(where comb leaves head)

figure 14-24
The occipital bone.

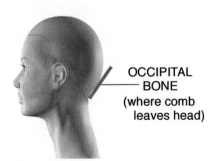

OCCIPITAL BONE
(where comb leaves head)

figure 14-25
The apex.

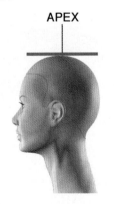

APEX

figure 14-26
The four corners.

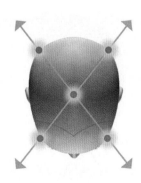

blending areas for these basic lengths vary with the haircut design and the shape of the head.

With the exception of a bald fade or a bi-level cut, tapering begins at the nape and side hairlines (including the sideburns), as indicated by the bottom dashed lines in the figures. The top lines depict the highest point of the tapered area and indicate transition areas into longer hair. Sections between dashed lines show where the gradual tapering and blending takes place. Notice the relationship of the tapering and blending areas in relation to the curves of the head. Longer styles usually require the least amount of close tapering.

Tapering is performed from the nape hairline to just below the occipital and just above the bottom of the ear when seen from the back (Figure 14-27). If the ears are exposed, tapering on the sides begins at the hairline and connects with the taper behind the ear before blending into longer side and back lengths. Medium-length styles do not have a scalped appearance, although the hair is cut closer to the head than in longer, fuller styles (Figure 14-28). Closer tapering is performed from the nape hairline to the occipital at a point that is about even with the tops of the ears.

In the sideburn areas, tapering should blend into the side section at the tops of the ears. Semi-short styles are tapered slightly higher to above the occipital. The hair is tapered to the bottom of the parietal ridge in the back and side sections (Figure 14-29). Short or close styles usually require close tapering up to the bottom of the crest or at a level within the crest, ending at the curvature of the head in this area (Figure 14-30). Fade styles are cut extremely close in the back and lower side areas, become gradually longer in the crest, and are longest in the top section. Very close cutting, including balding when desired, is performed from the nape to the bottom of the parietal ridge. Sides are cut using the next larger clipper blade to blend through the parietal area. The next larger blade is used in the parietal area to blend with the top section (Figure 14-31). Hair is cut against the grain, across the grain, or with the grain depending on the hair texture and growth pattern in the section being cut.

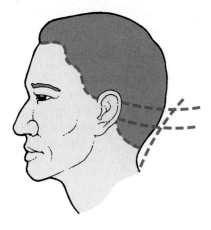

figure 14-27
Taper area for longer hairstyles.

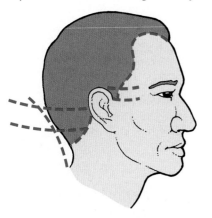

figure 14-28
Taper area for medium-length hairstyles.

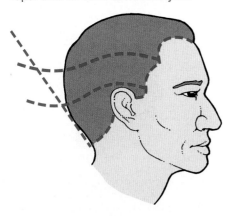

figure 14-29
Taper area for semi-short hairstyles.

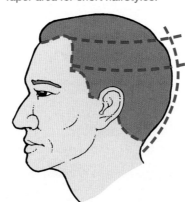

figure 14-30
Taper area for short hairstyles.

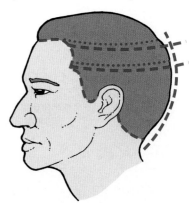

figure 14-31
Taper area for fade hairstyles.

UNDERSTAND DESIGN ELEMENTS USED IN HAIRCUTTING

Design is the foundation of all artistic applications and an understanding of its principles will help you develop a strong visual eye and the judgment needed to create successful designs for your clients. Barbers work with the three-dimensional design elements of line, form (shape), space, texture, and color.

Lines

A *line* is simply a series of connected dots that result in a continuous mark. Straight and curved lines are used in haircutting to create design, shape, and direction (**Figure 14-32**). *Curved* lines are either concave or convex in shape and may repeat, as in a wave pattern. The three types of *straight* lines used in haircutting are horizontal, vertical, and diagonal lines (**Figure 14-33**):

- **Horizontal lines** (hor-ih-ZAHN-tul LYNZ) are parallel to the horizon or floor and direct the eye from one side to the other.

  - *Horizontal cutting lines* build weight and are used to create a one-length look and low elevation or blunt haircut designs.

  - *Weight lines* are usually created at the perimeter or at the occipital area of a haircut (**Figures 14-34 and 14-35**).

- **Vertical lines** (VUR-tih-kuhl LYNZ) are perpendicular to the floor and are described in terms of up and down.

  - Vertical partings facilitate projecting the hair at higher elevations while cutting.

  - Vertical cutting lines remove weight within the cut and create layers.

  - Layers may be cut in from short to long, cut in from long to short, or cut uniformly depending on finger placement (**Figure 14-36**).

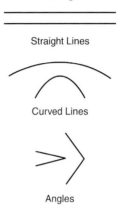

figure 14-32
Lines and angles.

Straight Lines

Curved Lines

Angles

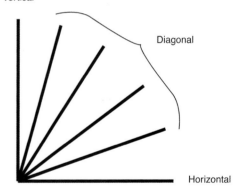

figure 14-33
Horizontal, vertical, and diagonal lines.

Vertical

Diagonal

Horizontal

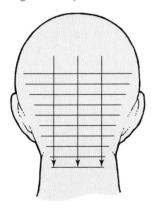

figure 14-34
Weight line at perimeter.

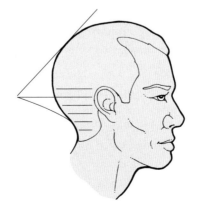

figure 14-35
Weight line at occipital.

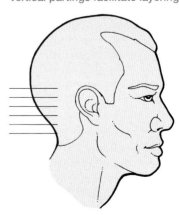

figure 14-36
Vertical partings facilitate layering.

figure 14-37
Diagonal line within top front sections.

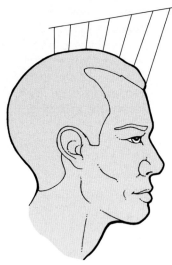

- **Diagonal lines** (dye-AG-ih-nul LYNZ) have a slanted direction and are used to create sloped lines within a haircut or at the perimeter to determine the design line (**Figure 14-37**).

  - When used at the perimeter, these lines are referred to as *diagonal forward* or *diagonal back*.

  - When used in the top section of a haircut design, a diagonal line produces increased length at one end and slopes down to a shorter length at the opposite end.

  - *Diagonal finger placement* may also be used to create a stacked, layered effect at the perimeter or to blend longer layers to shorter layers within a haircut.

- **Curved lines** (KURVD LYNZ) move in a semicircular or circular direction and can be shallow or deep. Curved lines soften a design and can be placed horizontally, vertically, or diagonally; when repeated in opposite directions, they create a wave pattern. The rounded portion of a concave line curves inward and the rounded portion of a convex line curves outward.

  - Concave and convex lines are often used at the perimeter of a hair design in the nape or back area and around the face.

  - Cutting the nape or back area into a rounded shape with the curve at the bottom of the design produces a convex line.

  - Cutting the nape area into a rounded shape with the curve at the top of the design and the ends of the curve ending at the corners of the nape produces a concave line (refer to **Figure 14-32**).

Form

Form (FORM) is the outline or shape of a hairstyle. The elements of width, length, and depth create a three-dimensional shape that can vary in terms of volume, proportion, and balance. Hairstyles should be proportionate to the client's overall body shape and size and balance with the features of his head, face, and neck.

- **Proportion** (pruh-POR-shun) measures or shows the comparative relationship between two or more design elements of a form. These elements influence the visual proportion of one section of the head form to another or between the head form and the facial features and/or the body. For example, if a client has a long neck and you shorten the natural hairline in the nape too high on the back of the head, the haircut will look out of proportion or *disproportionate* to the client's neck length and appear unbalanced.

- **Balance** (BAL-uns) is the equal or appropriate proportions that create symmetry and harmony in a design. Balance can be symmetrical or asymmetrical depending on the cutting lines and the ratio of length to width in the overall shape of the style. Hair density is an important design element when discussing balance because differences in the thickness of the hair can make one side appear heavier than the other and create an unbalanced or unfinished look.

Space

As it relates to art and design elements, space is considered either positive or negative. In hair design, the form (haircut or style) occupies *positive space* and the area that surrounds it is *negative space*. Barbers are usually more aware of the positive space (form) than the negative space; however, it is the negative space that brings the positive space into sharp focus. For example, when you face a client toward the mirror to check your work, his haircut (form) occupies positive space and the background you see in the mirror becomes negative space, allowing you to see areas of the form that need adjusting when checking for balance and proportion.

Design Texture

Design texture refers to the quality of a form's surface. Is the surface shiny or dull? Rough or smooth? Straight or wavy or curly? These conditions impact the degree to which light reflects off the surface of the hair and therefore affects the image or form we see. For example, wavy hair may appear to have light areas at the top (crest) of the wave and dark areas in the bottom (trough) of the wave, which may need special blending to appear more uniform in a close-cut hairstyle.

Color

Like texture, different colors reflect light differently. Dark colors tend to recede in a design and lighter colors appear to come to the foreground. These color differences create the illusions of more or less depth and volume in a form.

UNDERSTAND BASIC TERMINOLOGY USED IN HAIRCUTTING AND STYLING

Angles

An **angle** (ANG-gul) is the space between two lines or surfaces that intersect at a given point. Angles help to create strong, consistent foundations in haircutting and are used in two ways.

- *Angles* can refer to the degree of elevation at which the hair is held for cutting—a typical instruction, for example, would be "angle the hair section at a 45-degree projection from the head."

- *Angles* can also refer to the position of the fingers when cutting a section of hair (cutting line), as in "using a vertical parting, angle the fingers 45 degrees from the hairline to the occipital."

Directional Terms

Directional terms used in haircutting typically refer to how the tool is used relative to the direction of the way the hair grows.

- Cutting *against the grain* means to cut the hair in the opposite direction from which it grows.

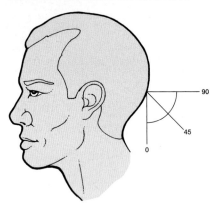

figure 14-38
Elevations relative to the head form.

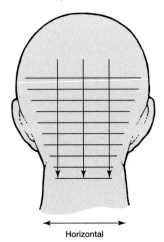

figure 14-39
Horizontal, zero elevation.

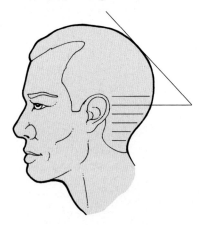

figure 14-40
Horizontal, 45-degree elevation.

- Cutting *with the grain* is cutting the hair in the same direction in which it grows.
- Cutting *across the grain* means the hair is cut in a direction that is neither with nor against the grain.
- Cutting with a circular motion may be required in whorl areas, where the hair does not grow in a uniform manner.

Cross-checking

Cross-checking (KRAWS-CHEK-ing) is the process of parting off subsections opposite from the elevation or direction at which they were cut to check the precision of cutting lines or blending. For example, a vertical subsection cut at a 90-degree projection can be cross-checked by parting off the subsections horizontally at 90 degrees.

Elevation and Projection

Elevation (el-uh-VAY-shun) is the angle or degree at which a section of hair is held from the head for cutting, *relative from where it grows*. Elevation, also known as **projection** (pruh-JEK-shun), is the result of lifting the hair section above 0 elevation, or natural fall. This projection of the hair while cutting produces graduation or layers and is usually described in terms of degrees (**Figure 14-38**).

- *0 elevation* is the lowest elevation and produces weight, bulk, and maximum length at the perimeter of a hair design.
    - 0 elevation is achieved by combing the hair straight down from where it grows and cutting it either against the skin (as in the nape or around-the-ear area) or as it is held straight down between the fingers to create the perimeter or design line (**Figure 14-39**).
    - The design line serves as a guide for all subsequent partings that will be brought to the perimeter for cutting.
    - 0-elevation cutting creates crisp, clean lines at the hairline on shorter hairstyles and achieves the standard *blunt cut* on longer hair.
- Holding the hair at *45 degrees* from where it grows is considered to be a *medium elevation*.
    - *Medium elevation*, or *graduation*, creates layered ends, or *stacking*, within the parting of hair from the 0-elevation distance to the 45-degree position. Movement and texture are created within the distance between the two degrees, depending on the length of the hair and the position of the angle in relation to the head form.
    - A horizontal parting and stationary guide at the perimeter is used to achieve the graduated or stacked effect (**Figure 14-40**).
    - Graduation can also be achieved by using a vertical parting projected at 45 degrees, with a diagonal finger placement of 45 degrees (**Figure 14-41**).
- A *90-degree elevation* is the most common projection used in men's haircutting and is considered to be a high elevation.

- A 90-degree elevation produces layering, tapering, and blended effects.

- When using a 90-degree elevation, the hair is held straight out from the head *from where it grows*.

- Either vertical and horizontal partings are used depending on the section of the head form being cut.

- A 90-degree elevation requires a traveling guide in order to move around and over the curves of the entire head.

- Lengths in various sections of the head form can vary, but the hair should still be blended overall.

A 90-degree elevation is used to create uniform layers in which each hair section is cut to the same length (**Figure 14-42a**) or to perform a taper that is shorter at the hairline and increasingly longer toward the top (**Figure 14-42b**).

- Compare **Figures 14-42a** and **14-42b**. In both cases the hair is positioned at 90 degrees using vertical partings in the back section. However, to create a tapered effect, the fingers, and therefore the cutting line, are positioned at a 45-degree angle to allow closer cutting to the head form in the nape area.

- If the haircut is started at the nape, the fingers will be positioned at a 45-degree angle from the hairline and will be gradually repositioned to a perpendicular position and then beyond a perpendicular as the hair is cut and blended over the curve of the head to the top section.

An elevation of *180 degrees* is often used to create layers when cutting long hair. A 90-degree stationary guide is used, usually in the top section, and the longer hair on the sides and back are elevated to the guide for cutting. It is important to remember that the hair being cut is at a 180-degree elevation, not the stationary guide. Refer to Chapter 16: Women's Haircutting and Styling.

A **part** (PART) is a line, created naturally or with a comb, that divides the hair at the scalp, separating one section of the hair from another. The position and direction of a *natural part* is determined by the direction or slant the hair takes as it leaves the follicle.

A client's natural part can easily be determined by combing clean, damp hair back toward the crown and then gently pushing the section forward: where the hair splits and falls to either side reveals the natural part. A *hard part* is created during the finishing steps of a haircut by shaving the scalp area of a natural or styled part line in the hair.

A **parting** (PART-ing), or subsection, is a smaller section of hair that is parted off from a larger section of hair.

- The use of partings is essential to maintain control of the hair in manageable proportions and to perform precision cutting.

- The direction of the parting line at the scalp should be consistent with the intended cutting line.

- Partings may be horizontal, vertical, or diagonal.

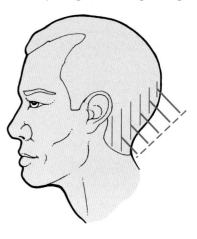

figure 14-41
Vertical parting with 45-degree angle.

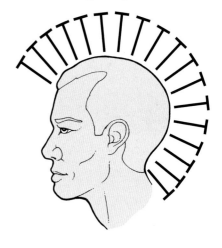

figure 14-42a
Uniform 90-degree layers.

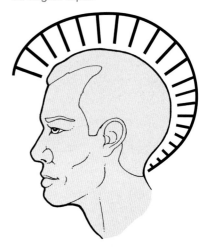

figure 14-42b
90-degree taper.

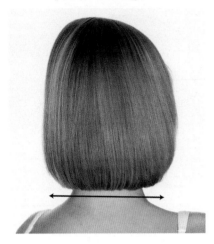

figure 14-43
Horizontal blunt cut design line.

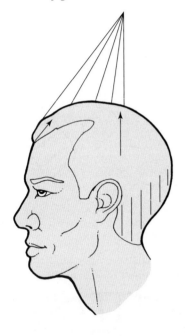

figure 14-44
Stationary guide.

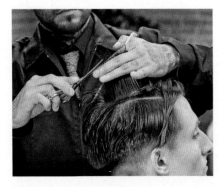

figure 14-45
Following the traveling guide.

- Partings are held horizontally, vertically, or diagonally, with a usual elevation range of 0 to 180 degrees.
- The way a parting is sectioned off from a larger section and projected for cutting determines the end result.
- Layering within a haircut is usually achieved using ¼-inch to ½-inch partings.

The **cutting line** (KUT-ing LYN) is established by the angle of the fingers or comb when securing a section of hair for cutting. Cutting lines are horizontal, vertical, or diagonal based on the position of the fingers or tool.

- The cutting tool used will follow the position and angle of the fingers or comb when cutting.
- Finger or comb placement should be checked before cutting to avoid
  - cutting in an unwanted line design (such as diagonal rather than horizontal);
  - losing the guide;
  - cutting off too much hair.

The **design line** (dee-ZYN LYN) is the outer perimeter line of the haircut. It may act as a guide depending on the overall design of the haircut and the method the barber uses to achieve it. A design line can be seen in the hanging length of a blunt cut or along the hairline of a short cut, wherever the perimeter of the haircut is located (**Figure 14-43**).

A **guide** (GUYD), also known as a *guideline* or *guide strand*, is a cut that is made by which subsequent partings or sections of hair will be measured and cut.

- Guides are classified as being either stationary or traveling.
- Both types of guides may originate at the outer perimeter (design line) of the hair or at an interior section such as the crown area.
- Most haircuts are achieved by using a combination of the two types of guides.
- A **stationary guide** (STAY-shun-ar-ee GUYD) is used for
  - achieving overall one-length-looking designs at the perimeter (blunt cut);
  - maintaining the length of a section while subsequent partings are brought from other sections to meet it for cutting; this produces either an overall longlayered effect or extra length within a section (**Figure 14-44**).
- A **traveling guide** (TRAV-ell-ing GUYD) moves along a section of hair as each cut is made **Figure 14-45**. Once the length of the initial guide has been cut, a parting is taken from in front of it or near it, combed with the original guide, and cut. Then a new parting is taken, combed with the second parting of hair, and cut against that guide. It is this use of the previous guide to cut a subsequent parting of hair that makes it a traveling guide.
  - Care must be taken not to recut the original or subsequent guides as you move along the section to cut a new parting.
  - When performed correctly, a traveling guide ensures even layering and blending of the hair from one section to another.

Layers (LAY-uhrz) are produced by elevating the hair beyond zero elevation for cutting.

- Layers can originate from the front, top (apex), crown, or perimeter (usually the design line).

- Layering can be angled (shorter on top and longer at the perimeter), uniform (even throughout), or fully tapered (longer on top and shorter at the perimeter).

- Layering is used to blend, to create fullness, or to create movement or texture in the hair.

A **taper** (TAYP-uhr), or *tapering*, means that the hair conforms to the shape of the head.

- The hair is shorter at the nape and hairline and longer in the crown and top areas.

- Most men's haircuts require some form of tapering.

- Blending of all of the hair lengths is extremely important.

A **weight line** (WAYT LYN) refers to the heaviest perimeter area of a 0-elevation or 45-degree cut.

- A weight line is achieved by using a stationary guide at the perimeter and may be cut in at a variety of levels on the head, depending on the style.

- Weight lines can be used in combination with a tapered nape area.

- The perimeter is the weight line in longer hairstyles that *look* to be one length.

Texturizing (TEKS-chur-yz-ing) is usually performed after the overall cut has been completed to create special effects such as wispy or spiky strands within the haircut or along the perimeter.

Tension (TEN-shun) is the amount of pressure applied while combing and holding a section of hair for cutting.

- Tension ranges from minimum to maximum, as a result of the amount of stretching employed when holding the hair between the fingers.

- The spacing between the teeth of the comb also influences the amount of tension you will be able to achieve when combing the hair. This is because the spacing between the teeth allows for more or less movement in the hair; for example, a fine-toothed comb facilitates more tension than a wide-toothed comb because the hair has less room to move or shift while the combing takes place.

- Use maximum tension on straight hair to create precise lines.

- Use minimal to moderate tension on curly and wavy hair as the hair may dry shorter than intended if maximum tension is used.

Thinning (THIN-ing) refers to removing excess bulk from the hair.

Outlining (OWT-lyn-ing) means marking the outer perimeter of the haircut in front of and around the ears and at the sides and nape of the neck; outlining at the front hairline is optional, depending on hair texture.

Overdirection (OH-ver-dih-REK-shun) creates a length increase in the design and occurs when the hair is combed away from its natural fall position rather than straight out from the head toward a guide.

Hairstyling (HAYR-sti-hyl-ing) is the art of arranging the hair in a particular style that is appropriately suited to the cut. Hairstyling may involve the use of styling aids such as hair spray, gel, tonic, oil sheen, pomade, or mousse; appliances in the form of blowdryers or irons; and implements such as brushes, combs, and clips.

A Word about Terminology

During the course of your barbering career, you will be introduced to a variety of haircutting terms. Terminology for the most part depends on who is presenting the information or technique and whether or not new terms have replaced formerly used terms. For example, *parting* and *subsection* are terms that are often used interchangeably.

Here are some important things to remember about terminology used in haircutting and styling:

- There are only so many angles and elevations that can be used in haircutting.

- Specific effects are created by using specific angles and elevations.

- History has a way of repeating itself in our industry and style trends tend to be cyclical in nature. For example, crew cuts and box fades can be traced back to the years of World War II, finger waves were a hit in the 1920s and 1930s, and braiding has probably been around since humans first walked the earth.

- Design variations occur when a new spin or twist is incorporated into a basic cut or style.

These examples simply reinforce why it is important that you become proficient in the basic skills, which will enable you to adapt to whatever the current terminology or trend might be.

Describe Haircutting Techniques

After reading this section, you will be able to:

 Explain basic cutting techniques using shears, clippers, and razors.

In Chapter 5, you were introduced to the correct holding positions for the comb, shears, clippers, and razor. The terms used to describe how we use these basic tools are *fingers-and-shear*, *shear-over-comb*, *freehand shear cutting*, *freehand clipper cutting*, *clipper-over-comb*, *razor-over-comb*, and *razor rotation*. It is important to note that most haircutting procedures require a combination of techniques and tools. The most important factors that determine the tools used to achieve the haircut are the client's desired outcome, the texture and density of the hair, and the barber's personal preference. As a professional barber you should be comfortable and skillful using all the tools of the trade.

IDENTIFY SHEAR CUTTING TECHNIQUES

The primary shear cutting techniques used in barbering are fingers-and-shear, shear-over-comb, shear-point tapering, and freehand shear cutting. Other shear techniques are used for texturizing or removing bulk in the hair (see Hair Thinning and Texturizing later in this chapter).

Fingers-and-Shear Cutting

The **fingers-and-shear** (FING-erz-AND-SHEER) technique may be used on many hair types, from straight to curly. The three basic methods for using fingers-and-shear techniques are cutting on top of the fingers, cutting below the fingers, and cutting palm-to-palm. Refer to Procedure 14-1 for fingers-and-shear cutting techniques.

Ⓟ 14-1 Fingers-and-Shear Cutting Techniques *pages 422–423*

- **Cutting above the fingers** (KUT-ing AH-bov THE FING-erz) is frequently used in men's haircutting to cut and blend layers in the top, crown, and horseshoe areas (see **Figure 14-46**). It is also used when cutting hair that is held out at a 90-degree elevation from a vertical parting, such as at the sides and back of the head form. Whether your finger position is perpendicular to the floor or angled at 45 degrees in these sections, the cutting should be performed on the outside (above) the fingers.

- **Cutting below the fingers** (KUT-ing BE-low THE FING-erz) is most often used to create design lines at the perimeter of the haircut (see **Figure 14-47**).

- **Cutting palm-to-palm** may be preferred by some practitioners. Care must be taken not to bend the hair or to project it higher than intended from the head form when using this technique. Also remember that the shears follow finger placement, so avoid curling the fingers inward when cutting unless you want a curved cutting line (**Figure 14-48**).

Shear-over-Comb Cutting

The **shear-over-comb** (SHEER-OH-ver-KOHM) technique is used to cut the ends of the hair and is an important method used in tapering. The comb is used to put the hair in a position to be cut and acts similarly to holding a section of hair between the fingers.

Most shear-over-comb cutting is performed in the nape, behind the ears, around the ears, and in the sideburn areas of a cut; however, an entire haircut can also be accomplished using this method.

Following are a few important guidelines for performing the shear-over-comb technique:

- Use vertical working panels when cutting back and side sections. Make sure panels overlap for better blending and to avoid missing sections of hair that need to be cut.

- After your first cut, make sure you can see the guide so you know where to cut to or cut from next.

- Use a diagonal comb placement when cutting areas behind and around the ears.

> ⚠ **CAUTION**
> The blades of the shears should rest flat and flush to the fingers for these positions. Angling the shear blades may cause injury to your fingers.

figure 14-46
Cutting above the fingers.

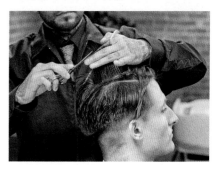

figure 14-47
Cutting below the fingers.

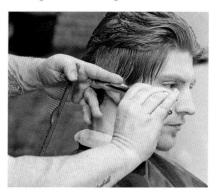

figure 14-48
Cutting palm-to-palm.

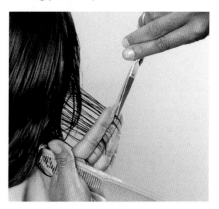

> ⚠ **CAUTION**
> Make sure you palm the shears when you use the comb and palm the comb when you cut with the shears.

figure 14-49
Hold the comb and shears
properly.

figure 14-50
Open and close the shears in tandem
with an upward movement of the comb.

figure 14-51
Roll the comb using a key-turning
motion.

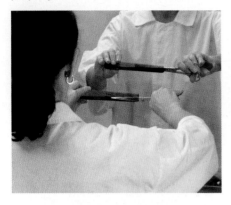

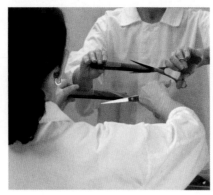

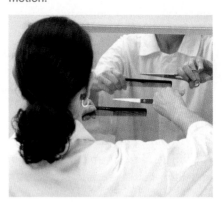

figure 14-52
Position the hair to be cut by rolling
the comb out.

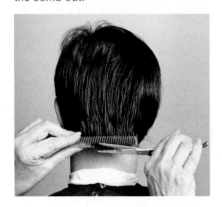

figure 14-53
Cut to center guide.

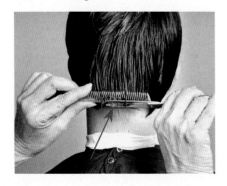

Take some time and practice the following exercises to help you master shear-over-comb cutting. You can practice in front of a mirror or facing a partner.

- Position the comb and shears parallel to each other. Practice aligning the still blade of the shears with the comb at the level where the teeth join the back of the comb (**Figure 14-49**).

- Move the comb upward, opening and closing the shears simultaneously with the movement of the comb (**Figure 14-50**).

- After several cutting movements, use a key-turning motion to roll the teeth of the comb away from you, as if you were combing through hair (**Figure 14-51**).

Once you have become comfortable with the exercises you can begin practicing on your mannequin.

- Start at the hairline in the center of the nape area.

- With the teeth of the comb pointing upward, comb into a section of hair at the hairline, rolling the comb out toward you. The hair should protrude from the teeth of the comb and be in a position for cutting. This is called **rolling the comb out** (ROHL-ing THE KOHM OUT) (**Figure 14-52**).

- Simultaneously move the shears and the comb through the center panel, cutting the hair in the process. Stop at the occipital area and comb the hair down toward the hairline.

- Begin the next panel by including some hair from the center section with the hair to the right or left of center. There should now be two lengths of hair in the comb: shorter hair from the center section and longer hair from the second section. The shorter hair from the center section becomes the guide for the second panel (**Figure 14-53**).

- Finish one vertical strip at a time before proceeding with the next section.

- The shear-over-comb technique is also used in **shear-point tapering** (SHEER-POYNT TAYP-uhr-ing) to thin out or customize difficult areas caused by hollows, wrinkles, whorls, or creases in the scalp. Dark and ragged hair patches can be minimized using the shear-point tapering technique, which uses the points of the shears to cut a few strands of hair at a time until the spot becomes less noticeable and blends in with the surrounding hair or hairline (**Figure 14-54**).

figure 14-54
Shear-point taper in the nape area.

figure 14-55
A comb can still be used to control hair for freehand cutting.

figure 14-56
Fine-tuning with freehand cutting.

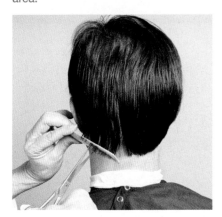

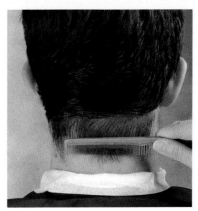

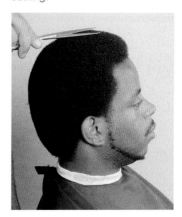

Freehand Shear Cutting

Freehand shear cutting (FREE-HAND SHEER KUT-ing) is a technique that may or may not utilize your fingers or a comb to control the hair while cutting against the skin. This will depend on your personal preference and the type of freehand cutting being performed. For example, combing a section of hair down and cutting against the skin is a form of freehand shear cutting (**Figure 14-55**); however, you may prefer to use the comb to control the hair section against the client's skin. A second method of freehand shear cutting is to consistently open and close the shears as you skim over the surface of the hair to cut any stray hairs protruding from the design. This technique can be used in the final stages of a haircut, beard trim, or other procedure to fine-tune your work and is especially effective for shaping or trimming tight curl textures (**Figure 14-56**).

IDENTIFY CLIPPER CUTTING TECHNIQUES

Clippers are versatile tools that can be used in several ways to cut a variety of hair textures and styles. The standard techniques are **freehand clipper cutting** (FREE-HAND KLIP-ur KUT-ing) and **clipper-over-comb** (KLIP-uhr-OH-ver-KOHM) cutting; however, you can also use clippers as you would shears to cut hair that is held between your fingers. This cutting method creates more texture in the hair ends than the blunt ends that shears produce. As a general rule, clipper cutting is followed up with shear-and-comb work to fine-tune the haircut and/or to perform arching or outline work.

Cutting and tapering the hair with clippers can be accomplished by cutting with the grain, against the grain, or across the grain. Compare the directions of hair growth and tool usage in **Table 14-1**.

Freehand Clipper Cutting

Freehand clipper cutting requires a steady hand and consistent use of the comb or hair pick while cutting. The use of the comb or pick is important because both implements are used to put the hair into a position to be cut and help to remove the excess hair cut from the previous section. This will provide you with a clearer view of the cutting results and any areas that may need reblending or cutting.

True freehand clipper cutting techniques tend to be used on two extremes of hair length.

table 14-1

DIRECTIONS OF HAIR GROWTH AND TOOL USAGE

Term	Action	Illustration
Cutting *with* the grain	Cut in the same direction of hair growth	
Cutting *against* the grain	Cut in the opposite direction of hair growth	
Cutting *across* the grain	Cut neither with nor against hair growth in transition areas	

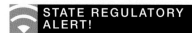

STATE REGULATORY ALERT!

Freehand clipper cutting, clipper-over-comb, and fingers-and-shear work are techniques that are frequently combined to perform a single haircut.

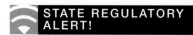

STATE REGULATORY ALERT!

The use of guards is not considered to be a form of freehand clipper cutting; nor is this technique usually acceptable for state board practical examinations.

- They are used for very short, straight, wavy, and curly lengths in which little clipper-over-comb work is performed.

  - For short hairstyles, detachable blade sizes generally range from size 0000 (close to shaving) to size 3½, which leaves the hair approximately ⅜ inch long. Some manufacturers now have 00000 blade sizes as well.

- Freehand clipper cutting techniques are used for longer, tightly curled hair lengths that require more sculpting.

  - Used for cutting tightly curled hair when a natural look is desired. The hair is picked out and put into position for cutting.

  - A keen eye for balance, shape, and proportion is important when sculpting the hair into shape.

figure 14-57
Lightly guide the clipper upward from the hairline into the hair about an inch above the hairline.

figure 14-58
Guide the blades through the ends of the hair.

figure 14-59
Remove the hair at lower nape area.

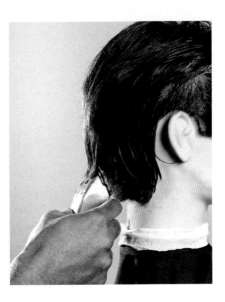

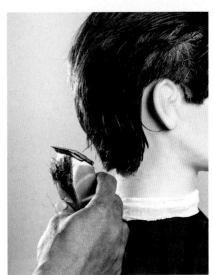

The freehand method is also used to taper hairlines at the nape, back, and sides. Refer to the following guidelines when practicing freehand clipper cutting. Remember to practice on a mannequin first.

- Start in the center nape area with the blades open.
- Gradually tilt the blade away from the head so the clipper rides on the heel of the bottom blade.
- Glide the clipper upward into the hair to about an inch above the hairline (**Figure 14-57**).
- Roll the clipper out as the blades cut through the ends of the hair (**Figure 14-58**).
- Note the removal of hair in the lower nape area (**Figure 14-59**).

Clipper-over-Comb Cutting

Clipper-over-comb cutting can be used for the entire haircut or to blend the hair from shorter tapered areas to longer areas at the top, crest, or occipital. Much like the shear-over-comb technique, the comb places the hair in a position to be cut and utilizes the same blending principles.

Refer to the following guidelines when practicing clipper-over-comb cutting; always remember to practice on a mannequin first.

- Begin in the back section and comb the hair down.
- Roll the comb out to put the hair in a position to be cut (**Figure 14-60**).
- Cut across the hair ends protruding from the comb with the clipper.

Arching with a Clipper or Trimmer

Many barbers prefer to use an outliner or trimmer with a fine cutting edge to finish sideburns and the outline around the ears and down the sides of the neck. This method of arching is efficient and precise due to the maneuverability of the smaller cutting head of the tool. If the desired result can

> **? DID YOU KNOW?**
> Detachable blades should not be confused with clipper attachment combs, most commonly known as *guards*. Guards are placed on top of a clipper blade, allowing for more hair length to remain while cutting.

figure 14-60
Roll the comb out to position hair for the clipper.

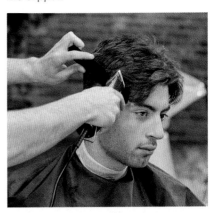

> **⏱ REMINDER**
> When using the clipper-over-comb technique to taper, be sure to tilt the comb away from the head to create a blended taper from shorter to longer sections.

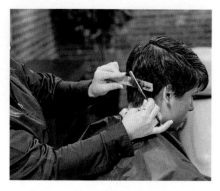

figure 14-61
Cutting using the razor-over-comb technique.

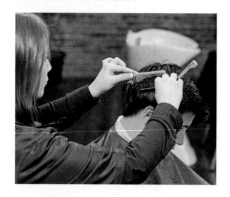

figure 14-62
Razor rotation involves a two-part continuous movement.

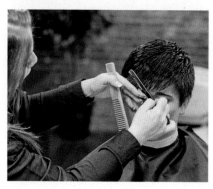

figure 14-63
Cutting using the fingers-and-razor technique.

> ⚠ **CAUTION**
> The use of a razor with a safety guard is recommended for the beginner.

be accomplished with a standard clipper, that method is equally acceptable. Refer to Procedures 14-2 and 14-3 for guidelines on arching techniques and the outline shave.

ⓟ 14-2   **Arching Techniques** *pages 424–427*

ⓟ 14-3   **Outline Shave** *pages 428–430*

RAZOR CUTTING

Razor cutting is another method used by barbers to cut or texturize the hair. The angle of the razor relative to the surface of the hair tapers the hair ends rather than the blunt ends produced by shear cutting. This advantage makes razor cutting an effective option for blending, softening, shortening, or releasing weight from the hair strands during a cut.

The basic razor cutting techniques are razor-rotation, razor-over-comb, and fingers-and-razor cutting. The hair sections being cut need to be kept uniformly damp to ensure that the blade cuts through the hair smoothly without pulling or snagging; dry cutting is uncomfortable for the client and can frizz the hair surface.

Razor Cutting Techniques

Razor-over-comb (RAY-zur-OH-ver-KOHM) cutting can be performed in two different ways using a freehand razor position. The first method is similar to shear- or clipper-over-comb cutting, where "rolling the comb out" projects the hair ends into position for cutting and vertical or diagonal razor strokes are used across the comb to remove length. The second method involves positioning the razor horizontally on top of the comb to cut the hair that extends through the teeth of the comb with short, precise strokes and medium pressure (**Figure 14-61**). This second method is often used to blend and taper sections or to soften weight lines.

Razor rotation (RAY-zur row-TAY-shun) is performed by using a rotating motion with the comb and razor as the hair is being cut. In the first movement, the razor follows the comb through the hair. In the second movement, the comb follows the razor and so on to taper, blend, thin, or remove weight (**Figure 14-62**). This method requires coordinated razor stroking and combing actions to maintain continuous movements through the hair.

Fingers-and-razor cutting (FING-erz-AND-RAY-zur KUT-ing) is performed by holding the hair section between your fingers and cutting either from the top to the bottom of the section or from one side to the other. This method can be used on vertically or horizontally parted sections to remove length, taper ends, or reduce weight in mid-shaft sections. Also known as **freehand slicing** (FREE-HAND sly-SING) with razor, this technique can be used to create more movement within a style or to soften perimeters (**Figure 14-63**).

Razor Strokes

Some barbers consider razor cutting to be the best method for tapering and blending the hair because the razor edge permits a smoother blend than what can be achieved with shears or clippers. When razor cutting a section, the cutting technique and angle of the razor strokes you use will determine how much hair is removed from the hair strands. It is important that you learn how to coordinate your razor and comb. A general rule is to taper a little at a time to avoid removing too much hair. Consider the following taper-blending methods used to achieve different effects.

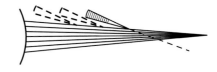

figure 14-64
Light taper-blending.

- In *light taper-blending* the razor is held almost flat against the surface of the hair. Note the small amount of hair that is cut when the blade is only slightly tilted and very little pressure is used (**Figure 14-64**).

- *Heavier taper-blending* is performed with the razor held up to 45 degrees from the surface of the hair strand. As the razor is tilted higher and a little more pressure is used, the depth of the cut increases (**Figure 14-65**).

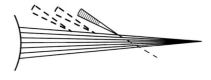

figure 14-65
Heavier taper-blending.

- In *terminal blending* the angle of the razor blade is increased to almost 90 degrees; this produces the least amount of tapering to the hair ends (**Figure 14-66**).

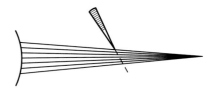

figure 14-66
Terminal blending.

Hair Textures and Razor Cutting

Some general guidelines to keep in mind when razor cutting different hair textures are as follows:

- Coarse, thick hair requires more strokes and heavier tapering than other textures to remove bulk.

- Medium-textured hair requires fewer razor strokes and lighter pressure than coarse, thick hair to blend or remove bulk; avoid overthinning the hair.

- Fine hair does not usually have any bulk to remove, although you might want to use the razor to create texture at the perimeter. Use a light stroke of the razor with very little pressure.

Razor Cutting Tips

- The hair must be clean and damp for best results and to avoid client discomfort. Maintain moisture content throughout the cut.

- Avoid tapering too close to the hair part or the scalp. Tapering the hair too closely to the hair part will cause the hair to stand up, making the part look ragged. Coarse hair that is cut too closely to the scalp will have short, stubby hair ends that can protrude through the top layer.

- Avoid over-tapering as it is difficult to correct a haircut after too much hair has been removed.

Razor Cutting Safety Precautions

- Handle the razor properly, keeping it closed whenever not in use.

- Be aware of the people around you when working with any sharp tool or implement.

  - A careless motion can cause injury to yourself or others.

  - Do not distract or startle anyone who is performing a service.

- Purchase and use only good-quality haircutting implements.
- Use changeable-blade razors and dispose of used blades in a sharps container.
- Replace dull razor blades during the cut if necessary.
  - A dull blade will pull the hair and cause pain or discomfort to the client.
  - Dull blades will also decrease the quality of the haircut.

Hair Thinning and Texturizing

Hair thinning is used to reduce the bulk or weight of the hair. You can use thinning (serrated) shears, regular shears, clippers, or a razor for this purpose. Regardless of the tool used, some general rules to follow when removing bulk from the hair are as follows:

- Make a careful observation of the hair to determine the sections that require some reduction in bulk or weight and cut accordingly.
- Avoid cutting top surfaces of the hair where visible cutting lines can be seen.
- Part off and elevate the hair to be cut to avoid cutting too deeply into the section.
- Avoid cutting too closely to the scalp or part lines.

Removing Bulk

Review the following methods that can be used to reduce bulky or thick areas within a hair design.

- **Thinning.** When thinning with serrated shears, the hair parting is combed and held between the index and middle finger.
  - Place the serrated shears about mid-shaft on the strands and make a cut (**Figure 14-67**).
  - Make subsequent cuts at about 1 inch from the first cut.
  - Do not cut twice in the same place.
- **Slicing and carving.** There are two slicing methods that can be used to remove bulk with regular shears.
  - **Figure 14-68** shows the slicing technique performed on the surface of the hair.
  - **Figure 14-69** shows the carving technique performed by elevating the hair at 45 to 90 degrees and gliding the open shears through the hair with a curving motion. This removes hair from the under-portion of the parting as the motion is continued to the hair ends.
- **Slithering.** In this procedure a thin parting of hair is held between the fingers. The shears are positioned for cutting and an up-and-down sliding motion along the hair section is combined with a slight closing of the shears each time they are moved toward the scalp (**Figure 14-70**).

Removing Weight from the Ends

Removing weight from the ends helps to taper or lighten the perimeter of graduated and blunt haircuts. This can be accomplished using thinning (serrated) shears by elevating the section and placing the shears at an angle

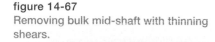

figure 14-67
Removing bulk mid-shaft with thinning shears.

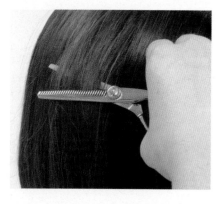

figure 14-68
Slicing on hair surface to remove bulk.

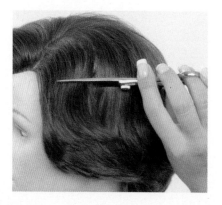

figure 14-69
Carving with shears to remove bulk.

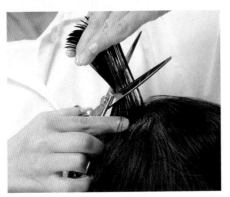

figure 14-70
Slithering.

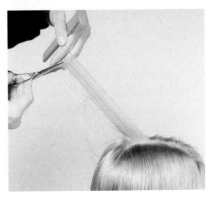

figure 14-71
Removing weight from the ends.

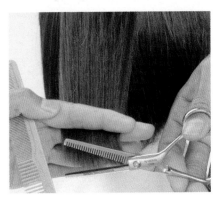

figure 14-72
Notching.

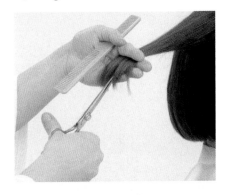

as the cuts are made or by using the comb to put the hair into position for cutting (**Figure 14-71**).

Point cutting or *notching* with regular shears can be used to reduce weight in the ends of the hair. For either of these techniques, the parting is held between the fingers, and the tips of the shears are used at vertical or diagonal angles to create points or notches in the hair (**Figure 14-72**). Typically, notching is a more aggressive type of point cutting that produces a chunkier effect at the hair ends.

Clippers and razors can also be used to remove weight from the ends of the hair as follows:

- Use the clipper-over-comb technique to put the hair ends in a position to be cut.

- Position the clipper blades under the ends of the hair.

- Use a *reverse* rotation technique with the clipper to comb through and cut the ends from one section to another.

- Razor-over-comb or freehand slicing techniques can be used to lighten hair ends with a razor.

Recognize Basic Haircut Styles

After reading this section, you will be able to:

LO**8**   Describe basic haircut styles.

As a barber, most of the haircuts you perform will result in some variation or combination of the basic haircuts discussed in this section; knowing how to perform these cuts provides the foundation from which to create customized hair designs for your clients. That said, it will be helpful to keep the following considerations in mind when discussing different haircut names and styles:

- Style names may refer to a particular haircut or a variation of a haircut, for example, taper cut or businessman's cut.

⏱ REMINDER
The haircut style will determine the point on the head at which the tapered area is blended into longer hair. Short styles, such as crew cuts and fades, have a high taper that is blended into the transition area of the crest; longer styles may be blended at or just below the occipital. There are as many variations as there are heads of hair to cut.

- Haircut style names may differ, or may be interpreted differently, from region to region. For example, a temple fade in the Midwest may be called a Philly fade on the East Coast and the quo vadis has been known to be called a Caesar cut in some parts of the country, when in fact, the traditional Caesar is a longer style.

- As with other expressions of fashion, haircut styles tend to be cyclical. This means that a basic style, often modified in some way, is reintroduced to the market and becomes popular again as a new trend. For example, the classic pompadour of the 1950s has returned in both its classic form and with variations or modifications that have produced a variety of pompadour fade styles.

Your familiarity with basic haircut style names will provide you with a frame of reference for discussing haircut options with your clients and the ability to perform the many variations you will encounter in the barbershop. Some classic haircut style names are the flat top, crew cut, high and tight, fade, taper, pompadour, Caesar, and quo vadis. Following is a discussion of these classic cuts and their variations.

- *Flat tops* are very short on the sides and back area, with slightly longer hair at the upper parietal and front sections and a flat top section. The top of the crest area should look squared off when viewed from the front (**Figure 14-73**). A high top fade is a variation of the flat top combined with elements of a fade. Flat tops require a steady hand and consistent horizontal comb placement when cutting through the top section to ensure a balanced, level cut. Following are a few tips for flat tops:

  - The squared off crest and top sections create the "flat" look.

  - Variations of the style and length of the top section will be determined by the client's preference, head shape, hair texture, and hair density.

  - A steady hand is needed when cutting the top section.

  - Clippers and shears are used to perform the cut.

- *Crew cuts* have short, semi-short, or medium-tapered side and back lengths with a top section that gradually increases in length from the crown to the front hairline (**Figure 14-74**). When viewed from the front, crew cuts are more rounded than flat tops in the crest area and should blend into the top section with a slight curvature that conforms to the contours of the head. Following are some basic guidelines for crew cuts:

  - The back and sides are cut relatively high to the bottom of the crest area.

  - Back and sides are tapered and blended to the crest and top sections.

  - A wide-toothed comb is used in the top section to provide a level guide.

  - The shears and comb are used to smooth out any uneven spots left by clipper work.

- *Brush* or *butch cuts* are variations of the crew cut. The sides and back are cut to a short crew-cut length, but the hair on top is uniformly cut at ¼ inch to ½ inch and follows the contours of the head. A brush cut is styled with the hair combed back over the top section to stand straight up while the butch cut may be styled forward or to the side.

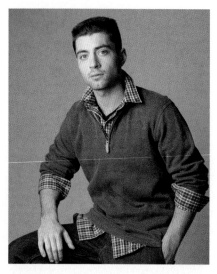

figure 14-73
Flat top.

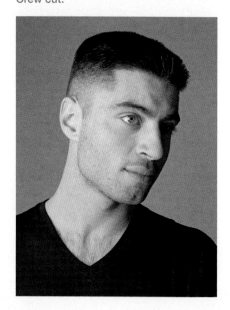

figure 14-74
Crew cut.

- *High and tight cuts* are cut extremely close or shaved on the sides and back to a level at the bottom, mid-point, or top of the parietal ridge, where visible hair should be seen blending with a short top section of no more than ¼ inch in length. Depending on the client's preferences, the line of demarcation at the top of the parietal ridge can either be left as is or be blended into the top section.

- The *fade style* derives its name from the fact that the hair is longest in the top section and gradually fades down to nothing at the hairline. Like the *high and tight cut*, the back and sides are cut extremely close, or shaved, with the hair becoming gradually longer at the parietal ridge and longest at the top (Figure 14-75). Like other basic styles discussed, there are many variations of fades that can be performed on a variety of hair textures. Following are some general guidelines for fade styles:

  - Cut the top section to the desired length.

  - Cut the nape up to the occipital to the desired length (bald, shadow, etc.).

  - The parietal ridge is the transition area between the sides and top sections; most of the blending and close tapering occurs in this area.

  - Be guided by the natural hair growth pattern to avoid creating gaps and patches.

- A *taper cut* is a well-blended, graduated cut that conforms to the head shape. A proper taper cut gradually increases in length from the hairline to the top section without any gaps or steps (Figure 14-76). Typically, the top section is left long enough to provide different styling options for parted and off-the-face styles. The basic taper cut may also be called a regular taper or standard haircut with variations that include the businessman's cut, Ivy League, Princeton, and precision cut. Taper cuts can vary in length and volume from short and close to long and full, but all tapers should conform to the natural head shape. When performing a taper cut, you will need to ask your client if he wants a natural taper at the nape or if he wants it blocked. Refer to Procedures 14-4 through 14-8 for guidelines on how to complete the precision cut, basic taper cut, razor cut, flat top and crew cut, and temple fade. Following are some general guidelines for taper cuts:

  - Use the fingers-and-shear technique in the top and crest sections.

  - Taper nape and side hairlines using freehand clipper or clipper-over-comb cutting.

  - Taper through the back and sides using clipper-over-comb or shear-over-comb techniques.

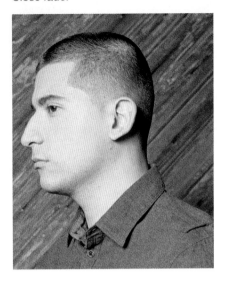

figure 14-75
Close fade.

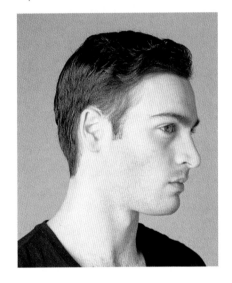

figure 14-76
Taper cut.

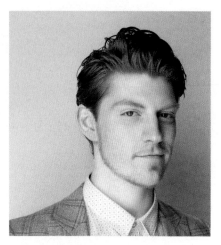

figure 14-77
Precision cut.

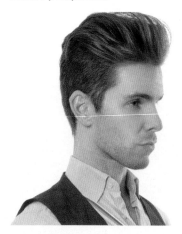

figure 14-78
Classic pompadour.

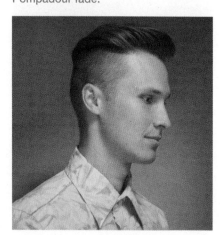

figure 14-79
Pompadour fade.

- A *precision cut* taper describes a variation in the cutting technique rather than a style description (**Figure 14-77**). The majority of the cut is performed using the fingers-and-shear cutting technique to taper and blend the hair from one section to another. A general rule to follow for using precision cutting on various hair textures is this: if the hair can be parted and picked up between the fingers to be put into a position for cutting, precision cutting can be performed. The hair should be clean and uniformly moist to enable you to maintain control of the hair while cutting and to produce the most precise cut.

- The *classic pompadour* is basically a medium to long taper cut with a long top section. Depending on the client's preferred length (short, medium, or long), the taper begins at the hairline and gradually increases in length through the back and sides to a long layered front and top section (**Figure 14-78**). Layering in the top section provides many styling options, from a slicked-back look to a full or spiky front section. Today's pompadour fade variation combines the very short nape, back, and side sections of a fade with the extra long top section of the classic cut. Compare **Figures 14-78** and **14-79** to see the blended lengths of the classic pomp and the demarcation between lengths of the pomp fade. Refer to Procedures 14-9 through 14-11 for guidelines on how to complete the pompadour fade, fade haircut with star design, and shadow fade cut. Following are some general guidelines for pompadour cuts:

  - Length increase in the top section can be achieved by using overdirection from the front to the crown or by using a diagonal cutting line that is shorter at the crown and increasingly longer toward the front.

  - When performing the classic pompadour, use vertical partings and steep, diagonal cutting lines to blend short sides to longer top lengths.

  - Be sure to have the client confirm what type of pompadour he desires: classic or pomp fade style.

Ⓟ 14-9 **Pompadour Fade** *pages 459–464*

Ⓟ 14-10 **Fade Haircut with Star Design** *pages 465–468*

Ⓟ 14-11 **Shadow Fade Cut** *pages 469–472*

- The *classic Caesar* style is cut with shears to create short, *uniform* layers from 1 to 2 inches throughout the head form (**Figure 14-80**). These short layers are often styled forward and down over the front hairline and may have a rounder appearance than other cuts. Today's versions of the Caesar may incorporate tapering or fading in the side and back areas with a uniform length in the top section that is styled forward. Following are some general guidelines for a Caesar:

  - Older clients may not be familiar with new variations of the Caesar cut, so you will have to explain the differences to them to confirm what type of Caesar they have in mind.

© iStock.com/jonathandowney.

© iStock.com/druvo.

figure 14-80
Caeser cut.

figure 14-81
Quo vadis.

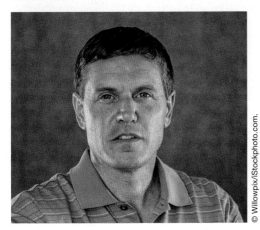

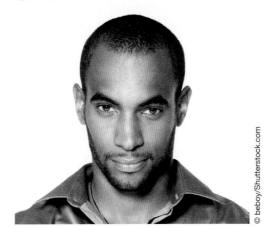

- The fingers-and-shear technique is used to cut the hair at 90-degree elevations to create uniform layers within the cut.

- The classic quo vadis is sometimes confused with the Caesar, so again, be sure your client confirms his expectations before you begin the cut.

- The *quo vadis* is another uniformly cut style; however, clippers are used to achieve its close, even-all-over length (**Figure 14-81**). This haircut style, which generally is suitable for most hair textures, conforms to the contours of the head and produces a more uniformly consistent appearance on medium to thick hair. Following are general guidelines for the quo vadis style:

- The even-all-over length will depend on the client's preferences.

- Select a blade size that will leave the hair at the desired length.

- Be guided by the natural hair growth pattern to avoid creating gaps and patches.

- Remember that cutting against the grain leaves the hair shorter than cutting with the grain.

Explain Haircut Finish Work

After reading this section, you will be able to:

LO**9**   Describe haircut finish work.

Once you have finished the haircut, you should include finishing work in your customer service routine. A neck or outline shave, an eyebrow trim, and the removal of stray hair from the ears or nostrils are standard procedures included in finishing work. Offering to perform these finishing touches after every haircut provides a professional barbershop experience for your clients and helps you build your client base and new referrals.

SHAVING THE OUTLINE AREAS

Performing a neck shave or outline shave as a feature of the haircut service contributes to the appearance of the finished cut and should follow outlining work performed with shears, clippers, or trimmers.

- The traditional *neck shave* consists of shaving the sides of the neck and across the nape with a razor.

- The *outline shave* starts at the bottom of the sideburns, arches around and behind the ears, down the sides of the neck, and across the nape. The front hairline is often included as part of the outline shave in many African American styles.

TRIMMING THE EYEBROWS

Eyebrow trimming may require a combination of techniques, depending on the length and density of brow hair.

- Shear-over-comb is the most popular technique for eyebrow trimming, but an outliner-over-comb technique can be used as well.

- Freehand shear cutting is sometimes required to cut individual stray hairs that extend beyond the natural arch of the brow and should be done carefully.

- Safety and protection of the client's eyes should always be the first consideration when using any eyebrow-trimming technique (Figure 14-82).

TRIMMING EXCESS NOSTRIL AND EAR HAIR

Outliners with T-shaped blades or nose hair trimmers are the safest tools to use for trimming excess hair from the nostrils.

- If you are using a T-bladed trimmer, simply grasp the tip of the nose between your thumb and index finger and gently tilt it up or to the side.

- Position the first few teeth of the blades on a slight diagonal to trim the hairs.

- Follow the manufacturer's directions when using nose hair trimmers, as there are several styles available on the market.

- Trimming excess hair in or around the ears is also performed with an outliner or trimmer; some barbers prefer a T-bladed tool because it is easier to maneuver in small tight areas.

- Always dust off residual hair in and around the ears after trimming.

DISCUSS HEAD SHAVING

The shaved head is one of today's fashion trends that many men choose regardless of the density or growth pattern of their hair (Figure 14-83). The hair and scalp are prepared with hot towels and lather followed by straight-razor shaving. Following are some guidelines for performing a head shave:

- Thoroughly analyze the scalp to identify moles and other hypertrophies.

- If you are precutting the hair, leave enough length for the razor to grab as the blade passes over the scalp.

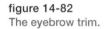

figure 14-82
The eyebrow trim.

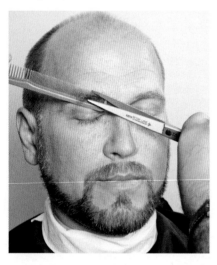

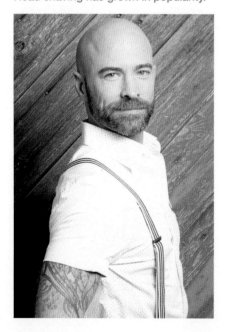

figure 14-83
Head shaving has grown in popularity.

- Keep the scalp moist and your stretching (nondominant) hand dry.
- Stretch the skin to create a smooth shaving surface.

Ⓟ 14-12 **The Head Shave** *pages 473–476*

Identify Styling Techniques

After reading this section, you will be able to:

LO ⑩ Describe basic styling techniques.

Hairstyling is the art of arranging the hair into an appropriate style following a haircut or shampoo service. Today, many haircuts require minimal hairstyling techniques due to the quality of the cuts, current styles, and the availability of effective styling aids such as gels, pomades, and styling sprays. Other haircuts require more styling attention, such as blowdrying or picking the style into place. In this section, the methods discussed for styling men's hair include natural drying, finger styling, scrunch styling, finger waving, blowdrying, and blow waving.

DESCRIBE BASIC STYLING TECHNIQUES

Many men prefer quick and easy styling routines. Review the following section to learn about some of these methods.

Natural Drying

As the name implies, *natural drying* is the term used when the hair is left to air-dry naturally. Typically, the hair is combed into place or arranged with the fingers and allowed to dry in place. Gels, pomades, or other styling products can be applied to hold the hair in place while it dries or can be applied after the hair is dry. Since it is not a good idea for both aesthetic and health reasons to let a client leave the shop with damp hair, use a heat lamp or blowdryer with diffuser to speed up the drying process.

Describe Finger Styling

When *finger styling* the hair, you will use your fingers to manipulate the hair into place instead of a comb or brush (**Figure 14-84**). Some clients prefer the more textured look that finger styling produces as opposed to the smoother looks achieved with combs or brushes. Using a blowdryer during the procedure is optional and will usually depend on the degree of dampness of the hair.

Scrunch Styling

Scrunch styling is actually a form of finger styling that is typically used on wavy to curly hair patterns with enough length to create a tousled look. A diffuser attachment on the blowdryer will allow only the heat to transfer while you lift and squeeze the hair between your fingers. Wavy and curly hair may require the application of a spray gel or a light

figure 14-84
Finger styling the hair.

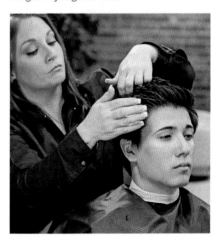

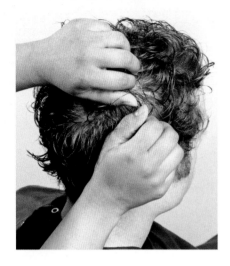

figure 14-85
Scrunch styling technique.

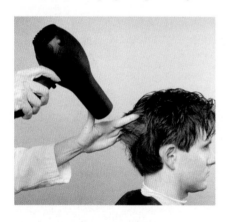

figure 14-86
Freeform blowdrying using the fingers.

FOCUS ON

Keep the air and the hair moving when blowdry styling to prevent burning the client's scalp.

pomade to reduce the frizzy hair ends that sometimes accompany these hair textures (**Figure 14-85**).

Finger Waving

Finger waving is a wet styling technique that involves the process of shaping and directing the hair into an S pattern using the fingers, comb, and styling lotion. Finger waving was popular for both men and women during the 1920s and 1930s and is still used today either to direct the hair into a flat, sleek, wave formation or to add volume and direction to a section of hair when dried (see Chapter 16: Women's Haircutting and Styling).

Practice Blowdry Styling

Blowdrying not only accelerates the hair drying process but also allows you to temporarily straighten or give direction to the hair to create a more finished look. **Blowdry styling** (BLOH-dry sti-hyl-ing) is the technique of drying and styling damp hair in one operation and has revolutionized the hair care industry. While some men may not wish to do more than comb their hair into place and let it dry, the use of a blowdryer offers some options for speed-drying and special-effects styling, such as blow waving. Refer to Procedure 14-13 for guidelines on blowdrying techniques.

Ⓟ 14-13   **Blowdrying Techniques** *pages 477–478*

The implements used with a blowdryer include combs, picks, and a variety of brushes. In most cases, the texture of the hair and the desired effect will dictate the type of implement to use. The blowdrying techniques discussed in this section are freeform, stylized or blow waving, and diffused.

Freeform Drying

Freeform blowdrying is a quick, easy method of drying the client's hair that is probably most like the techniques men use at home. This technique can build fullness into the style while allowing the hair to fall into the natural lines of the cut (**Figure 14-86**). Some barbers choose freeform blowdrying for the following reasons:

- It shows the client the ease with which the style can be duplicated.
- It demonstrates the quality of the haircut as the hair falls into place.
- The blowdrying service is accelerated.
- It allows the barber to check the accuracy of the work as the hair falls into place.

Stylized Drying

Stylized blowdrying creates a more finished appearance because each section is dried in a definite direction with the aid of a comb or brush followed by the dryer. Heat makes physical changes in the hair when using the blowdryer in this fashion and *sets* the hair in a particular direction for a look that is smoother and more precisely directed overall. Dry the hair underneath first to avoid missing damp sections and to speed up the drying process.

If you are using styling products, be sure to select one that allows manipulation of the hair, rather than one that sets the hair in place, while it is being dried and styled (Figures 14-87 to 14-89).

- When a comb or brush and the blowdryer are used to create wave patterns and direction in the hair, the technique is called *blow waving* or *air waving* (Figures 14-90 and 14-91).

Diffused Drying

Diffused drying is used when the client desires to maintain the natural wave pattern of the hair, as opposed to temporarily straightening it with the blowdryer and brush. A diffuser attachment on the blowdryer is an effective option when arranging or picking out very curly hair textures, manipulating sculpting with styling products, or when scrunching the hair (Figure 14-92).

figure 14-87
Styling the side section with blowdryer and brush.

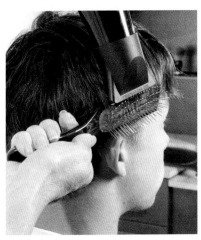

figure 14-88
Styling and drying the top section.

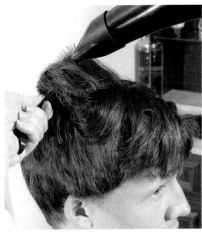

figure 14-89
Finish work over the surface of the hairstyle. Follow the brush with the dryer.

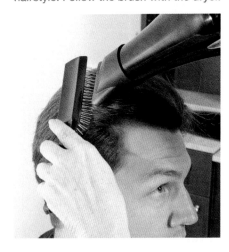

figure 14-90
Create a ridge or bend in the hair near the scalp with the comb.

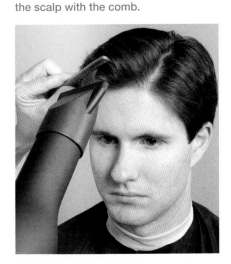

figure 14-91
Set the ridge with heat from the blowdryer.

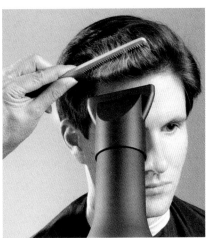

figure 14-92
Diffuser.

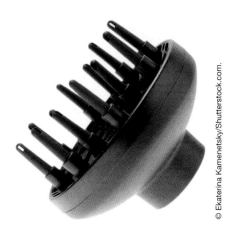

Building Volume

Occasionally, extra volume is needed in the crown, crest, or top areas of a style to create a more proportionate look. To build volume or to create an even contour throughout the hairstyle, use the blowdryer and brush in the following manner:

1. Lift the hair with the brush, bending the section as the blowdryer is directed at the base of the section and followed through to the ends. Avoid burning the scalp.

2. Follow the same procedure to build fullness on the sides. Use horizontal partings if the hair is to be styled down on the sides and vertical or diagonal partings if the hair will be brushed back.

BRAIDS AND LOCKS

The techniques associated with styling the hair into braids and locks is a form of natural hair care that originated in Africa thousands of years ago. Natural hair care has gained such popularity that an entirely new division of the hair care industry has developed. As a recognized professional segment of our industry, natural hair care is an active and exciting division that is currently advocating for education, licensing, and legislative changes to meet the needs of its educators, practitioners, and clients. Refer to Procedures 14-14 through 14-16 for guidelines on to complete braids and locks.

(P) 14-14 **Cornrow Braiding** *pages 479–482*

(P) 14-15 **Starting Locks with Nubian Coils** *pages 483–485*

(P) 14-16 **Cultivating and Grooming Locks** *pages 486–488*

Braids

While there are many variations of braids and braiding styles, on-the-scalp cornrows are one of the most popular styles worn today (**Figure 14-93**). Cornrows require working close to the scalp across the curves of the head. The braid may begin at the nape, top, or sides depending on the desired finished result.

Locks

Locks, also known as *dreadlocks*, are created from natural-textured hair that is intertwined together to form a single network of hair (**Figure 14-94**). **Hair locking** (HAYR lock-ing) is the process that occurs when coiled hair is allowed to develop in its natural state without the use of combs, heat, or chemicals. The more coil revolutions within a single strand, the faster the hair will coil and lock.

Cultivated locks are those that are intentionally guided through the natural process of locking. There are several ways to cultivate locks, such as double twisting, coiling, palm rolling, braiding, and wrapping with cord.

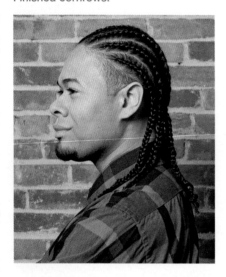
figure 14-93
Finished cornrows.

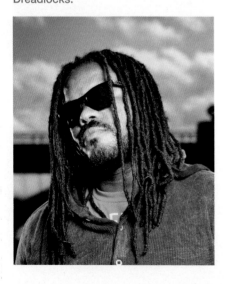
figure 14-94
Dreadlocks.

When consulting with a client who is considering locks, you should stress the following points:

- Once they are locked, locks can only be removed by cutting them off.

- The hair locks in progressive stages that can take from 6 months to a year to complete.

- General maintenance includes regular shop visits for cleaning, conditioning, and rerolling. Once the hair locks into compacted coils, it may be shampooed regularly and managed with a non-petroleum-based oil. Heavy oils should be avoided.

Two basic methods for locking men's hair, which is traditionally shorter at the beginning of the locking process, are the comb technique and the palm- or finger-rolling method (Figures 14-95 and 14-96).

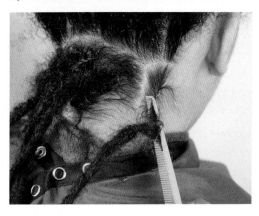

figure 14-95
Spiral the hair with the comb.

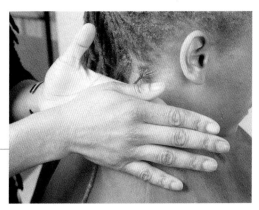

figure 14-96
Roll the hair or lock between the palms.

Discuss Safety Precautions for Haircutting and Styling

After reading this section, you will be able to:

LO**11** Discuss haircutting and styling safety precautions.

It is your responsibility as a barber to practice safety precautions daily in the performance of your work. Review the following reminders to meet the safety standards of a professional barber:

- Use all tools and implements in a safe manner.

- Use the right tool for the job.

- Always use a neck strip or towel as a barrier between the cape and the client's neck.

- Use smooth movements when raising or lowering chairs and seat backs.

- Properly clean, disinfect, and store tools and implements.

- Avoid applying dryer heat in one place on the head for too long.

- Keep metal combs away from the scalp when using heat.

- Keep the work area organized and cleaned and disinfected.

- Sweep the floor after every client and dispose of hair clippings appropriately.

Procedures 14-1 to 14-16

After reading and practicing Procedures 14-1 to 14-16, you will be able to:

LO**12** Demonstrate basic haircuts and styling techniques.

FINGERS-AND-SHEAR CUTTING TECHNIQUES

MATERIALS, IMPLEMENTS, AND EQUIPMENT

- ☐ All-purpose styling comb
- ☐ Hair clips
- ☐ Haircutting cape
- ☐ Haircutting shears

- ☐ Mannequin head and stand/clamp
- ☐ Neck strips
- ☐ Spray bottle with water

PREPARATION

1 Shampoo and condition the mannequin.

2 Set up the mannequin

3 Drape the mannequin for the haircut

PROCEDURES

A. CUTTING ABOVE THE FINGERS HORIZONTALLY

1 Palm the shears, comb through the top section of the hair, and create a part on the left side. Comb the hair over the top to the right.

2 At the front part of the crown, position the comb at about a 45-degree angle relative to the surface of the head. Use the first few teeth of the comb to part off a ¼-inch-thick parting.

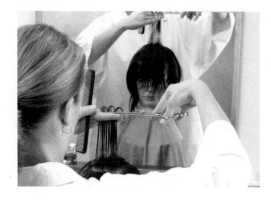

3 Comb the hair in front of the parting forward and away from you. With the teeth of the comb facing you, comb through the parting with the first two fingers of the opposite hand underneath the comb as you position the parting at a 90-degree elevation. Leave about an inch of hair extending beyond your fingers. The fingers and comb should be in a horizontal position parallel to the floor.

4 Palm the comb in the opposite hand while simultaneously positioning the shears at the tip of the fingers holding the hair section. Check the position of your fingers and shears for parallel placement.

5 Cut the hair projecting from between your fingers from the tips no further than the second knuckle.

B. CUTTING ABOVE THE FINGERS VERTICALLY ON THE **RIGHT SIDE**

6 Palm the shears, comb through the hair, and make a vertical part from the top of the crest to the hairline on the right side of the mannequin.

7 Part off a ¼-inch-thick vertical parting in front of the first parting.

8 With the teeth of the comb facing you in a vertical position, comb through the vertical section of hair with the fingers of the opposite hand following underneath the teeth of the comb to position the hair at a vertical 90-degree elevation. Your fingers and the comb should be in a vertical position with about an inch of hair extending beyond your fingers.

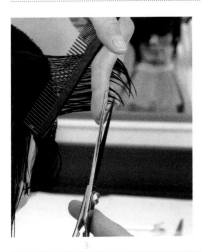

9 Palm the comb and cut the hair projecting from between your fingers from the tips no further than your second knuckle.

C. CUTTING BELOW THE FINGERS AT THE PERIMETER

10 Palm the shears and part off the hair into four sections from ear to ear and from front to nape. Use a clip to secure the hair at the sides.

11 Part off a ¼-to ½-inch horizontal parting along the hairline from each back section. Secure the hair remaining above the partings with clips.

12 Comb through the partings and leave about an inch of hair extending beyond your fingers. The fingers and comb should be in a horizontal position.

13 Palm the comb in the opposite hand while simultaneously positioning the tips of the shears just below the finger-tips holding the hair section. Cut the hair projecting from between your fingers from the tips no further than the second knuckle.

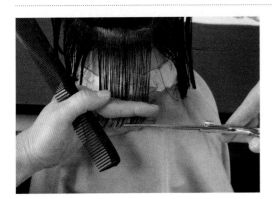

14 Turn your palm up while holding the section to practice palm-to-palm cutting.

ARCHING TECHNIQUES

HERE'S A TIP

Before beginning **arching** (ARE-ching), check to determine if one sideburn is longer than the other. Start on the side with the shorter sideburn to avoid unnecessary repetition of the procedure.

MATERIALS, IMPLEMENTS, AND EQUIPMENT

☐ All-purpose comb
☐ Haircutting cape
☐ Neck strips
☐ Outliner
☐ Razor and blade
☐ Shears

PREPARATION

1 Wash your hands.

2 Conduct a client consultation.

3 Drape the client for the haircut service.

4 Face the client toward the mirror and lock the chair.

PROCEDURES

A. ARCHING TECHNIQUE WITH SHEARS

1 Gently tug the client's ear down.

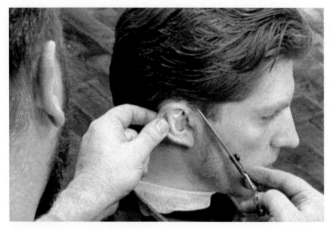

2 Start the outline on the right side as close to the natural hairline as possible.

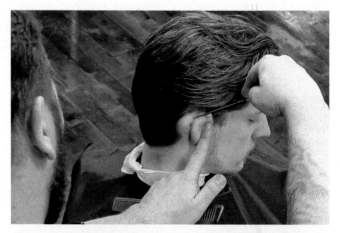

3 Start in front of the ear and cut a continuous outline around the ear and down the side of the neck.

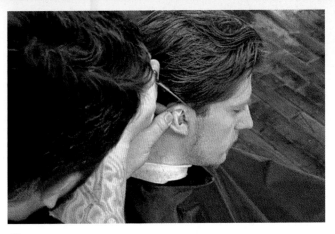

4 Reverse direction and arch back to the starting point.

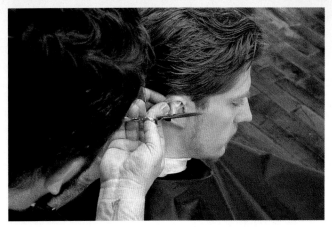

5 Square off and establish the length of the right sideburn.

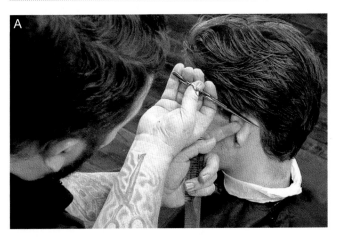

A

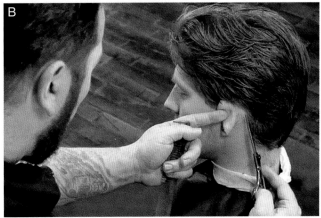

B

6 Repeat these steps on the left side using a backhand shear position to cut around the ear.

B. ARCHING TECHNIQUE WITH OUTLINER

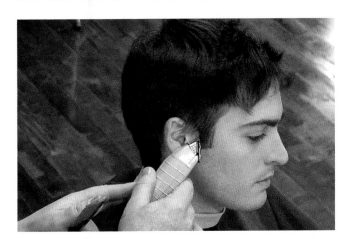

7 Use the first few teeth of the outliner T-blade to start the arching in front of the ear.

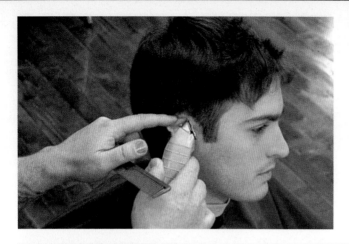

8 Arch around the ear using the T-blade in the same manner.

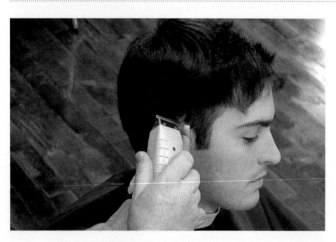

9 Continue arching around the ear; then reverse the direction.

C. ARCHING TECHNIQUE WITH RAZOR

10 Apply shaving cream to the bottom of the sideburn and around the ear.

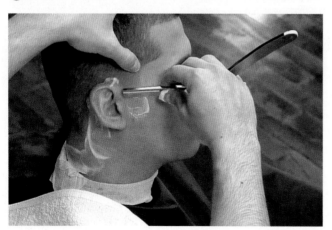

11 Shave the bottom of the sideburn using the freehand stroke.

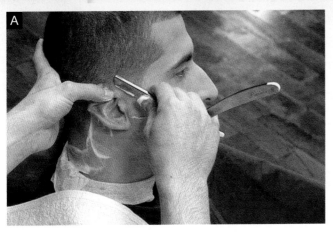
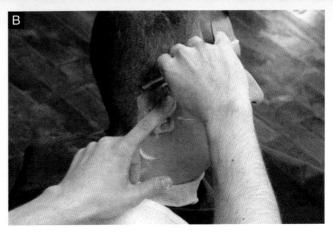

12 Gently bend or fold the ear out of the way to shave at the hairline in front of and over the ear.

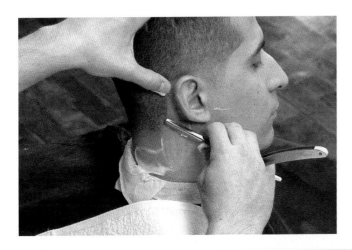

13 Shave in back of the ear to the corner of the nape.

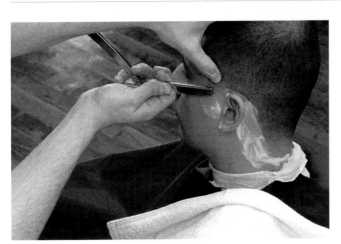

14 Repeat the procedure on the left side, using the backhand and reverse backhand strokes.

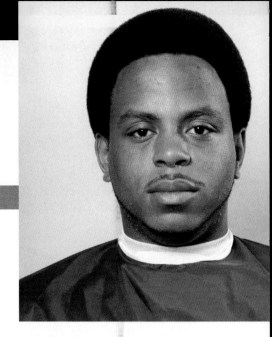

OUTLINE SHAVE

Note: An outline shave involves shaving the bottom of the sideburns, around and behind the ears, the nape area, and, when appropriate for the hairstyle, the front hairline. This procedure provides the steps for a complete outline shave.

MATERIALS, IMPLEMENTS, AND EQUIPMENT

☐ Disposable barber towels

☐ Haircutting cape

☐ Neck strips

☐ Shaving cream or gel

☐ Straight razor and blades

☐ Terry cloth towels

PREPARATION

1 Client should still be draped from the haircut service.

2 Disinfect razor and blades.

3 Wash your hands.

4 Loosen the cape and apply towel to neckline, leaving it loose enough for access to the nape when securing the drape.

PROCEDURE

1 Apply a light coating of lather at the front hairline.

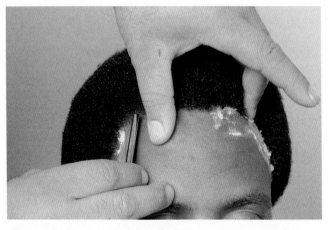

2 Stand at a slight diagonal to the client. Stretch the skin at the forehead and shave from the center along the front hairline to the temple area using the freehand stroke.

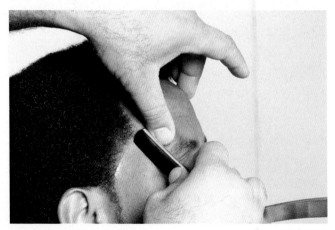

3 Shave from the temple along the hairline to the front of the sideburn.

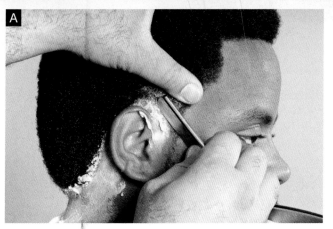

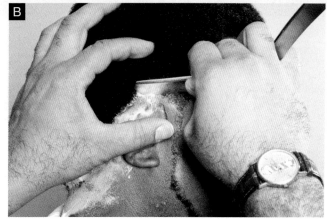

④ Apply lather around and behind the ear. Using the freehand stroke, begin shaving in front of the ear; then hold the ear away and shave around the ear.

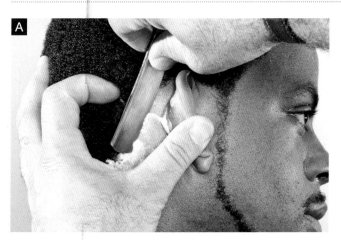

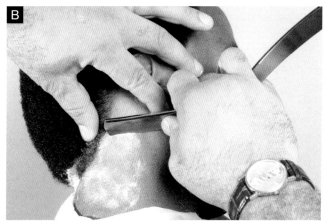

⑤ Shave behind the ear and down the side of the neck using the freehand stroke.

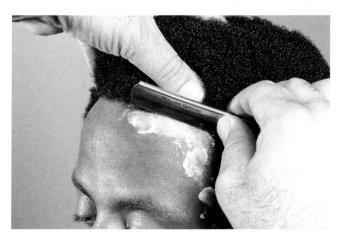

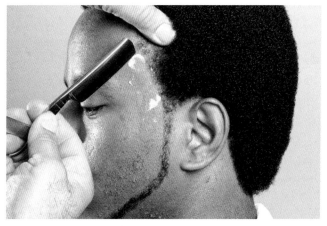

⑥ Move to the client's left side and reapply lather at forehead. Stretch the skin at the forehead area and repeat freehand strokes to the temple.

⑦ Use the backhand stroke to shave from the temple to the front sideburn area.

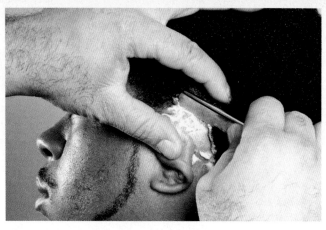

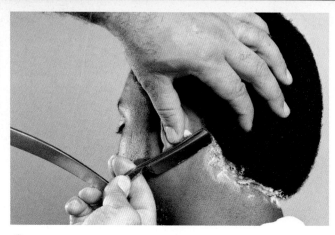

8 Apply lather around and behind the ear. Use the free-hand stroke to shave in front of and around the ear at the hairline, holding the ear away with the fingers.

9 Use the reverse backhand stroke to shave behind the ear and down the side of the neck.

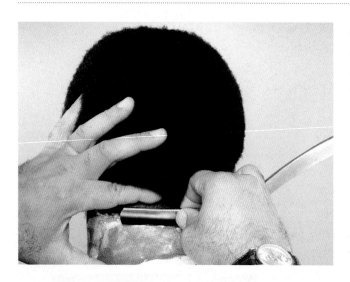

10 Shave the nape area with a freehand stroke.

11 Clean up the hairline with a warm, moist towel. Apply astringent, moisturizing cream, talc, or after-shave lotion as desired.

CLEAN-UP AND DISINFECTION

☐ Clean and disinfect the tools and implements.

☐ Clean and then disinfect the work area.

☐ Sweep up hair and deposit in closed receptacle.

☐ Deposit used blades in a sharps container.

☐ Dispose of single-use items. Place all used linens, towels, and capes in the laundry.

☐ Wash your hands.

PRECISION CUT

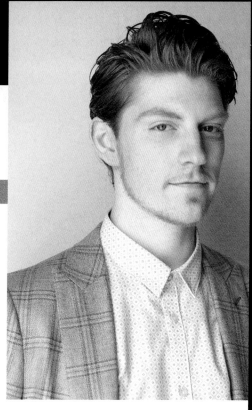

MATERIALS, IMPLEMENTS, AND EQUIPMENT

- □ All-purpose, taper, and flat top combs, picks, etc.
- □ Blowdryer
- □ Clipper disinfectant and coolant
- □ Clippers and outliner
- □ Disposable barber towels
- □ Hair clips
- □ Hand mirror
- □ Neck strips
- □ Shampoo and conditioner

- □ Shampoo cape and haircutting cape
- □ Shaving cream or gel
- □ Shears and blending shears
- □ Spray bottle with water
- □ Straight razor and blades
- □ Styling brushes
- □ Styling products
- □ Talc
- □ Terry cloth towels

PREPARATION

1. Wash your hands.
2. Conduct a client consultation.
3. Drape the client for wet service.
4. Shampoo and towel dry the hair.

5. Remove the waterproof cape; replace with a neck strip and haircutting cape.
6. Face the client toward the mirror and lock the chair.

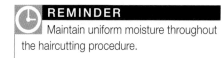

REMINDER
Maintain uniform moisture throughout the haircutting procedure.

PROCEDURE

A. TOP SECTION

1. Comb the hair down in the front, sides, and back. Standing behind the client, take a ¼-to ½-inch parting, depending on the density of the hair at the forward-most part of the crown.

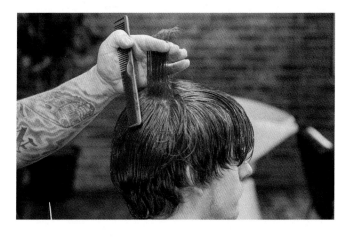

2. Comb the parting straight up at 90 degrees and hold it between the fingers of the left hand.

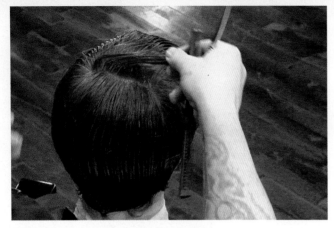

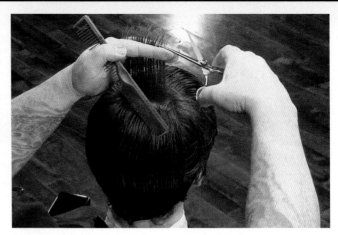

3 Bend the parting from right to left to determine at what length the hair will bend (bending point) to lie down smoothly over the head.

4 Use the bending point to establish and cut a guide length for the top section.

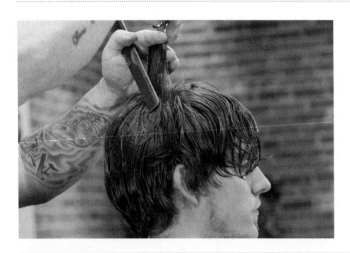

5 Part off a second parting at 90 degrees, comb through this parting while retaining the guide parting to see the guideline, and cut to the guide.

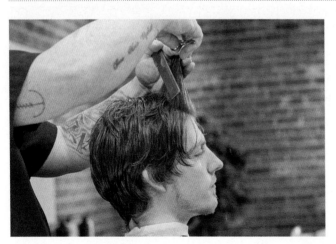

6 Complete the top section, moving forward toward the front with each parting and cut.

7 Comb the top section back. Move to the client's left side. Starting at the forehead, part off the top section of hair, front to back, with the thumb and middle finger.

8 Hold the original guide and a ½-inch parting at the crown at 90 degrees and cut. This establishes the guide for the crown and back sections.

HERE'S A TIP

To assist you in developing a rhythm for using a traveling guide in the top section, say the following to yourself as you go through the procedure: part on 1; comb forward on 2; pick up on 3; and cut on 4.

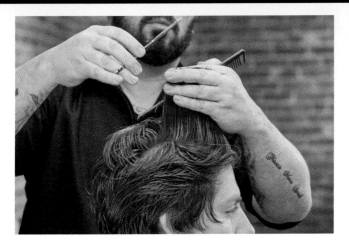

9 Work forward, still maintaining a side-standing position. Following the arc and contour of the head, and even off any length that does not blend with the traveling guide. This is a checkpoint for your work in the top section.

B. FRONT AND TEMPORAL SECTIONS

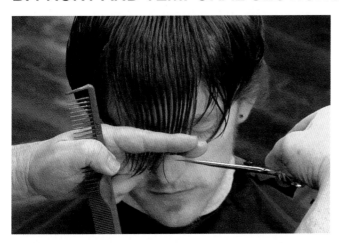

10 Comb the hair forward and move in front of the client. Comb the front section down at 0 elevation and cut a guide length in the center to establish the front design line. Cut right and then left of the center to the ends of the width of the eyebrows; this will act as a traveling guide for the temporal area.

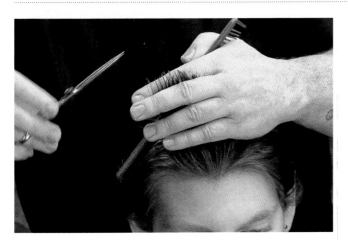

11 Move behind the client. Beginning on the right side, pick up the front hair of the temporal/crest region. A small amount of the previously cut top hair should be visible.

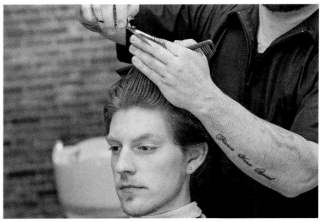

12 Hold the hair at 90 degrees and cut *to* the top guide.

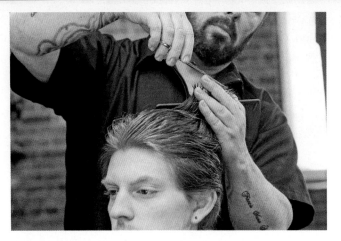

13 Continue cutting the crest area, working back to the center of the crown area. Cut hair only from the temporal region; do not pick up side hair.

14 Repeat this step on the left side of the client's hair. Cuts will be made *from* the top guide through the temporal region. The hair from the right and left crest areas should meet at the back center of the crown upon completion of this step.

C. RIGHT AND LEFT SIDES

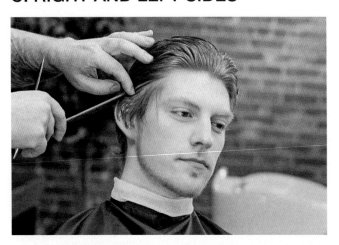

15 Comb client's hair straight down on the sides. Take a ¼-to ½-inch horizontal parting at the hairline, from the sideburn to the top of the ear and a diagonal parting of the same thickness from the right temple to the sideburn. Comb the remaining hair back or secure it with a hair clip.

16 Cut the design line either around the ears or to cover part of the ears at the desired length. If you are cutting around the ear, gently bend or slightly tug the ear down out of the way.

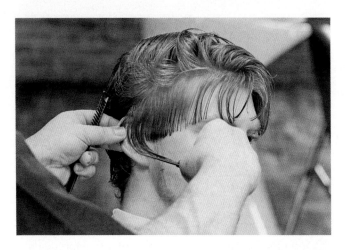

17 Move toward the front of the client facing the temporal and side areas.

18 Using the front and side design lines (which are acting as guides), cut the hair between these two points against the skin, cutting along the natural hairline.

19 Holding the hair between the fingers at the lowest elevation possible, check the design line cut.

20 Proceed cutting the remaining side hair section, repeating the partings as the density of the hair requires.

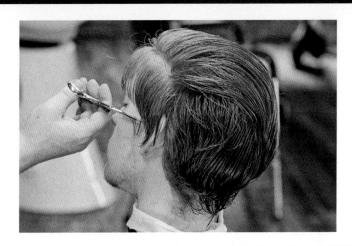

21 Repeat this procedure on the left side.

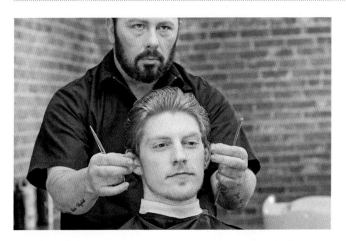

22 Check the length of the sides in the mirror for evenness.

23 Move behind the client. Pick up the hair in vertical partings, holding it straight out to the side at 90 degrees. The design/guide line should be visible at the tips of the fingers when you are working on the right side of the client's head.

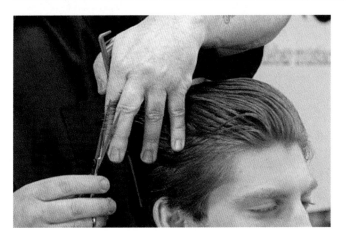

24 Make a straight, vertical cut from the design/guide line, cutting off any hair that extends past the guide. Continue cutting partings of hair while following the contour of the head until you reach the temporal/crest region to blend hair lengths.

25 Proceed until all the side hair is cut. Stop at the topmost point of the ear.

26 Repeat the steps on the left side. You may face the client to cut the left side or remain behind the chair.

27 The front, top, temporal, crown, and side areas are now cut.

D. BACK AND NAPE SECTIONS

28 Move behind the client. Section off a ¼-to ½-inch horizontal parting at the nape of the neck. Secure excess hair with a clip if necessary.

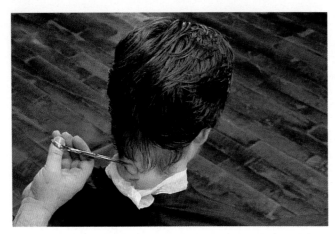

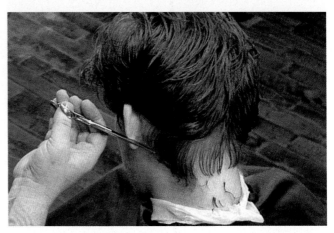

29 Starting in the center of the nape, cut the hair to the desired length; cut left and then right to the corners of the nape area and check the design line cut.

30 Move to the client's left side. Part off a ¼-to ½-inch section along the hairline. Cut hair in a downward direction behind the ear from the side design line guide to the left nape corner using a backhand shear position. Repeat this step on the right side using the freehand shear position.

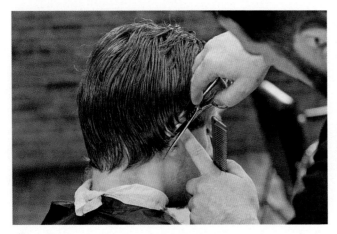

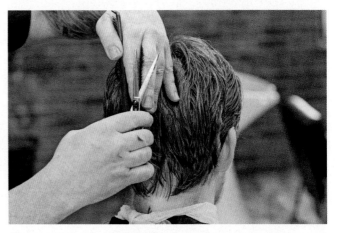

31 Part off a subsequent parting and comb hair down. Holding the design/guide line and parting between the fingers, cut hair at a low elevation or against the skin. Continue to take partings as the density requires, cutting the nape and behind-the-ear areas against the skin.

32 Starting at the hairline, pick up the hair in vertical partings at 90 degrees and blend through the back section up the crown and crest areas.

33 Proceed until the entire back section is cut and sides are blended to the back.

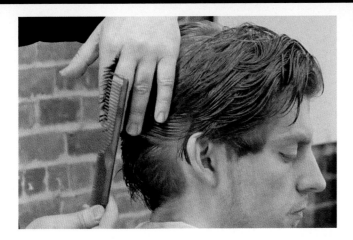

34 Check the entire haircut by combing the hair at 90 degrees, making sure that the hair blends from one section to another.

E. FINISHING WORK

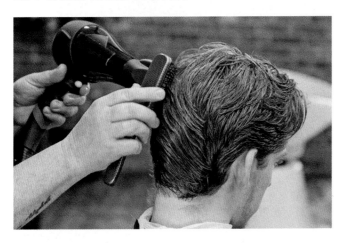

35 Dry and brush the client's hair into place using a directional nozzle, if needed.

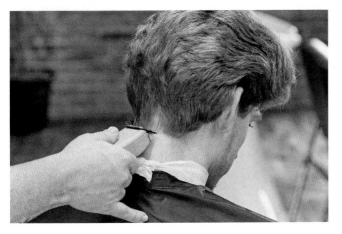

36 Check the perimeter and fine-tune the sideburns, sides, and nape with an outliner.

37 Complete the finish work by performing a neck shave after outlining the bottom of the sideburn and around-the-ear areas with a razor.

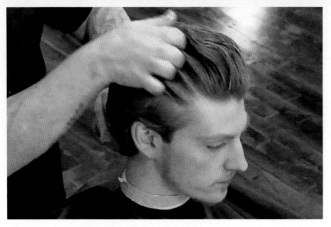

38 Offer a styling aid and arrange hair into the finished style.

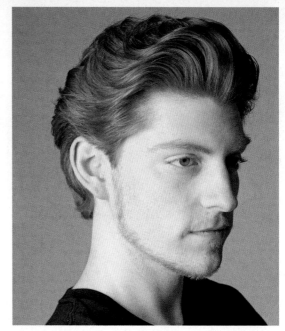

39 The haircut and style are now complete. Dust or vacuum stray hairs, making sure none remains on the client's face or neck.

CLEAN-UP AND DISINFECTION

☐ Clean and disinfect the tools and implements.

☐ Clean and disinfect the work area.

☐ Sweep up hair and deposit in a closed receptacle.

☐ Deposit used blades in a sharps container.

☐ Dispose of single-use items. Place all used linens, towels, and capes in the laundry.

☐ Wash your hands.

F. ALTERNATE START TO THE PRECISION CUT

Note: Some barbers prefer to begin the precision cut at the front section or with a side part established in the hair.

1 Comb the client's hair into the desired style with or without a side part. Start at the front hairline and project a parting of hair to 90 degrees. Cut to desired length and use this length as a traveling guide to cut the top section back toward the crown.

2 Pick up hair from the front temporal/crest area using the same procedure as in steps 11 to 14. Continue cutting all around the crest area through to the left side; or stop at the center of the crown and repeat the procedure on the left side, working from the front to the crown. Continue with sections C and D of Procedure 14-4.

BASIC TAPER CUT

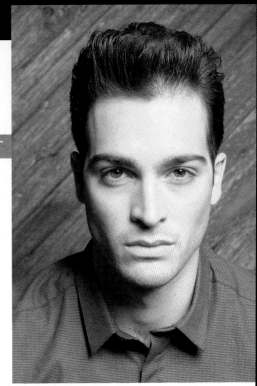

MATERIALS, IMPLEMENTS, AND EQUIPMENT

- ☐ All-purpose, taper, and flat top combs, picks, etc.
- ☐ Blowdryer
- ☐ Clipper disinfectant and coolant
- ☐ Clippers and outliners
- ☐ Disposable barber towels
- ☐ Hair clips
- ☐ Hand mirror
- ☐ Neck strips
- ☐ Shampoo and conditioner
- ☐ Shampoo cape and haircutting cape
- ☐ Shaving cream or gel
- ☐ Shears and blending shears
- ☐ Spray bottle with water
- ☐ Straight razor and blades
- ☐ Styling brushes
- ☐ Styling products
- ☐ Talc
- ☐ Terry cloth towels

PREPARATION

1. Clean your hands.
2. Conduct a client consultation.
3. Drape the client for wet service.
4. Shampoo and towel dry the hair. Blowdry the hair if the client prefers dry cutting.
5. Remove the waterproof cape; replace with a neck strip and haircutting cape.
6. Face the client toward the mirror and lock the chair.

PROCEDURE

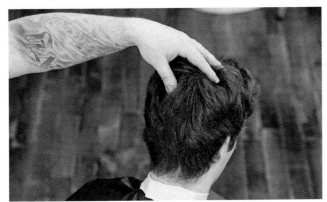

1. Comb the hair and tilt the client's head forward slightly.

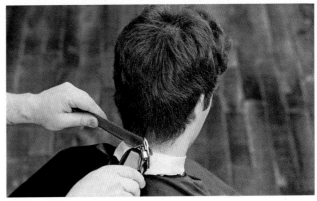

2. Use the clipper-over-comb or freehand clipper technique to establish a guide panel in the center back and cut to just below the occipital.

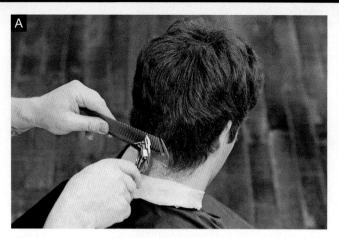 A

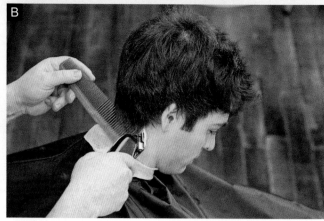 B

3 Roll the comb out to cut and blend the hair left and right of the center panel from the hairline to the occipital.

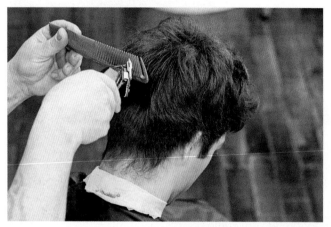

4 Continue to cut and blend through the back section up to the bottom of the crown area.

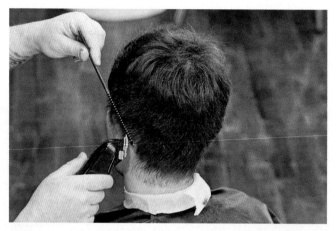

5 Move toward the client's side and use a diagonal comb placement to cut and blend the hair behind the ear into the back section.

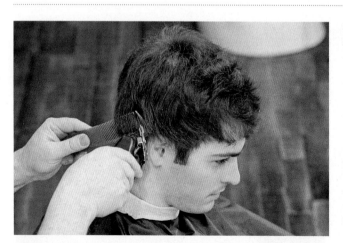

6 Repeat diagonal comb placement and blending on the opposite side.

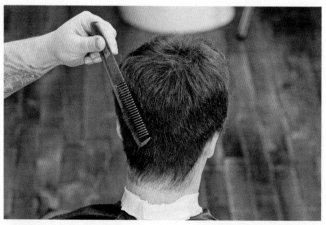

7 Check the entire back section for blending and balance.

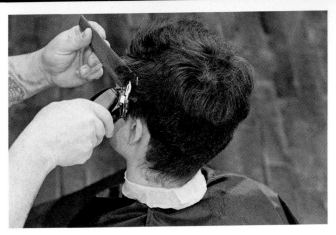

8 Taper around the ear and into the side section.

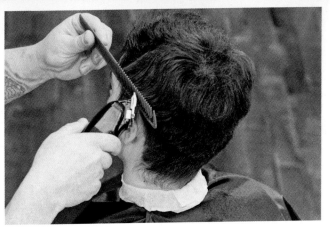

9 Continue to taper and blend toward the crest area.

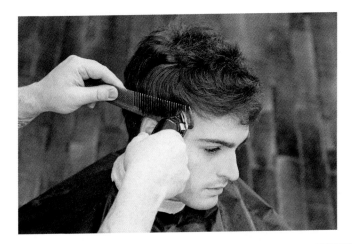

10 Repeat the tapering and blending procedure on the opposite side.

11 Check for balance on both sides of the head.

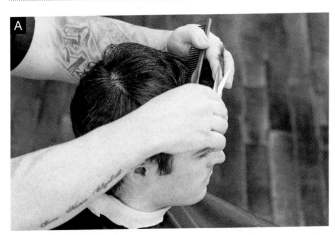

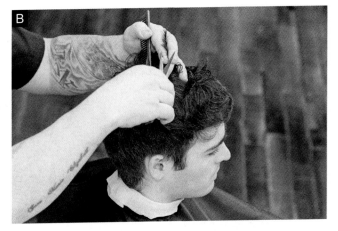

12 Comb through the top section. Using either the clipper-over-comb or fingers-and-shear technique, cut the top section from the front to the crown.

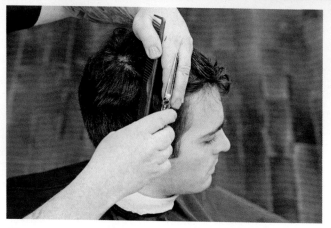

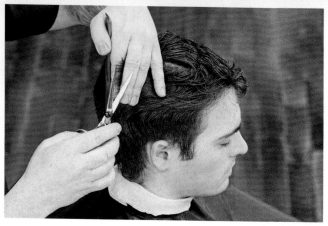

13 Pick up hair from the front of the top and temporal areas. Cut the hair from the crest area to the top guide.

14 Continue cutting and blending to the top section as you cut through the parietal ridge back to the crown.

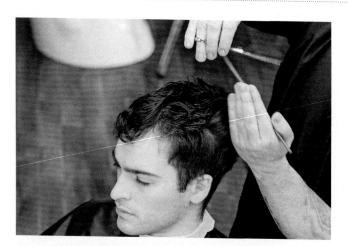

15 Repeat cutting through the top crest area on the opposite side until the cut hair meets at the center of the crown.

16 Check the blend through the entire cut, making sure the hair at the lower part of the crest blends into the side section. If the blend is off, the cut will appear to have gaps or steps.

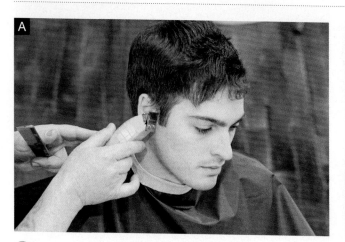

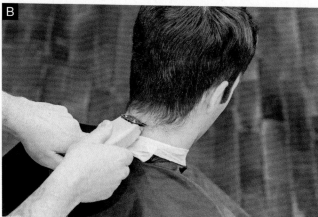

17 Perform the arching procedure over both ears with your preferred tool and use the outliner to remove stray hairs at the nape.

18 Perform a neck or outline shave as requested by the client.

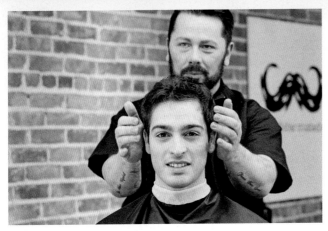

19 Style the hair and check for balance and proportion.

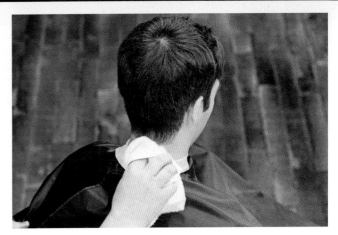

20 Dust hair clippings from client's neck, face, and ears.

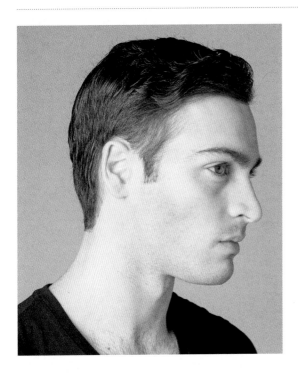

21 Finished taper cut.

CLEAN-UP AND DISINFECTION

□ Wash and disinfect the tools and implements.

□ Clean and disinfect the work area.

□ Sweep up hair and deposit in a closed receptacle.

□ Deposit used blades in a sharps container.

□ Dispose of single-use items. Place all used linens, towels, and capes in the laundry.

□ Wash your hands.

RAZOR CUT

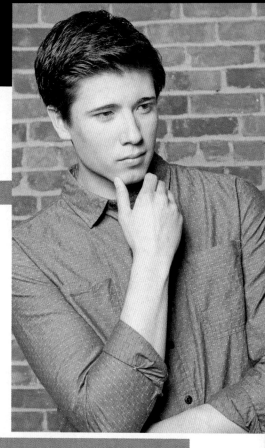

MATERIALS, IMPLEMENTS, AND EQUIPMENT

- ☐ All-purpose, taper, and flat top combs, picks, etc.
- ☐ Blowdryer
- ☐ Clipper disinfectant and coolant
- ☐ Clippers and outliners
- ☐ Disposable barber towels
- ☐ Hair clips
- ☐ Hand mirror
- ☐ Neck strips
- ☐ Shampoo and conditioner
- ☐ Shampoo cape and haircutting cape
- ☐ Shaving cream or gel
- ☐ Shears and blending shears
- ☐ Spray bottle with water
- ☐ Straight razor, blades, and guard
- ☐ Styling brushes
- ☐ Styling products
- ☐ Talc
- ☐ Terry cloth towels

PREPARATION

1. Wash your hands.
2. Conduct a client consultation.
3. Drape the client for wet service.
4. Shampoo and towel dry the hair.
5. Remove the waterproof cape; replace with a neck strip and haircutting cape.
6. Face the client toward the mirror and lock the chair.

> **✔ HERE'S A TIP**
> It is important to mist the hair with water to maintain moisture throughout the entire cutting process.

PROCEDURE

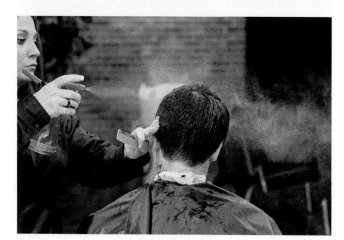
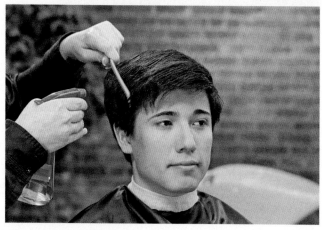

1. Re-dampen the client's hair and comb the hair forward to identify natural growth patterns.

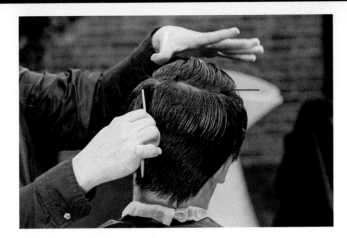

2 Section the hair into four sections. Create a horse-shoe shape around the top section and diagonal partings behind each ear to expose the back section for the next step.

3 Divide the back section into three vertical panels.

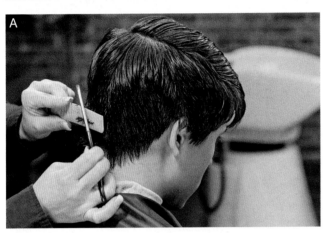

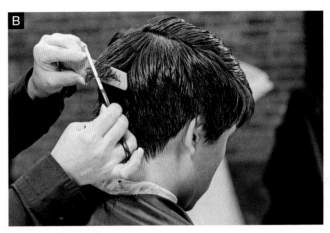

4 Begin in the center section at the hairline using the razor-over-comb technique with short strokes to gradually taper the hair toward the crown to establish a center panel and guide for the back section.

5 Comb the hair down after cutting the panel to check your work for blending and balance.

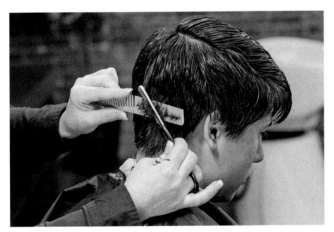

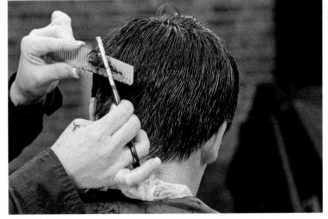

6 Moving just right of center, roll the comb out to position the guide and hair from the next panel for cutting.

7 Continue cutting through the back section right and left of the center panel.

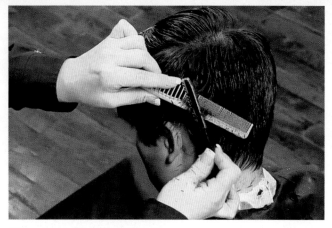

8 Use a slight diagonal comb placement when cutting and blending behind the ears.

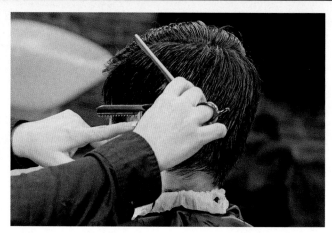

9 Move to the side and comb hair downward in direction of hair growth. Re-mist as necessary.

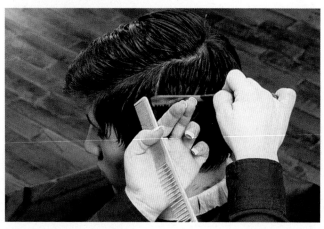

10 Part off a ¼-inch vertical section and hold the hair between your fingers; then taper from the crest down to the hairline.

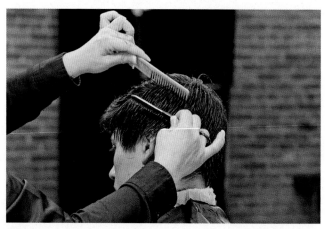

11 Comb the hair in the direction of hair growth and use the razor rotation technique to taper and blend the side with the back section.

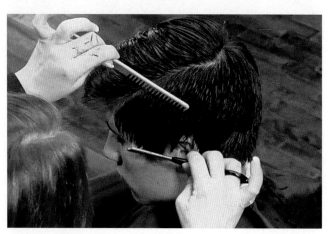

12 Comb the hair forward and taper lightly toward the face.

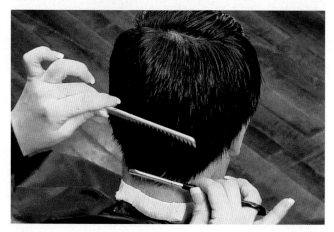

13 Trim the perimeter design line as needed.

14 Repeat steps 9 to 12 on the opposite side of the head before continuing to Step 15.

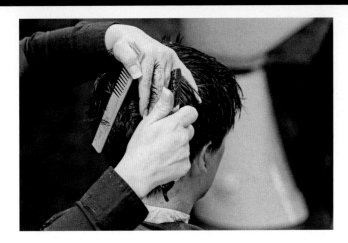

15 Comb the top section forward. Elevate the subsections to 90 degrees to blend the top, parietal, and crown areas using the freehand slicing technique.

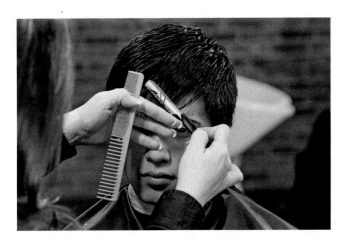

16 Hold the front section at a low elevation and trim using the freehand slicing technique.

17 Check your work. Repeat tapering and blending steps throughout the cut as needed.

18 Comb through the cut, redistributing the hair in a variety of directions to check for blending and evenness.

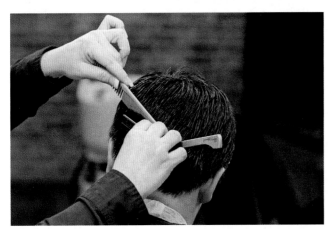

19 Perform light-taper blending with the razor-rotation technique to fine-tune your work.

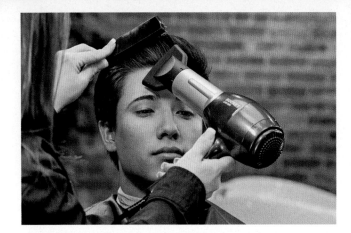

20 Consult with your client regarding a neck or outline shave and the use of styling aids. Style the hair as desired and dust off any stray hair clippings.

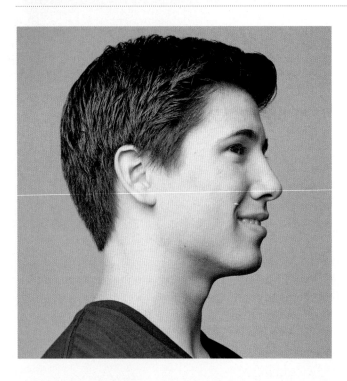

21 The haircut and style are now complete.

CLEAN-UP AND DISINFECTION

☐ Clean and disinfect the tools and implements.

☐ Clean and then disinfect the work area.

☐ Sweep up hair and deposit in a closed receptacle.

☐ Deposit used blades in a sharps container.

☐ Dispose of single-use items. Place all used linens, towels, and capes in the laundry.

☐ Wash your hands.

FLAT TOP AND CREW CUT

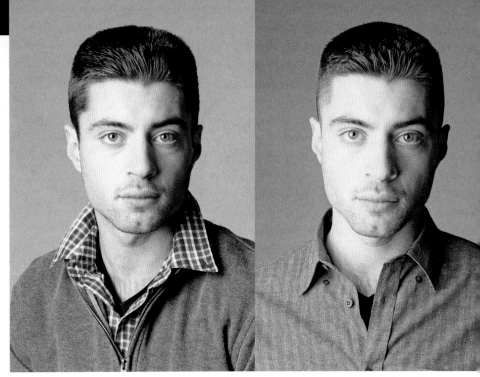

MATERIALS, IMPLEMENTS, AND EQUIPMENT

- ☐ All-purpose, taper, and flat top combs, picks, etc.
- ☐ Blowdryer
- ☐ Clipper disinfectant and coolant
- ☐ Clippers and outliners
- ☐ Disposable barber towels
- ☐ Hair clips
- ☐ Hand mirror
- ☐ Neck strips
- ☐ Shampoo and conditioner

- ☐ Shampoo cape and haircutting cape
- ☐ Shaving cream or gel
- ☐ Shears and blending shears
- ☐ Spray bottle with water
- ☐ Straight razor and blades
- ☐ Styling brushes
- ☐ Styling products
- ☐ Talc
- ☐ Terry cloth towels

PREPARATION

1. Wash your hands.
2. Conduct a client consultation.
3. Drape the client for wet service.
4. Shampoo and towel dry the hair.
5. Remove the waterproof cape; replace with a neck strip and haircutting cape.
6. Face the client toward the mirror and lock the chair.

A. FLAT TOP

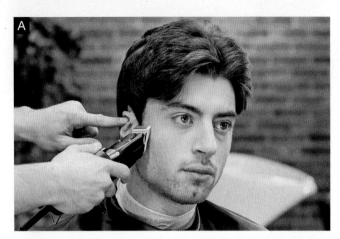
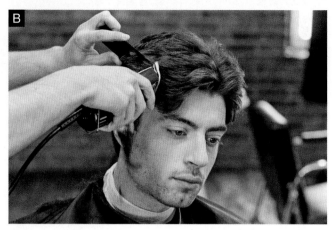

1 Start on your preferred side using a clipper blade and the freehand clipper technique, or select a blade size or adjustment of your choice and use clipper-over-comb to cut from the hairline to the parietal ridge.

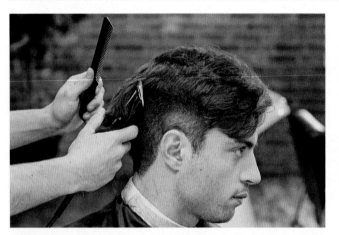
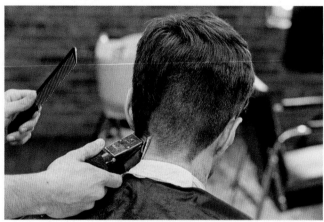

2 Cut through the sides to the back section.

3 Taper and blend through the back section.

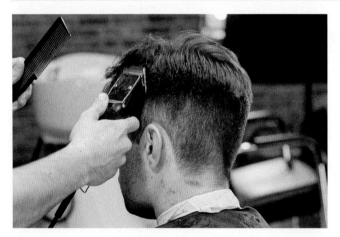
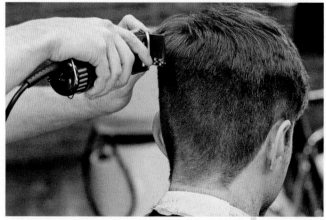

4 Continue cutting and blending to the opposite side.

5 Check and fine-tune blending through the parietal ridge.

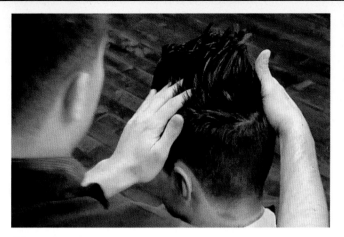

6 Work gel, pomade, or styling wax through the top section.

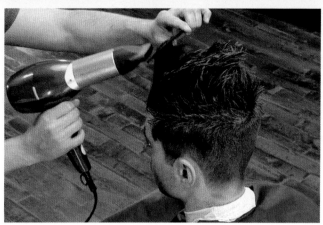

7 Blowdry the hair up and back from the scalp to position the hair to stand straight up.

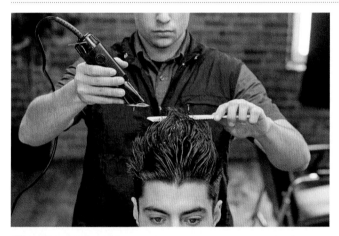

8 Stand in back of the client and use clipper-over-comb to begin cutting the crown area.

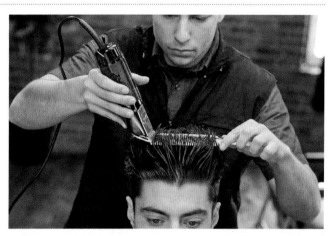

9 Using the length at the front of the crown as a guide, use a horizontal comb placement as you cut over the top toward the front.

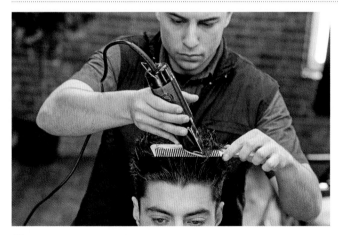

10 Due to the curve of the head, the hair will be gradually longer as you cut toward the front section.

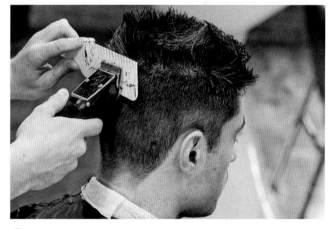

11 Blend and round the corners of the crown area into the top section.

12 Continue cutting and blending the upper crest area into the top section as you work toward the front on both sides. Be sure you are cutting to a previously established guide.

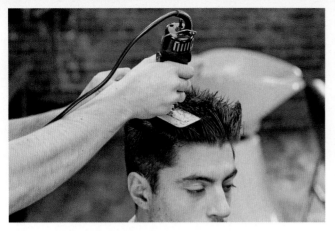

13 Fine-tune the blend from the crest to the top section by angling the comb from shorter to longer hair. This means the comb will rest closer to the head in the crest areas and farther away from the head in the top section.

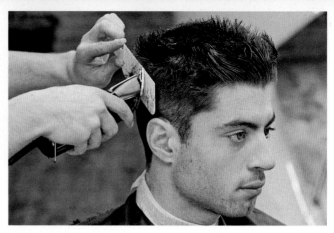

14 Reblend the hair around the entire crest area and into the top section.

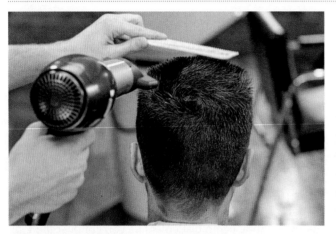

15 Reapply styling aid; re-comb and style the hair.

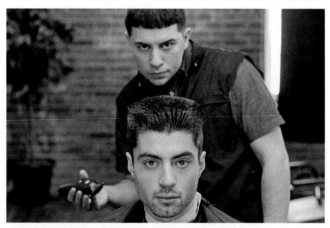

16 Check the cut for balance and blending; fine-tune as necessary.

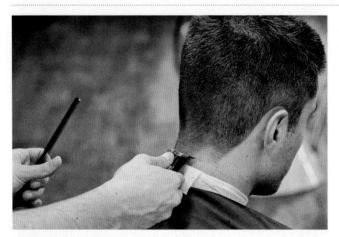

17 Perform finish work with an outliner and offer a neck or outline shave.

18 Dust or vacuum stray hairs, making sure none remains on your client's face or neck.

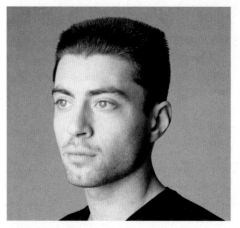

19 Finished flat top style.

B. CREW CUT

Note: When modifying a flat top to a crew cut, the crew cut is rounded in the top section and cut closer at the crown with a gradual length increase toward the front.

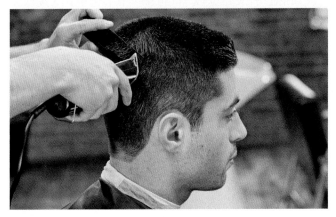

20 Using the clipper-over-comb technique, blend and round out the crest area at the crown.

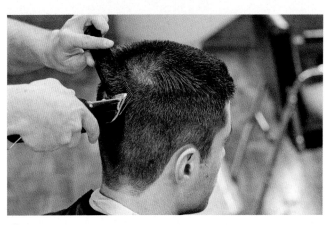

21 Use the shortened crown section as a guide for cutting the top section.

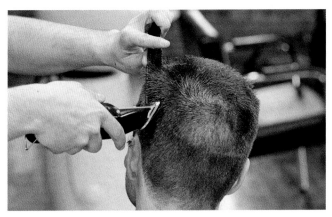

22 Use a diagonal comb placement to cut and blend through the side and back areas up through the crest.

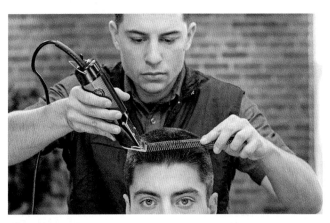

23 Shorten and blend the top and front sections to the desired length.

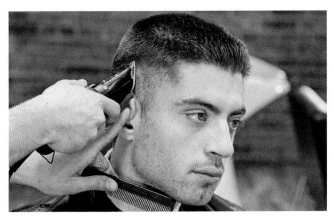

24 Starting on your preferred side, use the freehand clipper technique to cut from the hairline to the bottom of the crest to shorten the sides.

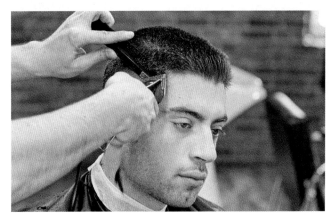

25 Switch to the clipper-over-comb technique to blend the transition areas.

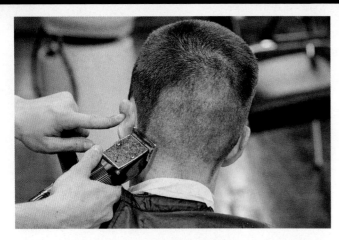

26 Continue cutting and blending around the entire head.

27 Check your work and reblend transition areas as needed.

28 Complete detail work at the hairline and offer a neck or outline shave.

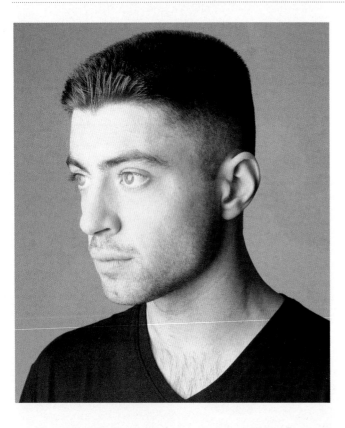

29 Finished crew cut style.

CLEAN-UP AND DISINFECTION

☐ Clean and disinfect the tools and implements.

☐ Clean and then disinfect the work area.

☐ Sweep up hair and deposit in a closed receptacle.

☐ Deposit used blades in a sharps container.

☐ Dispose of single-use items. Place all used linens, towels, and capes in the laundry.

☐ Wash your hands.

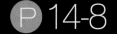

TEMPLE FADE

Note: There are many variations of temple fades. Close cut sideburn areas with longer temple and crest areas blend into either short or longer top sections. This procedure describes a temple fade variation that blends into a short top length.

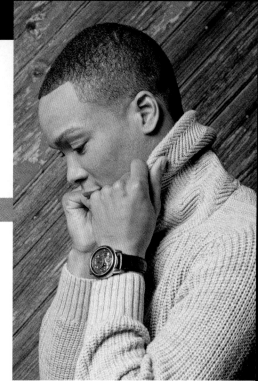

MATERIALS, IMPLEMENTS, AND EQUIPMENT

- ☐ All-purpose, taper, and flat top combs, picks, etc.
- ☐ Clipper disinfectant and coolant
- ☐ Detachable blade and adjustable clippers
- ☐ Disposable barber towels
- ☐ Hand mirror
- ☐ Neck strips
- ☐ Outliner

- ☐ Shampoo cape and haircutting cape
- ☐ Shaving cream or gel
- ☐ Shears
- ☐ Straight razor and blades
- ☐ Styling brushes
- ☐ Styling products
- ☐ Talc
- ☐ Terry cloth towels

PREPARATION

1. Wash your hands.
2. Conduct a client consultation.
3. Drape the client for wet service.
4. Shampoo, towel dry hair, and blowdry the hair.
5. Remove the waterproof cape; replace with a neck strip and haircutting cape.
6. Face the client toward the mirror and lock the chair.

PROCEDURE

1. Start by assessing the client's hair texture, density, and growth pattern.

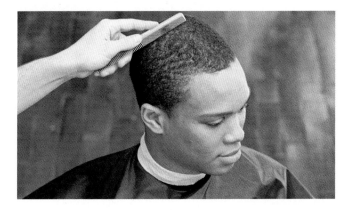

2. Comb or pick the hair out. Determine the length for the top section and the shortest length for back section.

3. Select the appropriate blade size, guard, or adjustable setting that will leave the hair in the top section at the desired length.

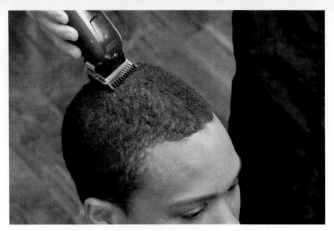

4 Cut a center panel in the top section to establish a guide. Cut with or against the grain, depending on the density, curl pattern, and desired length.

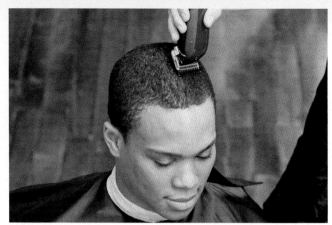

5 Cut left and right of the center panel to blend the top section.

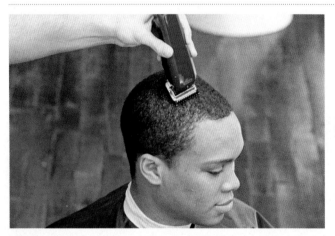

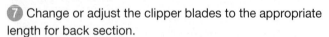

6 Blend into and around the crest areas.

7 Change or adjust the clipper blades to the appropriate length for back section.

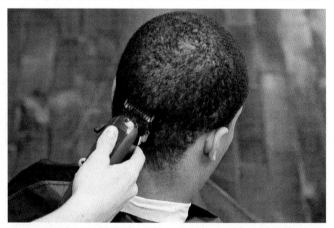

8 Starting at the hairline in the center of the back section, cut against the grain up to the occipital area to create a guide for the back.

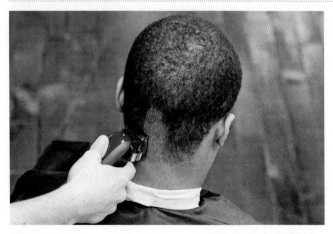

9 Cut panels left and right of the center panel to this guide.

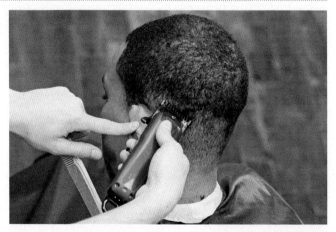

10 Cut the hair behind the ears on a slight diagonal to blend into the back section.

11 Repeat on the opposite side and blend behind the ear into the back section.

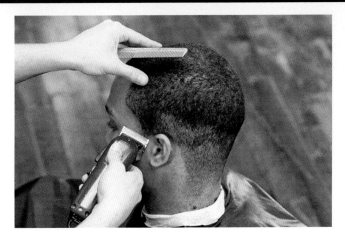

12 Move to the side of your client and adjust the clipper blades to the open position.

13 Begin cutting from the hairline at the bottom of the sideburn. Adjust the clipper blade or guard as necessary to taper from the hairline into the side section.

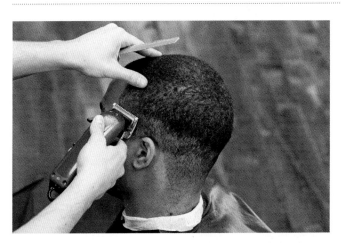

14 Taper and blend the hair toward the temple area and into the side.

15 Repeat the tapering and blending steps on the opposite side.

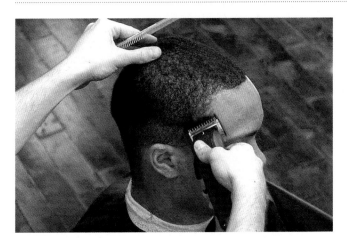

16 Move toward the front. Taper and blend the front side section into the temple area, either by changing the blades or by opening the adjustable clipper as the hair gets longer.

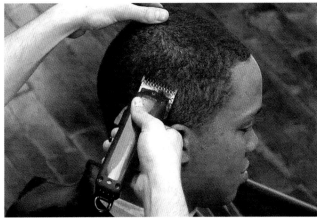

17 Continue blending from the side into the crest and back sections.

18 Repeat the tapering and blending steps on the opposite side and throughout the cut. Change the guards or blades as necessary to achieve the desired blend.

19 Check and fine-tune your work to make sure the sides blend with the crest and back section.

20 Remember to dust the hair clippings from your client, as needed, throughout the haircut.

21 Check your work in the mirror.

22 Finish with an outliner to detail the hairline. To avoid injuring the client's skin, do not apply pressure when using outliners; let the teeth of the tool do the work.

23 Perform an outline shave if requested.

24 Use the mirror to check sideburn lengths.

25 Finished temple fade.

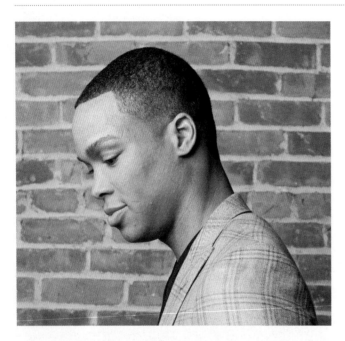

CLEAN-UP AND DISINFECTION

☐ Clean and disinfect the tools and implements.

☐ Clean surfaces and chair.

☐ Sweep up hair and deposit in a closed receptacle.

☐ Dispose of single-use items. Place all used linens, towels, and capes in the laundry.

☐ Wash your hands.

POMPADOUR FADE

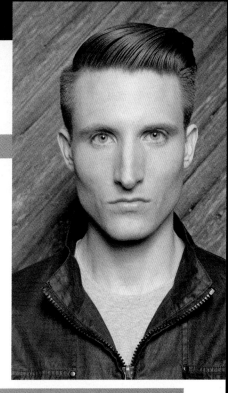

MATERIALS, IMPLEMENTS, AND EQUIPMENT

- All-purpose, taper, and flat top combs, picks, etc.
- Blowdryer
- Clipper disinfectant and coolant
- Clippers and outliners
- Disposable barber towels
- Hair clips
- Hand mirror
- Neck strips
- Shampoo and conditioner
- Shampoo cape and haircutting cape
- Shaving cream or gel
- Shears and blending shears
- Spray bottle with water
- Straight razor and blades
- Styling brushes
- Styling products
- Talc
- Terry cloth towels

PREPARATION

1. Wash your hands.
2. Conduct a client consultation.
3. Drape the client for wet service.
4. Shampoo and towel dry the hair.
5. Remove the waterproof cape; replace with a neck strip and haircutting cape.
6. Face the client toward the mirror and lock the chair.

PROCEDURE

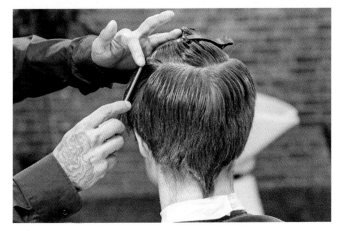

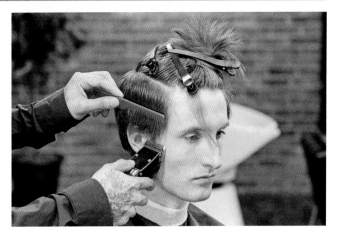

1. Re-dampen the top section with water, if necessary.
2. Part off the top section, following the curve of the head at the top of the parietal ridge and secure with clips.
3. Select the appropriate blade size to leave the hair in the back and sides at the desired length.

4. On your preferred side, use the freehand clipper technique to establish a guide in the side section. Rock the clipper out at the point on the head where you will later create transition areas from shorter to longer sections.

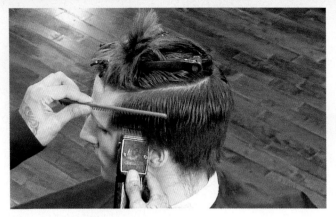

5 Repeat the cutting procedure on opposite side.

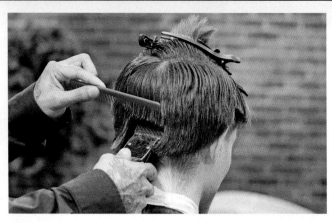

6 Establish a guide in the center back section from the nape to the mid-occipital area.

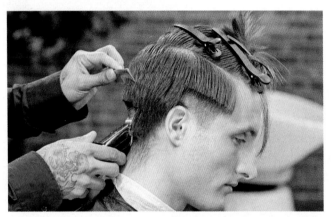

7 Cut the panels left and right of center through the back section; then blend and connect to the side guides.

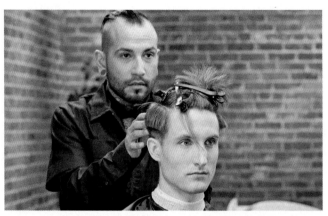

8 Go back over previously cut areas to fine-tune your work and check side lengths for evenness and balance.

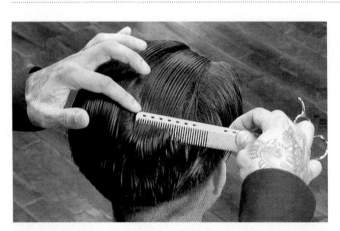

9 Dampen the top section. Comb hair back toward the crown, allowing the hair to fall naturally over the curves of the head.

10 Stand at the back of your client. Part off a ¼-to ½-inch parting in the center of the top section from the front to crown.

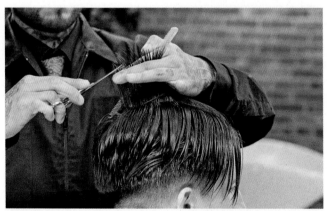

11 Stand at the client's side. Starting at the forward-most part of the crown, project the hair at 90 degrees to establish a guide length for the top section.

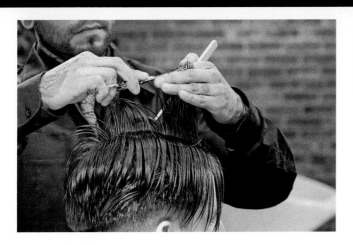

12 Using the guide from the crown, use a diagonal finger placement and slight overdirection to gradually leave the hair longer as you move toward the front.

13 Comb through the section and check your work.

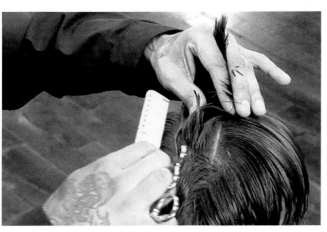 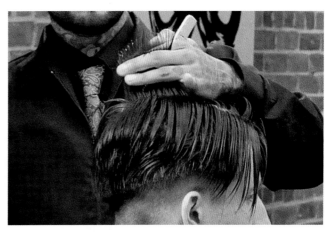

14 While maintaining a side position, create a ¼-inch parting parallel to the center guide. Comb and overdirect the parting to the center top guide for cutting.

15 Continue overdirecting the hair from the parietal area up to the top guide and cut until the length no longer reaches the top guide. Be sure to maintain clean sections and even tension, and cut flush to this guideline at all times.

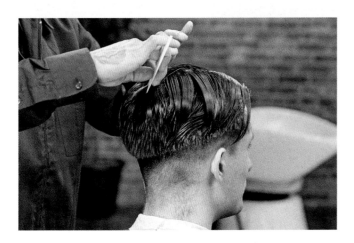

16 Move behind the client and comb the hair back. Create a ¼-inch parallel parting just to the right of the center panel on the right side. Return to the side standing position.

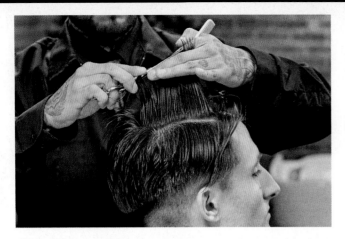

17 Comb through both the parallel parting and center panel to create a slight overdirection of the parting to the center top guide. Cut the parting to the guide.

18 Continue cutting the hair from the parietal area up to the top.

19 Move behind the client and comb through the top sections to check the hair horizontally and blend as needed.

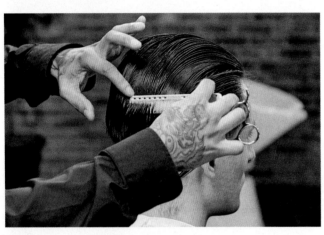

20 Comb through the top section and just above the occipital area; take a vertical parting from the center back.

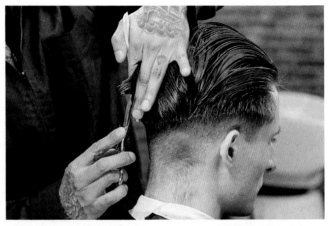

21 Project the parting to 90 degrees; using the shortest length at the occipital as a guide, cut and blend the shorter back area with the longer crown section.

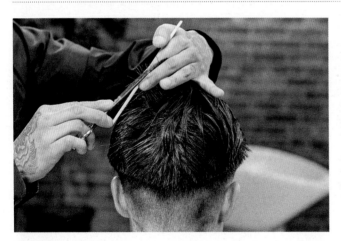

22 Pivot through the crown section as you cut and blend the hair from the back into the left-side area.

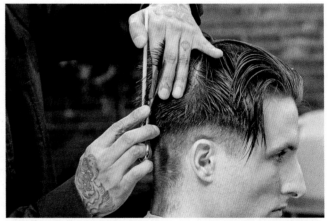

23 Return to the center back to cut and blend toward the right side.

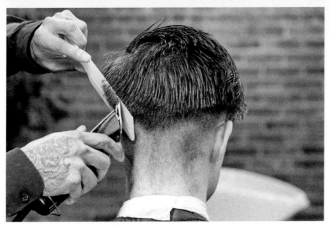

24 Use the clipper-over-comb or freehand technique with the appropriate clipper blade size to fade and blend shorter lengths to longer lengths in the top sections.

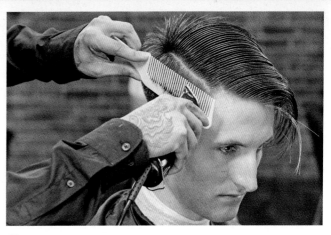

25 Move to the side sections and blend through the parietal ridge as needed.

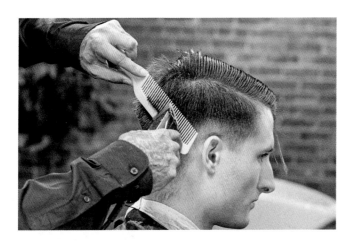

26 Finish blending the back section using a combination of clipper-over-comb, shear-over-comb, or freehand clipper techniques as you prefer.

27 To fine-tune your work, dampen the hair and recheck the blending from the hairline through the parietal ridge and around the head.

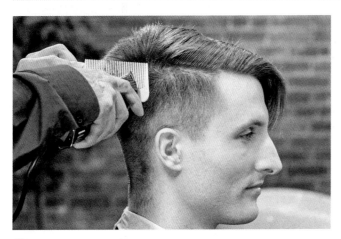

28 Tighten the blend and fade at the sides and back according to the desired length, hair texture, and growth pattern as necessary.

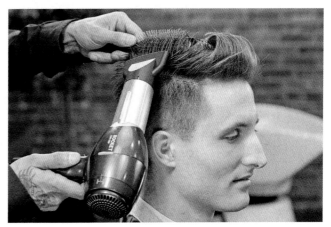

29 To style, re-mist the hair if necessary and apply a light gel product. Overdirect the hair over the curve of the head while drying. Be sure to follow the brush with the dryer heat from the scalp to the ends. While applying the heat, roll the hair and turn the ends under to create a finished look.

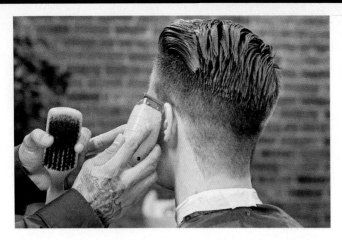

30 Reapply styling product as needed and comb the hair into place.

31 Use an outliner to define the hairline and perform a neck shave if requested by your client.

32 Perform final cleanup, remove any stray hair clippings, and show your client the results in the mirror.

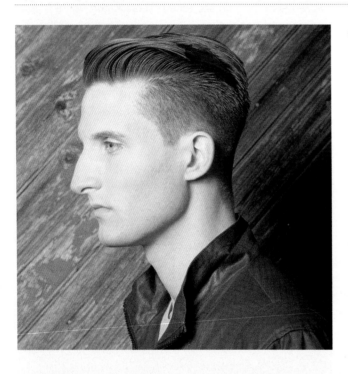

33 Finished pompadour fade.

CLEAN-UP AND DISINFECTION

☐ Clean and disinfect the tools and implements.

☐ Clean surfaces and chair.

☐ Sweep up hair and deposit in closed receptacle.

☐ Dispose of single-use items. Place all used linens, towels, and capes in the laundry.

☐ Wash your hands.

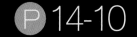

FADE WITH STAR DESIGN

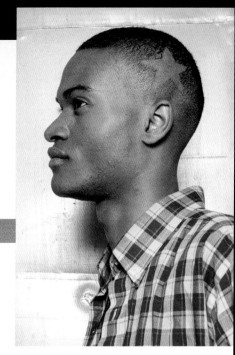

Following are important general notes for this procedure:

☐ Do not cut the hair too low when doing design work as you will need the length for blending around the design.

☐ The star represents the two arms, two legs, and head of the body.

MATERIALS, IMPLEMENTS, AND EQUIPMENT

☐ All-purpose, taper, and flat top combs, picks, etc.

☐ Blowdryer

☐ Clipper disinfectant and coolant

☐ Clippers and outliners

☐ Disposable barber towels

☐ Hair clips

☐ Hair pattern pencils

☐ Hand mirror

☐ Neck strips

☐ Shampoo and conditioner

☐ Shampoo cape and haircutting cape

☐ Shaving cream or gel

☐ Shears and blending shears

☐ Spray bottle with water

☐ Straight razor and blades

☐ Styling brushes

☐ Styling products

☐ Talc

☐ Terry cloth towels

PREPARATION

1. Wash your hands.

2. Conduct a client consultation.

3. Drape the client for wet service.

4. Shampoo and towel dry the hair.

5. Remove waterproof cape; replace with a neck strip and haircutting cape.

6. Face client toward the mirror and lock the chair.

PROCEDURES

A. THE DESIGN: BASIC 5-POINT STAR DESIGN ★

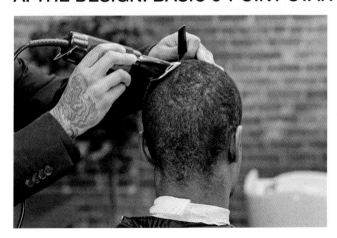

1. To begin, cut all hair to a uniform length (quo vadis or even-all-over cut).

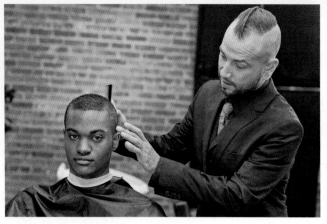

2 Decide the placement and size of the star based on the shape of the head and client's desires.

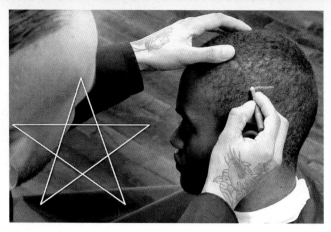

3 Use a hair pencil to draw the design on your client's head.

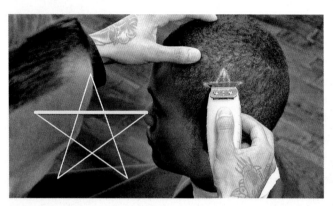

4 Use outliner with T-blade to establish the shape guidelines. Cut in a horizontal line to the desired width of the "arms" of the star.

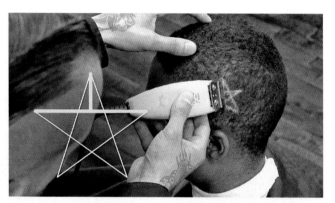

5 Find the center point of the horizontal line. Cut in a vertical line that is half the length of the horizontal line to create a shape similar to an upside-down "T." The vertical line becomes the center point of the "head" of the star; the horizontal line becomes the "arms."

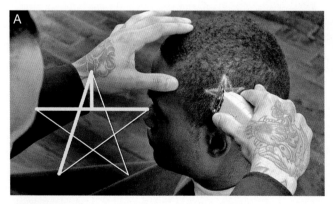

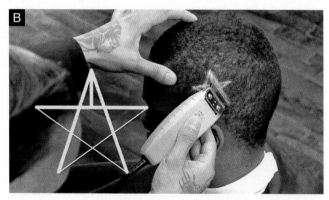

6 Using the top point of the vertical line as the center guide, you will cut in an upside-down "V" the same *length* as the *width* of the horizontal line.

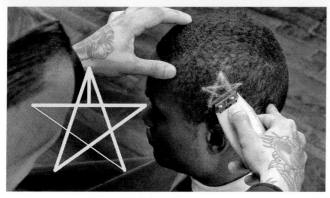

⑦ Position the T-blade on an angle from the ends of the left line of the "V" to the end of the horizontal line on the right to create the left "leg."

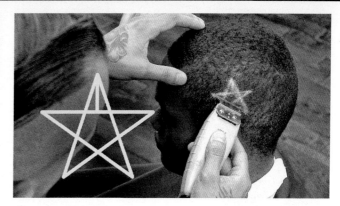

⑧ Position the T-blade on an angle from the ends of the right line of the "V" to the end of the horizontal line on the left to create the right "leg."

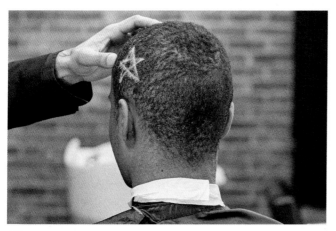

⑨ Star outline is now complete.

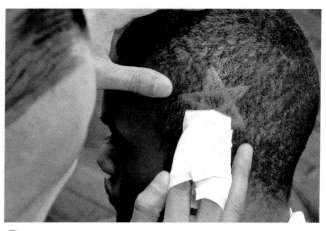

⑩ Gently remove pencil residue to check star outline.

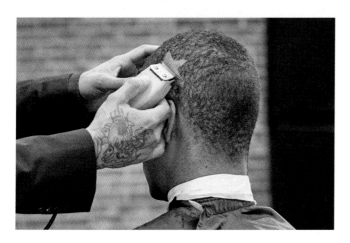

⑪ Use T-blade and/or razor to cut remaining hair within the design.

Design Option: Trace a neat line around the points of the star to add more depth to the design.

B. FADING AND BLENDING

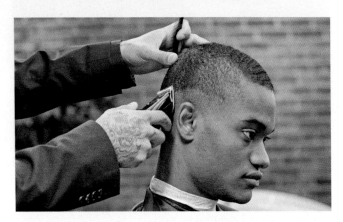

12 Fade the back and sides to desired length and level of blending areas.

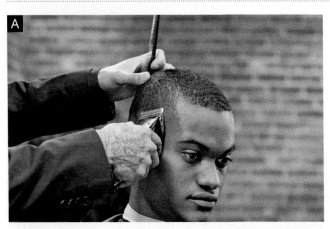

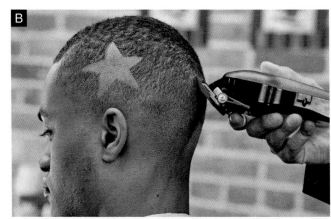

13 Blend transition areas without lines or gaps from the faded areas into the longer top section.

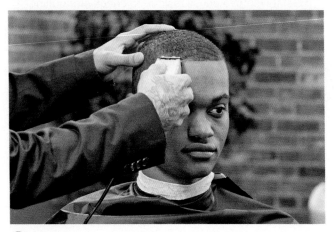

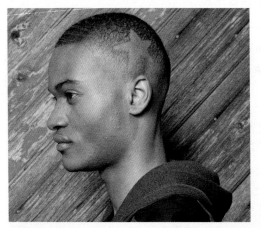

14 Outline the cut and complete neck shave or outline shave as requested by the client.

15 Finished fade with star design style.

CLEAN-UP AND DISINFECTION

☐ Wash and disinfect tools and implements.

☐ Clean surfaces and chair.

☐ Sweep up hair and deposit in closed receptacle.

☐ Dispose of single-use items. Place all used linens, towels, and capes in the laundry.

☐ Wash your hands.

SHADOW FADE CUT

This procedure should be performed using an adjustable-blade clipper with and without guards.

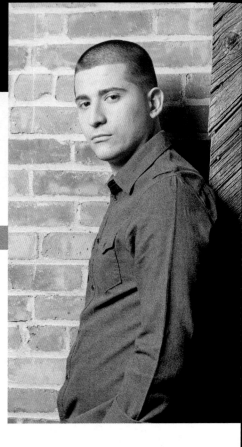

MATERIALS, IMPLEMENTS, AND EQUIPMENT

- All-purpose, taper, and flat top combs, picks, etc.
- Blowdryer
- Clipper disinfectant and coolant
- Clippers and outliners
- Disposable barber towels
- Hair clips
- Hand mirror
- Neck strips
- Shampoo and conditioner

- Shampoo cape and haircutting cape
- Shaving cream or gel
- Shears and blending shears
- Spray bottle with water
- Straight razor and blades
- Styling brushes
- Styling products
- Talc
- Terry cloth towels

PREPARATION

1. Wash your hands.
2. Conduct a client consultation.
3. Drape the client for wet service.
4. Shampoo and towel dry the hair.
5. Remove the waterproof cape; replace with a neck strip and haircutting cape.
6. Face the client toward the mirror and lock the chair.

PROCEDURE

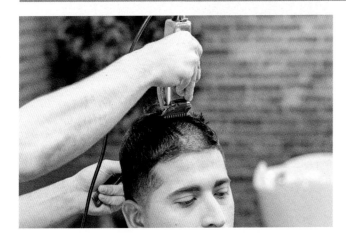

1. Determine the length to be left in the top section and select the appropriate clipper blade or guard and adjustable blade level. Start at the front hairline and cut the center guide back to the crown.

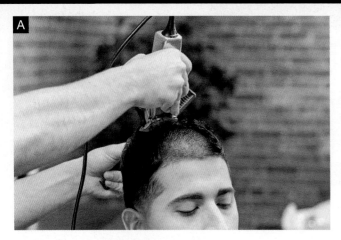

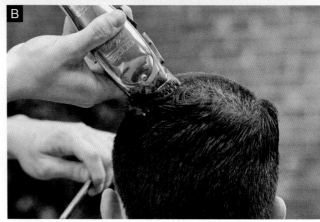

② Cut the sections right and left of center from the front through the top section and into the crown (A and B).

③ Move to the back section and adjust the clippers to the open blade position. Start at the hairline at the center of the nape, cutting against the grain to the mid-occipital area to establish a horizontal guide.

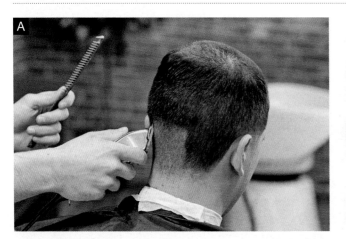

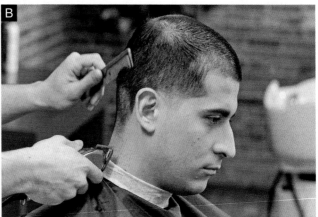

④ Cut the sections left and right of the center panel through the back section to the guide (A and B).

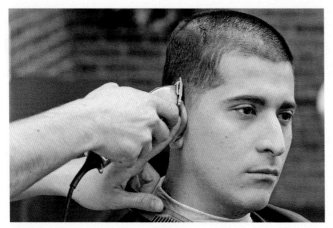

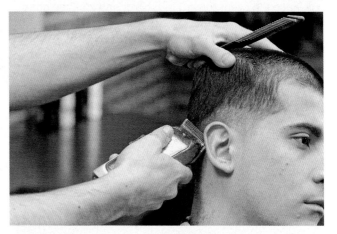

⑤ Move to the side and cut from the hairline to the top, middle, or bottom of the crest area as desired by the client.

⑥ Cut the remaining hair on the side to this guide, connecting it with the guide in the back section.

⑦ Cut around the ear and blend into the previously cut back section, cutting up and/or across, as the growth pattern allows. Repeat this procedure on the opposite side.

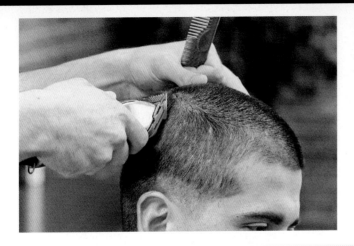

8 When the back and sides are cut, attach the guard and close the blades halfway. Blend the hair at the top of the parietal ridge into the top section around the entire head, leaving the middle transition area.

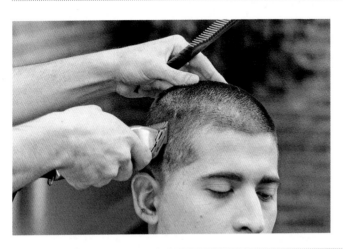

9 Adjust the blades to the closed position and repeat the blending technique through the middle parietal section.

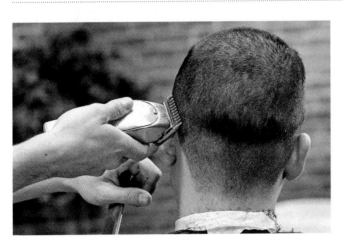

10 Attach a No. 0 guard and adjust the blades to the half-closed position. Blend around the entire parietal ridge to remove the weight line of the remaining hair.

REMINDER

Cutting against the grain achieves a closer cut than cutting with the grain. Procedure 14-11 shows one method to achieve a shadow fade cut. Be guided by your instructor for different techniques and fade style variations.

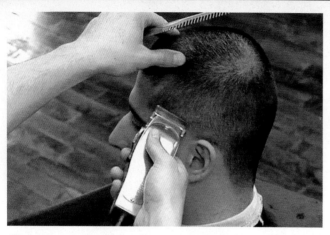
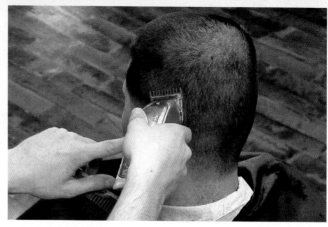

11 Adjust the blades to the closed position and blend any remaining weight around the entire head.

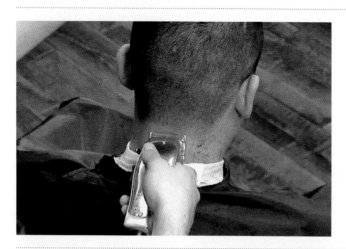

12 Remove the guard; with the blades in the open position, taper and blend the hairline along the perimeter.

13 Finish with the trimmer and/or outline shave to define the hairline.

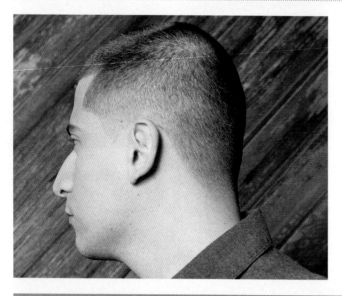

14 The haircut is now complete. Dust or vacuum stray hairs, making sure none remains on the client's face or neck.

CLEAN-UP AND DISINFECTION

□ Clean and disinfect the tools and implements.
□ Clean and then disinfect the work area.
□ Sweep up hair and deposit in a closed receptacle.
□ Deposit used blades in a sharps container.

□ Dispose of single-use items. Place all used linens, towels, and capes in the laundry.
□ Wash your hands.

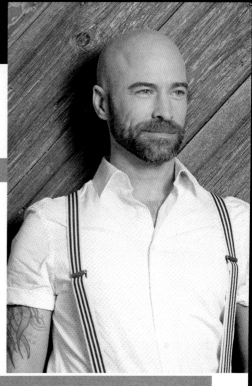

THE HEAD SHAVE

MATERIALS, IMPLEMENTS, AND EQUIPMENT

- ☐ All-purpose, taper, and flat top combs, picks, etc.
- ☐ Clipper disinfectant and coolant
- ☐ Clippers and outliners
- ☐ Disposable barber towels
- ☐ Hand mirror
- ☐ Neck strips
- ☐ Shampoo and conditioner

- ☐ Shampoo cape and haircutting cape
- ☐ Shaving cream or gel
- ☐ Spray bottle with water
- ☐ Straight razor and blades
- ☐ Talc
- ☐ Terry cloth towels
- ☐ Witch hazel or skin toner

PREPARATION

1. Wash your hands.
2. Conduct a client consultation.
3. Drape the client for a haircut.
4. Face the client toward the mirror and lock the chair.

PROCEDURE

1. Examine the scalp for any abrasions, primary or secondary lesions, or scalp disorders.

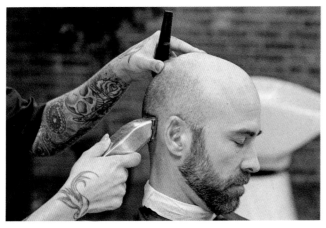

2. Remove excess hair length with the clippers if necessary; enough hair needs to remain for the razor to remove it without injuring the surface of the scalp.

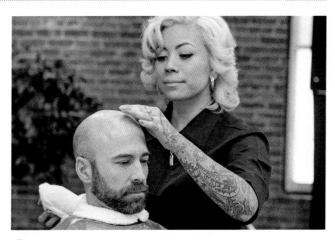

3. Drape the client for a wet service and shampoo the remaining hair; reexamine the scalp.

4. Remove the shampoo cape. Re-drape the client with a haircutting cape and towels under and over the drape. Tuck a wiping cloth into the neckline of the drape.

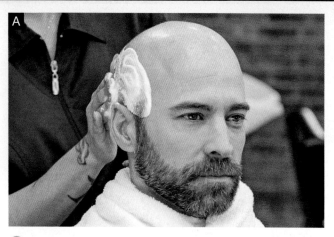

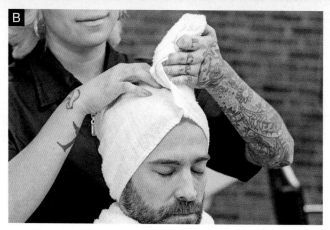

5 Apply shaving cream or gel and lather. Follow with two or three steamed-towel treatments to soften the remaining hair.

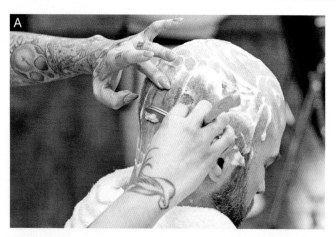

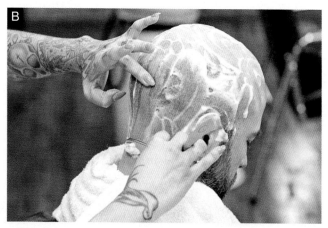

6 Re-lather the client's scalp and lock the chair. Start in the back section using a freehand stroke to shave with the grain of the hair from the crown to the nape. Use your opposite hand to stretch the skin taut as needed for each area to be shaved. Follow the curve of the head as you shave the entire back section.

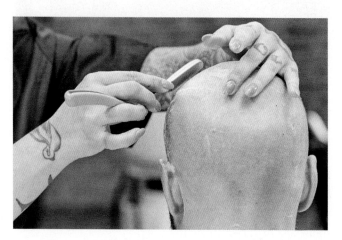

7 Move in front of the client and tip his head forward slightly. Continue shaving from the crown to the front hairline, reapplying lathering agent as needed. Remember to keep the skin moist to facilitate shaving.

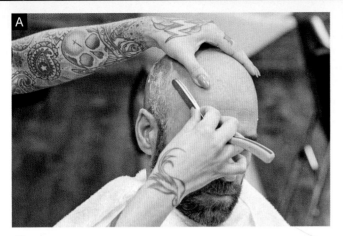

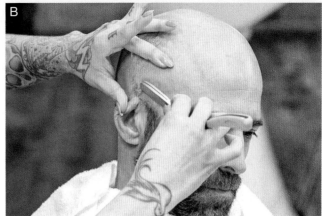

8 When the top section is completed, work down the sides. Just below the crest, hold the ear out of the way with the left hand, finish shaving the side, and carefully shave in front of and around the ears.

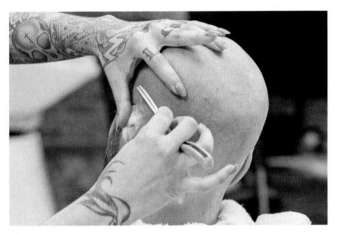

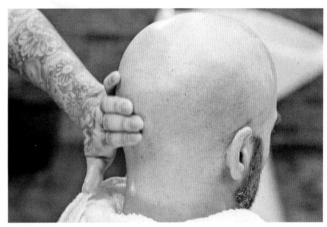

9 Repeat the shaving procedure on client's left side.

10 Check for any missed areas and re-shave as necessary.

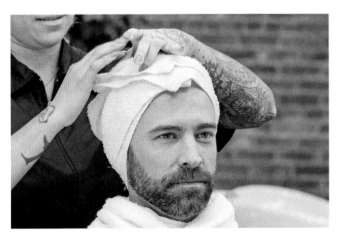

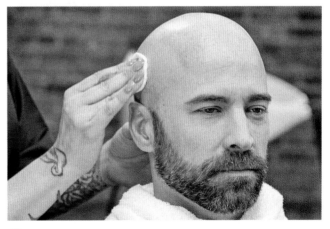

11 Wrap a warm towel around the client's head; then use it to remove any remaining lather.

12 Apply witch hazel or skin toner, and follow with a cool-towel application for 2 to 3 minutes.

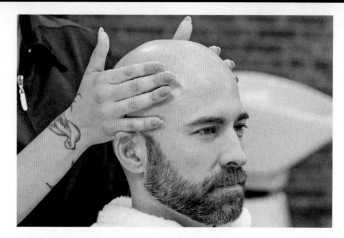

13 Apply moisturizing cream or oil as requested.

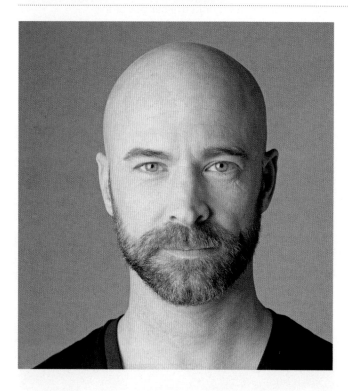

14 Finished head shave.

CLEAN-UP AND DISINFECTION

☐ Clean and disinfect the tools and implements.

☐ Clean and then disinfect the work area.

☐ Sweep up hair and deposit in a closed receptacle.

☐ Deposit used blades in a sharps container.

☐ Dispose of single-use items. Place all used linens, towels, and capes in the laundry.

☐ Wash your hands.

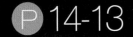

BLOWDRYING TECHNIQUES

MATERIALS, IMPLEMENTS, AND EQUIPMENT

☐ All-purpose, taper, and flat top combs, picks, etc.

☐ Blowdryer and diffuser

☐ Disposable barber towels

☐ Hand mirror

☐ Neck strips

☐ Shampoo and conditioner

☐ Shampoo cape and haircutting cape

☐ Spray bottle with water

☐ Styling brush

☐ Talc

☐ Terry cloth towels

PREPARATION

1. Wash your hands.

2. Conduct a client consultation.

3. Drape the client for wet service.

4. Shampoo and towel dry the hair.

5. Remove the waterproof cape; replace with a neck strip and haircutting cape.

6. Face the client toward the mirror and lock the chair.

PROCEDURES

A. FREEFORM

1. Hold the dryer 6 to 10 inches from the hair at an angle with the nozzle pointing downward.

2. Dry the layers underneath first, moving the dryer briskly from side to side to dry the hair.

3. As the hair underneath is dried, release the next layered section from the comb or brush and dry.

4. Comb or brush the hair down after each section is dried.

5. Dry the sides in the same manner.

6. Dry the top loosely and comb or brush into desired style.

B. STYLIZED

1. Begin in the back section, lifting a section of hair with the comb or brush.

2. Follow the movement of the comb or brush with the dryer to apply a concentrated stream of heated air to the section. Dry from scalp to ends.

3. Repeat the process until the hair is dry in that section.

4. Move to the next section and sides to repeat the process.

C. BLOW WAVING

1. Use the blow-waving technique to create lift or direction in the top section.

2. Work from the natural part, parting off a section with the comb or brush.

3. Elevate the hair to create the desired fullness and follow with the blowdryer.

4. To create definite direction in the front section, insert the comb or brush about 1½ inches from the hairline.

5. Draw the comb or brush a little to the back and then toward the hairline in one motion. This will create a ridge or bend in the hair that will set it in a different direction.

6. Apply dryer heat across the section until a soft ridge has been formed.

7. Repeat to subsequent sections in the top and crest areas as needed.

8. Apply a suitable styling aid to finish the styling service.

D. DIFFUSED

1. Pick the hair out into the basic shape of the desired style.

2. Begin drying in the back section, working toward the crown and sides.

3. Gently pick the hair out as the dryer is moved from section to section.

4. Dry the sides in the same manner.

5. Dry the top section forward from the crown, picking the hair out as each area is dried.

6. Apply a suitable styling aid to complete the styling service.

CLEAN-UP AND DISINFECTION

☐ Clean and disinfect the tools and implements.

☐ Clean and then disinfect the work area.

☐ Sweep up hair and deposit in a closed receptacle.

☐ Deposit used blades in a sharps container.

☐ Dispose of single-use items. Place all used linens, towels, and capes in the laundry.

☐ Wash your hands.

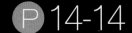
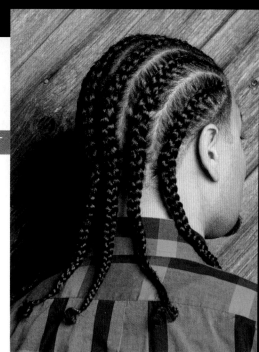

CORNROW BRAIDING

MATERIALS, IMPLEMENTS, AND EQUIPMENT

- ☐ Blowdryer and diffuser
- ☐ Disposable barber towels
- ☐ Essential oil scalp product
- ☐ Hair clips
- ☐ Hand mirror
- ☐ Neck strips
- ☐ Oil sheen spray
- ☐ Rubber bands
- ☐ Shampoo and conditioner
- ☐ Shampoo cape and haircutting cape
- ☐ Tail comb, wide-toothed comb, pick, etc.
- ☐ Terry cloth towels

PREPARATION

1. Wash your hands.
2. Conduct a client consultation.
3. Drape the client for wet service.
4. Shampoo and condition the client's hair.
5. Remove the waterproof cape; replace with towels under and over the haircutting cape.
6. Face the client toward the mirror and lock the chair.

PROCEDURES

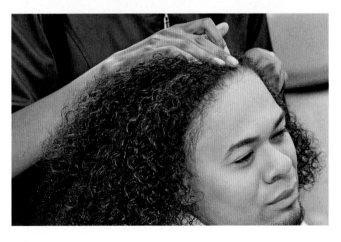

1. Start with clean, damp hair. Apply and massage essential oil to the scalp.
2. Determine the correct size and direction of the cornrow base.

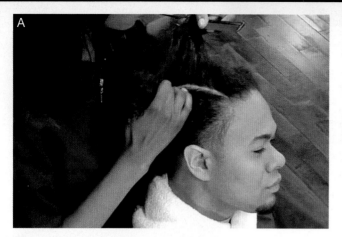

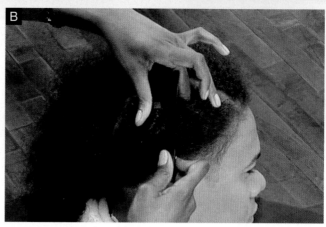

3 Use a tail comb to part off the top section of hair on the right side from front to nape. Secure the section with a clip.

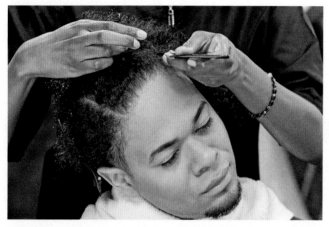

4 Use the mirror to determine where to section off the left side of the top section and secure with a clip.

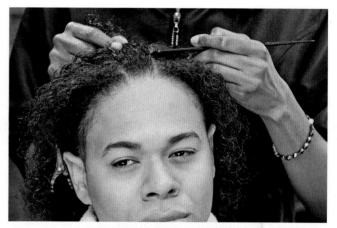

5 Create two parallel partings in the center of the top section to form a neat row for the cornrow base.

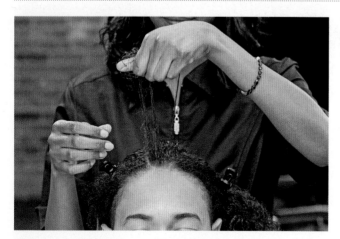

6 Divide the parting into three strands.

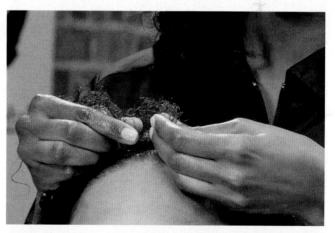

7 Place your fingers close to the base and cross the left strand under the center strand.

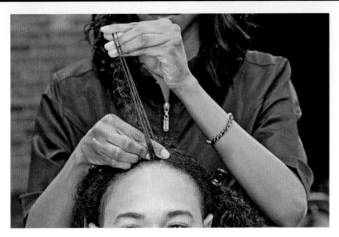

8 Cross the right strand under the center strand.

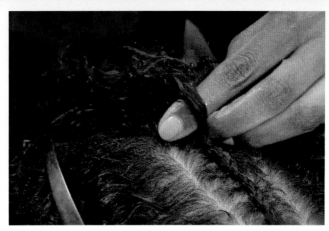

9 With each crossing under, pick up hair from the base of the panel and add it to the outer strand before crossing it under the center strand.

10 When you have finished the braid, secure the hair ends with a small rubber band.

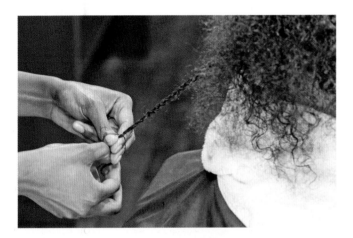

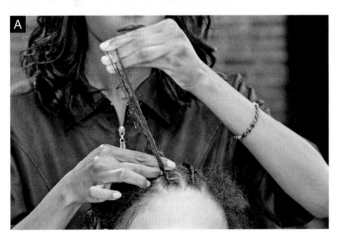

11 Braid subsequent panels left and right of the center braid in the same manner.

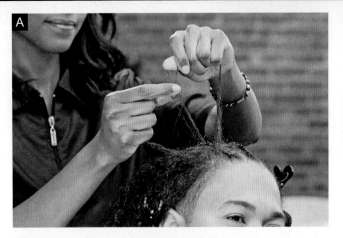

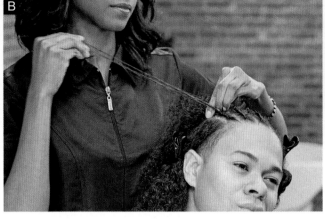

12 Once you have completed the top three braids, complete the braids on the left and right side of the head, maintaining even tension and following the curvature of the head.

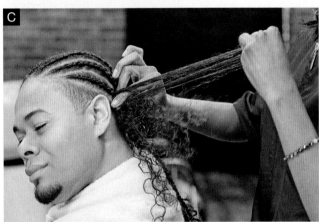

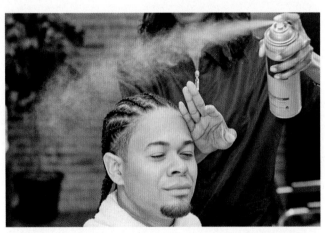

13 Finish with oil sheen or an appropriate styling aid for a finished look.

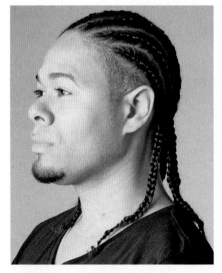

14 Finished cornrow braids.

CLEAN-UP AND DISINFECTION

☐ Clean and disinfect the tools and implements.

☐ Clean and then disinfect the work area.

☐ Sweep up hair and deposit in closed receptacle.

☐ Dispose of single-use items. Place all used linens, towels, and capes in the laundry.

☐ Wash your hands.

STARTING LOCKS WITH NUBIAN COILS

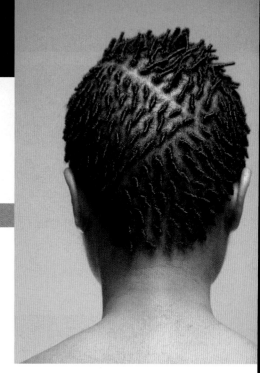

MATERIALS, IMPLEMENTS, AND EQUIPMENT

- ☐ Barber's comb
- ☐ Four butterfly clips
- ☐ Holding gel
- ☐ Hood dryer
- ☐ Leave-in conditioner
- ☐ Long duckbill clips
- ☐ Natural botanical oil
- ☐ Shampoo cape
- ☐ Sulfate-free moisturizing shampoo
- ☐ Wide-tooth comb

PREPARATION

1. Wash your hands.
2. Conduct a client consultation.
3. Drape the client for wet service.
4. Shampoo and condition the client's hair.
5. Remove the waterproof cape; replace with towels under and over the haircutting cape.
6. Face the client toward the mirror and lock the chair.

PROCEDURE

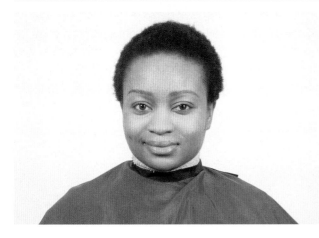

1. Drape the client for a shampoo service. If necessary, comb and detangle the hair.
2. Cleanse the hair with sulfate-free shampoo; then condition and rinse.
3. Spray a leave-in conditioner and detangle with a wide-tooth comb.
4. Apply a natural botanical oil to the scalp and massage the oil into the scalp.
5. Detangle and divide the hair into two sections.
6. Clip the hair for control.

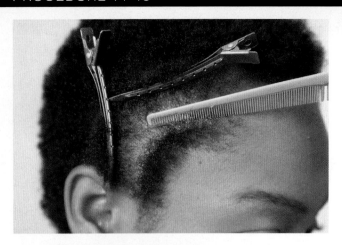

7 To create movement, start at the hairline and create a crescent-shape part with the smaller end of the comb. Apply gel to the tip of the comb.

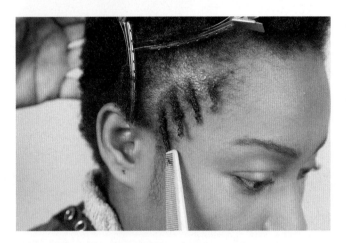

8 Comb the gel through the entire parted section. At the base, start to rotate or roll-comb with a clockwise rotation, down the hair shaft to the end. The hair is curled toward the end and the coil lies flat on the scalp.

9 Using the comb, twirl the hair and place the coil end in the direction you would like the hair to lie.

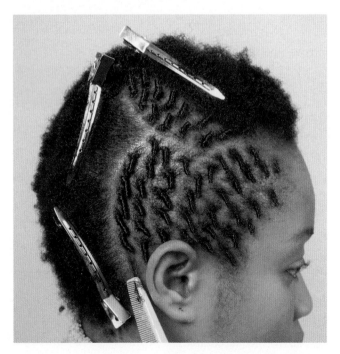

10 As you move up and around the head, create a sculpting movement that features the head contour.

11 The movement can be made in multiple directions with dimension. For example, the entire back will move forward from the center back toward the front on both sides, while the top will move upward and forward. Positioning the comb and directing the hair upward will give a different directional movement to the top crown.

12 Once the right back section to front section is complete, start on the right side, twirling the comb toward the front of the head in a counterclockwise rotation.

13 The coil style has one continuous movement from front to back.

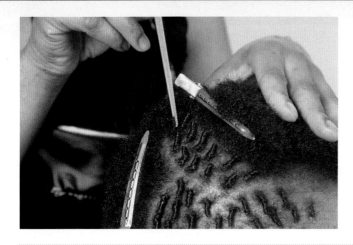

14 Continue the coil movement at crown, keeping the contours and directions of coil uniform, directing from back to front in an upward and forward direction. The coils will lie flat and point upward.

15 While front coils are still damp, fine-tune their direction and make a soft bang.

16 Place the client under the dryer. Add oil for more sheen.

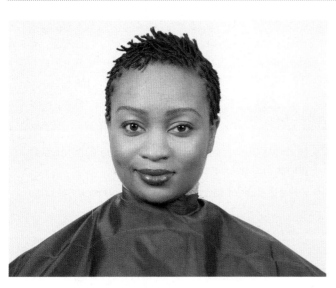

17 Finish the style.

CLEAN-UP AND DISINFECTION

☐ Clean and disinfect the tools and implements.

☐ Clean and then disinfect the work area.

☐ Sweep up hair and deposit in closed receptacle.

☐ Dispose of single-use items. Place all used linens, towels, and capes in the laundry.

☐ Wash your hands.

CULTIVATING AND GROOMING LOCKS

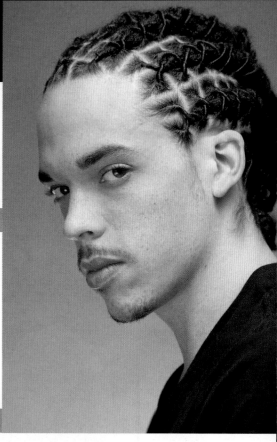

MATERIALS, IMPLEMENTS, AND EQUIPMENT

☐ Box of small two-pronged roller clips

☐ Five butterfly clips

☐ Herbal rinse

☐ Hood dryer

☐ Natural botanical oil and light moisturizing conditioner

☐ Shampoo cape

☐ Steamer

☐ Sulfate-free shampoo

☐ Tapered barber's comb

☐ Water-soluble gel

PREPARATION

1. Wash your hands.

2. Conduct a client consultation.

3. Drape the client for wet service.

4. Shampoo and condition the client's hair.

5. Remove the waterproof cape; replace with towels under and over the haircutting cape.

6. Face the client toward the mirror and lock the chair.

PROCEDURE

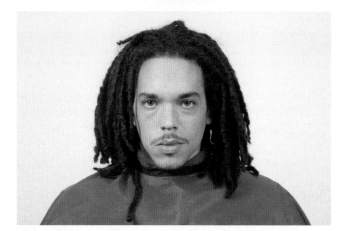

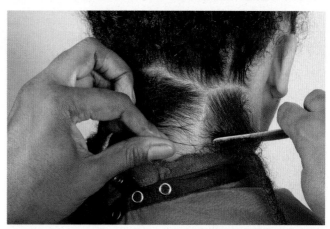

1. Drape the client for a shampoo service.

2. Cleanse the hair and scalp with a sulfate-free conditioner.

3. Add light moisturizing conditioner, steam, and then rinse the locks.

4. Apply oil to the scalp and entire length of the lock, and massage the scalp.

5. Starting at the base of the neck, use the larger end of the barber's comb to square off new growth of locked hair, creating a clean part.

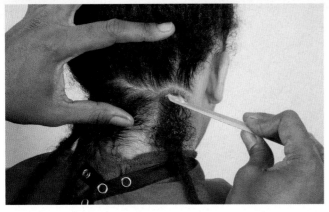

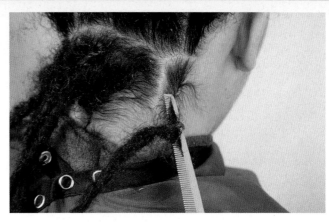

6 With the smaller end of comb, apply gel to the comb. Place a small amount of gel at the new growth base of each lock.

7 Pull down all the loose hair together into the lock with a comb and gel. This step compacts the loose hair and builds the lock base. Rotate the comb once.

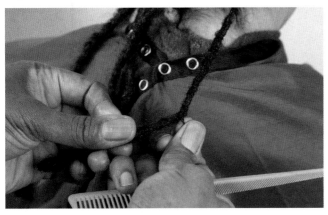

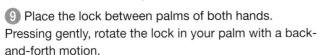

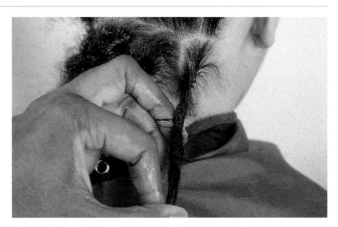

8 Remove the comb, and, using two fingers (index finger and thumb), push loose hair together and smooth and then roll hair between fingers.

9 Place the lock between palms of both hands. Pressing gently, rotate the lock in your palm with a back-and-forth motion.

10 Move down the entire length of the lock, palm rolling to smooth the loose hair into the lock.

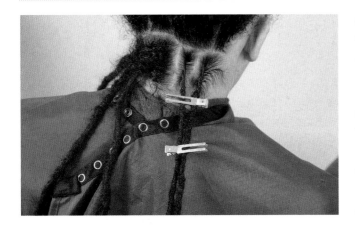

11 Clip off each section at the base if needed and along the length of the lock with a small clip or a large duck tail, as you complete palm rolling the locks. Continue grooming the entire head and place under a dryer to dry the locks completely.

12 Once you complete the entire back section, continue to the right and left sides of the head and save the crown section for last.

13 Place the client under the hood dryer until locks are completely dry.

15 Remove the clips and then apply natural botanical oil on the locks for additional shine.

16 Place the client under a hood dryer for 30 to 40 minutes until the locks are completely dry.

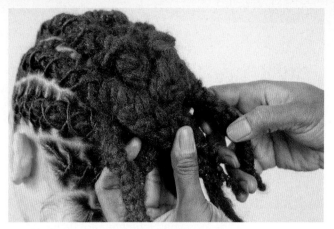

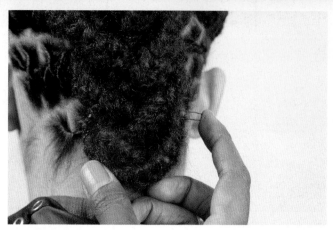

17 For dimensional styling, gather several locks and braid damp hair to create crimped locks; or, after removal from the dryer, cornrow the entire head of locks with 8 to 10 cornrows. Secure the ends with elastic bands.

18 Take the braided locks and create a fishtail braid. Secure with elastic band and tuck the fishtail under. Secure with hair pins.

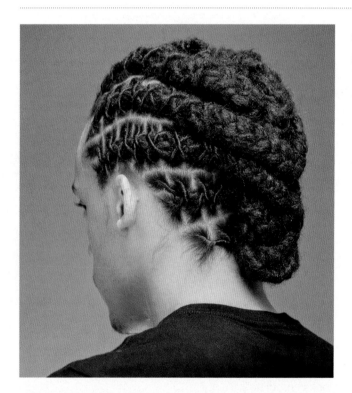

19 Spray locks with oil shine.

20 Finish the style.

CLEAN-UP AND DISINFECTION

☐ Clean and disinfect the tools and implements.

☐ Clean and then disinfect the work area.

☐ Sweep up hair and deposit in closed receptacle.

☐ Dispose of single-use items. Place all used linens, towels, and capes in the laundry.

☐ Wash your hands.

REVIEW QUESTIONS

1. Explain what a good haircut and style should accomplish.

2. What should a client consultation be able to tell you about the client's desired haircut and style?

3. List seven facial shapes.

4. What anatomical features influence haircutting and styling and what are the physical considerations that help to determine the best haircut and style for an individual?

5. Explain the process of envisioning.

6. List the sections of the head form as they apply to men's haircutting.

7. List design elements used in haircutting and styling.

8. List and define the basic haircutting terms used in haircutting and styling.

9. List cutting techniques used in men's haircutting.

10. Explain why the hair should be in a damp condition for razor cutting.

11. Describe the razor-rotation technique.

12. Explain the braiding technique used to create cornrows.

13. Define *hairlocking*.

14. Why do state barber boards most often require a licensure candidate to perform a taper cut during the practical exams?

CHAPTER GLOSSARY

angle (ANG-gul)	p. 397	the space between two lines or surfaces that intersect at a given point; in haircutting, the hair is held away from the head to create an angle of elevation
arching (ARE-ching)	p. 424	method used to cut around the ears and down the sides of the neck
balance (BAL-uns)	p. 396	the equal or appropriate proportions that create symmetry and harmony in a design
blowdry styling (BLOH-dry sti-hyl-ing)	p. 418	technique of drying and styling damp hair in one process
clipper-over-comb (KLIP-uhr-OH-ver-KOHM)	p. 405	cutting over a comb with the clippers
crest (KREST)	p. 393	the widest area of the head, also known as the parietal ridge, temporal region, hatband, or horseshoe
cross-checking (KRAWS-CHEK-ing)	p. 398	the process of parting off subsections opposite from the elevation or direction at which they were cut to check the precision of cutting lines or blending
curved lines (KURVD LYNZ)	p. 396	lines that move in a semicircular or circular direction
cutting above the fingers (KUT-ing AH-bov THE FING-erz)	p. 403	cutting of the hair is performed on the outside of the fingers; used with horizontal or vertical 90-degree projections of hair
cutting below the fingers (KUT-ing BE-low THE FING-erz)	p. 403	cutting of the hair is below or performed on the inside of the fingers; used in 0- and 45-degree elevation cutting
cutting line (KUT-ing LYN)	p. 400	the position of the fingers when cutting a section of hair

cutting palm-to-palm	p. 403	cutting of the hair is performed with the palms of both hands facing each other; an alternative method used in layering vertical or horizontal sections of hair
design line (dee-ZYN LYN)	p. 400	usually the perimeter line of a haircut
diagonal lines (dye-AG-ih-nul LYNZ)	p. 396	lines positioned between horizontal and vertical lines
elevation (el-uh-VAY-shun)	p. 398	angle or degree at which a subsection of hair is held, or elevated, from the head when cutting; also referred to as projection
envision (EN-vijg-ohn)	p. 386	the ability to picture or see something in your mind
facial shape (FAY-shul SHAYP)	p. 387	oval, round, inverted triangular, square, oblong, diamond, and pear-shaped are the seven facial shapes
fingers-and-razor cutting (FING-erz-AND-RAY-zur KUT-ing)	p. 408	cutting technique performed by holding the hair section between the fingers and cutting either from the top to the bottom of the section or from one side to the other; also known as *freehand slicing* with a razor
fingers-and-shear (FING-erz-AND-SHEER)	p. 403	technique used to cut hair by holding the hair into a position to be cut
form (FORM)	p. 396	the outline or shape of a design
freehand clipper cutting (FREE-HAND KLIP-ur KUT-ing)	p. 405	generally interpreted to mean that guards are not used in the cutting process
freehand shear cutting (FREE-HAND SHEER KUT-ing)	p. 405	cutting with shears without the use of fingers or a comb to control the hair
freehand slicing (FREE-HAND sly-SING)	p. 408	method of removing bulk from a hair section with the shears
guide (GUYD)	p. 400	section of hair, located at either the perimeter or the interior of the cut, that determines the length the hair will be cut to; also referred to as a guideline; usually the first section that is cut to create a shape
hair locking (HAYR lock-ing)	p. 420	the process that occurs when coiled hair is allowed to develop in its natural state without the use of combs, heat, or chemicals
hairstyling (HAYR sti-hyl-ing)	p. 402	the art of arranging the hair in a particular style that is appropriately suited to the cut
horizontal lines (hor-ih-ZAHN-tul LYNZ)	p. 395	lines parallel to the horizon
layers (LAY-uhrz)	p. 401	graduated effect achieved by cutting the hair with elevation or overdirection; the hair is cut at higher elevations, usually 90 degrees or above, which removes weight
outlining (OWT-lyn-ing)	p. 401	finish work of a haircut with shears, trimmers, or razor
overdirection (OH-ver-dih-REK-shun)	p. 402	combing a section away from its natural falling position, rather than straight out from the head, toward a guideline; used to create increasing lengths in the interior or perimeter
parietal ridge (puh-RY-ate-uhl RIJ)	p. 393	widest area of the head, also known as the crest, hatband, horseshoe, or temporal region

part (PART)	p. 399	a line, created naturally or with a comb, that divides the hair at the scalp, separating one section of the hair from another
parting (PART-ing)	p. 399	a line dividing the hair of the scalp that separates one section of the hair from another or creates subsections from a larger section of hair
projection (pruh-JEK-shun)	p. 398	angle or elevation that hair is held at from the head for cutting
proportion (pruh-POR-shun)	p. 396	a design principle that measures or shows the comparative relationship between two or more design elements of a form
razor-over-comb (RAY-zur-OH-ver-KOHM)	p. 408	texturizing technique in which the comb and the razor are used on the surface of the hair
razor rotation (RAY-zur row-TAY-shun)	p. 408	texturizing technique similar to razor-over-comb, done with small circular motions
reference points (REF-err-ence POYNTZ)	p. 393	points on the head that mark where the surface of the head changes or the behavior of the hair changes, such as ears, jawline, occipital bone, and apex; used to establish design lines that are proportionate
rolling the comb out (ROHL-ing THE KOHM OUT)	p. 404	a method used to put the hair into position for cutting by combing into the hair with the teeth of the comb in an upward direction
shear-over-comb (SHEER-OH-ver-KOHM)	p. 403	haircutting technique in which the hair is held in place with the comb while the shears are used to remove length
shear-point tapering (SHEER-POYNT TAYP-uhr-ing)	p. 404	haircutting technique used to thin out difficult areas in the haircut, such as dips and hollows
stationary guide (STAY-shun-ar-ee GUYD)	p. 400	guideline that does not move, but all other hair is brought to it for cutting
taper (TAYP-uhr)	p. 401	haircuts in which there is an even blend from very short at the hairline to longer lengths as you move up the head; *to taper* is to narrow progressively at one end
tension (TEN-shun)	p. 401	amount of pressure applied when combing and holding a section, created by stretching or pulling the section
texturizing (TEKS-chur-yz-ing)	p. 401	removing excess bulk without shortening the length; changing the appearance or behavior of hair through specific haircutting techniques using shears, thinning shears, clippers, or a razor
thinning (THIN-ing)	p. 401	removing bulk from the hair
traveling guide (TRAV-ell-ing GUYD)	p. 400	guideline that moves as the haircutting progresses; used when creating layers or graduation; also referred to as moving or movable guidelines
vertical lines (VUR-tih-kuhl LYNZ)	p. 395	lines that are straight up and down
weight line (WAYT LYN)	p. 401	a visual line in the haircut, where the ends of the hair hang together; the line of maximum length within the weight area: heaviest perimeter area of a 0-degree (one-length) or 45-degree (graduated) cut

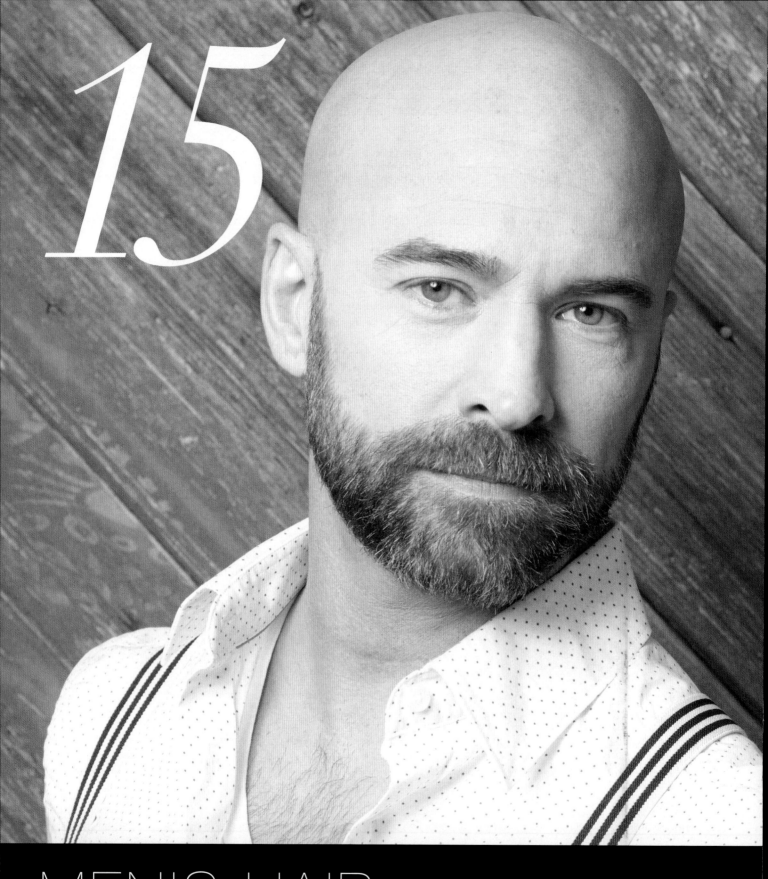

15

MEN'S HAIR REPLACEMENT

LEARNING OBJECTIVES

After completing this chapter, you will be able to:

LO❶
Discuss the reasons why men may purchase a hair replacement system.

LO❷
Understand the factors that influence hair replacement services.

LO❸
Discuss selling hair replacement systems.

LO❹
Discuss alternative hair replacement methods.

LO❺
Identify the types of hair used in hair replacement systems.

LO❻
Define stock and custom replacement systems.

LO❼
Recognize supplies needed to service hair replacement systems.

LO❽
Describe how to clean and service a hair replacement system.

LO❾
Describe how to fit and cut in a hair replacement system.

Introduction

After reading this section, you will be able to:

LO❶ Discuss the reasons why men may purchase a hair replacement system.

figure 15-1
Before hairpiece.

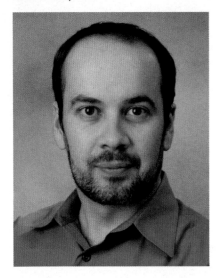

figure 15-2
After hairpiece.

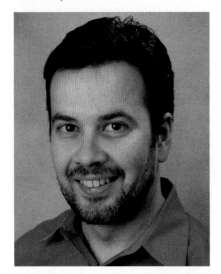

❓ DID YOU KNOW?

Ancient Greek physicians used onions applied directly to the scalp, while ancient Egyptians used castor oil, spider webs, and egg yolk to promote a cure for baldness.

From early Assyrian, Egyptian, and Roman times, hairpieces and wigs have been worn in an attempt to cover balding pates, as a part of ceremonial ritual, or in conformance with the prevailing fashion. False beards and mustaches, dreadlocks, full-bottom wigs, partial wigs, periwigs, side rolls, bobbed wigs, clubs, and queues all have played a role in history, from ancient times to the present. During the eighteenth century, the word **toupee** (too-PAY) was used to describe the front section of hair, also known as the foretop. This section of hair was grown long enough to cover the front part of the wig, which was placed farther back on the head in order to blend the natural hair with the artificial wig hair. Over time, the foretop was combed higher and extended back toward the crown until it became one long tail of hair. Over the years, the term *toupee* evolved to mean a small wig for men that covered the top or crown of the head, and still later the term *hairpiece* was adopted. Today, the industry uses the terms **hair replacement system** or **hair solution**. These changes in terminology are the result of new bonding technologies and continued improvements in the base designs of hair replacement products. The days of your father's toupees or *rugs* are over. No longer is the hairpiece placed on the wig stand at night, to be applied to the scalp in a morning ritual. In keeping with these changes in the industry, the terms *hair replacement system* and *hair solution* will be used interchangeably throughout this chapter.

For centuries, barbers were involved with the making and styling of wigs. Today, the care and fitting of men's hair replacement systems in the barbershop continues the traditions established so long ago. Although not all barbers choose to specialize in these services, the professional who can design, fit, and custom-cut a hair replacement system can open the door to increased clientele and financial gain.

Men wear hair replacement systems for a variety of personal reasons. Some men choose to cover their thinning or bald areas because they feel it makes them look younger. Others just might prefer to know how they look with more hair. Regardless of the motivation, men have several options when it comes to deciding how to achieve the *look* they want (**Figures 15-1** and **15-2**).

Hair replacement options range from topical applications of drugs such as minoxidil to hair replacement systems to surgical hair transplantation and scalp reduction. This chapter focuses primarily on men's hair replacement systems, with a brief discussion of other alternatives available to men with hair loss conditions.

why study
MEN'S HAIR REPLACEMENT?

Barbers should study and have a thorough understanding of hair replacement systems because:

> The thinning-hair market is one of the fastest growing categories in the industry, second only to haircoloring.

> Having an understanding of hair replacement helps to solve the problem in the marketplace. Given a choice most men would choose a healthy head of hair.

> A specialist in hair replacement systems can look to increased clientele and financial gain.

Mastering the Art of the Consultation

After reading this section, you will be able to:

LO ❷   Understand the factors that influence hair replacement services.

> **⚠ CAUTION**
>
> The loss of one's hair can be a very touchy and personal subject and should be approached very carefully. During your consultation, ask your client if he could change anything about his hair what would it be. This question can open up the conversation if he is looking for answers to his hair loss.

When discussing hair replacement with your client, you should be sure to take a very personal and private approach. The nature of hair loss is a very sensitive subject and should be discussed in private. If you have an office, take the client into the office away from other patrons; if not, make sure that it is just you and the client in the room. Be sure and discuss every option that is available in the industry, including surgery and low-light laser therapy; by offering all of these solutions, you instill confidence in the client that you have his best interest in mind. Take the time to explain the finer points of hair restoration, upkeep, bonding methods, and different hair solutions. Once you have decided what the best solution is for your client, give him your professional advice on what system will be best for his needs and budget. You can determine how many systems your client will need by his lifestyle, age, as well as the amount of money he is willing to spend. Create incentive programs with different types of systems and bonding methods. Give the client a choice as to how many systems and services he will receive in a year's period. Only after all this information has been discussed and all questions have been answered, should you ask for the sale.

Selling Hair Replacement Systems

After reading this section, you will be able to:

LO ❸   Discuss selling hair replacement systems.

In order to sell men's hair solutions, it is important to know why men buy them. As discussed in the first part of this chapter, men wear hair replacements for a variety of personal reasons. When a man expresses an interest in wearing a hair solution to his barber, he will not appreciate a hard-sell approach. His interest has already been made evident, and he is simply looking for guidance and purchasing information at this stage. It is the barber's responsibility to educate the client about the possibilities and options available to him.

Just as a hard-sell approach should be avoided, the barber should never promise what cannot be delivered, nor raise the client's expectations to an unreasonable level. For example, it is not professionally ethical to convince an elderly man that he can recapture the appearance of his 40s with a hair solution. It simply cannot be done. The color of the hair solution is also an important consideration. Dark, opaque colors are not recommended for any age group, especially older persons. It is better to recommend a salt-and-pepper blend or medium brown shade. The more natural looking the color, the less obvious the hair solution will appear.

SOCIAL MEDIA MARKETING TECHNIQUES

Use today's technology to reach your consumers. In today's world it is extremely important to master social media marketing. Take a look at the pages and websites from other successful businesses and see what they do to set themselves apart. If you need help in this area, you can hire a site developer or social media coordinator to help increase your online presence.

Start a fan page on a social networking platform, with before-and-after pictures of clients. It is best to do a picture without showing the model's face; and remember to always get permission to use the photos before you post them. Update your status on a daily basis with information about how hair replacement works, links to important articles, and any promotions you may be running.

HAIR REPLACEMENT SYSTEM DISPLAY

One or two correctly styled hair solutions displayed in the shop will alert clients to the fact that hair solution services are performed there. Make certain that the sample is clean and nicely styled. It should be large enough to cover the average balding area of a man, since most clients will be men with an average amount of hair loss, and many may want to try it on.

REFERRALS AND WORD OF MOUTH

Referrals and word of mouth may be a slower approach, and are not to be relied on exclusively for new business, but they still are very effective forms of advertising. Personal referrals are the best evidence of pleased and satisfied clients.

WINDOW DISPLAYS

Window displays can add to increased hair replacement sales. Before-and-after illustrations in the shop window let the walk-by and drive-by traffic know that hair replacement systems can be obtained through the barbershop. These illustrations can also offer encouragement to those clients whom you feel cannot be approached directly with the idea of wearing a

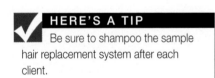

HERE'S A TIP
Be sure to shampoo the sample hair replacement system after each client.

hair solution. As they become more comfortable with the idea of a hair replacement or see other men in the shop receiving these services, they may feel more inclined to explore their own options.

PERSONAL APPROACH

The personal approach may certainly be used to suggest a hair replacement system to a client; however, it must be a tactful approach. Wait for an opening during the consultation or haircutting service, when the client brings up his hair loss condition in the conversation; then offer him the opportunity to try on a hair solution. A quick demonstration may convince him of his improved appearance and lead to a sale.

PRINT ADS

Print ads include all printed advertising, from coupons to billboards. It is important to advertise hair replacement services because not all barbershops pursue this market.

In some communities, newspaper advertising is inexpensive and profitable. If a model is used, be sure to secure a model release for any photos that might be used in the ads. Even if the model is your best friend, do not assume that a release is unnecessary.

PERSONAL EXPERIENCE

If you wear a hair replacement yourself, you can develop an excellent promotional approach. Often, nothing is more convincing than your own before-and-after demonstration. The fact that you wear a hair solution with assurance and complete ease can make a very strong impression on prospective hair replacement clients.

Understand Alternative Hair Replacement Methods

After reading this section, you will be able to:

LO④ Discuss alternative hair replacement methods.

In addition to hair replacement systems and hair solutions that can be applied in a barbershop, two other approaches are available: nonsurgical and surgical hair replacement options. It is important that you be aware of all replacement options available in order to fully gauge the client's needs.

NONSURGICAL ALTERNATIVE OPTIONS

Hair solutions are just one of the nonsurgical alternatives. The use of cover-up hair fibers has become a popular alternative that is quick and easy. The hair fibers are just shaken on to the hair and sprayed with a hair spray to hold them for the day.

Topical Medications for Hair Replacement

A 2 percent solution of **minoxidil** (MIN-ox-ih-dil) applied twice daily has been shown to be moderately effective for about 50 percent of the men using it. Clinical studies conducted by Pharmacia & Upjohn (a subsidiary of Pfizer and the maker of Rogaine-branded minoxidil) revealed that 26 percent of the men reported average-to-dense hair growth, and 33 percent reported minimal hair growth, after 4 months of treatment with Rogaine. Women's study results showed minimal regrowth in 40 percent of the women tested over an 8-month period. Minoxidil is available for both men and women in a 2 percent formula (regular strength) and for *men only* in a 5 percent formula (extra-strength).

Finasteride (fin-ASTER-eyed) is an oral medication that is prescribed only for men to stimulate hair growth. Although it is considered more effective and convenient than minoxidil, its potential side effects include weight gain and loss of sexual function.

Low-Light Laser Therapy

Low-light laser therapy, also known as laser hair enhancement, was approved by the FDA in 2007 for the promotion of healthy hair growth. Studies associated with this nonsurgical procedure report hair growth as a result of cold-beam, red-light laser treatments that stimulate or increase blood circulation and cell regeneration in the hair follicles. This service can be offered in the barbershop by purchasing a low-light laser machine from a manufacturer, providing your clients with another option for hair replacement.

SURGICAL HAIR RESTORATION

The three types of surgical hair restoration available are hair transplants, scalp reduction, and flap surgery.

1. **Hair transplantation** (HAYR TRANZ-plant-ay-shun) is strictly a medical procedure that should be performed only by licensed medical professionals. The process consists of removing hair from normal-growth areas of the scalp, such as the back and sides, and transplanting it into the bald areas under a local anesthetic. Small sections of hair ranging from single strands to larger plugs of 7 to 10 hairs are surgically removed, including the hair follicle, papilla, and hair bulb, and reset in the bald area. With today's technological advances in hair restoration, micrographs have replaced the larger plug sections of the past few decades. The transplanted hair usually grows normally in its new environment, while the area from which the hair was removed heals and shrinks in size to a very tiny scar.

   The surgeon must select the hair to be transplanted with care, taking into consideration color, texture, and type. Placement of the hair in the direction of natural growth to permit proper care and complementary styling is also an important factor. Transplanted hair can last a lifetime if the service is performed properly. If the doctor is skilled and the individual cares for the hair as directed, hair transplants can be very successful as a method of permanently eliminating baldness.

2. **Scalp reduction** (SKALP REE-duk-shun) is a process by which the bald area is removed from the scalp and surrounding scalp areas with hair growth pulled together to fill in the spot.

3. **Flap surgery** (flap SIR-jer-ee), like scalp reduction surgery, removes the bald scalp area. A flap of hair-bearing skin is then attached to what was the bald area.

Learn about Hair Replacement Systems

After reading this section, you will be able to:

LO**5** Identify the types of hair used in hair replacement systems.

LO**6** Define stock and custom replacement systems.

The quality of a hair replacement system varies with the kind of hair used in its manufacture and the way in which it is constructed. The barber is often the one to measure, fit, cut, and style the system once it has been received from the supplier.

HUMAN HAIR

Human hair is a desirable choice for a quality hair solution, although synthetic fibers can simulate the look and feel of human hair as well. The advantages of human hair include a more natural look and texture, durability, and the ability to tolerate chemical processes such as permanent waving and haircoloring. Some of the disadvantages associated with a human hair solution are that it reacts to climate changes, fades with exposure to light, requires styling maintenance, and can become damaged just as natural hair can.

Human hair solutions are usually cleaned with shampoo and conditioner formulated for hair replacement systems. Always follow the manufacturer's directions. In today's market, human hair has become the most popular choice when it comes to hair replacement. The combination of human hair and new base designs results in a natural-looking hair replacement system that is virtually undetectable.

Most of the human hair used in hair solutions is imported and must be prepared for use. The process usually includes chemical cleaning with an acid solution, sorting, and **hackling** (HAK-ling) (the process used to comb through the hair strands to separate them). However, most of the cuticle is removed in the processing of the hair. This means the hair becomes more like a fabric, so it should be treated as such. No harsh solvents or acetones should be used to clean the hair.

SYNTHETIC HAIR

Synthetic hair is used in the production of full wigs and some hair solutions. It is challenging to make synthetic hair that matches the texture of human hair, which makes it difficult to blend the piece with the client's natural hair.

Synthetic fibers also possess a high gloss, which makes them more noticeable, and they tend to matte and tangle easily when blended with human or animal hair. Overall, synthetic hair replacement systems can usually be cleaned with cleaner solutions, are less costly than human hair, and do not oxidize or lose their style.

MIXED HAIR

Mixed-hair products, such as human hair blended with synthetic or animal hair, are often used in the manufacture of theatrical or fashion wigs. Horse and yak hair, as well as angora and sheep's wool, are some of the materials used in the manufacture of wigs and hair solutions. Angora has a finer texture than yak hair and may be used at the front hairline to create a softer and more natural look.

UNDERSTAND BASES AND CONSTRUCTION

Hair replacement systems may be machine-made, handmade, or made by a combination of both methods. They are typically available with hard, soft, mesh, net, polyurethane, or combination bases. The materials used in base construction include silk, nylon, and plastic mesh; lace; thin (onion) skin; or a combination of materials. Some professionals prefer a doubled base material for increased strength and a more exact fit (**Figure 15-3**).

Knotting refers to the way the hair is attached to the base of the hair solution. Knotting methods include single knotting, V-looping, and single hair injection into the base. The single-knot method is frequently used and, although durable, may come untied during the cleaning process. Double-knotted hair helps the hair to remain intact through use and cleaning,

figure 15-3
Base constructions—left to right: full skin base; thin skin and French lace; bio-lace, French lace, and skin; polyurethane and monofilament.

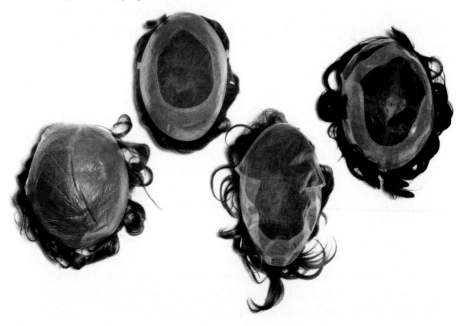

but may not produce as natural a look as other knotting methods. Plastic or nylon-mesh bases resist shrinkage and wrinkling when cleaned in water-based solutions or shampoos.

Root-turning (ROOT-TURN-ing) refers to sorting the hair strands so that the cuticle points toward the hair ends in its natural direction of growth. When a manufacturer states that a hair solution is root-turned, it means that the hair has been attached to the base with the cuticle of the hair strands in this natural position. Hair that has been root-turned minimizes tangling and matting because the cuticle scales are flowing in the correct direction.

New construction techniques with more natural-looking materials are constantly evolving in the manufacture of hair replacement systems. The new generation of manufacturing techniques has completely changed the industry, resulting in hair replacement systems that can look and feel quite natural.

UNDERSTAND STOCK AND CUSTOM HAIR REPLACEMENT SYSTEMS

Hair replacement systems are available from manufacturers and distributors in stock sizes and colors, which allows the barber to maintain an inventory of these products. Stock systems, or *pre-custom systems*, as the industry now refers to them, can be used as samples to show prospective hair replacement clients what a replacement system might look like or may be customized to fit the client if one happens to be the correct color.

Custom hair solutions are tailored to the client's head shape and hair replacement needs. This customization requires the barber to create a template or pattern and a color-matching sample for the supplier to use as a guide in the production of the hair solution.

A template or contour analysis should be done prior to fitting any hair solution. This analysis will help to determine whether the client has the option of purchasing a stock product or requires a custom-made hair solution.

Obtaining Hair Replacement Systems

After reading this section, you will be able to:

 Recognize supplies needed to service hair replacement systems.

It is advisable for the barber who is interested in servicing or supplying hair replacement systems to study this area of the industry in detail. Decisions will have to be made about manufacturers, supplies, products, and equipment; naturally, this should be done with as much knowledge as possible.

The selection of a hair replacement manufacturer to work with is an important decision that should be based on the manufacturer's ability to meet the barber's needs in terms of cost, time, and product quality. The following sample questions may help to guide the selection of a manufacturer to provide hair replacement goods to the barbershop.

- What hair materials are used in the construction of the hair solution: human, synthetic, or mixed?
- What chemical treatments have been applied?
- If the hair is human hair, is it graded in terms of strength, elasticity, and porosity?
- Will the manufacturer stand behind their product?
- What is the life expectancy of the hair solution?
- Does the manufacturer have the ability to create custom colors?
- Is technical training offered about the manufacturer's products?

SUPPLIES FOR HAIR REPLACEMENT SERVICES

Most barbershops will already have many of the tools and implements required for hair solution services (**Figure 15-4**). The few supplies that are not standard items, like special adhesives or solvents, can be obtained from a barber or hair replacement supply company. Be guided by the following checklist when purchasing hair solution service supplies.

- Adhesive remover
- Alcohol
- Blowdryer
- Client record cards
- Clippers
- Comb
- Double-sided adhesive tape
- Envelopes
- Grease pencil

figure 15-4
Supplies for hair solution services.

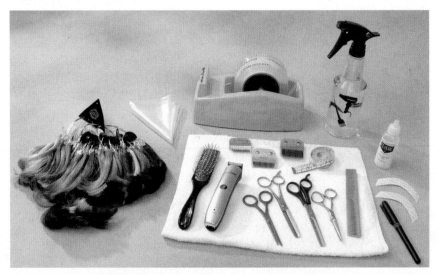

- Hair density chart
- Hairnet
- Haircutting shears
- Manufacturer's color ring
- Measuring tape
- Plastic wrap
- Razor
- Roller picks
- Scissors (for cutting pattern)
- Small brush
- Spirit gum/adhesive
- Styling or wig block
- Thinning shears
- T-pins
- Transparent tape
- Wig cleaner

MEASURE FOR HAIR REPLACEMENT SYSTEMS

Once the client consultation has been performed and an understanding has been reached about the type of hair solution to be purchased, a preliminary haircut should be performed.

To achieve a natural look, the client's hair should be allowed to grow fairly long to make it easier to blend it with that of the hair solution. When performing the preliminary cut, the hair should be lightly trimmed, leaving a long neckline and length close to the ears at the sides. Make sure to trim the front section as well. After the preliminary cut is finished, gently twist a small section of the hair from the client's crown and cut with thinning shears to create a sample. This color will be used in the front, top, and crown areas of the hair replacement. Wrap adhesive tape around the base of the hair sample to keep it in place. Take a separate hair sample from the temple, side, and back area if the client has gray hair to ensure the correct blend of gray at the blending area of the system.

The sizes of men's hair solutions are commonly measured in inches. For example, a 6-inch by 4-inch piece would be 6 inches long from front to back and 4 inches wide. In the manufacturer's code, the larger number refers to the length unless otherwise indicated. Tape measurements alone can be used for ordering stock hair solutions. Custom pieces, however, require a pattern or template of the client's head form in the area of hair loss. Refer to Procedure 15-1 to learn how to measure and create a template for a client.

Ⓟ 15-1 **Making a Template** *pages 509–510*

CREATE A PLASTER MOLD FORM

Today, some manufacturers prefer plaster of paris models of the client's head form. These models are made after creating the pattern but, instead of tape, plaster is applied while the client holds the plastic wrap in place. The plaster forms a hard mold that allows the manufacturer to create a perfect fit when creating the base. The manufacturer then pours a foam mold into the cast to create a permanent mold for the client to use again and again. Refer to Procedure 15-2 for instruction in creating a plaster mold.

Ⓟ 15-2   **Making a Plaster Mold Form** *pages 511–513*

DISCUSS WAYS TO AFFIX HAIR REPLACEMENT SYSTEMS

Full Head Bonding

Full head bonding (FUL head BAHND-ing) is the process of attaching a hair replacement system to the head with an adhesive bonding agent. This allows the replacement system to adhere to all areas of the head rather than just being held in place with double-sided tape. Barbers can ask their suppliers about which copolymer should be used for full head bonding. The adhesives used with hair replacement systems are water soluble. Be sure to remind clients to always allow the adhesive to dry for a few minutes after shampooing and before styling. Refer to Procedure 15-3 for instruction in applying bonding agents.

Ⓟ 15-3   **Full Head Bonding** *pages 514–516*

Partial Hair Replacement Systems

For a small degree of hair loss, a partial lace fill-in may be all that is required. Partial hair solutions can be made for the front or crown areas of the head. The measuring, application, and cutting techniques are the same as those used for full hair solution styles. Be sure to shave the area to be covered so the spirit gum will adhere better to the scalp and the hair solution.

Lace-Front Hair Solution

A **lace-front** (LAYS-front) hair solution is recommended when the hair is worn in an off-the-face style. It is scarcely visible from the front view and provides the required lightness for a natural-looking hairstyle. Remember that reinforced areas of a lace-front hair solution vary with the design of the foundation and the manufacturer's specifications. Never apply tape directly to the lace. Refer to Procedure 15-4 A and B to practice applying and removing a lace-front hair solution.

Ⓟ 15-4   Applying and Removing Hair Replacement Systems
pages 517–518

Facial Hair Replacement Solutions

Facial hair solutions are attached with spirit gum. Mustaches, sideburns, and beards may all be attached in the same manner. Clean the facial area and apply spirit gum to the appropriate section. Wait until the gum is tacky, position the piece, and gently press down with a lint-free cloth. Trim the piece to the desired style.

Full Wigs

While most men might not choose to wear a full wig, many women enjoy the coverage, convenience, and instant style changes they can achieve with wigs. Ready-to-wear wigs are usually made of the synthetic fiber Kanekalon.

Full, ready-made wigs are constructed on a stretch cap made of lightweight elastic. The wig has permanent elastic bands at the sides designed to hold it in place. It should fit comfortably, but tightly enough to maintain its position without slipping, shifting, or lifting. Wigs come in a wide variety of colors and in many styles.

Cleaning and Styling Hair Replacement Systems

After reading this section, you will be able to:

LO⑧ Describe how to clean and service a hair replacement system.

LO⑨ Describe how to fit and cut in a hair replacement system.

The life of a hair replacement system depends on its construction and the overall treatment it receives. Manufacturers furnish instructions on the care of their hair solutions that both the barber and client should follow carefully. Clients should have at least two hair solutions to ensure that one will always be in good condition while the other one is being serviced and maintained.

CLEANING SYNTHETIC HAIR REPLACEMENT SYSTEMS

Synthetic hair solutions should always be cleaned with a solvent. Attach the hair solution to a plastic foam head mold with T-pins and immerse it in lukewarm water with the recommended solvent. Do not use hot water, which would cause the hair solution to shrink or become matted and tangled. Swish the hair solution around in the shampoo solution. Rinse with clean, lukewarm water. Permit the hair solution to dry naturally, pinned on the mold overnight; if time does not permit, place it under a dryer with cool air. Some hair solutions may be dry-cleaned, so always follow the manufacturer's instructions. Refer to Procedures 15-6 and 15-7 for instruction in cleaning hair replacement systems and wigs.

Ⓟ 15-6   **Cleaning Human Hair Replacement Systems** *pages 521–522*

Ⓟ 15-7   **Cleaning Wigs** *page 523*

BASIC HAIR REPLACEMENT SYSTEM CARE

- Use the manufacturer's tape, antiseptic, cleaner, and softeners.

- When the hair solution is not being worn, it should be placed on an appropriate block.

- Some hair solutions should be removed for showering and swimming.

- Clean the hair solutions after the first week of wear, and then every 3 to 4 weeks, or as needed.

- Never fold hair solutions.

- Always follow the manufacturer's recommendations for removing hair solutions.

- Apply light styling products and spray sparingly and with even distribution.

- Set hair solutions with plain water.

RECONDITION HAIR REPLACEMENT SYSTEMS

Reconditioning treatments should be given as often as necessary to prevent dryness or brittleness of the hair. Reconditioning treatments may also be used to liven up hair solutions that look dull and lifeless.

A small amount of reconditioner may be used, as directed by the manufacturer. If a slight color adjustment is necessary due to fading or yellowing, a suitable temporary color rinse is recommended. Select the rinse carefully so that the color matches that of the client's hair. Refer to Procedure 15-8 for further instruction.

P 15-8   **Coloring Hair Replacement Systems** *page 524*

PERMANENT WAVING HAIR REPLACEMENT SYSTEMS

Permanent waving a hair solution requires time, creativity, and careful attention to detail. The objective is to create a natural look that blends the system with the client's natural hair. The hair system is attached to a wig or styling block with T-pins and should be custom wrapped according to the contours of the client's head.

The rod placement does not rest on the scalp of the hair system as it would in a perm procedure on natural hair. Instead, the rods are *floated* to eliminate weight and rod marks on the base. Floating is accomplished by using roller picks to support the rod above the base of the hair system. The picks are inserted at both ends of the rod and are held in place by the rubber band of the perm rod. After the hair system has been rolled and secured with the roller picks, use the following guidelines to complete the process. Refer to Procedure 15-9 for instruction in permanent waving hair replacement systems.

P 15-9   **Permanent Waving Hair Replacement Systems** *page 524*

General Recommendations and Reminders

- Comb hair solutions carefully to avoid matting, loss of hair, or damage.

- Use a wide-tooth comb to avoid weakening or damaging the foundation.

- Never rub or wring cleaning fluids from the hair solution. Let it dry naturally.

- Be careful not to cut too much hair when cutting, tapering, and blending a hair solution.

- Take accurate measurements to assure a comfortable and secure fit.

- Recondition hair solutions as often as necessary to prevent dryness, brittleness, or dullness of the hair.

- Brush and comb hair solutions with a downward movement.

- To avoid damage to the foundation, never lighten or cold-wave a hair solution.

- If coloring is necessary, it must be done with care.

UNDERSTAND CUTTING, TAPERING, AND BLENDING HAIR REPLACEMENT SYSTEMS

The following steps outline one method that can be used to cut in a hair replacement system:

- **Top section.** Remove excess length using the clipper-over-comb or fingers-and-shear method at a 90-degree elevation. Work forward from front of crown to forehead. Repeat this step using shears to blend the top section (**Figures 15-5A** and **15-5B**).

- **Sides.** Comb the side hair down and blend with the natural hairline from temple to sideburn to the ear (**Figure 15-6**). Taper and blend from the side hairline to crest. Taper gradually using a slide cutting method so the replacement system will be undetectable when blended with the client's natural hair.

figure 15-6
Comb the sides down and blend to the hairline.

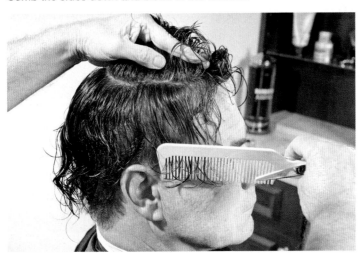

figure 15-5
(A) Remove excess hair from top section
(B) Blend the top section.

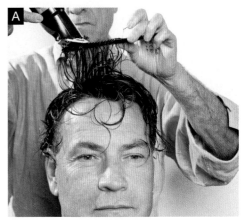

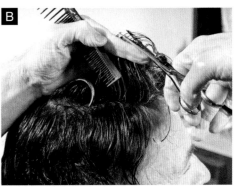

HERE'S A TIP

If any part of the system appears heavy, use the first couple of teeth on thinning shears close to the base of the system to remove bulk. Be sure to make very narrow partings in order to keep it looking natural. Be careful not to overcut.

figure 15-7
Blend the back section with thinning shears.

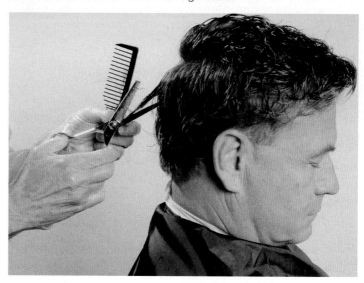

- **Back.** Cut any excess hair length from the replacement. Use thinning shears to blend the ends of the replacement with the client's natural hair (**Figure 15-7**).

Refer to Procedure 15-5 for instruction in customizing a stock hair solution.

Ⓟ 15-5 **Customizing a Stock (Pre-Custom) Hair Replacement System** *pages 519–520*

Congratulations! You have just completed cutting and customizing a hair replacement system (**Figures 15-8A and 15-8B**).

figure 15-8
Hair replacement system—(A) front view; (B) back view.

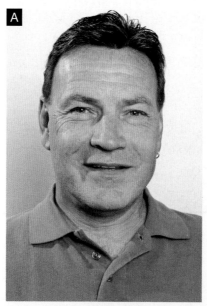

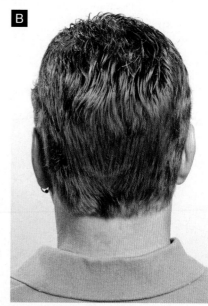

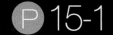

MAKING A TEMPLATE

☐ Grease pencil

☐ Permanent marker

☐ Plastic wrap

☐ Tape measure

☐ ¾-inch transparent tape (preferably the dull-finish type for easy writing)

PREPARATION

1. Perform a client consultation.

2. Perform a preliminary haircut.

3. After the preliminary cut is finished, tape the hair samples to the template form or follow the manufacturer's directions on sending in hair samples.

PROCEDURE

Measuring

For a front hairline to look natural, it should not be too low on the forehead. The original, natural hairline should be followed as closely as possible. The following procedure is a standard method of measuring for a hair solution.

1. Place four fingers above the eyebrow with the last finger resting on the bridge of the nose. Make a dot with a grease pencil on the forehead directly in line with the center of the nose to indicate where the hair solution is to begin. Take caution when using this method as hand sizes are different. Use this as your guide to find the natural hairline.

2. Place the tape measure on the dot. Measure the length to where the back hair begins and mark the tape measure. Be sure to measure back to where substantial growth begins and disregard sparse hair between the forehead and bald crown areas.

3. The next measurement is across the top, directly over the sideburns. This is the place where the front hairline of the hair solution blends in with the client's own hair at the sides of the head. Measure across the crown area if it is noticeably different from the front width. These measurements can be used to order a stock hair solution.

Creating a Template

To create a template for a custom hair solution, assemble the measuring tape, plastic wrap, ¾-inch transparent tape (preferably the dull-finish type for easy writing), and grease pencil or permanent marker.

4 Trim excess or stray hairs.

5 Place approximately 2 feet of plastic wrap on top of the client's head and twist the sides tightly until they conform to the contour of the head.

6 Find the desired hairline by looking at the forehead and finding the curve; this is where the natural hairline should be. Each person's natural hairline is different. Some men may want to have more of a recession than others; you should discuss this preference during the client consultation. Use your four fingers above the eyebrows if need be as noted in point 1 above. Make a dot on the pattern to indicate the new hairline. Place additional dots as follows:

- Two dots on each side where the front hairline is to meet the client's own hairline
- Two dots in back of the head on each side of the balding spot
- One dot at the center back edge of the bald spot to determine the length of the area to be covered

7 Connect the dots with a permanent marker to outline the balding area. Ignore minor irregularities and sparse areas.

8 While the client holds the plastic wrap, place a strip of tape no more than 4 to 5 inches in length just below the areas you marked. Place the tape in different directions going from front to back and side to side to ensure good coverage. Feel for any soft spots and add more tape if need be. The template should feel like a hard shell in order to hold its shape.

9 Mark the front part of the template *F* and the back *B.* Mark the direction of any swirls at the crown that influence the flow of the hair stream or the location of a part line. Then remove the template and cut around the edge with scissors. After cutting the outline, replace the template over the balding area. Make sure this area is covered exactly. Although it is better to have a foundation that is slightly smaller than one that is too large, accuracy is very important.

10 Attach samples of the client's hair to the template or client card for color matching by the manufacturer.

11 Create a client record card, which can also serve as an information sheet when ordering stock and custom hair solutions. Send the measurements, template, and hair samples to the manufacturer with any special instructions.

CLEAN-UP AND DISINFECTION

☐ Clean and disinfect the tools and implements.

☐ Clean and disinfect the work area.

☐ Sweep up hair and deposit in a closed receptacle.

☐ Dispose of single-use items. Place all used linens, towels, and capes in the laundry.

☐ Wash your hands.

MAKING A PLASTER MOLD FORM

MATERIALS, IMPLEMENTS, AND EQUIPMENT

- ☐ Black and white eyeliner pencils
- ☐ Permanent marker
- ☐ Plaster gauze strips
- ☐ Plastic bowl for mixing
- ☐ Scissors or shears
- ☐ Tape
- ☐ Towels
- ☐ Waterproof cape

PREPARATION

1 Clean and then disinfect the work area.

2 Drape the client.

3 Cut six plaster gauze strips at 9 or 10 inches and eight plaster gauze strips at 4 inches.

PROCEDURE

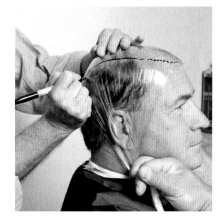

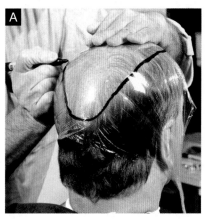

1 Stretch the plastic wrap over the client's head, twist the sides, and have the client hold the ends so the wrap conforms to his head.

2 Mark the pattern and add details.

3 Apply towel around the client's neck.

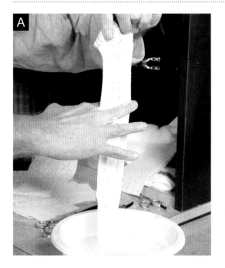

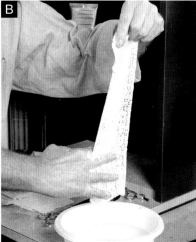

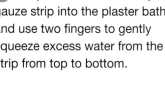

4 Mix plaster and water. Dip a gauze strip into the plaster bath and use two fingers to gently squeeze excess water from the strip from top to bottom.

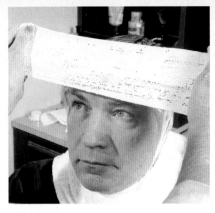

5 Apply the first strip from front to back.

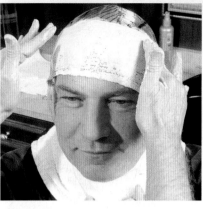

6 Smooth out the strip following the contour of the head from the front around to the temple areas.

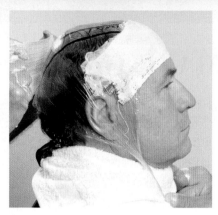

7 Apply the second strip from back to front, making sure to smooth the strip to the contour of the head.

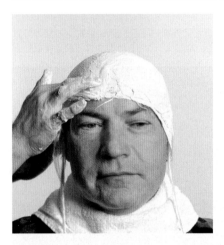

8 Apply shorter strips across the top of the head.

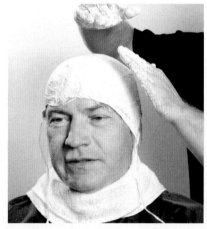

9 Repeat the process to create second and third layers of the gauze strips.

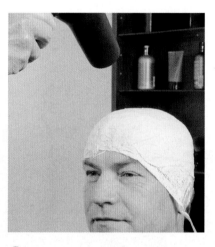

10 Blowdry to set the plaster until completely dry.

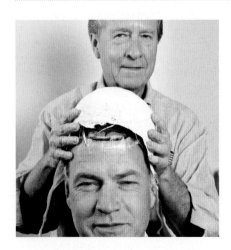

11 When the mold is dry, gently remove it by lifting it off the client's head. If any hair sticks to the plaster, mist the area with water to remove. It is extremely important to smooth out the gauze strips to fit the contour of the head.

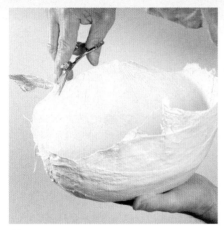

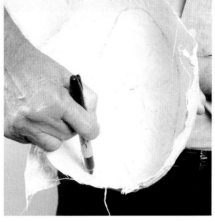

12 Trim excess plaster from the mold.

13 The inside of the mold should have a faint outline of the pattern. Trace over the outline with a permanent marker. Write the client's name and date on the outside of the plaster mold.

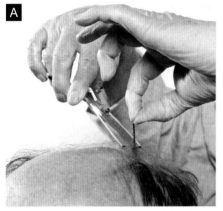

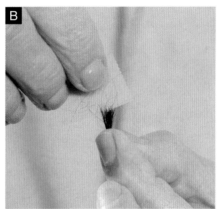

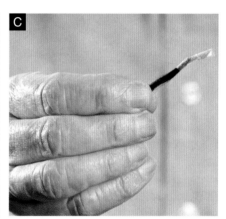

14 Gently twist a small section of hair from the client's crown and cut with thinning shears to create a sample. This color will be used in the front, top, and crown areas of the hair replacement system. Wrap tape around the base of the hair sample to keep it in place. Take separate hair samples from the temple, side, and back areas, as they tend to have more gray hair.

15 Shampoo and condition the client's hair.

Note that the plaster mold will need to cure for 24 hours before it is shipped to the manufacturer.

CLEAN-UP AND DISINFECTION

☐ Clean and disinfect the tools and implements.

☐ Clean and disinfect the work area.

☐ Sweep up hair and deposit in a closed receptacle.

☐ Dispose of single-use items. Place all used linens, towels, and capes in the laundry.

☐ Dispose of leftover plaster mixture; use paper towels to wipe the mixture from the bowl before washing and deposit in the trash.

☐ Wash your hands.

DID YOU KNOW?

When hair replacement systems first became popular, the hair along the track was braided with a wire and the hair replacement system was sewed into the braid. When removed, it had to slowly be cut out.

FULL HEAD BONDING

MATERIALS, IMPLEMENTS, AND EQUIPMENT

☐ Eyeliner pencil

☐ Makeup sponges

☐ Safety data sheet for adhesive

☐ Soft-bond adhesives

☐ Towels

☐ Waterproof cape

PREPARATION

When preparing to do a full head bond, follow *all* the manufacturer's directions for using the adhesive.

1 Perform a patch test with any adhesive 24 hours before applying.

2 Clean and then disinfect the work area.

3 Wash your hands.

4 Drape the client and shampoo the hair and scalp with a pH-balanced shampoo.

5 Towel dry and change the drape to a haircutting cape.

6 Always make sure the base of the hair replacement system is dry before applying.

PROCEDURE

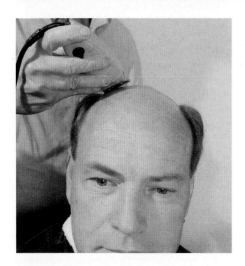

1 Trim the client's scalp with edgers.

2 Rinse excess hair from the scalp.

3 Dry the hair again after the client's scalp is rinsed. Do not touch the client's scalp with your hands after this step.

4 Select the correct adhesive for the hair replacement system.

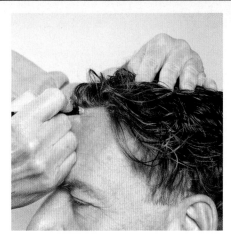

5 Place the hair replacement system on the client's head. With an eyeliner pencil, mark exactly where the hair replacement system needs to be placed on the front hairline, temples, and back of the head to ensure proper placement. Remember to never bond on a client's wrinkle or too far back on the client's scalp.

6 Shake the adhesive product well before applying.

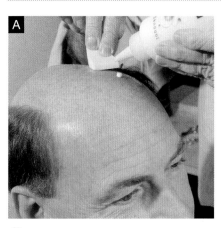
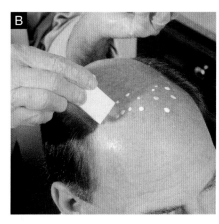
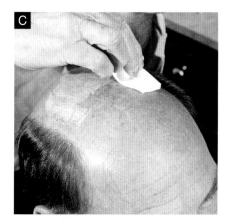

7 Apply a small amount of adhesive in a circular motion onto the client's clean scalp. Use a makeup sponge to distribute the adhesive evenly over the scalp. The adhesive will appear white until it dries completely to a clear state.

8 When the first coat is dry, apply a second coat and let it dry. Repeat these steps for a total of four times, remembering to use small amounts of adhesive.

9 Once the adhesive is completely dry, it is time to apply the hair solution.

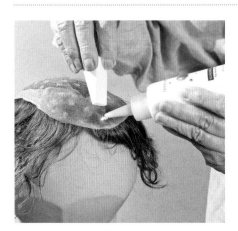

10 Apply one coat of adhesive to the base of the hair replacement system. Do not apply adhesive to any lace present in the hair replacement system.

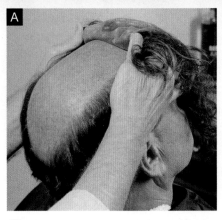

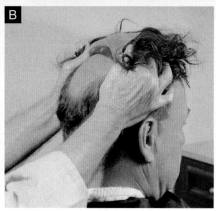

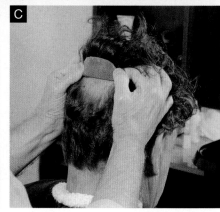

11 Stand behind the client and hold the hair solution in both hands. Place the hair replacement system at the front hairline and start rolling the hair solution back, placing it on your marks and applying pressure without stretching the hair solution. Make sure not to wrinkle the base of the hair solution.

12 Once the hair replacement system is fully on, use the back of a comb to check around the perimeter of the hair replacement system for wrinkles. Smooth out any minor inconsistencies.

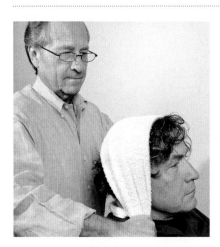

13 Take a towel and place it over the hair replacement system. Stretch both ends of the towel and pull down tightly to ensure an even fit.

The hair replacement system is now ready to be cut. After cutting and blending, remember to tell the client to allow 24 to 48 hours before shampooing.

CLEAN-UP AND DISINFECTION

☐ Clean and disinfect the tools and implements.

☐ Clean and disinfect the work area.

☐ Sweep up hair and deposit in a closed receptacle.

☐ Dispose of single-use items. Place all used linens, towels, and capes in the laundry.

☐ Wash your hands.

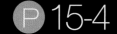
APPLYING AND REMOVING HAIR REPLACEMENT SYSTEMS

A. APPLYING A LACE-FRONT HAIR SOLUTION

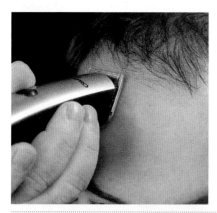

1 Clean the bald area with rubbing alcohol or with soap and water.

2 Remove hair on the scalp where the tape or lace is to be attached.

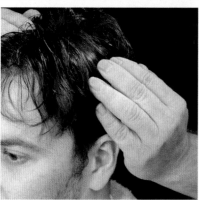

3 Attach strips of two-sided tape to reinforced parts of the foundation, usually near the front, on the sides, and at the back of the hair solution. Note that reinforced areas vary with the design of the foundation and the manufacturer's specifications. Never apply tape directly to the lace.

4 Adjust the hair solution to the desired position using the four-finger method. Press it down into place with the back of a comb to ensure that oils from the fingers do not stain the tape.

B. REMOVING A LACE-FRONT HAIR SOLUTION

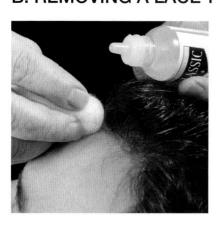

1 Before removing a lace-front hair solution, dampen the lace with acetone or solvent in order to loosen it from the scalp.

2 Do not pull or stretch the lace.

3 To apply solvent, use a piece of cotton or a brush.

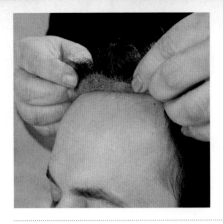

4 After the lace becomes loosened, use the fingertips to remove the tape from the scalp.

5 Do not pull off the hair solution by tugging on the hair.

6 Clean the reinforced areas with a small brush dipped in acetone or other solvent.

C. APPLYING A NON-LACE-FRONT HAIR SOLUTION

1 Before adjusting a hair solution to the scalp, trim the front hairline and clean the entire bald area with a piece of cotton dampened with rubbing alcohol, or soap and water; then dry thoroughly.

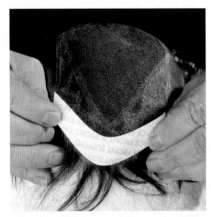

2 Apply two-sided tape in a V-shape on the front reinforced area of the foundation. This tape holds the hair solution close to the scalp. Place additional pieces of tape on the reinforced parts of the foundation at the sides and back of the hair solution.

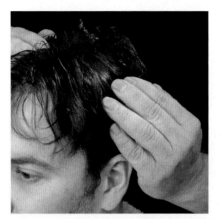

3 Place four fingers above the eyebrow to locate the hairline. Position the hair solution at the hairline using the center of the nose as a guide. When the hair solution is in the proper position, press down firmly on the various taped areas.

D. REMOVING A NON-LACE-FRONT HAIR SOLUTION

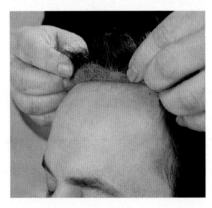

1 Reach up under the hair solution with the fingertips at the front section and detach the tape from the scalp.

2 Make sure the tape stays on the foundation so that it can be reactivated with spirit gum.

CLEAN-UP AND DISINFECTION

☐ Clean and disinfect the tools and implements.

☐ Clean and disinfect the work area.

☐ Sweep up hair and deposit in a closed receptacle.

☐ Dispose of single-use items. Place all used linens, towels, and capes in the laundry.

☐ Wash your hands.

CUSTOMIZING A STOCK (PRE-CUSTOM) HAIR REPLACEMENT SYSTEM

MATERIALS, IMPLEMENTS, AND EQUIPMENT

- ☐ Canvas block and stand
- ☐ Plastic and tape template
- ☐ Razor blade
- ☐ Scissors
- ☐ Shampoo and conditioner
- ☐ T-pins or tipped straight pins
- ☐ Towels

PREPARATION

1 Clean and disinfect the work area.

2 Drape the client.

3 Perform a client consultation.

PROCEDURE

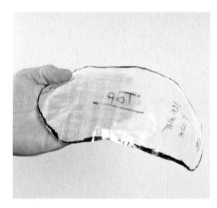

1 To customize a stock hair replacement system, use the plastic and tape template.

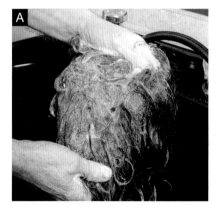

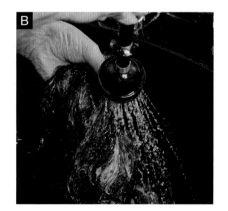

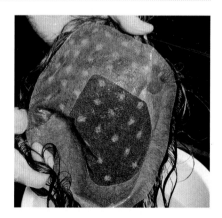

2 Shampoo the hair replacement system and rinse thoroughly.

3 Condition the hair replacement system and rinse lightly, leaving a small amount of conditioner in the hair replacement system.

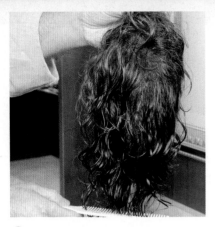

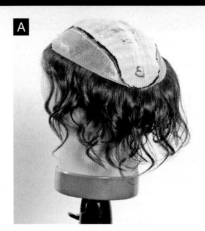
A

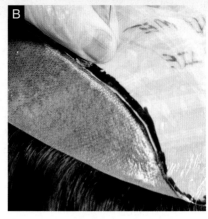
B

④ After swishing the hair replacement system through the water a few times, remove it and comb gently.

⑤ Towel-blot the hair replacement system and invert it.

⑥ Drag the hair replacement system over the back of the canvas block, making sure all the hair is behind the front edge of the hair replacement system. Invert the template and place it on the hair replacement system, making sure to use as much of the natural hairline of the hair replacement system as possible. Secure the template and hair replacement system to the block with pins.

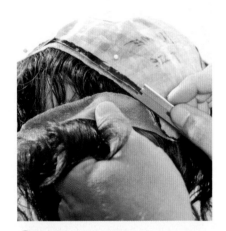

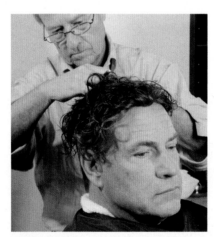

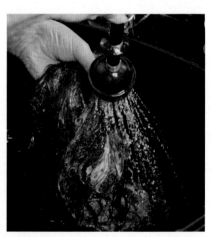

⑦ Use the tip of the razor blade to carefully cut the base, using the template as a guide. Cut all the way around the base, but do not cut the hair.

⑧ After the base has been cut, remove the pins from the canvas block and check for fit.

⑨ Rinse out excess conditioner and lay the hair replacement system to the side.

CLEAN-UP AND DISINFECTION

☐ Clean and disinfect the tools and implements.

☐ Clean and disinfect the work area.

☐ Sweep up hair and deposit in a closed receptacle.

☐ Dispose of single-use items. Place all used linens, towels, and capes in the laundry.

☐ Discard used razor blade in a sharps container.

☐ Wash your hands.

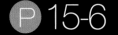

CLEANING HUMAN HAIR REPLACEMENT SYSTEMS

Hair solutions must be kept clean just as natural hair must be kept clean. Cleaning should be performed carefully to help maintain the life of the hair solution. Use the following guidelines and the manufacturer's recommendations to clean a hair solution.

MATERIALS, IMPLEMENTS, AND EQUIPMENT

- ☐ Brush
- ☐ Manufacturer's recommended cleaning solution
- ☐ Mixing bowl
- ☐ T-pins
- ☐ Tape removal solvent
- ☐ Towels
- ☐ Wide-toothed comb
- ☐ Wig block

PROCEDURE

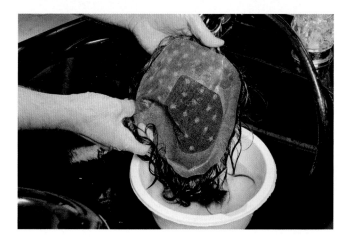

1 Remove all the old tape and clean any reinforced areas by lightly dabbing with the recommended solvent.

2 Put enough cleaner in a glass bowl so that the hair replacement system can be submerged. Invert the hair replacement system with the inside up and place into the cleaning solution. Soak for 3 to 5 minutes. Swish the hair replacement system back and forth (or dip it up and down) in the cleaning solution until all residue is removed from the hair and foundation. If the cleaning solution darkens, replace it with fresh solution and repeat the swishing process.

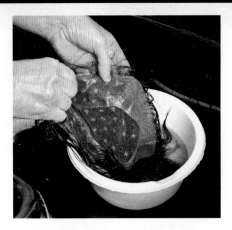

3 Gently tap the edge of the hair replacement system with a small brush or your fingers until the adhesive has been removed. Do not rub or scrub.

4 Place a towel on a flat surface and place the hair replacement system on the towel with the inside facing up. Gently press out the cleaner with the towel.

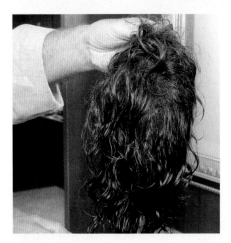

5 Hold the hair replacment system by the front section and comb gently.

6 Fasten the hair replacement system to the **wig block** (WIG BLAHK) with T-pins, style with a blowdryer, and store until the client picks it up, or dry the hair replacement system and reattach to the client's scalp.

CLEAN-UP AND DISINFECTION

☐ Clean and disinfect the tools and implements.

☐ Clean and disinfect the work area.

☐ Dispose of single-use items. Place all used linens, towels, and capes in the laundry.

☐ Dispose of used cleaning solution and solvents per the manufacturer's recommendation.

☐ Wash your hands.

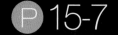

CLEANING WIGS

Cleaning a ready-made wig is a fairly quick and easy process. Use the guidelines provided and the manufacturer's cleaning instructions for this process.

MATERIALS, IMPLEMENTS, AND EQUIPMENT

☐ Brush

☐ Manufacturer's recommended cleaning solution

☐ Mixing bowl

☐ T-pins

☐ Towels

☐ Wide-toothed comb

☐ Wig block

PROCEDURE

1 Brush the wig thoroughly to remove all surface dirt and residue.

2 Mix a solution of warm water and wig solution in a bowl.

3 Dip the entire wig into the solution; swish it around in the solution.

4 Rinse the wig in clean, cold water.

5 Blot it dry with a towel.

6 Turn the wig inside out and dry it with a towel.

7 Pin the wig to a head mold or wig block of the correct size.

8 Carefully brush the hair into place.

9 Permit the wig to dry naturally, pinned to the form.

10 If necessary, use cool air to dry the wig quickly.

11 When dry, brush into the proper style.

CLEAN-UP AND DISINFECTION

☐ Clean and disinfect the tools and implements.

☐ Clean and disinfect the work area.

☐ Dispose of single-use items. Place all used linens, towels, and capes in the laundry.

☐ Wash your hands.

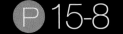
COLORING HAIR REPLACEMENT SYSTEMS

Permanent haircoloring products (aniline derivatives) can be used only on hair solutions made of 100 percent human hair. Use the following procedure and manufacturer's recommendations when coloring a hair solution with permanent haircoloring products.

PROCEDURE

1. Clean the hair solution with a solvent.

2. Cover the head form block with plastic material to prevent staining from the coloring product.

3. Secure the hair solution firmly with T-pins or straight pins in the front, back, and sides.

4. Give a strand test on a small section of hair to determine the color desired. If using a tint with peroxide, apply it on a dry hair strand.

5. Mix the desired shade of haircoloring product.

6. Apply with a haircoloring brush.

7. Comb the color product lightly, being careful not to saturate the foundation.

8. Test every 5 minutes until the desired shade is obtained.

9. After processing, rinse thoroughly with warm water. Shampoo and condition the hair replacement system according to the manufacturer's directions.

10. Comb and set into the desired style.

PERMANENT WAVING HAIR REPLACEMENT SYSTEMS

PROCEDURE

1. Select a mild permanent wave solution appropriate for bleached or damaged hair types. Remove the T-pins from the hair replacement system—you should not use metal with a perm on human hair—and carefully apply the solution.

2. Take a test curl every minute until processing is complete.

3. Rinse the hair replacement system for 10 to 15 minutes. The hair replacement system does not require the application of a neutralizing solution.

4. Thoroughly blot each rod with paper towels to absorb as much water as possible.

5. Leave the rods in the hair solution and cover loosely with a plastic cap for 24 hours. At this time you can secure the hair replacement system with the T-pins.

6. On day 2, remove the cap and allow the hair replacement system to dry for another day. Remove the rods only when the hair is completely dry.

REVIEW QUESTIONS

1. Explain why some men might choose to wear a hair replacement system.

2. What two types of hair are used to make men's hair replacement systems?

3. List the steps of measuring for a hair replacement system.

4. What important information should be labeled on a template?

5. List the steps for applying a hair replacement system with tape.

6. What type of product is used in a full head bonding application?

7. What type of product is used to clean hair replacement systems?

8. Name two medications that may be prescribed to encourage hair growth.

9. Name the oral and topical medications that should not be prescribed for women.

10. List three surgical methods of hair replacement.

CHAPTER GLOSSARY

finasteride (fin-ASTER-eyed)	p. 498	an oral medication prescribed for men only to stimulate hair growth
flap surgery (flap SIR-jer-ee)	p. 499	a surgical technique that involves the removal of a bald scalp area and the attachment of a flap of hair-bearing skin
full head bonding (FUL head BAHND-ing)	p. 504	the process of attaching a hair replacement system to all areas of the head with an adhesive bonding agent
hackling (HAK-ling)	p. 499	process used to comb through the hair strands to separate them
hair replacement system	p. 494	formerly called a *hairpiece*; also known as a *hair solution*
hair solution	p. 494	any small wig used to cover the top or crown of the head and integrated with the natural hair
hair transplantation (HAYR TRANZ-plant-ay-shun)	p. 498	any form of hair restoration that involves the surgical removal and relocation of hair, including scalp reduction and flap surgery
lace-front (LAYS-front)	p. 504	popular hair solution style used for off-the-face styles
minoxidil (MIN-ox-ih-dil)	p. 498	topical medication used to promote hair growth or reduce hair loss
root-turning (ROOT-TURN-ing)	p. 501	refers to sorting the hair strands so that the cuticle points toward the hair ends in its natural direction of growth
scalp reduction (SKALP REE-duk-shun)	p. 499	the surgical removal of a bald area, followed by the pulling together of the scalp ends
toupee (too-PAY)	p. 494	outdated term used to describe a small hair replacement that covers the top or crown of the head
wig block (WIG BLAHK)	p. 522	also known as *styling*; a head-shaped form made of plastic, foam, or other materials used as a stand for a wig or hair replacement system

PART 4

ADVANCED BARBERING SERVICES

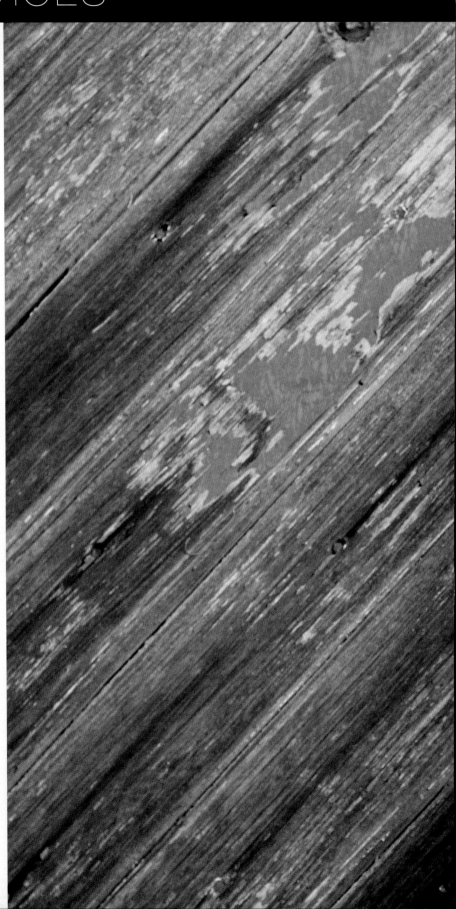

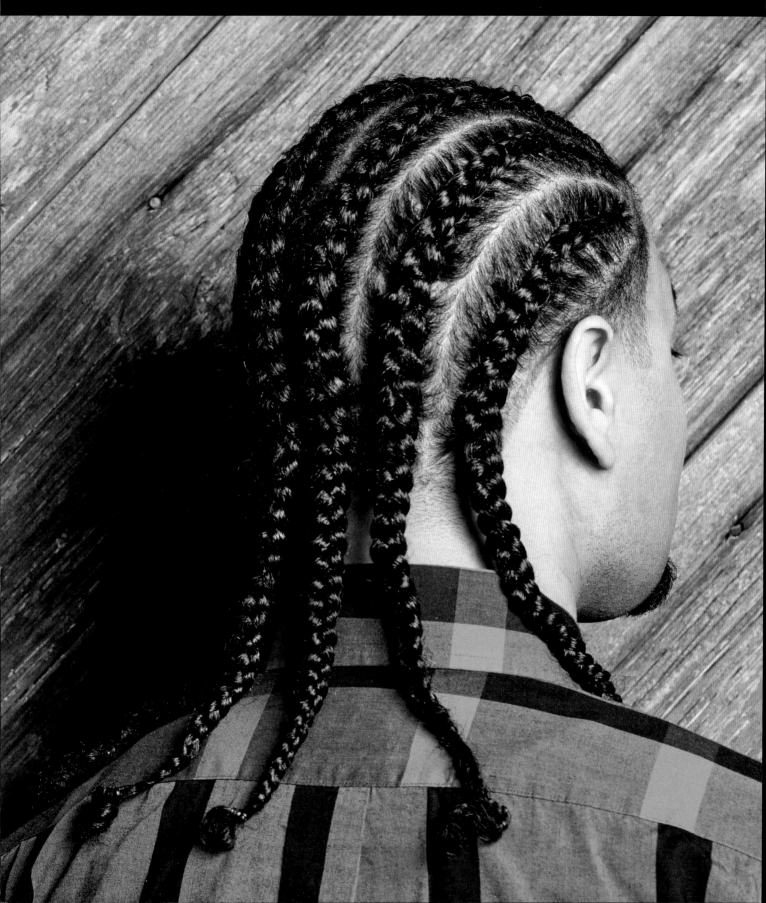

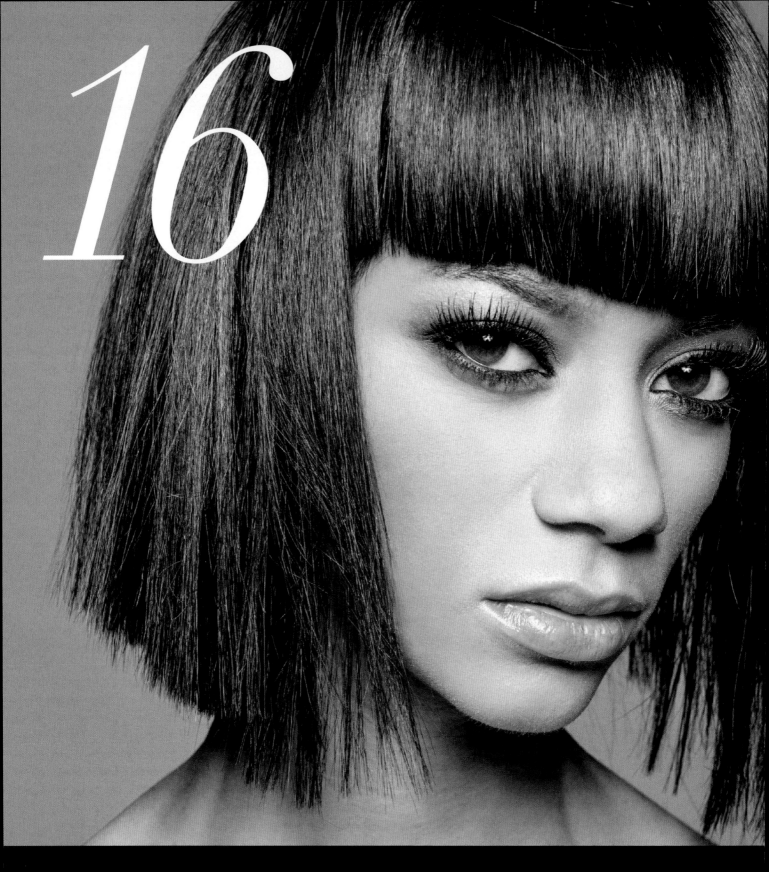

16

WOMEN'S HAIRCUTTING AND STYLING

LEARNING OBJECTIVES

After completing this chapter, you will be able to:

LO❶
Identify the differences between men's and women's haircutting.

LO❷
Describe four basic women's haircuts.

LO❸
Explain wave formation in curly hair textures.

LO❹
Discuss other haircutting techniques.

LO❺
Explain different hairstyling techniques.

LO❻
Demonstrate a blunt cut.

LO❼
Demonstrate a graduated cut.

LO❽
Demonstrate a uniform-layered cut.

LO❾
Demonstrate a long-layered cut.

Introduction

In general, the concept of a barbershop implies a male domain. However, many women seek haircutting services from a barber. One should never assume that a barbershop is just for men. There are women today that walk into a barbershop and request a service. Perhaps they saw the way their husband, son, or friend had their hair cut and they want that same level of detail. A professional barber should be willing and able to accommodate the request of any client, male or female.

Many cosmetology salons maintain a fairly equal ratio of male to female clients. If you choose to work in a cosmetology salon, it is a must to be proficient in cutting and styling women's hair. This chapter will guide you to build upon the basic foundations of cutting and styling men's hair and apply that knowledge to women's cuts and styles. With a few variations, the same terminology will be used to accomplish four basic haircuts in this chapter:

- blunt cut
- graduated cut
- uniform-layered cut
- long-layered cut

Since a women's service does not usually end with the haircut, this chapter will introduce some basic styling techniques. Styling women's hair tends to be a more involved process than styling men's hair and includes techniques such as:

- wet setting
- hair wrapping
- styling with a blowdryer
- styling with a curling iron

This chapter addresses only those techniques that can be accomplished using a blowdryer, thermal irons, or hair wrapping. For information and procedures regarding wet setting, finger waving, and pin curls, refer to *Milady's Standard Cosmetology* textbook and MiladyPro.com.

why study
WOMEN'S HAIRCUTTING AND STYLING?

Barbers should study and have a thorough understanding of women's haircutting and styling because:

➤ Being able to provide hair care services to women will enable you to expand your client base and increase your financial earnings.

➤ Knowledge and skill in women's haircutting will help to apply your men's haircutting skills in new ways.

➤ Barbers need to know how to perform basic hairstyling techniques after completing a woman's haircut in order to meet her styling expectations.

Discuss Men's versus Women's Haircutting

After reading this section, you will be able to:

LO**1** Identify the differences between men's and women's haircutting.

There are some basic differences between cutting women's hair and cutting men's hair:

- Short, tapered men's cuts usually appear more angular in their overall form; women's short cuts often appear more rounded and softer-looking.

- In women's haircutting, curved design lines, feathering, or texturizing at the perimeter is often used to soften the look of a short cut.

- Women's cuts tend to require more styling than men's cuts to achieve the final look.

- Women's cuts and styles often require manipulating longer lengths of hair than men's cuts and styles.

HAIRCUTTING REMINDERS

Remember these rules when cutting women's hair to ensure that you provide the best service for your client:

- Start with clean, conditioned hair.

- Pay attention to the client's head position during a haircut.

- Your body position should be comfortable and easy to maintain, following correct ergonomics.

- Pay attention to your finger placement. Comb through and practice the finger placement you will use before actually cutting the hair.

- Take consistent, clean partings to produce precise results.

- Keep the hair damp when cutting.

- Work with the natural growth patterns, not against them.

- Use the appropriate amount of tension when combing and holding sections of hair. The amount of tension will depend on the hair texture.

- Comb through partings or subsections *from the scalp* to support tension.

- Always work with a guide or guideline. If you cannot see the guide, do not cut! Cross-check to find where you left off.

- The mirror is one of your most important tools, use it to check length and proportion.

- Plan for the shrinkage factor that results when the hair dries or when cutting wavy and curly hair textures.

- Always check and cross-check your work.

> **DID YOU KNOW?**
> Cross-checking is the process of checking your work. Part off subsections opposite to the direction at which they were cut to check for precision of line or blending. For example, if you have cut the hair vertically, cross-check it by holding it out horizontally. Make sure when cross-checking that the hair is elevated and overdirected in the same manner as it was cut. For example, a vertical subsection cut at a 90-degree projection can be cross-checked by parting off the subsections horizontally at 90 degrees.

Define Four Basic Women's Haircuts

After reading this section, you will be able to:

LO**❷**   Describe four basic women's haircuts.

The art of women's haircutting is made up of the variations and combinations of four basic haircuts:

- blunt
- graduated
- uniform layered
- long layered

As with men's haircutting, a variety of elevations (**Figure 16-1**) and hand positions are used to create these effects. Review Chapter 14 if necessary.

BLUNT HAIRCUT

Listed are the characteristics of a blunt cut (0-degree elevation):

- The **blunt cut** (BLUNT KUT) is also known as a *one-length cut* because all the hair strands end at one level to form a heavy weight line at the perimeter.
- Blunt cuts *look* like all the hair is the same length, but the hair is actually all falling to one point and is of varying lengths.
- The head should be held in an upright position to avoid shifting the hair out of its natural fall position. If the head is positioned forward, an undercut will be created.
- The design line at the perimeter may be cut in horizontal, diagonal forward, or diagonal back lines (**Figures 16-2 to 16-4**). **Figures 16-2** through **16-4** illustrate the technical pattern of the blunt cuts with different design lines.

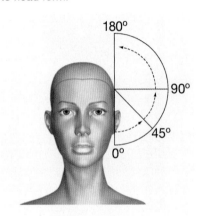

figure 16-1
Hair that falls at 0 elevation in natural fall elevated up to 180 degrees relative to head form.

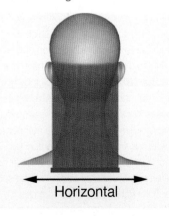

figure 16-2
Horizontal cutting line.

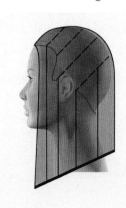

figure 16-3
Diagonal forward cutting line.

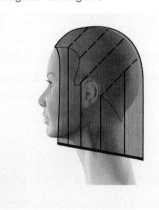

figure 16-4
Diagonal cutting line.

Haircutting Tips for a Blunt Cut

- Shampoo and condition the hair before cutting.

- Maintain uniform moisture in the hair while cutting—re-wet as needed.

- Work with the natural growth patterns of the hair.

- Keep the client's head upright and parallel to the floor.

- Take clean partings and subsections, parallel to the design line.

- Comb through the subsections twice from scalp to ends before cutting, and cut parallel to the part.

- Follow the comb with the fingers to maintain control of the hair parting.

- Cut with uniform minimal to moderate tension, depending on hair texture and elasticity.

Ⓟ 16-1   **Blunt Cut** *pages 544–547*

GRADUATED HAIRCUT

Listed are the characteristics of a graduated cut (45 degrees):

- A **graduated cut** (GRAJ-ooayt-ud KUT) has a wedge or stacked shape that is created by cutting with tension at low to medium elevations.

- The most common elevation for a graduated cut is 45 degrees.

- Graduated cuts build weight and volume along the perimeter of the hairstyle.

- The graduated haircut can be accomplished with either horizontal or vertical partings.

- The horizontal method is described in the following procedure, with references to the vertical parting technique noted as applicable.

- See **Figure 16-5** for a technical illustration of a graduated cut.

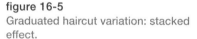
figure 16-5
Graduated haircut variation: stacked effect.

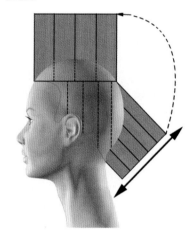

Haircutting Tips for a Graduated Cut

- Shampoo and condition the hair before cutting.

- Graduation makes fine hair of average density appear thicker and fuller.

- Maintain the same elevation around the perimeter when cutting design lines (guides).

- Maintain even, uniform tension and moisture throughout the haircut when cutting at a 45-degree angle away from the head.

- Blend from one subsection to another.

- Work with the natural growth patterns of the hair.

- Comb through the subsections twice from scalp to ends before cutting.

- Hold the hair that is being cut at a 45-degree elevation from the head and always use a traveling guide.

- Follow the comb with the fingers to maintain control of the hair parting.

Ⓟ 16-2   **Graduated Cut** *pages 548–553*

figure 16-6
Traveling guidelines.

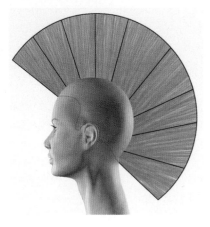

UNIFORM-LAYERED CUT (90 DEGREES)

Listed are the characteristics of a uniform-layered cut (90 degrees):

* In a **uniform-layered cut** (YOO-nih-form-lay-UHRD KUT), all of the hair strands are cut to the same length at a 90-degree elevation, straight out from where the hair grows.

* A traveling guide is used on the interior sections to create layers within the entire haircut.

* When finished, the cut will look soft and textured and conform to the head shape without weight lines or corners.

* A uniform-layered cut can be used to cut short- or long-layered haircuts.

* Hold the hair that is being cut at a 90-degree elevation from *where it grows*, and always use a traveling guide.

* See **Figure 16-6** for a technical illustration of a uniform-layered cut.

Haircutting Tips for a Uniform-Layered Cut

* Shampoo and condition the hair before cutting.

* Maintain uniform moisture in the hair while cutting—re-wet as needed.

* Take clean partings and subsections.

* Comb through the subsections twice from scalp to ends before cutting.

* Follow the comb with the fingers to maintain control of the hair parting.

* Either exterior (perimeter) or interior guides can be cut first; depending on how you are taught, either is acceptable.

* Avoid cutting into the perimeter (exterior) guide when layering.

* Always check design lines for blending the perimeter of the cut.

* Work with the natural growth pattern, wave formation, and density of the hair.

* Always make sure the hair blends from one section to another.

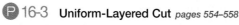

P 16-3   **Uniform-Layered Cut** *pages 554–558*

figure 16-7
180-degree long-layered technical.

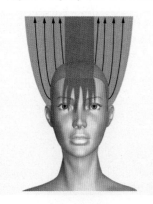

LONG-LAYERED CUT (180 DEGREES)

Listed are the characteristics of a long-layered cut (180 degrees):

* A **long-layered cut** (LAWNG-lay-UHRD KUT) consists of increased layering that is achieved by cutting the hair at a 180-degree elevation.

* This cut produces progressively longer layers from the top to the perimeter; the hair on top of the head is shorter than the hair closer to the perimeter/exterior guide.

* Sometimes a long-layered haircut begins with a stationary guide in the top section of the head.

* **Figure 16-7** depicts the technical pattern of a long-layered cut.

Haircutting Tips for Long-Layered Cuts

- Shampoo and condition the hair before cutting.

- Maintain uniform moisture in the hair while cutting—re-wet as needed.

- Take clean partings and subsections.

- Work with only as much hair as is comfortable and controllable. Create thinner working subsections of hair if the combination of length and density becomes unmanageable.

- Either exterior (perimeter) or interior guides can be cut first; depending on how you are taught, either is acceptable.

- If in doubt about what the remaining hanging length of the hair will be when it is cut to the top guide, cut in the design line at the perimeter first.

- Avoid cutting into the perimeter (exterior) guide when layering.

- Always check design lines for blending the perimeter of the cut.

- Work with the natural growth pattern, wave formation, and density of the hair.

- Always make sure the hair blends from one section to another.

- Comb through subsections from scalp to ends with even tension.

- Avoid steps and gaps between the layers. Blend sections from long to short.

P 16-4 **Long-Layered Cut** *pages 559–564*

table 16-1

TEXTURE AND DENSITY

Texture	Density		
	Thin	**Medium**	**Thick**
FINE	Limp, needs weight.	Great for many cuts, especially blunt and low elevation. Razor cuts are good.	Usually needs more texturizing. Suitable for many haircuts.
MEDIUM	Needs weight. Graduated shapes work well.	Great for most cuts. Hair can handle texturizing.	Many shapes are suitable. Texturizing usually necessary.
COARSE	Maintains some weight. Razor cuts not recommended.	Great for many shapes. Razor cuts appropriate if hair is in good condition.	Very short cuts do not work. Razors may frizz and *expand* hair. Maintain some length to weigh hair down.

Discuss Curly Hair Textures

After reading this section, you will be able to:

LO❸ Explain wave formation in curly hair textures.

Curly hair types range from large, loose curl patterns to tight, springy curls. Any of the four cutting elevations can be used on curly hair; however, the results will be different from those achieved on straighter hair. For example, curly hair tends to graduate naturally due to the elasticity and curl pattern. Use less elevation if strong angles are desired.

The trough and crest formation of the waves in curly hair textures needs to be taken into account when performing a haircut. Depending on the amount of curl, cutting the hair parting in the trough of the wave may cause the hair ends to flip out from the head form. Conversely, cutting just after the crest of the wave as it dips toward the trough may encourage the hair to fall inward toward the head form (**Figure 16-8**).

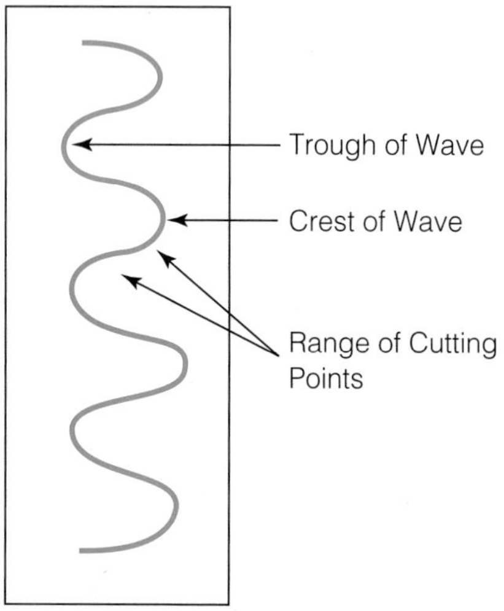

Knowing where to cut on the wave is helpful when cutting all lengths of curly hair and should be considered when analyzing the hair texture. It is most important when cutting shorter hairstyles, especially maintenance cuts on regular customers, because the amount of hair to be cut may have to be adjusted according to the wave pattern at any given time. For example, a client with wavy to curly hair has a standing appointment every four weeks. Assume that the hair grows at an average of ½ inch per month. If the hair was cut at a point just after the crest of the wave during the previous haircut service, those hair ends may now be part of the trough that develops as the hair curls naturally. Be careful not to automatically cut ½ inch of hair during the next visit because it may encourage the curl to wave out from the head form. Cutting a little less or a little more will place the cut line at the crest of the wave again and encourage the hair to curl toward the head form instead of away from it.

figure 16-8
Crest and trough formation of waves.

Trough of Wave

Crest of Wave

Range of Cutting Points

TECHNIQUES FOR CUTTING NATURAL CURLY STYLES

Depending on the overall length of the hair, short natural cuts on extremely curly hair can be created by using the freehand clipper or fingers-and-shear cutting technique. The hair is tapered at the perimeter and may be tapered, rounded, or wedged from the sides to the top section. When using clippers, the hair should be clean and dry. Fingers-and-shear cutting is usually performed on clean damp hair.

The decision to use clippers or shears will depend on the density and texture of the hair. Thick, coarse hair types are easier to cut with the clippers. Curly hair of medium density and a softer curl may be easier to cut with shears. The rule for fingers-and-shear cutting on extremely curly hair is that if a parting can be made and held between the index and second finger, fingers-and-shear cutting can be performed.

Haircutting Tips for Clipper Cutting Curly Hair

• Observe the density and curl pattern closely. Sometimes extremely curly hair give the illusion that the scalp will not be seen if the hair is cut close, but in reality, it may continue to curl in upon itself in small tufts, leaving partings throughout the hair and scalp exposed.

• Use your comb as a guard around the hairline to avoid cutting the hair too close to the head.

• After each cut with the clipper, comb or pick the hair to check the effect.

• Create flattering and proportionate design forms throughout the parietal and apex sections.

Explore Various Cutting Techniques

After reading this section, you will be able to:

LO④ Discuss other haircutting techniques.

In addition to the basic haircutting elevations, other techniques that can be used to create different effects in the appearance and behavior of the hair include:

• overdirection

• razor cutting

• texturizing

OVERDIRECTION

Overdirection occurs when the hair is combed away from its natural fall position. This technique of shifting the hair into a different position can be used to:

• Increase the lengths in a perimeter design line

• Blend short and long lengths along a perimeter design line or interior section (**Figure 16-9**)

RAZOR CUTTING

Razor cutting produces an angle at the ends of the hair that results in softer shapes with more movement and visual separation than shear cutting. Generally, haircuts that can be accomplished with shears can also be performed with a razor.

When cutting hair with a razor, the *hair must be damp*.

Review **Figures 16-10** to **16-14** for razor applications on longer hair.

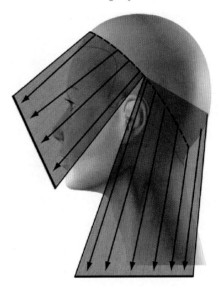

figure 16-9
Overdirection in long-layered haircut.

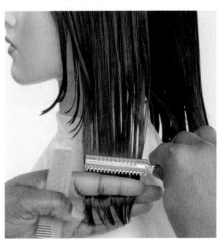

figure 16-10
Razor cutting parallel to subsection.

figure 16-11
Razor cutting at 45-degree angle.

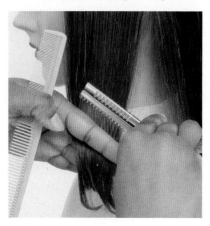

figure 16-12
Incorrect razor angle.

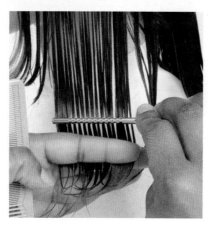

figure 16-13
Hand position in vertical section.

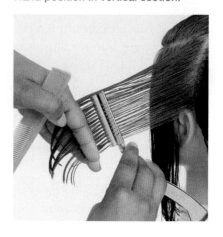

figure 16-14
Hand position on horizontal section.

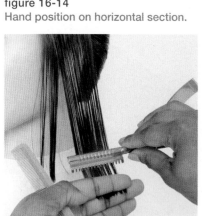

figure 16-15a
Point cutting with steeper shears angle.

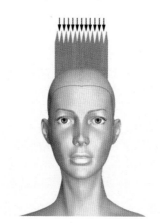

figure 16-15b
Point cutting.

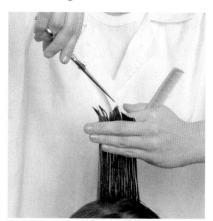

figure 16-16
Notching.

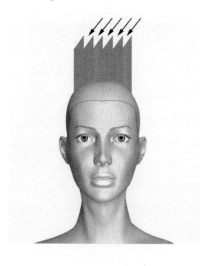

TEXTURIZING

Texturizing techniques can be used to remove excess bulk, add volume, create movement, or create wispy and spiky effects. The most commonly used texturizing techniques are:

- **Point cutting** is performed at the ends of the hair using the tips of the shears at a steep shear angle in relation to the hair parting (Figures 16-15a and 16-15b).

- **Notching** creates a chunkier effect than point cutting and is produced by positioning the shears at a flatter angle to the ends of the hair (Figure 16-16).

- Freehand notching is also accomplished with the tips of the shears but is usually performed within the interior sections of the haircut.

- **Slithering** is the process of thinning the hair to graduated lengths with the shears, which produces volume and movement. The hair is cut using a sliding shears movement with the blades kept partially opened (Figure 16-17).

figure 16-17
Slithering.

figure 16-18
Slicing with shears.

figure 16-19
Carving a twisted section of hair to remove the bulk.

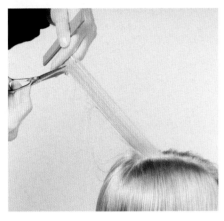

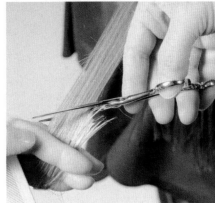

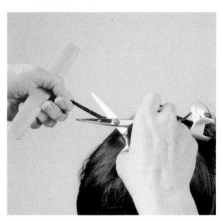

- **Slicing** also removes bulk and adds movement in the hair. The blades are kept open, and only the portion of the blade near the pivot is used for cutting (Figure 16-18).

- **Carving** is a version of slicing that creates separation in the hair. The shears are moved throughout the hair with an open and closing movement that carves out sections of hair (Figure 16-19). Carving the ends of the hair will create texture and separation at the perimeter.

Discuss Hairstyling

After reading this section, you will be able to:

 5   Explain different hairstyling techniques.

As with haircutting, the first step in the hairstyling process is the client consultation. During the consultation, guide the client toward the most suitable hairstyle for her face shape, hair texture, and lifestyle. Keep styling magazines accessible for easy reference during the consultation. Hairstyling techniques include:

- wet hairstyling
- blowdry styling
- thermal styling
- natural dry styling

Discussion and procedures for hair wrapping and molding, blowdry styling, curling irons, pressing combs, and flat irons are included in this chapter. For finger waving, pin curls, and roller-set procedures, refer to *Milady Standard Cosmetology* textbook.

WET HAIRSTYLING

Wet hairstyling is accomplished by hair wrapping, hair molding, finger waving, pin curls, and roller sets. The tools needed include:

- rollers
- pin-curl clips
- sectioning clips
- all-purpose combs
- brushes
- setting lotion

What are various methods of wet hairstyling?

- **Finger waving** is the process of shaping and directing the hair into an S-shaped pattern through the use of fingers, comb, and setting lotion.

- **Pin curls**

  Are the basis for patterns, lines, waves, and curls used in a variety of hairstyles. They are wound from the hair ends into a spiral or circle creating a flattened curl formation against the head. Pin curls are secured with a hair clip, dried, and styled.

- **Roller sets**

  Rollers set a pattern in the hair that will form the basis for a hairstyle. Wet hair is wrapped around rollers, which are available in a variety of materials, shapes, and sizes:
  - Plastic rollers are used for most wet roller sets.
  - Hot rollers are used on dry hair.
  - Velcro rollers are used on wet or dry hair.

- **Natural dry styling**

  Once the hair is towel-dried, it is combed into place or arranged into a style with the hands and fingers. It is then allowed to dry naturally. Natural dry styling requires minimal manipulation of the hair.

> **⚠ CAUTION**
>
> Be careful of the type of brush used on damp hair as some bristle styles can snag, damage, or stretch the hair during the brushing process. If the use of a brush is preferred or necessary to perform hair wrapping or molding techniques, choose a brush with wide-spaced bristles.

HAIR WRAPPING

Hair wrapping (HAYR RAP-ing) is a technique used to keep curly hair smooth and straight while retaining a beautiful shape (**Figure 16-20**). Curly hair can be wrapped around the head to give it a smooth, rounded contour, resulting in an effect that is similar to that attained with rollers. When wrapping hair, very little volume is attained because the hair at the scalp is not lifted. If height is desired, you can place large rollers directly at the crown, with the remainder of the hair wrapped around the head.

Wrapping can be done on wet or dry hair. When wrapping dry hair, use a silicone shine product instead of using a gel; this will provide a glossy comb out. On curly hair, wet wrapping creates a smooth, sleek look. When working with very curly hair, press it first, and then do a dry hair wrapping.

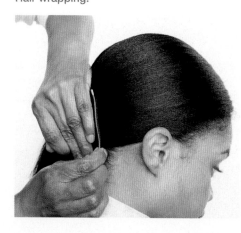

figure 16-20
Hair wrapping.

Ⓟ 16-5 **Hair Wrapping** *pages 565–567*

HAIR MOLDING

Hair molding (HAYR MOHLD-ing) is the process of combing the hair straight down over the client's head, followed by drying, and finishing with thermal irons. Like hair wrapping, hair molding also uses the client's head as a form or tool.

BLOWDRY STYLING

Blowdry styling (BLOH-dry sti-hyl-ing) is the technique of drying and styling damp or wet hair in one step. A blowdryer, brush, and styling products (optional) are used to style the hair (in a manner similar to that used in men's styling). Blowdrying can also prepare the hair for thermal iron curling or straightening. Combined with the foundation of a good haircut, blowdry styling is a quick and relatively simple option.

Ⓟ 16-6   Blowdrying Blunt or Long-Layered, Straight to Wavy Hair into a Straight Style *pages 568–570*

THERMAL STYLING

Thermal styling (THUR-mul sti-hyl-ing) uses *heat* to produce curls or waves (curling irons) or straightened hair (pressing combs or flat irons).

Thermal Waving

Thermal waving is performed with Marcel irons or electric thermal (curling) irons. There are two important factors to consider when creating curls with a curling iron:

1. The barrel size of the iron determines the size of the wave or curl.

2. The projection of the hair from the scalp will determine where the curl sits in relation to its base, and hence the amount of volume achieved.

    The differences between a Marcel iron and a curling iron are:

* A curling iron has a spring mechanism that holds the clamp tight to the barrel.

* A Marcel iron has a clamp that is controlled manually by the user; it does not have a spring.

    Understanding of the three parts of a curl will help explain the relationships between hair projection, bases, and volume:

1. The **base** is the stationary foundation of the curl on which the barrel (or roller) is placed.

2. The **stem** (STEM) is the hair between the scalp and the first arc of the circle; it gives the hair direction and mobility.

3. The **circle** (SUR-kul) forms the curl as the hair is wrapped around the barrel or roller. The ultimate size of the curl along the length of the hair shaft depends on how it is wrapped (**Figure 16-21**).

    A hair section that is wrapped in a spiral along the curling iron barrel will have a more uniform curl formation than a hair section that is

figure 16-21
Parts of a curl.

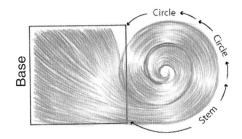

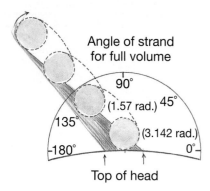

figure 16-22
On-base roller: full volume.

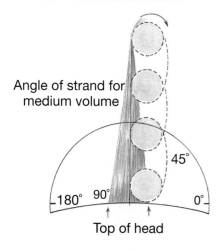

figure 16-23
Half-base roller: medium volume.

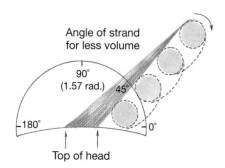

figure 16-24
Off-base roller: less volume.

repeatedly wrapped around itself over one section of the barrel. There are three kinds of bases used in thermal (and roller) styling:

1. **On-base** (also known as *no-stem*)
   - Roller placement sits directly on the base and produces a full-volume curl.
   - On-base placement is achieved by slightly overdirecting the hair beyond 90 degrees in front of the base (**Figure 16-22**).

2. **Half off-base** (also known as *half-base* or *half-stem*)
   - Roller placement sits halfway on and halfway behind the base after rolling the hair parting at 90 degrees (**Figure 16-23**).
   - This gives less volume than an on-base placement, but more volume than an off-base placement.

3. **Off-base** roller (also known as *long stem*)
   - Placement produces the least amount of volume and sits completely off the base.
   - The hair is held at 45 degrees from the base and rolled down to the scalp (**Figure 16-24**).

Thermal Straightening

Thermal hair straightening, also known as **hair pressing** (HAYR PRES-ing), temporarily straightens hair by using heated pressing combs or irons. Pressings generally last until the next shampoo, although high humidity and other weather conditions can cause the hair to partially revert to its natural condition. Following a shampoo and blowdry, the hair is prepared for the pressing service with an application of a pressing cream or oil. These products make the hair softer and help prevent the hair from burning or scorching. In some cases, environmental conditions may determine what type of press to use:

1. **Soft press**
   - Removes 50 to 60 percent of the curl.
   - Accomplished by applying the pressing comb once to each side of the hair section.

2. **Medium press**
   - Removes 60 to 75 percent of the curl.
   - Performed in the same manner as the soft press, but with more pressure.

3. **Hard press**
   - Removes 100 percent of the curl.
   - Involves two applications of the pressing comb on each side of the hair section.

Safety Precautions for Thermal Curling and Pressing Irons

- Use thermal irons only after receiving instruction on their use.
- Keep irons clean.
- Always test the temperature of the iron before using it on a client.

- Do not overheat irons.

- Handle and remove heated irons and stoves carefully.

- Do not place heated stoves near a station mirror as the heat can cause breakage.

- Place a hard rubber comb between the client's scalp and the iron.

- Never use a metal comb when performing thermal styling services.

- Place heated stoves and irons in a safe place to cool.

Ⓟ 16-7   **Hair Pressing** *pages 571–572*

FLAT IRONS

Electric flat irons are used to temporarily straighten hair. They can also be used to give direction to straighter hair texture styles while imparting a glossy, finished look to the hair.

- Flat irons are available in many sizes from mini-irons for short hair lengths or tight styling areas to larger irons suitable for long-hair styling.

- Flat irons should only be used on clean, dry hair because heat applied to hair that has oil or styling product buildup can damage the hair and the iron.

- The application of a leave-in thermal styling product is recommended before drying the hair to protect the hair from heat damage.

- Excessive heat damages the hair, so care needs to be taken to monitor the temperature of the flat iron.

- Test the temperature by placing a piece of misted tissue paper between the heating plates. If the temperature is safe to apply to the hair, the moisture in the paper will evaporate without leaving any evidence of scorching.

Safety Precautions for Flat Irons

- Use flat irons only after receiving instruction on their use.

- Keep irons clean.

- Choose the right size of iron to achieve desired results.

- Start with clean, conditioned, and thoroughly dried hair.

- Always test the temperature of the iron before using it on a client.

- Do not overheat irons.

- Section the hair according to the density of the hair and the size of the iron.

- Handle and remove heated irons carefully.

- Place a hard rubber comb between the client's scalp and the iron.

- Never use a metal comb when performing thermal styling services.

- Place heated irons in a safe place to cool.

Ⓟ 16-8   **Flat Iron Pressing** *pages 573–574*

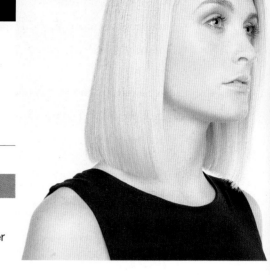

BLUNT CUT

After reading and practicing this procedure, you will be able to:

LO❻ Demonstrate a blunt cut.

MATERIALS, IMPLEMENTS, AND EQUIPMENT

☐ Blowdryer

☐ Classic styling brush

☐ Cutting comb

☐ Haircutting cape

☐ Haircutting shears

☐ Neck strip

☐ Sectioning clips

☐ Shampoo and conditioner

☐ Shampoo cape

☐ Spray bottle with water

☐ Towels

☐ Wide-tooth comb

PREPARATION

1 Wash your hands.

2 Conduct client consultation.

3 Drape client for wet service.

4 Shampoo and towel-dry hair. Blowdry the hair if dry cutting is preferred.

5 Remove waterproof cape.

6 Escort the client back to the styling chair.

PROCEDURE

1 Face the client toward the mirror and lock the chair.

2 Drape your client for a haircut.

3 Secure a neck strip around the client's neck. Place a haircutting cape over the neck strip and fasten in the back. Fold the neck strip down over the cape so that no part of the cape touches the client's skin.

4 Detangle the hair with the wide-tooth comb.

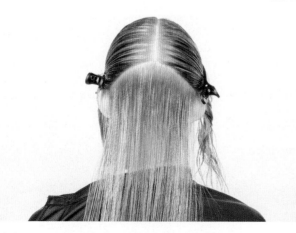

5 Take a central profile parting from the front hairline through to the nape; take two diagonal forward partings from the occipital to behind the ear. (The depth of the section may vary due to hair density.)

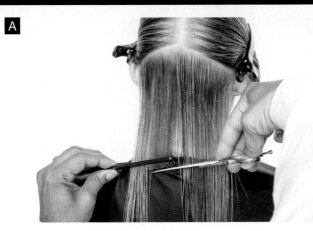

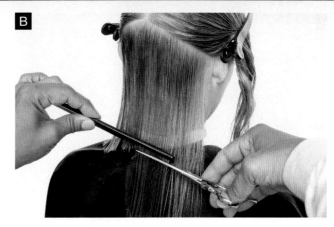

6 Tilt the head slightly forward. Starting in the center, using the fine teeth, comb the hair into natural fall (0 elevation) and cut line parallel to the diagonal forward parting. Repeat on the opposite side, starting cut from the outer corner to the center creating a slight arc-shaped line. Check balance.

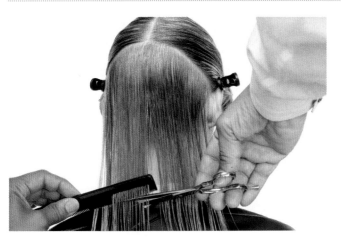

7 Take another set of diagonal forward partings from the top of the occipital to the top of each ear. Take a center part that runs from the top occipital to the nape, dividing the head into two. The head position will move up slightly, but the natural fall distribution and 0 elevation remain consistent. Cut parallel to parting and follow the length of your guide.

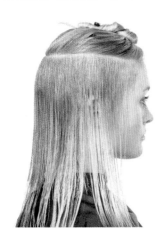

8 With the client's head upright, take a horseshoe section from just below the crown to the front hairline. Starting in the rear of the horseshoe section, using the wide teeth, comb the hair into natural fall over the previously cut hair. Cut the line along the comb following your guide beneath, till you reach the sides just below the ear.

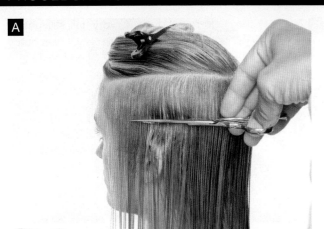

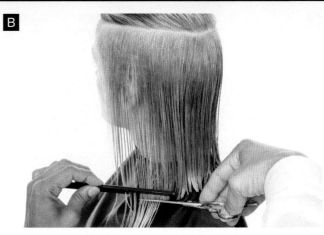

9 On the sides just behind the ear, continue to comb the hair into natural fall, cutting the hair parallel to the horseshoe parting. Pay close attention to the protrusion of the ear and tap the hair above the comb before you cut to release any tension.

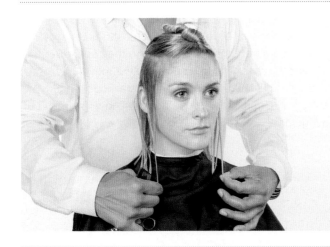

10 Repeat on the opposite side. Before moving on, stand behind the client and check the lengths on both sides while looking in the mirror. Make any needed adjustments.

11 Take another subsection from the horseshoe above the crown to the front hairline. Starting at the back, comb the hair to natural fall and cut at 0 elevation following your guide. When you reach the sides continue the same technique as Step 9.

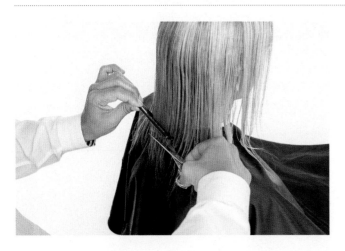

12 Release the remainder of the section, comb hair to natural fall, paying close attention to any cowlicks or movement at the crown. Starting at the back continue combing the hair to natural fall and cutting at 0 elevation following your guide.

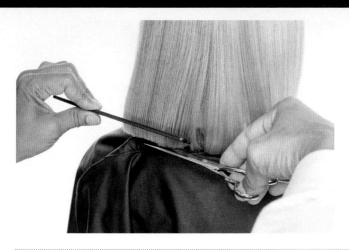

13 To check the line for accuracy, blowdry hair straight and smooth sectioning the hair the same way it was cut, using classic styling brush. Do not use a round brush; it creates a bend in the ends of the hair making it difficult to check the line.

14 Once the hair is dry, check the line in the mirror. You should see an even, horizontal line all the way around the head. Using the wide teeth, comb the hair to natural fall and clean up the bob line. (Avoid cutting the line shorter.)

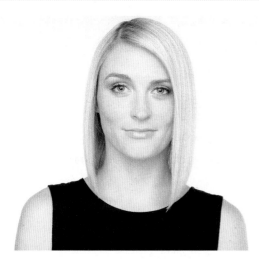

15 Finished look.

CLEAN-UP AND DISINFECTION

☐ Clean and disinfect tools and implements.

☐ Clean and disinfect work area.

☐ Sweep up hair and deposit in closed receptacle.

☐ Dispose of single-use items. Place all used linens, towels, and capes in the laundry.

☐ Wash your hands.

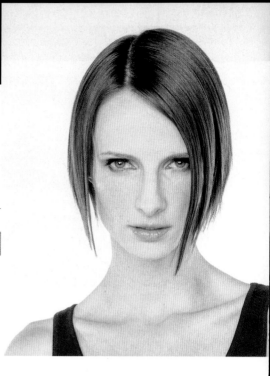

GRADUATED CUT

After reading and practicing this procedure, you will be able to:

LO❼ Demonstrate a graduated cut.

MATERIALS, IMPLEMENTS, AND EQUIPMENT

- □ Blowdryer
- □ Cutting or styling comb
- □ Haircutting cape
- □ Haircutting shears
- □ Neck strip
- □ Sectioning clips
- □ Shampoo and conditioner
- □ Shampoo cape
- □ Spray bottle with water
- □ Towels
- □ Wide-tooth comb

PREPARATION

1. Wash your hands.
2. Conduct client consultation.
3. Drape client for wet service.
4. Shampoo and towel-dry hair. Blowdry the hair if dry cutting is preferred.
5. Remove waterproof cape.
6. Escort the client back to the styling chair.

PROCEDURE

1. Face the client toward the mirror and lock the chair.
2. Drape your client for a haircut.
3. Secure a new neck strip around the client's neck.
4. Place a haircutting cape over the neck strip and fasten in the back. Fold the neck strip down over the cape so that no part of the cape touches the client's skin.

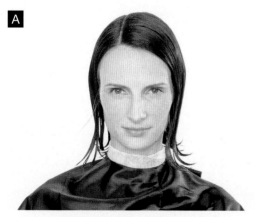

A

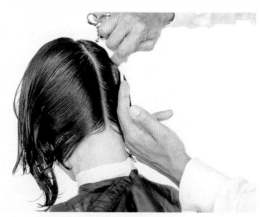

B

5. Begin your first section by taking the parting from the client's natural side part back to the crown. Then take a central parting from the crown to the nape.

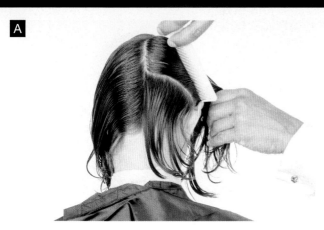

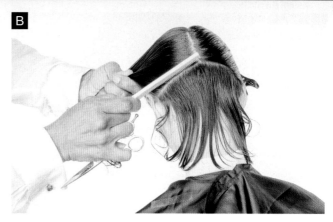

6 At the occipital bone, take a diagonal forward parting from the central parting to the middle of each ear. Then take a pivoting diagonal forward subsection, elevate it to 45 degrees, and cut parallel to your parting. Both your finger angle and elevation should be at 45 degrees.

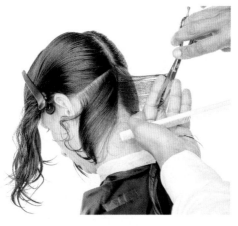

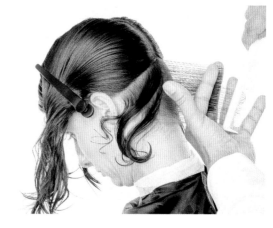

7 Make sure that your section is no longer than 2 to 3 inches in length or your graduation will sit too low. This will serve as your traveling guide.

8 Continue taking pivoting diagonal forward subsections, using the previously cut subsection as a traveling guide. Both your elevation and finger angle are held at 45 degrees. Elevate and cut parallel to your parting.

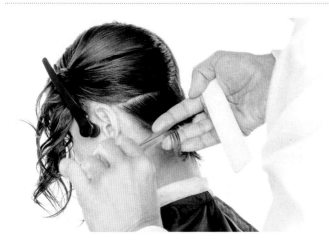

9 Once you have reached your last subsection, you should be parallel to your diagonal forward parting; continue to elevate to 45 degrees following your traveling guide.

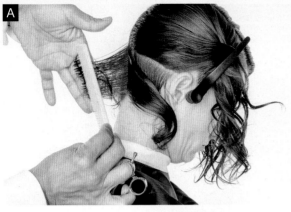

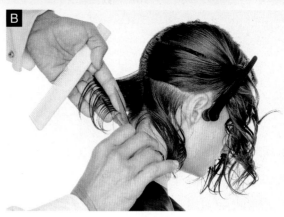

10 Repeat the same steps and technique on the opposite side. (Note the change in hand position. The tips of your fingers will now be palm up, pointing down.) Once completed, cross-check the balance from the outer edges on both sides.

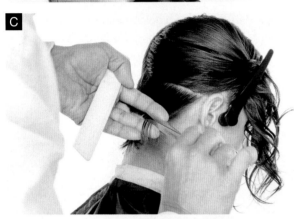

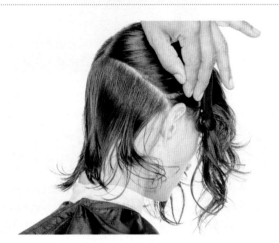

11 To begin the next section, take a diagonal forward parting from above the occipital bone extending to the top of each ear. Each side is then subsectioned and cut as before, using pivoting diagonal forward subsections to work your way through the section.

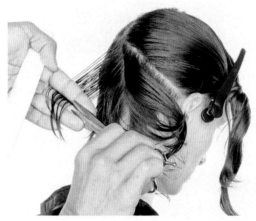

12 To maintain the same level of graduation as the first section, comb the hair parallel to your parting, and, using a small piece of the length of hair, cut from the first section as a guide, cut in a stationary guide at a 45-degree elevation.

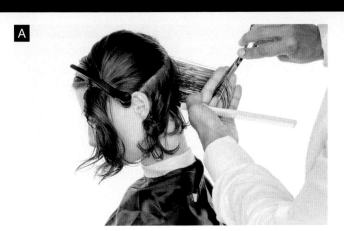

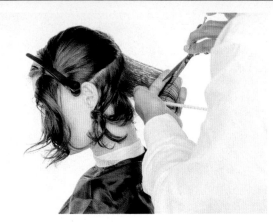

13 Repeat the steps on the opposite side; once completed, check for visual balance.

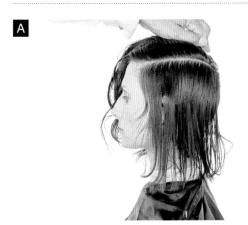

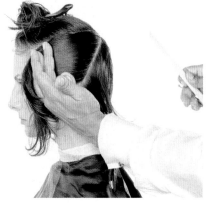

14 The next section will be a horseshoe section, taken from just below the crown to the recession area on both sides. This section will be subdivided and cut using traveling diagonal forward subsections, combed at natural fall, and then elevated to 45 degrees and cut parallel to the horseshoe parting.

15 The elevation will decrease to one finger's depth just behind the ear, where you transition to the sides, and the bob line begins. From the ear forward, the hair is held in the comb to release tension, and cut at 0 elevation parallel to the horseshoe parting.

16 Repeat the same steps on the opposite side.

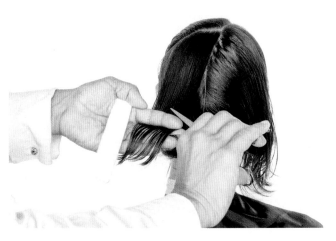

17 Continue taking sections from the horseshoe, until the natural side part is reached, and all remaining hair has been cut following your guide.

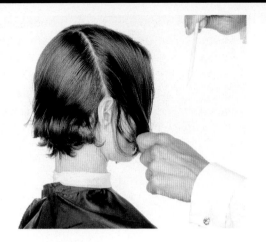

18 In preparation for layering, create a radial section by taking a radial parting from the crown to the top of each ear. Take a ½-inch-wide central vertical subsection from the crown to the occipital.

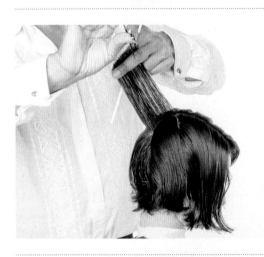

19 The hair in this section is elevated to 90 degrees and overdirected back. Your guide will be taken from the perimeter of the graduation for the length. You will point cut following the head shape. (Do not cut below occipital or you will cut into your graduation.)

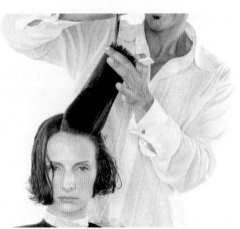

20 Pivoting subsections are combed to 90 degrees, overdirected back, and, using a traveling guide, cut parallel to the head. When you have completed the radial section, repeat on the opposite side.

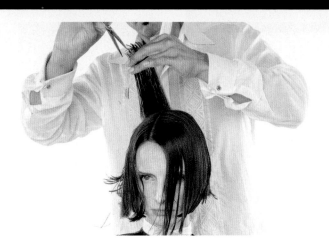

21 When you reach the sides, take a horizontal subsection from the natural side part, elevate to 90 degrees, overdirect back, and point cut following your guide from the radial section. (Make sure to keep your elbows up to avoid cutting into the perimeter.) Remember to begin at the natural side part and overdirect the section back to a stationary guide at the radial section.

22 In the front, length is maintained by overdirecting back to a stationary guide at the radial section. Repeat the same steps on the opposite side.

23 Once the hair is dry, detail the perimeter, starting at the nape use the points of your shears for softness, or blunt cut for a stronger line. At the sides, clean up your line at the perimeter. (Avoid cutting too much hair, remember that you are just detailing.)

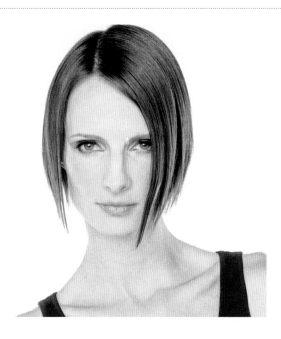

24 Finished look.

CLEAN-UP AND DISINFECTION

☐ Clean and disinfect tools and implements.

☐ Clean and disinfect work area.

☐ Sweep up hair and deposit in closed receptacle.

☐ Dispose of single-use items. Place all used linens, towels, and capes in the laundry.

☐ Wash your hands.

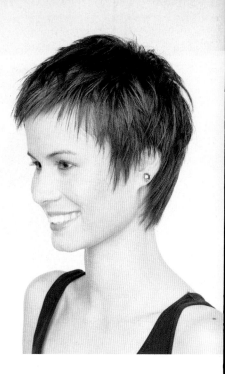

UNIFORM-LAYERED CUT

After reading and practicing this procedure, you will be able to:

LO⑧ Demonstrate a uniform-layered cut.

MATERIALS, IMPLEMENTS, AND EQUIPMENT

- ☐ Blowdryer
- ☐ Cutting or styling comb
- ☐ Haircutting cape
- ☐ Haircutting shears
- ☐ Neck strip
- ☐ Sectioning clips

- ☐ Shampoo and conditioner
- ☐ Shampoo cape
- ☐ Spray bottle with water
- ☐ Towels
- ☐ Wide-tooth comb

PREPARATION

1. Wash your hands.
2. Conduct client consultation.
3. Drape client for wet service.
4. Shampoo and towel-dry hair. Blowdry the hair if dry cutting is preferred.
5. Remove waterproof cape.
6. Escort the client back to the styling chair.

PROCEDURE

1. Face the client toward the mirror and lock the chair.
2. Drape your client for a haircut.
3. Secure a neck strip around the client's neck. Place a haircutting cape over the neck strip and fasten in the back. Fold the neck strip down over the cape so that no part of the cape touches the client's skin.
4. Detangle the hair with the wide-tooth comb.

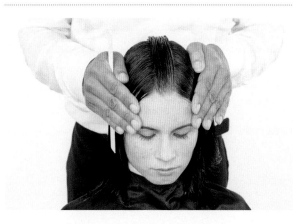

5. To create a guide, take a ½-inch-wide profile section from the front hairline to the nape. Cut palm-to-palm until you have reached the apex and then switch hand position.

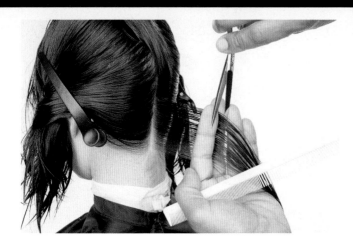

6 Starting at the nape, elevate the hair to 90 degrees and cut 3 inches in length working in small increments following the head shape.

A

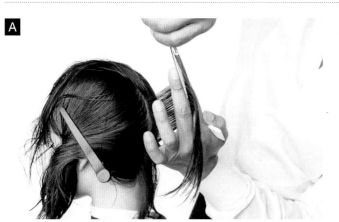

B

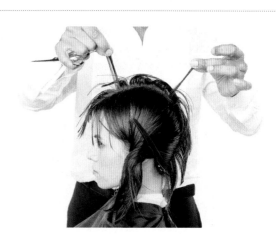

7 Above occipital, switch hand position and cut to the second knuckle to avoid corners forming on the line. Follow the guide to the front hairline. Once you have cut the center guide, check the length for balance and remove any corners.

8 After completing the guide, make a horseshoe section from recession to recession and below the crown. Make sure your section is clean and balanced at both sides of the recession.

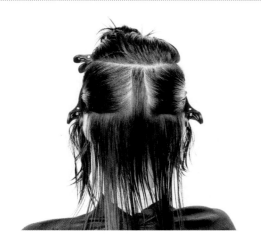

9 Take a horizontal parting from the occipital to the back of each ear and clip the section above your horizontal line. At the back, take a center section from the occipital to the nape, dividing your first initial profile section guide into half.

10 Starting at the center back, take a slight diagonal forward parting through to the nape, incorporating your guide from the profile section.

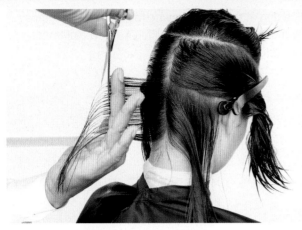

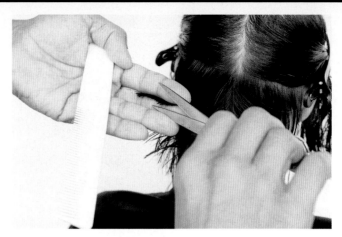

11 Elevate the hair to 90 degrees and cut parallel to the parting for your subsection following the guide. If you cannot see your guide, take a smaller subsection. (Hand position is palm-to-palm when cutting the left side.)

12 Cross-check horizontally; on every fourth section (any overdirection should be corrected section by section), the line should go round because you are following the head shape.

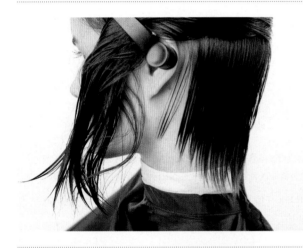

13 Continue taking slight diagonal forward subsections, elevating at 90 degrees, and cutting parallel to your parting for your subsection until you have reached the back of the ear. Switch hand position and repeat on the opposite side.

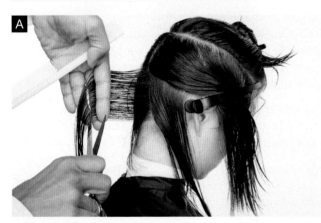

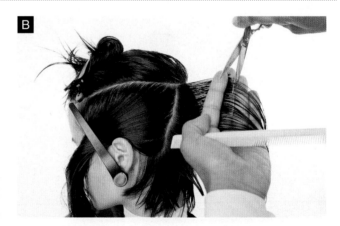

14 Release the lower portion of the horseshoe and cut palm-to-palm below the horseshoe on both sides. Continue taking slight diagonal forward subsections, elevating to 90 degrees, and cutting parallel to your parting. Follow your guide until you have completed the side and then repeat on the opposite side.

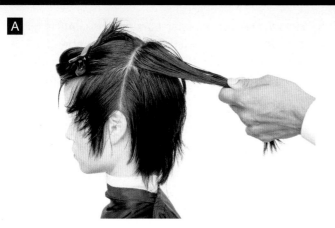

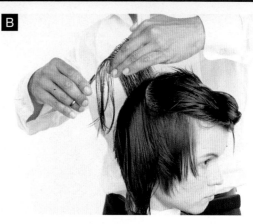

15 Release the horseshoe section and then take a radial section from above the crown to the top of each ear separating the hair from front to back. Switch hand position and cut above your fingers for the remainder of the haircut.

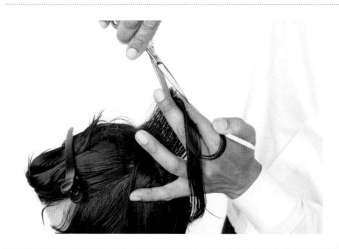

16 Pivoting wedge-shaped sections are taken from below your radial section following your guide; elevate the hair to 90 degrees and cut until you have completed both sides. (Remember to cross-check.)

17 At this point, you should have a guide from the top, sides, and behind the radial section allowing you to stay consistent and follow the head shape.

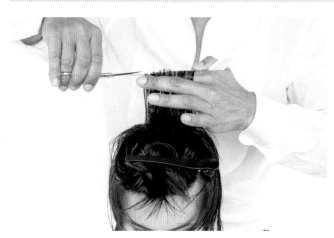

18 Continue taking horizontal subsections elevated to 90 degrees and cut to the traveling guide, until you have reached the front hairline. Repeat the same technique on the opposite side.

19 Dry the haircut with your hands or a paddle brush avoiding the sides. Once the haircut is dry, texturize the interior to remove weight by using deep point cutting.

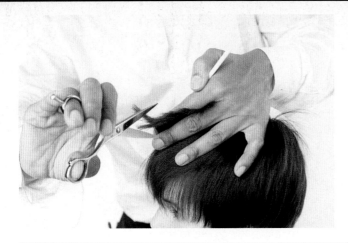

20 Hold the section 2 inches from the ends, and enter the section parallel so you do not remove any length; work in 1-inch panels. (Do not angle your shears and close the blade on the way out to avoid cutting your fingers.)

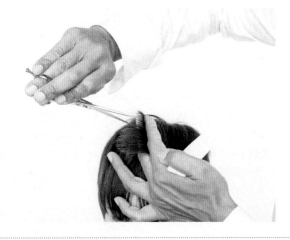

21 Use your mirror, and visually look at the balance. Detail the bang area (utilize the short-textured bangs technique) and perimeter with point cutting and carving.

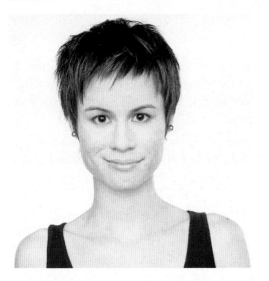

22 Finished look.

CLEAN-UP AND DISINFECTION

☐ Wash and disinfect tools and implements.

☐ Clean and disinfect work area.

☐ Sweep up hair and deposit in closed receptacle.

☐ Dispose of single-use items. Place all used linens, towels, and capes in the laundry.

☐ Wash your hands.

P 16-4

LONG-LAYERED CUT

After reading and practicing this procedure, you will be able to:

LO❾ Demonstrate a long-layered cut.

MATERIALS, IMPLEMENTS, AND EQUIPMENT

□ Blowdryer

□ Cutting or styling comb

□ Haircutting cape

□ Haircutting shears

□ Neck strip

□ Sectioning clips

□ Shampoo and conditioner

□ Shampoo cape

□ Spray bottle with water

□ Towels

□ Wide-tooth comb

PREPARATION

1 Wash your hands.

2 Conduct client consultation.

3 Drape client for wet service.

4 Shampoo and towel-dry hair. Blowdry the hair if dry cutting is preferred.

5 Remove waterproof cape.

6 Escort the client back to the styling chair.

PROCEDURE

1 Face the client toward the mirror and lock the chair.

2 Drape your client for a haircut.

3 Secure a neck strip around the client's neck. Place a haircutting cape over the neck strip and fasten in the back. Fold the neck strip down over the cape so that no part of the cape touches the client's skin.

4 Detangle the hair with a wide-tooth comb.

A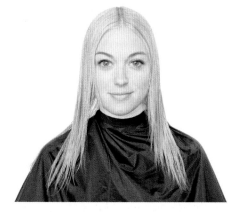

B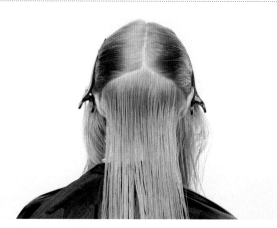

5 Begin by taking a central profile parting from the front hairline through to the nape, and then take two slight diagonal forward subsections (½ inch wide) from the occipital to behind the ear. (The thickness of the section may vary depending on hair density.)

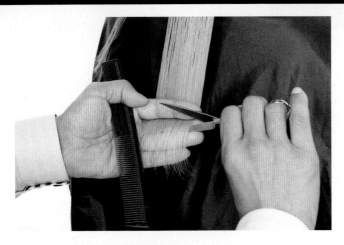

6 Tilt the head slightly forward. Starting in the center back, comb the hair to natural fall at 0 degrees. Cut (length) the line parallel to the parting. This will serve as your guide for the perimeter. The perimeter guide can be cut by holding it with either your fingers or a comb.

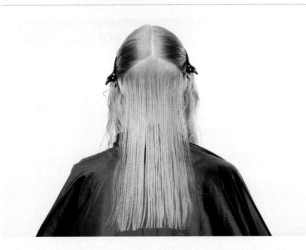

7 Take another ½-inch-wide set of slight diagonal forward subsections from the top of the occipital to the top of each ear. The head position will move up slightly, but the natural fall distribution and 0 elevation will remain. Cut parallel to the parting and follow the length of your guide.

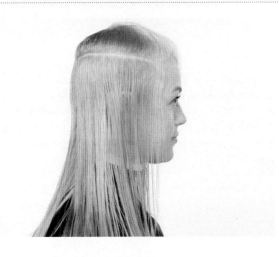

8 With the client's head upright, take a horseshoe section from below the crown to the front hairline. Starting at the back of the head, comb the hair into natural fall with 0 elevation, and cut the line following your guide.

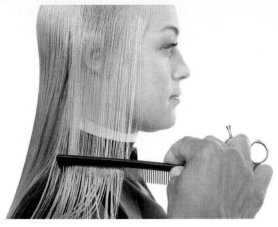

9 On the sides, comb the hair to natural fall, and over-direct to behind the shoulder and cut the line square to your guide. To do this, you will stand to the side to comb the hair into natural fall. Then step to the back and cut the line square.

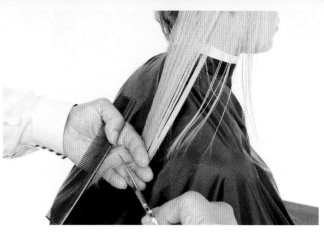

10 Repeat the same technique on the opposite side. Continue cutting the hair in the horseshoe until you've reached the profile part (at the apex of the head) or run out of hair to cut.

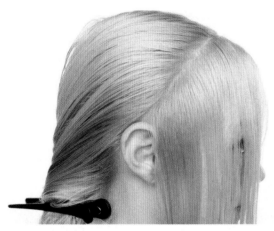

11 On the sides, take a diagonal back parting, from the profile part to the top of each ear.

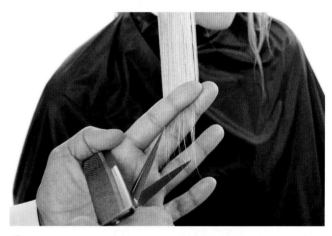

12 Standing to the front side of your client, comb the hair parallel to your diagonal back parting, elevate to a 45-degree angle from the face. Starting at the bottom corner, cut the hair in small increments to the length of the chin.

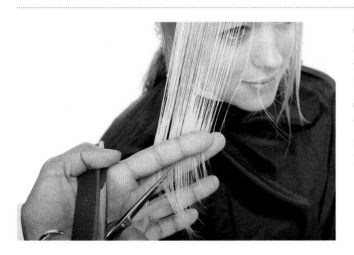

13 To keep the length on the sides from front to back, avoid cutting the corner at the sideburn area or just in front of the ear. Clients with long hair want to see their length at the front and back.

14 Take another diagonal back parting; this time extend to behind the ear (incorporating the hair from your first diagonal back subsection). Comb the hair parallel to the parting, elevate to 45 degrees, and follow your guide.

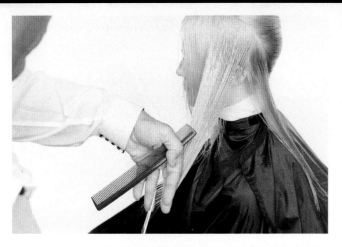

15 Although you are sectioning out and taking hair behind the ear, this hair will not be cut. You will only be cutting hair from your corner, not what is behind the ear; avoid overdirecting any hair beyond that point.

16 Continue taking the diagonal back subsections, elevating to 45 degrees until you have reached the profile parting; at that point, you will be combing the hair at natural fall because you are cutting parallel to your line.

17 Repeat the same technique on the opposite side, paying close attention to body position, balance, and your corner.

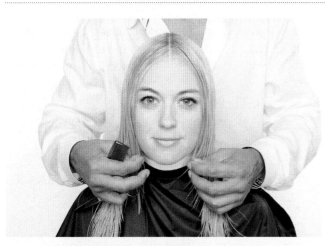

18 Once the sides are completed and you have checked your balance, take two diagonal forward partings from the top of the occipital to the back of each ear. The hair below your diagonal partings will be sectioned out of the way.

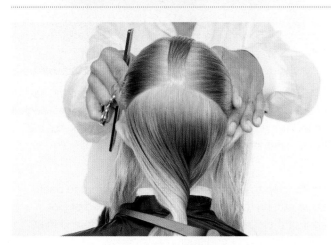

19 Starting at the front hairline, take a ½-inch profile section to the occipital, using your length from the chin as a guide.

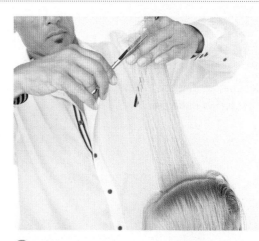

20 Elevate profile section to 90 degrees, and as you work toward the occipital, you will be overdirecting with your finger angle the length from the back at the occipital. The layered profile section will serve as a stationary guide for your interior layers.

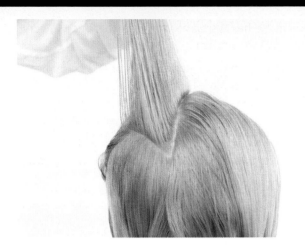

21 Below the crown and above the occipital, take a diagonal back line, elevate to 90 degrees, and overdirect to your center stationary guide. You should stand in front of the guide and overdirect the sections to your body keeping your elbows up.

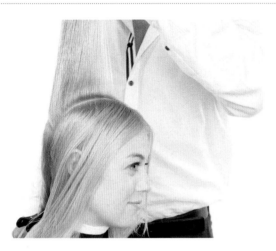

22 Continue taking diagonal back subsection, elevate up at 90 degrees, and overdirect to the stationary center guide. Continue until you have reached the front hairline section. Make sure you are combing the hair diagonally back and up into the center.

23 Repeat on the opposite side with the same technique. Remember to switch body position; stand on the opposite side and in front of your guide.

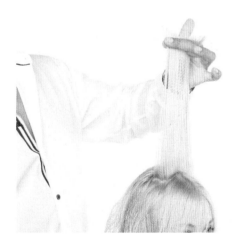

24 Cross-check the haircut by taking a horizontal section at the top and looking for an increase in length. Remember when the hair travels to a stationary guide it increases in length. The line should still be consistent, a short to long angle.

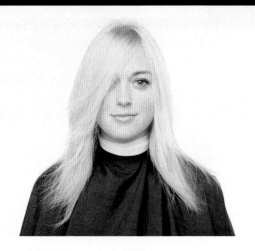

25 Section the hair the same way it was cut and blowdry using a large round brush.

26 Once the hair is dry, detail the interior and perimeter using deep point cutting. Hold the section 3 inches from the ends and enter the hair parallel (use the entire length of the blade) so you do not remove any length.

27 Work in 1-inch panels. (Do not angle your shears and close the blade on the way out to avoid cutting your fingers.)

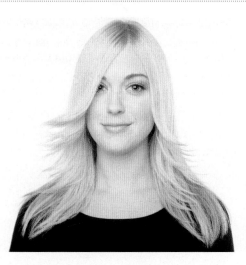

28 Finished look.

CLEAN-UP AND DISINFECTION

☐ Clean and disinfect tools and implements.

☐ Clean and disinfect work area.

☐ Sweep up hair and deposit in closed receptacle.

☐ Deposit used blades in a sharps container.

☐ Dispose of single-use items. Place all used linens, towels, and capes in the laundry.

☐ Wash your hands.

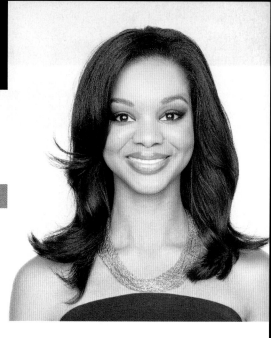

P 16-5

HAIR WRAPPING

□ Boar-bristle paddle brush
□ Bobby pins
□ Conditioner
□ Duckbill clips
□ Haircutting cape
□ Hairnet

□ Hood dryer
□ Neck strip
□ Shampoo
□ Shampoo cape
□ Styling product (light oil is optional)
□ Wide-tooth comb

PREPARATION

1 Wash your hands.

2 Conduct client consultation.

3 Drape client for wet service.

4 Shampoo the client's hair, and condition if necessary. Blowdry the hair.

5 Remove waterproof cape.

6 Escort the client back to the styling chair.

PROCEDURE

1 Face the client toward the mirror and lock the chair.

2 Drape the client with a neck strip and haircutting cape.

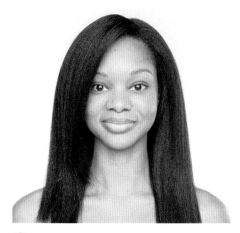

3 Press dry hair.

4 Remove any tangles with a wide-tooth comb, starting at the ends and working up to the scalp.

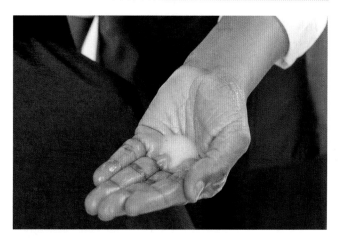

5 Apply a light oil or styling aid to dry hair before wrapping.

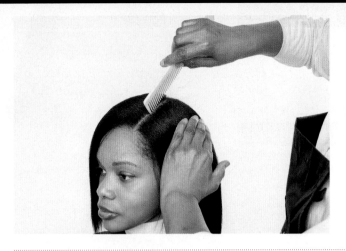

6 Create a parting from the recession area to the crown. Start combing the hair flat and to the right of the parting and hold it down with your hand.

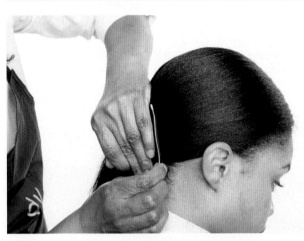

7 Starting on the heavy side of the part, using a natural bristle paddle brush, begin to wrap hair smooth to head shape counterclockwise, or in desired style direction. Use duckbill clips or large bobby pins to keep the hair in place while wrapping.

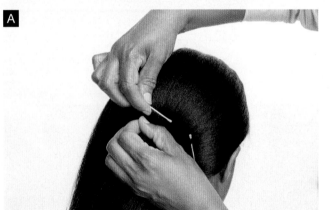

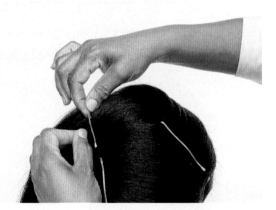

8 Continue wrapping the hair in a clockwise direction around the head. Follow the comb or brush with your hand or use your fingers, smoothing down the hair and keeping it tight to the head as you proceed.

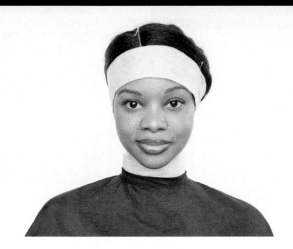

9 When all the hair is wrapped, stretch a neck strip or hairnet around the head so that it overlaps at the ends.

10 Place the client under a hooded dryer until the hair is completely dry, usually 45 minutes to 1 hour, depending on the hair length. If you have been working on dry hair, leave the hair wrapped for about 17 minutes. The longer the hair is wrapped, the smoother it will be.

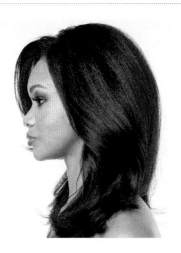

11 Finished look.

CLEAN-UP AND DISINFECTION

☐ Clean and disinfect tools and implements.

☐ Clean and disinfect work area.

☐ Dispose of single-use items. Place all used linens, towels, and capes in the laundry.

☐ Wash your hands.

BLOWDRYING BLUNT OR LONG-LAYERED, STRAIGHT TO WAVY HAIR INTO A STRAIGHT STYLE

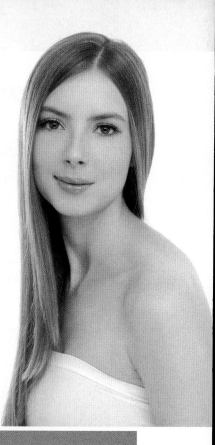

MATERIALS, IMPLEMENTS, AND EQUIPMENT

- ☐ Blowdryer with attachments
- ☐ Conditioner
- ☐ Haircutting cape
- ☐ Neck strip
- ☐ Paddle brush
- ☐ Round brush

- ☐ Sectioning clips
- ☐ Shampoo
- ☐ Shampoo cape
- ☐ Styling and finishing products
- ☐ Towels
- ☐ Wide-tooth comb

Thom Carson Photography

PREPARATION

1. Wash your hands.
2. Conduct client consultation.
3. Drape client for wet service.

4. Shampoo and towel-dry hair.
5. Remove waterproof cape.
6. Escort the client back to the styling chair.

PROCEDURE

1. Face the client toward the mirror and lock the chair.
2. Place a clean neck strip on the client.
3. Drape your client with a cutting or styling cape. Place a cape over the neck strip and fasten in the back.
4. Fold the neck strip over the cape so no part of the haircutting cape touches the client's skin.
5. Remove any tangles with a wide-tooth comb, starting at the ends and working up the scalp.
6. Apply a light gel or a straightening gel.

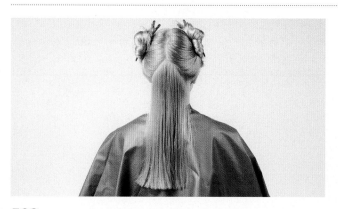

7. Attach the nozzle or concentrator attachment to the blowdryer for more controlled styling. Part and section the hair so that only the section you are drying is not in clips.

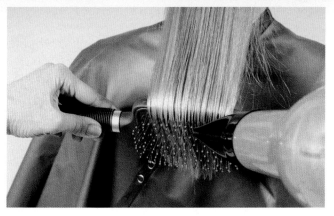

8 Using 1-inch subsections, start your first section at the nape of the neck and use a classic styling brush to dry the hair straight and smooth. Place the brush under the first section and hold the hair low.

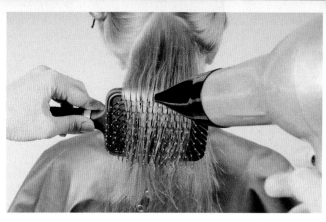

9 Follow the brush with the nozzle of the dryer, while bending the ends of the hair in the desired direction, either under or flipped outward. Continue using the same technique, working up to the occipital area in 1-inch sections.

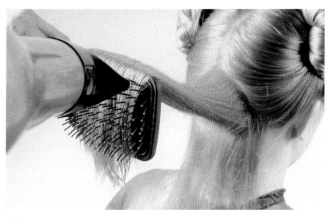

10 To keep the shape flat and straight, use low elevation. For more lift and volume, hold the section straight out from the head or overdirect upward.

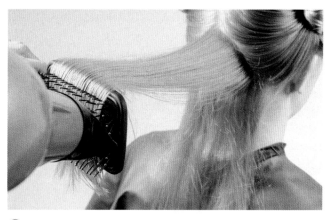

11 Work up to the crown, continuing to take 1-inch sections. On the longer sections toward the top of the crown, you can switch to a paddle brush, using the curve of the brush to add bends to the ends of the hair.

12 After each section is blown dry, follow by using the cooling button on the blowdryer to help set each section and to keep it smooth. For a fuller look, switch to a round brush.

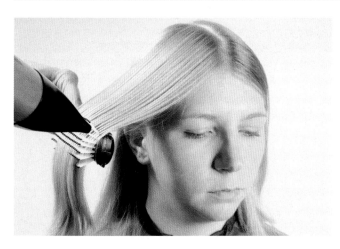

13 Continue by subdividing the hair on the side, and start with the section above the ear. Continue working in 1-inch sections. Hold at a low elevation and follow with the nozzle of the dryer facing toward the ends. Bend the ends under by turning the brush under for a rounded edge, or outward for a flipped edge.

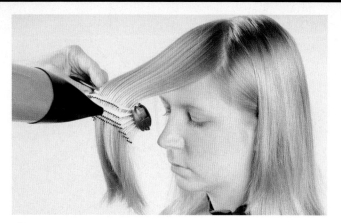

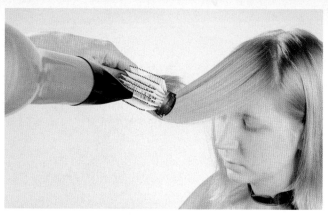

14 Work in the same manner across the top of the head. If there is a bang, dry it in the desired direction. To dry the bang straight and onto the forehead, point the nozzle of the dryer down over the bang and dry it straight, using your fingers or a classic styling brush to direct the hair.

15 To direct the bang away from the face, brush the bang back and push the hair slightly forward with the brush, creating a curved shaping.

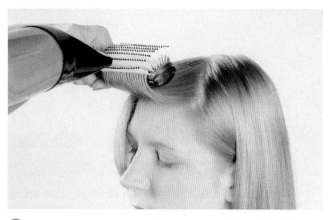

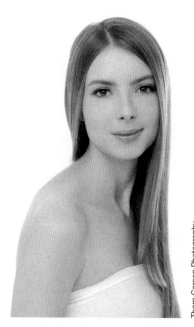

17 Finished look.

16 Place the dryer on a slow setting and point the nozzle toward the brush. When dry, the bang will fall away from the face and slightly to the side, for a soft look.

Thom Carson Photography

CLEAN-UP AND DISINFECTION

☐ Clean and disinfect tools and implements.

☐ Clean and disinfect work area.

☐ Dispose of single-use items. Place all used linens, towels, and capes in the laundry.

☐ Wash your hands.

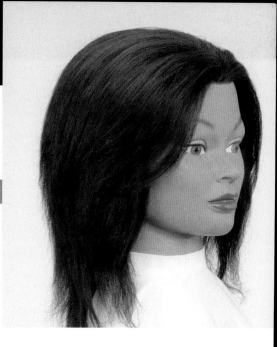

HAIR PRESSING

MATERIALS, IMPLEMENTS, AND EQUIPMENT

- ☐ Blowdryer with attachments
- ☐ Brush
- ☐ Clips
- ☐ Comb
- ☐ Electric heater (stove)
- ☐ Haircutting cape
- ☐ Neck strip

- ☐ Pressing comb
- ☐ Pressing cream, wax, or oil
- ☐ Shampoo
- ☐ Shampoo cape
- ☐ Styling pomade
- ☐ Towels

PREPARATION

1. Clean and then disinfect work area.
2. Conduct client consultation and hair analysis.
3. Wash your hands.
4. Drape client and perform shampoo service. Towel-blot the hair.
5. Drape client with chair cloth and neck strip. Heat the pressing comb.

PROCEDURE

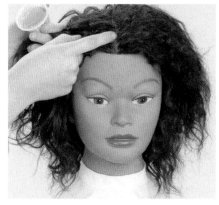

1. Blowdry the hair. Apply pressing cream, wax, or oil.

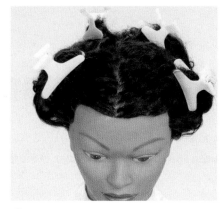

2. Comb and part off the hair into four sections.

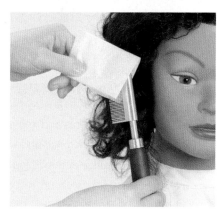

3. Test the temperature of the heated pressing comb by using a paper neck strip or end paper. If the paper scorches, the iron is too hot and will burn the hair.

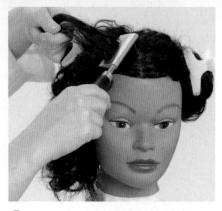

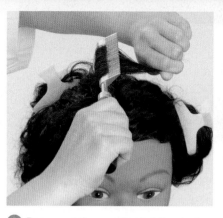

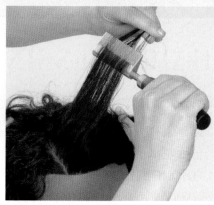

4 Divide the first section into 1-inch subsections. Apply additional pressing cream, wax, or oil to the subsection as needed.

5 Hold the first subsection away from the scalp and insert the teeth of the comb into the top side of the hair section.

6 Draw out the comb slightly, making a quick turn so that the back of the comb does the actual pressing.

7 Press the comb slowly through the hair until the ends pass through the teeth of the comb.

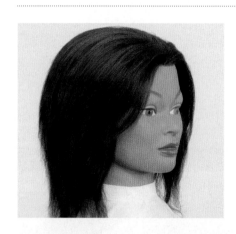

8 Continue this procedure until all the hair is pressed. Add pomade if desired.

9 Style and comb the hair or finish with thermal irons according to the client's wishes.

CLEAN-UP AND DISINFECTION

☐ Clean and disinfect tools and implements.

☐ Clean and disinfect the chair and workstation.

☐ Dispose of single-use items. Place all used linens, towels, and capes in the laundry.

☐ Wash your hands.

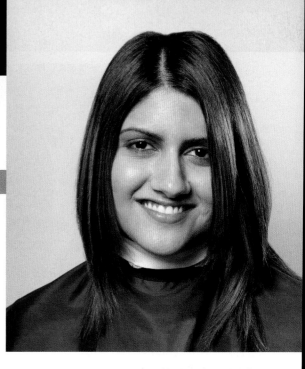

FLAT IRON PRESSING

MATERIALS, IMPLEMENTS, AND EQUIPMENT

- ☐ Blowdryer with attachments
- ☐ Brush
- ☐ Clips
- ☐ Electric flat iron
- ☐ Finishing spray
- ☐ Haircutting cape
- ☐ Leave-in thermal styling spray

- ☐ Neck strip
- ☐ Shampoo
- ☐ Shampoo cape
- ☐ Styling comb
- ☐ Tail comb
- ☐ Towels

PREPARATION

1 Clean and then disinfect work area.

2 Conduct client consultation and hair analysis.

3 Wash your hands.

4 Drape client and perform shampoo service.

5 Towel-blot hair and apply leave-in thermal styling spray.

6 Drape client with styling cape and neck strip. Heat the flat iron.

PROCEDURE

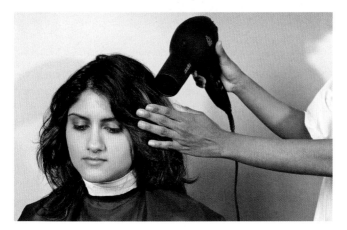

1 Blowdry and style hair according to the cut.

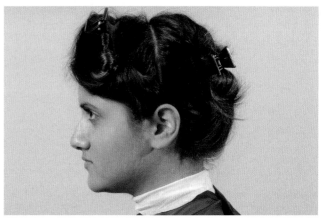

2 Comb and part off the hair into four sections. Divide the first section into subsections based on the density of the hair.

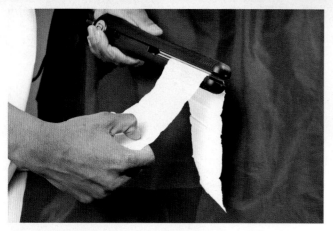

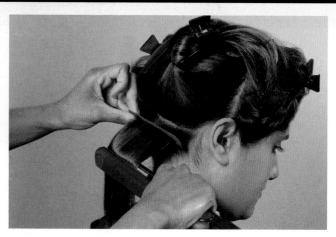

3 Test the temperature of the heated iron by using a paper neck strip or end paper. If the paper scorches, the iron is too hot and will burn the hair.

4 Hold the first subsection away from the scalp and grasp the section between the plates of the flat iron.

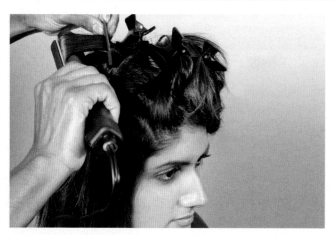

5 Insert the comb under the top side of the hair section to protect the scalp.

6 Draw the iron smoothly through the subsection, recomb, and reapply the flat iron as necessary to sufficiently straighten the hair.

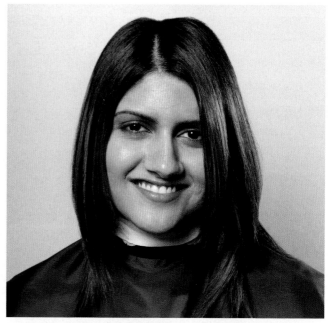

7 Repeat this process through each section until all the hair has been flat ironed. To increase lift in the top or crest sections, comb and elevate the subsection before ironing.

8 Comb and style the hair. Finish with styling spray or other preferred product.

CLEAN-UP AND DISINFECTION

☐ Clean and disinfect tools and implements.

☐ Clean and disinfect work area.

☐ Sweep up hair and deposit in closed receptacle.

☐ Deposit used blades in a sharps container.

☐ Dispose of single-use items. Place all used linens, towels, and capes in the laundry.

☐ Wash your hands.

REVIEW QUESTIONS

1 List the four basic cuts and the elevations or projections used to achieve them.

2 Explain overdirection.

3 List wet hairstyling methods.

4 Define *on-base*, *half off-base*, and *off-base* curl placement. Explain the effects of each.

5 What is thermal hairstyling?

6 List the tools used in thermal hairstyling.

CHAPTER GLOSSARY

base	p. 541	the stationary foundation of the curl on which the barrel (or roller) is placed
blowdry styling (BLOH-dry sti-hyl-ing)	p. 541	technique of drying and styling damp hair in one process
blunt cut (BLUNT KUT)	p. 532	haircut in which all the hair comes to one point at 0 elevation to form a weight line
circle (SUR-kul)	p. 541	also known as the *curl*; part of a curl that forms a complete circle
graduated cut (GRAJ-ooayt-ud KUT)	p. 533	graduated, wedge, or stacked shape at the perimeter of a haircut, usually cut at 45 degrees
hair molding (HAYR MOHLD-ing)	p. 541	styling method that uses the head as a tool to set the hair in a straight position
hair pressing (HAYR PRES-ing)	p. 542	temporarily straightening hair by using heated pressing combs
hair wrapping (HAYR RAP-ing)	p. 540	method where the hair is wrapped around the head for drying and styling purposes
half off-base	p. 542	position of a curl one-half off its base; provides medium volume and movement
long-layered cut (LAWNG-lay-UHRD KUT)	p. 534	hair is cut at a 180-degree elevation to create short layers at the top and increasingly longer layers at the perimeter
off-base	p. 542	position of a curl off its base; provides maximum mobility and minimum volume
on-base	p. 542	position of a curl directly on its base; provides maximum volume
stem (STEM)	p. 541	the section of a curl between the base and the first arc of the circle; gives the curl direction and movement
thermal styling (THUR-mul sti-hyl-ing)	p. 541	methods of curling or straightening dry hair using thermal irons and/or pressing combs
uniform-layered cut (YOO-nih-form-lay-UHRD KUT)	p. 534	haircut in which all the hair is cut at the same length using a 90-degree elevation

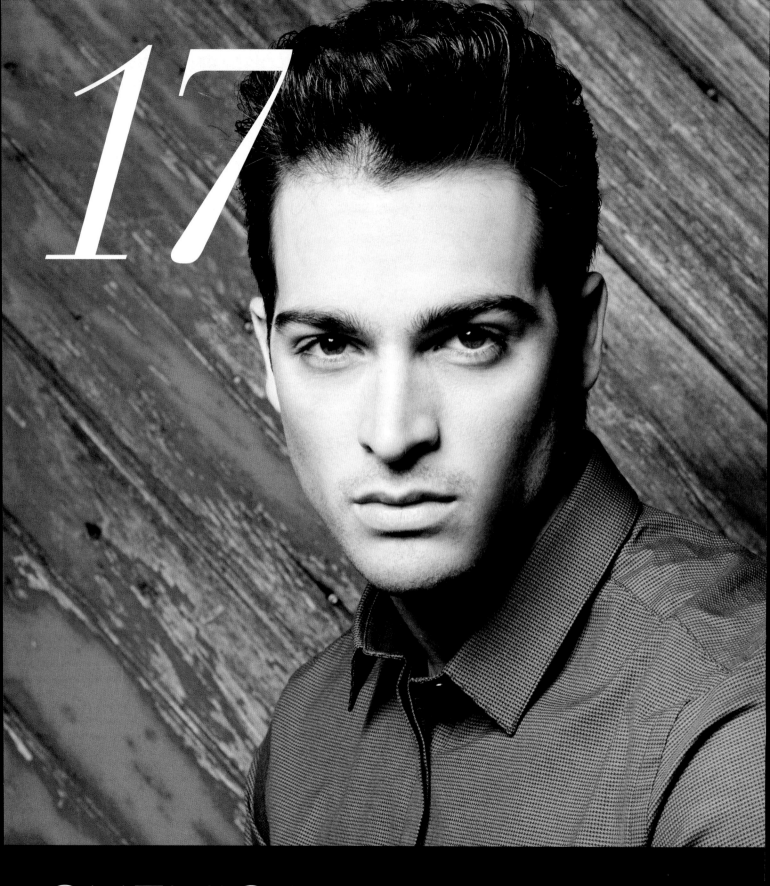

17

CHEMICAL TEXTURE
SERVICES

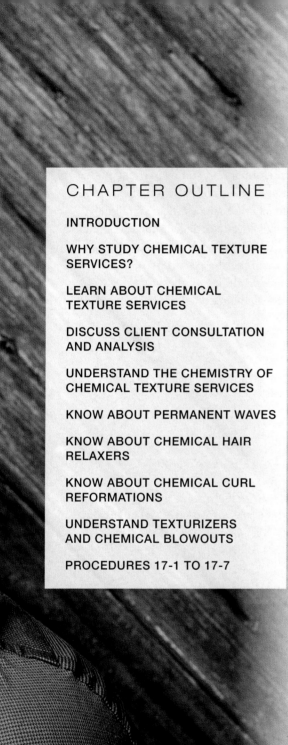

LEARNING OBJECTIVES

After completing this chapter, you will be able to:

LO❶
Describe how permanent waves, relaxers, and curl reformation services change the appearance of the hair.

LO❷
List topics to discuss during a client consultation.

LO❸
Identify six characteristics of the hair and scalp that are analyzed before performing chemical texture services.

LO❹
Describe how the ingredients in permanent waves, relaxers, and curl reformation services are chemically similar and chemically different from each other.

LO❺
Explain the physical and chemical actions of permanent waving, chemical relaxing, and curl reformation processes.

LO❻
Identify types of perm rods and end wrapping techniques.

LO❼
Define *on-base*, *half off-base*, and *off-base* rod placement.

LO❽
Identify two types of chemical relaxers.

LO❾
Explain the difference between *base* and *no-base* relaxers.

LO❿
List three strand tests to be performed before a chemical relaxing process.

LO⓫
Explain the three steps of a curl reformation process.

LO⓬
Describe the intended outcomes of texturizer and chemical blowout services.

Introduction

Clients that come to you for a service may want to change the curliness or straightness of their natural hair to achieve a certain look. Sometimes a client will want a style that is not possible with their natural wave pattern. **Chemical texture services** (KEM-uh-kul TEKS-chur SER-vicez) such as permanent waving (also known as chemical waving), curl reformations, and relaxers chemically change the hair's natural wave pattern of existing hair growth. For example, a permanent wave can be used to permanently change a client's straight hair to a curly texture and clients with naturally overly curly hair may straighten their hair by having it chemically relaxed. When new hair growth occurs, retouch applications are required to maintain the altered texture and structure of the hair. Chemical texture services are practical, versatile, and lucrative services that provide clients with alternatives in haircut designs and styling.

why study
CHEMICAL TEXTURE SERVICES?

Barbers should study and have a thorough understanding of chemical texture services because:

> The more knowledge and skills you have, the more services you can offer your clients in the barbershop, adding to your versatility as a barber.

> Knowing how to perform permanent waves, chemical relaxers, and curl reformations increases the amount of money you can make in the barbershop.

> Knowing when to suggest a chemical texture service will help build loyalty with your clients and confidence with your professional skills.

> Chemical services may cause damage, hair loss, and harm to clients and yourself if not used properly. To avoid these situations, it is important that you understand how to use the chemicals safely.

Learn about Chemical Texture Services

After reading this section, you will be able to:

LO① Describe how permanent waves, relaxers, and curl reformation services change the appearance of the hair.

Chemical texture services are services that use chemicals to change the natural straightness or curliness of hair into a new, wave pattern.

Permanent, or chemical, waving is a process used to chemically restructure natural hair into a different wave pattern. Most permanent waving services are performed to change straight or wavy hair into curly hair. Permanent waving:

- increases the fullness of fine, softer hair
- redirects resistant growth patterns until new growth occurs
- provides greater styling control

Permanent waving requires:

- permanent wave rods
- end papers
- thio-based waving lotion
- neutralizer

Chemical hair relaxing chemically rearranges the basic structure of overly curly hair into a straighter hair form. The relaxing process includes a:

- chemical relaxer (sodium hydroxide or thio based)
- neutralizer (neutralizing shampoo or H_2O_2 based)

A properly performed chemical relaxing service should leave the hair in a soft, relaxed form that can be wet set, wrapped, or thermal styled.

A **curl reformation**, also known as a soft-curl perm, Jheri® curl, or simply a *curl*, is a process used to restructure very curly hair into a larger curl pattern. Curl reformation services require:

- a thio-based relaxing product to partially straighten the hair
- permanent wave rods
- end papers
- thio-based wrap/waving lotion
- neutralizer
- hair moisturizer/conditioner

A curl reformation is a combination of a thio-based chemical relaxer and a permanent wave.

Chemical texturizing services require maintenance and periodic reapplications as new growth appears. The barber who develops the ability to perform chemical texture services has additional skills to establish a loyal following of satisfied clients, repeat customers, and new referrals.

Discuss Client Consultation and Analysis

After reading this section, you will be able to:

LO❷ List topics to discuss during a client consultation.

LO❸ Identify six characteristics of the hair and scalp that are analyzed before performing chemical texture services.

The consultation with the client takes only a few minutes but it is time well spent. It helps:

- establish your credibility as a professional

- inspire the client's confidence

- make the entire chemical texture service experience more satisfactory for both the client and the barber

Open communication between the barber and the client helps assure a successful chemical texture service outcome. This can be accomplished by asking open-ended questions to determine the client's desires and past experience with texture services.

Discuss these topics during client consultation:

- *The desired hairstyle and amount of curl or straightening:* Pictures, magazines, and stylebooks can help figure out what the client likes and dislikes, making the desired outcome clear to both client and barber.

- *The current type and condition of the client's hair:* Can what the client desires be achieved on their hair, considering the current condition and type of the hair they have?

- *The client's lifestyle:* Do they have leisure time or a demanding schedule that requires a low-maintenance style?

- *How the hairstyle relates to overall personal image:* Is the client concerned about current fashion trends?

- *Previous experience:* Was the last chemical texture service satisfactory? If not, what were the problems?

Keep the information learned during the consultation in the form of a written record that includes the client's address and home and business contact information. See **Figure 17-1** for an example of an organized client record card.

In addition to determining the client's desires, the barber also needs to have a clear understanding of what the finished style will look like. This is key to a successful texture service because the desired finished look will help determine the degree of curl or relaxation that is needed.

UNDERSTAND SCALP AND HAIR ANALYSIS

Before proceeding with any chemical texture service, it is important to correctly and carefully analyze the client's scalp and hair condition. The analysis should be used to determine whether the scalp and hair should receive a chemical texture service and the types of products to be used.

The scalp should be examined for:

- cuts

- abrasions or scratches

- open sores

- scalp disease

figure 17-1
Client record card.

PERMANENT WAVE RECORD

Name . . . . Tel . . . .

Address . . . .

City . . . . State . . . . Zip . . . .

DESCRIPTION OF HAIR

Length	Texture	Type	Porosity	
☐ short	☐ coarse	☐ normal	☐ very	☐ slightly
☐ medium	☐ medium	☐ resistant	porous	porous
☐ long	☐ fine	☐ tinted	☐ moderately	☐ resistant
		☐ highlighted	porous	
		☐ bleached	☐ normal	

CONDITION

☐ very good ☐ good ☐ fair ☐ poor ☐ dry ☐ oily

Tinted with . . . .

Previously permed with . . . .

TYPE OF PERM

☐ alkaline ☐ acid ☐ body wave ☐ other . . . .

No. of rods . . . . Lotion . . . . Strength . . . .

RESULTS

☐ good ☐ poor ☐ too tight ☐ too loose

Date	Perm Used	Stylist	Date	Perm Used	Stylist
. . . . . .	. . . .	. . . . . .	. . . . . .	. . . .	. . . . . .
. . . . . .	. . . .	. . . . . .	. . . . . .	. . . .	. . . . . .
. . . . . .	. . . .	. . . . . .	. . . . . .	. . . .	. . . . . .
. . . . . .	. . . .	. . . . . .	. . . . . .	. . . .	. . . . . .
. . . . . .	. . . .	. . . . . .	. . . . . .	. . . .	. . . . . .

Any of these conditions can make a chemical process uncomfortable and dangerous to a client. Do not proceed with the service if abrasions or signs of scalp disease are present. Refer the client to a physician as necessary.

The hair analysis includes observing and determining the hair's:

* porosity

* texture

* elasticity

* density

* length

* direction of growth

HAIR POROSITY

How does porosity affect chemical texturizing services?

The processing time for chemical texturizing services depends more on hair porosity than on any other factor. Generally, the more porous the hair, the less the processing time. The porosity level of the hair determines the speed with which moisture will be absorbed into the hair and is directly related to the condition of the cuticle layer. Hair porosity is classified as resistant, normal, or porous. These classifications help determine the most appropriate strength of a chemical product to use on different hair types.

- *Resistant* hair has a tight, compact cuticle layer that resists penetration of chemical solutions. This hair type requires a more alkaline solution to raise the cuticle and permit uniform saturation and processing.
- *Normal* porosity means that the hair is neither resistant nor overly porous. Chemical texture services performed on this hair type will usually process as expected.
- *Porous* hair has a raised cuticle layer that easily absorbs chemical solutions. This hair type requires a less alkaline solution to help prevent damage to the hair.

Do not proceed with the service if the hair shows signs of breakage or overporosity.

DID YOU KNOW?
Porosity is best evaluated on clean, dry hair. Roughness indicates a raised cuticle and a higher porosity level.

Porosity Level Mini-Procedure

To accurately test the porosity level:

1. Start by using these four different areas:
   - at the front hairline
   - temple
   - near the crown
   - nape
2. Grasp some strands of dry hair.
3. Hold the ends firmly with the thumb and index finger of one hand, and slide the fingers of the other hand from the ends toward the scalp.
4. If the fingers do not slide easily, or if the hair ruffles up as your fingers slide down the strands, the hair is porous. The more ruffles that form, the more porous the hair; the fewer ruffles that form, the less porous it is.
5. If the fingers slide easily and no ruffles are formed, the cuticle layers lie close to the hair shafts. This type of hair is the least porous and most resistant, and may require a longer processing time (Figure 17-2).
6. Keep in mind the porosity may be different from the base area to the ends of the hair. If drastically different, the client may need a product, such as a light spray moisturizer, to even out the porosity before proceeding with the service.

figure 17-2
Porosity test.

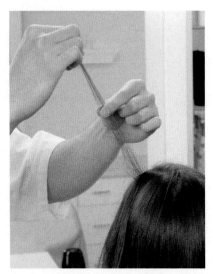

HAIR TEXTURE

How does hair texture affect chemical texturizing services?

- While hair porosity is important in determining the processing time, hair texture also plays a part in the decision. For example, coarse, porous hair will usually process faster than fine, resistant hair.

- Hair texture describes the diameter of a single strand of hair as being coarse, medium, or fine:

    - *Coarse* hair usually requires more processing than medium or fine hair and may also be more resistant to chemical processes.
    - *Medium* hair is the most common hair texture. It is considered normal and does not usually pose any special processing problems.
    - *Fine* hair is typically more fragile, easier to process, and more susceptible to damage from chemical services. Generally, fine hair will process faster and more easily than medium or coarse hair types.

HAIR ELASTICITY

How does hair elasticity affect chemical texturizing services?

- Hair elasticity is an important factor to consider because it is an indication of the strength of the cross-bonds in the hair.

- The greater the degree of elasticity, the longer the wave will remain in the hair because less relaxation of the hair occurs; thus the elasticity of the hair determines its ability to hold a curl.

- Hair elasticity is classified as normal or low:

    - *Normal* elasticity is indicated by wet hair that can stretch up to 50 percent of its original length and then return to that length without breaking. Hair with normal elasticity usually holds the curl from wet sets and permanent waves.
    - *Low* elasticity is indicated by wet hair that does not return to its original length when stretched and may not be able to hold curl patterns.

Test for Elasticity Mini-Procedure

To test for elasticity:

1. Take a few strands of damp hair.

2. Hold them between the thumb and forefinger of each hand.

3. Slowly stretch the strands between your fingers (**Figure 17-3**).

    a. The more they can be stretched without breaking, the more elasticity the hair has.

    b. If the elasticity is good, the hair slowly contracts after stretching.

    c. Hair with poor elasticity will break quickly and easily when stretched.

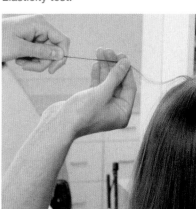

figure 17-3
Elasticity test.

d. Signs of poor elasticity include limpness, sponginess, and hair that tangles easily. Generally speaking, such hair will not develop a firm, strong wave and may result in breakage.

e. There are special waving solutions available for hair with poor elasticity; if used in combination with smaller-diameter rods, it may result in a satisfactory permanent wave or curl reformation process.

HAIR DENSITY

How does hair density affect chemical texturizing services?

Hair density measures the number of hairs per square inch and indicates how thick or thin the hair is. Think of walking through a forest that has many trees—the forest is very "dense" and it is difficult to walk through. On the other hand, think about walking across a field with very few trees—the field is not very dense. Hair density is important to consider when performing chemical texture services because it helps determine the number of blockings or subsections that will be best for the service that is performed. For example, in permanent waving, smaller blocks (subsections) and larger rods may be required for thick density hair. If the hair density is thin, however, smaller-diameter rods are required to form a good wave pattern close to the head. Avoid large blockings on thin hair growth in permanent waves as the strain may cause breakage. In chemical relaxing, subsections may need to be very small according to the density for proper saturation. Hair density can also indicate the amount of product that will be needed. If a client has a lot of hair, more product may be needed.

HAIR LENGTH

How does hair length affect chemical texturizing services?

In permanent waving and curl reformation processes, hair length may determine the wrapping technique to use. For example, while hair of average length may be wrapped normally, hair that is 6 inches or longer may not sit close enough to the scalp to develop a good, strong wave pattern in that area. In addition, the weight of long hair may relax or stretch the curl to the extent that the majority of the wave pattern remains mid-shaft and on the hair ends with very little lift in the scalp area. Like hair density, the length of the hair will also help determine the amount of product that will be needed for the chemical texturizing process. For example, clients with long hair may require additional waving solution, relaxer, or neutralizer to complete the process.

HAIR GROWTH PATTERN

How does hair growth pattern affect chemical texturizing services?

The direction of the natural hair growth creates hair streams, whorls, and cowlicks that can influence the finished style and reappear as new growth occurs. The direction of hair growth must be considered when selecting the wrapping pattern and rod placement for permanent waves or curl reformations and for the direction of combing and smoothing when using chemical relaxers. When wrapping a permanent wave or curl reformation, wrapping in the opposite direction of a strong growth pattern may cause breakage.

Understand the Chemistry of Chemical Texture Services

After reading this section, you will be able to:

LO**4** Describe how the ingredients in permanent waves, relaxers, and curl reformation services are chemically similar and chemically different from each other.

LO**5** Explain the physical and chemical actions of permanent waving, chemical relaxing, and curl reformation processes.

Chemical texture services create permanent changes in the structure and appearance of the hair. As you learned earlier, hair is composed of three layers: cuticle, cortex, and medulla.

- *Medulla:* Because the medulla is considered to be empty space and may be present only in medium to coarse hair types, the cuticle and cortex are the two layers most affected by chemical texture services.

- *Cuticle:* The cuticle is the tough, outermost layer that protects the cortex from damage. The degree to which hair is resistant to chemical changes depends on the strength of the cuticle. The alkaline solutions and substances used in chemical texture services soften and swell the cuticle, allowing for penetration into the cortex (Figure 17-4).

- *Cortex:* The cortex gives the hair its strength, flexibility, elasticity, and shape. These characteristics are derived from the millions of polypeptide chains found in the keratin that makes up the cortex of the hair.

Restructuring keratin and polypeptide chains in the cortex: As you learned earlier, amino acids form proteins, and chemical reactions among proteins produce peptide linkages.

Hair develops and maintains its natural form by means of the physical and chemical cross-bonds in the cortex layer. The physical bonds, hydrogen and salt, are weaker bonds and are easily broken by shampooing and rinsing. Chemical bonds (disulfide) are broken or rearranged through the chemicals used in permanent waving, curl reformations, and relaxers.

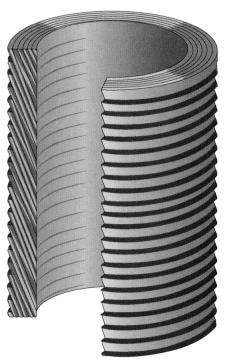

figure 17-4
The cuticle layer.

Alkaline substances used in chemical texture products break the chemical bonds and allow for the softening and expansion of the hair. During this process, cystine (formed by disulfide or sulfur bonds) is altered slightly to become cysteine. Cysteine is an amino acid obtained by the reduction of cystine. This chemical action is important because it changes the chemical rearrangement of the inner structure of the hair as it assumes a new shape and form. For example, in permanent waving and curl reformation, the hair will take the shape and curl of the perm rod. In relaxing, the naturally curly hair is "relaxed" into a straighter, less curly form as it is manually "smoothed."

After the hair has assumed the desired shape (curly on a perm rod or smoothed into a straighter form), it must be neutralized so that the hydrogen and sulfur cross-bonds in the cortical layer are permanently reformed. Cysteine is changed back to the cystine state during the process of oxidation and neutralization, which hardens the S bonds of the hair into the newly constructed shape. Both physical and chemical actions cause the bonds within the cortex to be rearranged and restructured during chemical texturizing services.

DEFINE THE PRINCIPLE ACTIONS OF CHEMICAL TEXTURIZING SERVICES

Chemical texture services involve two principal actions on the hair: physical and chemical (**Figures 17-5 to 17-8**). These actions are compared in **Table 17-1**.

figure 17-5
Polypeptide chains are formed when amino acids link together.

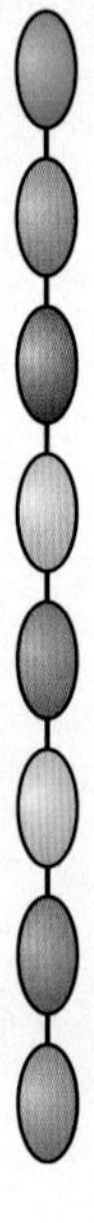

figure 17-6
Keratin proteins are long, coiled peptide chains.

figure 17-7
Side bonds cross-link polypeptide chains together.

figure 17-8
A correct permanent wave service only alters the side bonds.

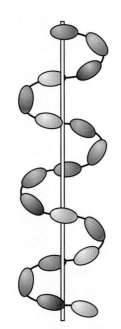

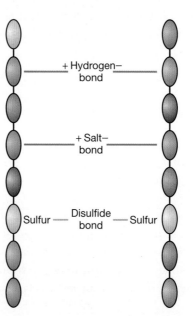

+ Hydrogen–
bond

+ Salt–
bond

Sulfur —— Disulfide
bond —— Sulfur

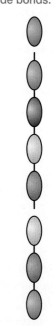

table 17-1

PHYSICAL AND CHEMICAL ACTIONS OF CHEMICAL TEXTURE SERVICES

Actions	Permanent Waving	Chemical Relaxing	Curl Reformation
Physical	• shampooing • rinsing • wrapping the hair around perm rods	• combing or smoothing relaxer through the hair • shampooing • rinsing • conditioning	• combing or smoothing rearranger through the hair for partial relaxation of the natural curl • rinsing • wrapping the hair on rods

Chemical	• Waving lotion/solution:
	  • first, this softens and swells the cuticle layer
	  • second, it breaks the disulfide bonds, called *reduction*
	• Neutralizer:
	  • rehardens the newly arranged disulfide bonds
	  • neutralizes any remaining waving lotion in the hair through oxidation
		Relaxer is either thio based or sodium hydroxide based:
		
		Thio relaxers:
		• Thio relaxing products also require the use of a neutralizer to chemically oxidize the hair.
		• The reducing agent has a higher strength than that used in permanent waving. Most **thio relaxers** (THY-oh re-LAX-uhrz) have a pH above 10 and are manufactured in cream form for better adhesion and control.
		• Relaxer softens and swells the hair and breaks apart the disulfide bonds. This action permits the removal of curl from the hair as the bonds are rearranged into a straighter position through the physical actions of combing and smoothing the hair.
		• The hair is then rinsed and neutralized with an oxidizing agent, such as hydrogen peroxide, that rebuilds the disulfide bonds broken by the relaxer.
		
		Hydroxide relaxers:
		• These are strong alkalis that can swell the hair up to twice its normal diameter.
		• **Hydroxide relaxers** (hy-DRAHKS-yd re-LAX-uhrz) can have a pH as high as 13.5. At these high concentrations, the hydroxide product permanently breaks the disulfide bonds to the point where they can never be reformed. This process is known as **lanthionization** (lan-THEE-ohn-iz-ay-shun) and occurs as the disulfide bonds are converted to lanthionine bonds when the relaxer is rinsed and the hair is still at a high pH level.
		• Hydroxide relaxers are *not* compatible with thio relaxers because they use a different chemistry.
		• Hydroxide relaxing products are neutralized through the physical actions of the shampooing and rinsing process because the disulfide bonds that have been broken by this type of relaxer cannot be reformed through oxidation.
			• Rearranger:
			  • relaxes the natural curl by softening and swelling the cuticle, allowing for penetration into the cortex
			  • ammonium thioglycolate in cream form (thicker consistency)
			  • combed through the hair
			• Waving lotion (booster):
			  • ammonium thioglycolate in lotion form (thinner consistency)
			  • applied as hair is wrapped on perm rods
			• Neutralizer:
			  • rehardens newly arranged disulfide bonds
			  • neutralizes any remaining waving lotion in the hair through oxidation

Know about Permanent Waves

After reading this section, you will be able to:

LO**6** Identify types of perm rods and end wrapping techniques.

LO**7** Define *on-base*, *half off-base*, and *off-base* rod placement.

Permanent waving is a process that involves two principal actions on the hair:

1. *physical* action of wrapping the hair on perm rods

2. *chemical* changes caused by the waving solution and neutralizer

Permanent waves are performed on hair that has been freshly shampooed and is uniformly damp. A spray water bottle must be used to maintain even wetness throughout the hair during the wrapping procedure.

UNDERSTAND THE CHEMICAL PERM WRAP

Perm Rods

In permanent waving, the size, shape, and type of curl are determined by the size, shape, and type of perm rod and the method used to wrap the hair. The size and shape of the rod determines the size of the curl (**Figure 17-9**).

The proper selection of perm rods is essential for successful permanent waving. The most commonly used rods are made of plastic.

Perm Rod Diameter

- The diameter of the rod controls the size of the curl.
- These diameters usually vary from ⅛ inch to 1½ inches.
- The hair used in the subsection must be wrapped at least 1½ times around the rod to create a curl formation.

Perm Rod Lengths

- Rods are available in lengths that typically measure from 1¾ inches to 3½ inches.
- Perm rod lengths are known as:
  - short
  - medium
  - long

Perm Rod Shapes
Concave rods

- Concave rods are the most commonly used perm rod.
- Concave rods have a smaller diameter in the center, which gradually increases to a larger diameter at both ends.
- This shape produces a tighter curl in the center and a larger curl on the sides of the hair parting resulting in a more natural wave (**Figure 17-10**).
- Concave rods are used when a definite wave pattern, close to the head, is desired.

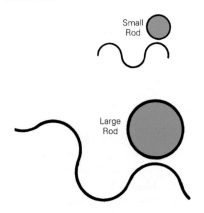

figure 17-9
The size of the rod determines the size of the curl.

Small Rod

Large Rod

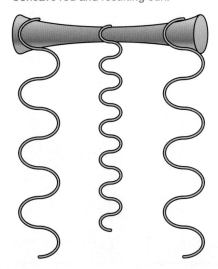

figure 17-10
Concave rod and resulting curl.

Straight rods

- Straight rods have a uniform circumference and diameter along the rod's length.

- This type of rod creates a consistently sized wave from one side of the hair parting to the other (**Figure 17-11**).

- Large, straight rods are usually used for a body wave that serves as a foundation for further styling.

Bender rods

- Bender rods are made of stiff wires covered by soft foam that permits bending into a variety of shapes.

- These rods measure about 12 inches in length and have a uniform diameter (**Figure 17-12**).

Circle or loop rods

- The circle tool or loop rod is a plastic-coated tool that also measures about 12 inches with a uniform diameter along the length of the rod.

- These rods are secured by fastening the ends together to form a circle (**Figure 17-13**).

End Papers or End Wraps

- **End wraps** are absorbent papers used to control the ends of the hair when wrapping and winding the hair on perm rods.

- End papers should extend beyond the ends of the hair to keep them smooth and straight, and to prevent "fishhooks." A fishhook is a flaw in the wrapping that results in the tip of the hair bending in the opposite direction to that of the rest of the curl.

- End papers are especially effective in helping to smooth out the wrapping of uneven hair lengths. For very uneven lengths, you may use multiple end wraps up the hair strand to control the hair.

End Paper Wrapping Techniques

The most common end paper–wrapping techniques are the bookend wrap, the single flat wrap, and the double flat wrap.

- The **bookend wrap** uses one paper folded in half over the ends of the hair (**Figure 17-14**). It can be used with short rods or short lengths of hair. Be careful to distribute the hair evenly over the entire length of the rod and avoid bunching the ends together toward the center of the rod.

- The *single flat* or *single end wrap* uses one paper placed over the top of the hair parting being wrapped (**Figure 17-15**). Because there is paper on only side of the hair, it may be difficult to control the hair using this method.

- The *double flat* or *double-end wrap* uses two end papers, one placed under and one over the parting of hair being wrapped. Both papers should extend beyond the hair ends (**Figure 17-16**).

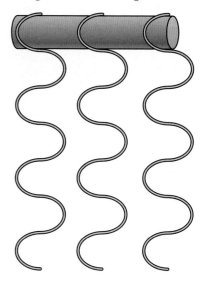

figure 17-11
Straight rod and resulting curl.

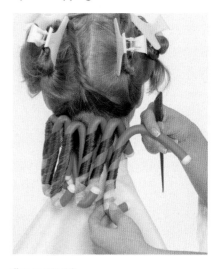

figure 17-12
Spiral wrapping with soft bender rods.

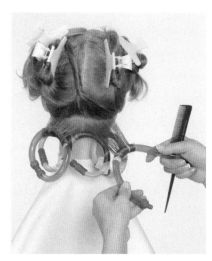

figure 17-13
Circle tools.

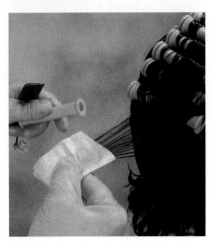

figure 17-14
Bookend wrap rodding a reformation curl.

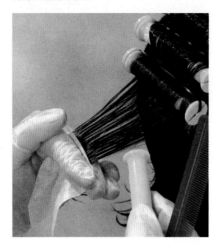

figure 17-15
Single flat wrap rodding a reformation curl.

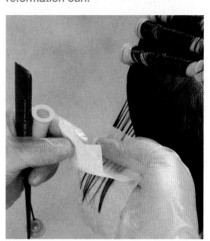

figure 17-16
Double-end wrap rodding a reformation curl.

Bookend Wrapping Mini-Procedure

1. Part and comb subsection up and out until all the hair is evenly directed and distributed (see **Figure 17-17**).

2. Hold the subsection between the index and middle fingers. Fold and place the end paper over the subsection, forming an envelope (see **Figure 17-18**).

3. Hold the subsection smoothly and evenly. Slide the paper envelope a small fraction beyond the hair ends (see **Figure 17-19**).

4. With your right hand, pick up the rod (see **Figure 17-20**).

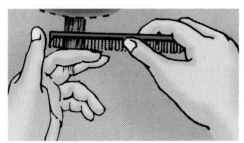

figure 17-17
Bookend wrap step 1.

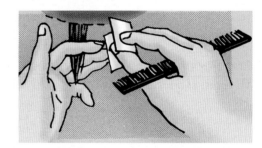

figure 17-18
Bookend wrap step 2.

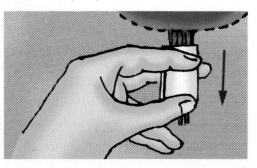

figure 17-19
Bookend wrap step 3.

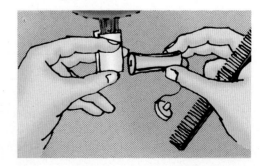

figure 17-20
Bookend wrap step 4.

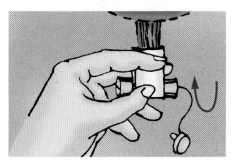

figure 17-21
Bookend wrap step 5.

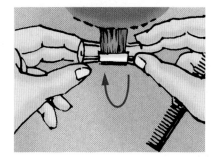

figure 17-22
Bookend wrap step 6.

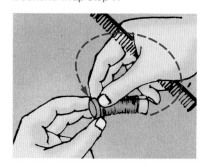

figure 17-23
Bookend wrap step 7.

5. Place the rod under the folded end paper, parallel to the parting. Draw the end paper and rod toward the hair ends until they are visible above the rod, and start winding the end paper and hair under toward the scalp (see **Figure 17-21**).

6. Wind the hair smoothly, without tension, on the rod (see **Figure 17-22**).

7. Fasten the band evenly across the wound hair at the top of the rod (see **Figure 17-23**).

Single Flat Wrap Mini-Procedure

1. Place the end paper on top of the subsection and hold it flat to prevent bunching (see **Figure 17-24**).

2. Place the rod under the subsection, holding it parallel with the parting. Then, draw the end paper and rod downward until the hair ends are covered (see **Figure 17-25**).

3. Roll the end paper and subsection under, using the thumb of each hand to keep the strands smooth. Wind the subsection on the rod to the scalp without tension. Fasten the band across the top of the rod in the same manner as the bookend paper wrap (see **Figure 17-26**).

figure 17-24
Single flat wrap step 1.

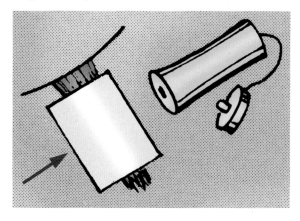

figure 17-25
Single flat wrap step 2.

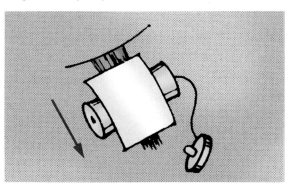

figure 17-26
Single flat wrap step 3.

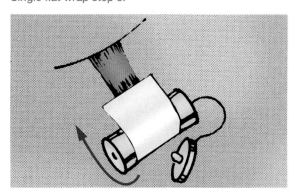

Double Flat Wrap Mini-Procedure

figure 17-27
Double flat wrap step 1.

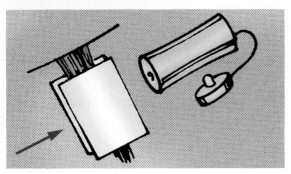

1. Place one end paper beneath the hair subsection and the other on top (see **Figure 17-27**).

2. Place the rod under double-end papers, parallel with the parting. Draw both papers toward the hair ends (see **Figure 17-28**).

3. Wind the subsection smoothly on the rod to the scalp without tension. Then fasten the band across the top of the rod in the same manner as the bookend wrap (see **Figure 17-29**).

figure 17-28
Double flat wrap step 2.

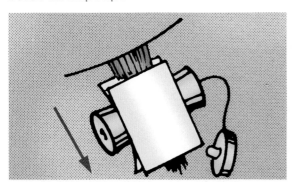

figure 17-29
Double flat wrap step 3.

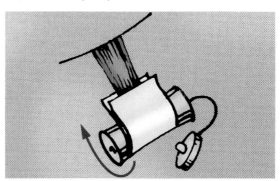

The *elastic band* secures the hair and the rod into the desired position to prevent the curl from unwinding during the procedure.

Sectioning

Perm wraps begin with sectioning the hair into panels. The size, shape, and direction of these panels will vary depending on the wrapping pattern and the type of tool being used. Each panel is further divided into subsections called **base sections**. The base sections are actually partings taken from the subsection that measure *almost* the same length and width as the rod or perming tool.

The number of base sections and the rod sizes will vary with each client depending on the sectioning pattern used and the texture, density, and elasticity of the hair (**Table 17-2**). The average base section, or parting, should be slightly shorter than the length of the rod. If the rod is shorter than the length of the blocking, the hair will slip off the ends of the rod during winding and result in an uneven curl formation.

The texture, elasticity, porosity, and condition of the client's hair all help determine how the hair should be sectioned and subsectioned, which rods to use, and where the application of waving solution should begin. Be guided by your instructor.

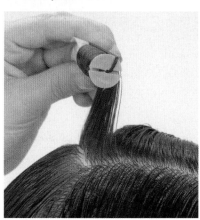

figure 17-30
On-base placement.

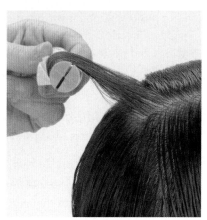

figure 17-31
Half off-base placement.

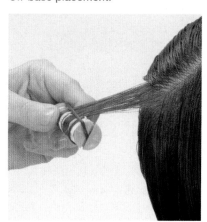

figure 17-32
Off-base placement.

table 17-2

SUGGESTED BASE SECTIONS AND ROD SIZES

Texture	Density	Elasticity	Base Section	Diameter of Rod
Coarse	Thick	Good	Narrow	Large
Medium	Average	Normal	Smaller	Medium
Fine	Thin	Poor	Smaller	Small
Damaged	Average	Very Poor	Smaller	Large

Base Control

Base control *refers* to the position of the perm rod or tool in relation to its base section and is determined by the angle at which the hair is wrapped. Rods can be wound *on-base, half off-base (half-base),* or *off-base:*

* In *on-base* placement, the hair is projected about 45 degrees beyond perpendicular (90 degrees) to its base section and the rod is placed *on* the base section (**Figure 17-30**). On-base placement results in greater volume at the scalp area and maximum movement.

* *Half off-base* placement results from wrapping the hair at an angle of 90 degrees to its base section (**Figure 17-31**). At this elevation of the hair, the rod is positioned half off its base section. Half off-base placement results in medium volume and movement.

* *Off-base* placement is achieved by wrapping the hair at a 45-degree angle below perpendicular to its base section (**Figure 17-32**). The rod is positioned completely off its base section and creates the least amount of volume and movement in the style.

Base Direction

Base direction refers to the directional pattern in which the hair is wrapped. Although wrapping with the natural direction of hair growth causes the least

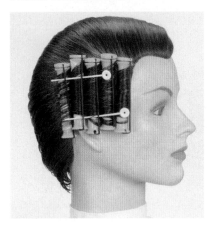

figure 17-33
Vertical base direction.

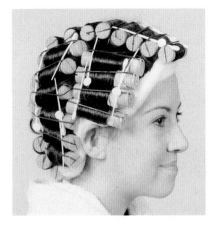

figure 17-34
Horizontal base direction.

figure 17-35
Croquignole perm wrap.

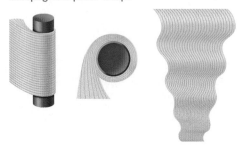

figure 17-36
Spiral perm wrap.

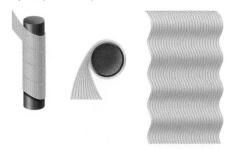

amount of stress on the hair, wrapping forward, backward, or to the side can create special effects in the final hairstyle. Be careful not to wrap the hair opposite a strong growth pattern as it may result in breakage.

Base direction also refers to the horizontal, vertical, or diagonal partings and positioning of the rod on the head, as pictured in Figures 17-33 and 17-34.

Wrapping/Rodding Techniques

The two basic methods used to wrap the hair around the perm rod are:

Croquignole

When using the **croquignole perm wrap** (KROH-ken-yohl) technique, the hair is wound from the hair ends toward the scalp. This overlapping of the hair layers with each revolution of the rod increases the size of the curl as it nears the scalp area, with a tighter curl at the ends (Figure 17-35).

Spiral

* A spiral wrap can be accomplished in two ways:
    * from the hair ends toward the scalp, or
    * from the scalp toward the hair ends.

In both cases, the rod or perm rod is positioned vertically as the hair parting is "rocked" or spiraled along the length of the rod. Straight rods are usually used for a spiral wrap and tend to produce a more uniform curl when the hair is spiraled properly along the rod (Figure 17-36). A spiral wrap is performed at an angle that positions the hair in a spiral pattern along the length of the rod. This technique produces a uniform curl formation from the scalp to the ends and is especially appropriate for long hair designs.

To form a uniform wave, the hair must be wrapped smoothly and neatly on each rod without stretching. The hair should not be stretched or wrapped too tightly because that could interfere with the penetration and expansion process of the waving solution and the contraction process of the neutralizer. Tight wrapping can also result in hair breakage due to the amount of tension put on the hair.

Water versus Lotion Wrapping

Water Wrap

A *water wrap* is the action of wrapping the hair around rods when it is moist with water. It is important to keep all of the hair moist throughout the wrapping process. If some of the hair has dried, remoisten it using a spray bottle. Although most perms are wrapped in this manner, always follow the manufacturer's directions.

Lotion Wrap

A **lotion wrap** is the application of permanent wave solution to one working panel or section of hair just before wrapping the hair on rods to pre-soften resistant hair. This technique is usually used with alkaline (cold) waves to make it easier to wrap resistant, straight hair types—it "jump starts" the processing action. Once the hair is wrapped, the remaining solution is applied to the entire head. Always follow the manufacturer's instructions.

Permanent Waving Wrapping Patterns

Once the client consultation has been completed, the barber should have a definite plan of action designed to achieve the desired results. This plan should include the selection of the permanent waving product, rod size(s), and wrapping pattern that will be used for the service. The parting technique most often used is a straight part. However, zigzag partings, known as the *weave technique,* can be used for an entire perm or to create smooth transitions from wrapped areas to non-wrapped areas within a partial perm.

There are four common wrapping patterns used in permanent waving:

* *Basic wrap*
  In this wrapping pattern, all the rods within a panel are positioned in the same direction on equal-size bases (**Figure 17-37**). All base sections are horizontal and slightly smaller than the length of the rod and even to the width of the rod. The base control is usually half off-base, although other bases may be used.

* *Curvature perm wrap*
  This wrapping pattern is one of the best to use for men's styles as it produces a more natural-looking wave pattern. The movement curves within sectioned-out panels with partings and bases following the natural curvature of the head and distribution of the hair (**Figure 17-38**).

* *Bricklay perm wrap*
  The base sections are offset from each other row by row to prevent noticeable splits in the hair (**Figure 17-39**). The bricklay pattern will blend hair from one area to another and may be preferred for men's styling over the basic perm wrap pattern.

* *Piggyback perm wrap*
  The piggyback perm wrap uses two perm rods for each parting of hair for even curl formation on long and/or dense hair. The first rod is placed about midway between the scalp and hair ends. This section is wrapped toward the scalp and leaves a tail of hair that extends from the mid-shaft point to the hair ends. The "tail" is then wrapped from the ends to the midway point and secured and positioned across the first rod (**Figure 17-40**). In this way, the second rod is "piggybacking" the first rod.

P 17-2 **Chemical (Permanent) Wave and Processing Using a Basic Permanent Wrap** *pages 614–618*

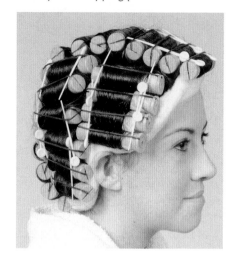

figure 17-37
Basic perm wrapping pattern.

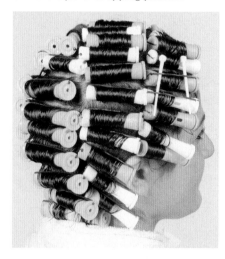

figure 17-38
Curvature perm wrapping pattern.

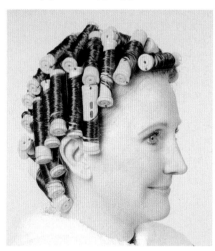

figure 17-39
Bricklay perm wrapping pattern.

figure 17-40
Piggyback wrap.

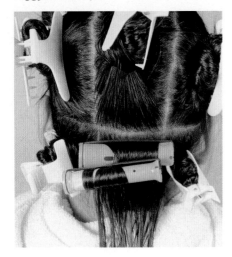

TYPES OF PERMANENT WAVES

Permanent wave chemistry is constantly being refined and improved. Different formulas designed for a wide variety of hair types are available from today's manufacturers. Waving lotions and neutralizers for both acid-balanced and alkaline perms are available with new conditioners, proteins, and natural ingredients that help protect and condition the hair during and after perming.

Stop-action processing is incorporated into many waving lotions to ensure optimum curl development. The curling takes place within a fixed time, without the risk of overprocessing or damaging the hair. Special pre-wrapping lotions have also been developed to compensate for hair with varying degrees of porosity.

Alkaline Perms (Cold Waves)

The first **alkaline or cold waves** (AL-kuh-line WAYVZ) were developed in 1941. The main active ingredient or reducing agent in alkaline perms is **ammonium thioglycolate (ATG)** (uh-MOH-nee-um THY-oh-GLY-kuh-layt). This chemical compound is made up of ammonia and thioglycolic acid. The pH of alkaline waving lotions generally falls within the range of 9.0 to 9.6, depending on the amount of ammonia. These high pH levels cause the hair shaft to swell and the cuticle layer to lift, allowing penetration into the cortex. This permanent wave may require a plastic cap for processing. Always read the manufacturer's directions carefully before proceeding with the service.

The benefits associated with alkaline perms are strong curl patterns, fast processing time (5 to 20 minutes), and room temperature processing. Alkaline perms are generally used when perming resistant hair types, when a strong or tight curl is desired, or when the client has a history of early curl relaxation.

True Acid Waves

True acid waves (TROO AS-ud WAYVZ) were first introduced in the early 1970s. These perms have a pH range between 4.5 and 7.0 and use **glyceryl monothioglycolate (GMTG)** (GLIS-ur-il mon-oh-THY-oh-GLY-kuh-layt) as the primary reducing agent. This lower pH is gentler on the hair and typically produces a softer curl and less damage than alkaline cold waves. Most true acid waves require the addition of heat from a hair dryer to accelerate the processing and are considered to be *endothermic* perm products. **Endothermic waves** (en-duh-THUR-mik WAYVZ) require the use of an outside heat source to activate chemical reactions and processing. It should be noted that although a pH of 7.0 is neutral on the pH scale, a pH of 5.0 is neutral for hair. Since every step in the pH scale represents a 10-fold change in pH, a pH of 7.0 is 100 times more alkaline than the pH of hair. Even pure water will cause the hair to swell and expand.

REMINDER

Repeated exposure to GMTG has been known to cause allergic sensitivity in practitioners and clients. Watch clients closely for signs of allergy or irritation. If problems develop, suggest they see a dermatologist.

- The benefits of true acid waves are:

  - softer curl patterns
  - slower, but more controllable processing time (usually 15 to 25 minutes)
  - gentler treatment for delicate hair types

- Generally, true acid perms should be used when:

  - "perming" is sufficient delicate, fragile, or color-treated hair
  - a soft, natural curl or wave pattern is desired
  - style support, rather than strong curl, is desired

Acid-Balanced Waves

Most of today's acid waves have a pH between 7.8 and 8.2. Modern acid waves are **acid-balanced** waves that have a 7.0 or neutral pH. Acid-balanced waves process at room temperature and do not require the heat of a hair dryer for processing. Although GMTG is the primary reducing agent in acid-balanced waves, these waving products usually contain some ATG.

- All acid-balanced waves have three chemicals:

  - permanent waving solution
  - activator
  - neutralizer

- The permanent waving solution usually contains ATG and the activator GMTG. These products must be added together just prior to use.

- Acid-balanced waves process more quickly and produce firmer curls than true acid waves.

Exothermic Waves

Like acid-balanced perms, all **exothermic waves** (ek-soh-THUR-mik WAYVZ) have three components:

- permanent waving solution
- activator
- neutralizer

The activator in an exothermic wave, however, contains an oxidizing agent (usually hydrogen peroxide) that causes a rapid release of heat when mixed with the waving solution. The chemical reaction that releases heat and causes the waving solution to become warm can usually be felt when holding the bottle of solution. This rise in temperature increases the rate of the chemical reaction, which in turn shortens the processing time.

Ammonia-Free Waves

Ammonia-free waves use *alkanolamines* to replace ammonia and are gaining in popularity because of their low odor. Ammonia-free does not mean free of damage, so although these new products may not smell as strong as ammonia, they can still have a high alkaline pH. Processing takes place at a lower pH. Alkanolamines evaporate slowly, which is why they do not give

> **⚠ CAUTION**
> Accidentally mixing the contents of the activator tube with the neutralizer instead of the permanent waving solution will cause a violent chemical reaction that can cause injury, especially to the eyes.

off odors, and maintain the same pH level throughout the entire processing time. This constant pH level can ultimately be more damaging to the hair than are waves containing ammonia.

Thio-Free Waves

Thio-free waves use *cysteamine* or *mercaptamine* as the primary reducing agent. When used at high concentrations, these thio compounds with a pH range of 7.0 to 9.6 can be just as damaging as regular thio formulations.

Low-pH Waves

Sulfates, sulfites, and bisulfites offer an alternative to ATG but are weak and do not produce a firm curl. Sulfite perms are usually marketed as *body waves* and have a pH range of 6.5 to 7.0.

Strengths of Waving Solutions

Although the strength of a waving solution can be adjusted by increasing the amount of the active ingredient, today's wide range of waving products virtually eliminates the need to do so. Be cautioned that if the strength of a solution is adjusted through the addition of ammonia, the pH level should not exceed 9.6.

Most manufacturers market three or more strengths of permanent waving products:

- *Mild:* for damaged, porous, or tinted hair
- *Normal:* for normal hair with good porosity
- *Resistant:* for resistant hair with less porosity

Pre-wraps

Some permanent waving product packages contain a **pre-wrap solution** that is applied to the hair before wrapping on rods. In most cases, the pre-wrap is simply a leave-in conditioner that helps equalize the porosity of the hair to ensure even penetration of the waving lotion and to protect the hair from unnecessary damage. Always follow the manufacturer's directions.

Perm Selection

For a successful permanent waving service, it is essential to select the proper waving product for the client's hair type and desired result. After a thorough client consultation, the barber should be able to determine which type of permanent waving product is best suited to the client's hair condition. Most resistant hair types require an alkaline wave; alkaline or acid-balanced perms can be used on most normal hair types; and acid-balanced or true acid perm formulas are the best choice for most tinted, highlighted, or delicate hair types. Use Table 17-3 as a general guide to the selection of the most common types of permanent waves.

table 17-3

PERMANENT WAVE SELECTION

Perm Type	Active Ingredient	Wrapping Method	Process	Recommended Hair Type	Results	Advantages	Disadvantages
Alkaline/cold wave pH: 9.0 to 9.6	Ammonium thioglycolate (ATG)	Lotion wrap or water wrap	Room temperature	Coarse, thick, or resistant	Firm, strong curls	Processes quickly at room temperature	Unpleasant ammonia odor; may damage delicate hair
Exothermic wave pH: 9.0 to 9.6	Ammonium thioglycolate (ATG)	Water wrap	Exothermic	Coarse, thick, or resistant	Firm, strong curls	Faster processing time	Unpleasant ammonia odor; may damage delicate hair
True acid wave pH: 4.5 to 7.0	Glyceryl monothioglycolate (GMTG)	Water wrap	Endothermic	Extremely porous or very damaged	Soft, weak curls	Low pH produces minimal swelling	Requires heat from hair dryer; will not produce firm, strong curls
Acid-balanced wave pH: 7.8 to 8.2	Glyceryl monothioglycolate (GMTG)	Water wrap	Room temperature	Porous or damaged	Soft curls	Minimal swelling; processes at room temperature	Repeated exposure may cause allergic sensitivity in clients and stylists
Ammonia-free wave pH: 7.0 to 9.6	Monoethanolamine (MEA) or aminomethylpropanol (AMP)	Water wrap	Room temperature	Porous to normal	Medium to fine curls	No unpleasant ammonia odor	Overall strength varies with different manufacturers
Thio-free wave pH: 7.0 to 9.6	Mercaptamine or cysteamine	Water wrap	Room temperature	Porous to normal	Medium to fine curls	May be gentler, depending on formula	Overall strength varies with different manufacturers
Low-pH wave pH: 6.5 to 7.0	Ammonium sulfite or ammonium bisulfite	Water wrap	Endothermic	Normal, fine, or damaged	Weak curl or body wave	Minimal swelling	Requires heat from hair dryer; produces weak curls

figure 17-41
S pattern.

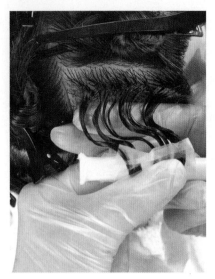

figure 17-42
Underprocessed hair.

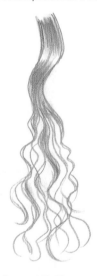

figure 17-43
Overprocessed hair.

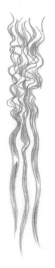

PERMANENT WAVE PROCESSING AND WAVE FORMATION

The strength of any permanent wave is based on the concentration of its reducing agent. In turn, the amount of processing time is determined by the strength of the permanent waving solution and the porosity level of the hair. Most of the processing takes place within the first 5 to 10 minutes, so the amount of processing should be determined by the strength of the solution and not by how long the perm processes. If the hair is not sufficiently processed after 10 minutes, it may require reapplication of the solution. The next time the client receives a perm service, a stronger solution may be used. Conversely, if the client's hair has been overprocessed, a weaker solution should have been used.

As the hair is processing, the waves form a deep-ridged pattern. The wave has reached its peak when it forms a firm letter S shape (Figure 17-41). The S pattern reaches a desirable peak only once during the perm process. Shortly after the S is well formed, the hair may become frizzy unless processing is stopped. Frizziness indicates that the processing time has reached its absolute maximum. Beyond this point, the hair becomes overprocessed and damaged.

Different conditions and hair textures will cause the quality of wave patterns to vary. Hair of good texture will show a firm, strong pattern, whereas hair that is weak or fine will not produce a firm pattern.

Underprocessing

* This is when hair has not been sufficiently softened to permit the breaking and rearrangement of the disulfide bonds.

* This results in a limp or weak wave formation with undefined ridges within the S pattern.

* The hair retains little or no wave formation and is unable to hold the desired curl (Figure 17-42).

* Reapplication of the permanent waving solution is necessary to complete the process.

Overprocessing

* The hair can also appear to be too weak to hold a curl (Figure 17-43).

* Any solution that can process the hair properly can also overprocess it.

* Solution left on the hair too long results in overprocessing and if too many disulfide bonds are broken, the hair may not have enough strength to hold the desired curl.

* Signs that the hair has been overprocessed include:
  * a weak curl formation
  * a very curly appearance when wet but completely frizzy when dry
  * an inability to be combed into a suitable wave pattern

* In hair that has been overprocessed, the elasticity of the hair has been damaged to the point where it is unable to contract into the wave formation.

* Overprocessed hair usually feels harsh after being dried and should be given reconditioning treatments.

Test Curls

Test curls help determine how the client's hair will react to the permanent waving process. A test curl provides information about how to obtain the best possible results out of the perm service. Test curls are performed by wrapping one parting of hair in three different areas of the head: the top, side, and nape (**Figure 17-44**).

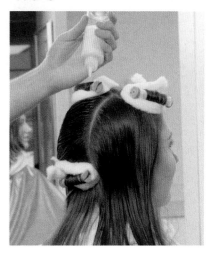

figure 17-44
Applying wave lotion to test curls.

Test curls enable the barber to observe the following aspects of the hair:

* speed of wave formation

* degree of wave formation

* exact time when peak of wave formation is reached

* identification of resistant areas

* appropriateness of product selection

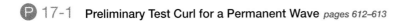

Ⓟ 17-1   **Preliminary Test Curl for a Permanent Wave** *pages 612–613*

NEUTRALIZATION

Permanent waving neutralizers are actually oxidizers that stop the action of permanent wave solutions and rebuild the disulfide bonds broken during processing. This process is known as **neutralization** (noo-truh-ly-ZAY-shun). The most common neutralizer is hydrogen peroxide with a concentration range between 5 volume (1.5 percent) and 10 volume (3 percent). Other types of neutralizers are sodium bromate and sodium perborate.

Neutralization has two important functions:

1. Rebuild the disulfide bonds that were broken and rearranged by the waving solution.

2. Deactivate any waving solution that remains in the hair after rinsing.

   If the hair is not properly neutralized, the curl will relax or straighten within one to two shampoos. As with waving solutions, there may be slightly different procedures recommended for individual products. To achieve the best possible results, always read the directions carefully.

   Proper rinsing is key to a perm. The rinsing process must last for at least 5 minutes, adding an additional minute for every inch the hair is longer than 5 inches. After thoroughly rinsing the permanent wave solution from the hair, it should be blotted until no excess water is absorbed into the towel. This is an important step in the neutralization process because excess water left in the hair prevents even saturation of the neutralizer and dilutes its properties.

Neutralizer Application

* The neutralizer should be applied to the top and bottom of each rod to assure saturation and even distribution of the product.

* Always give clients a towel to protect their eyes from excess or dripping neutralizer. A fresh cotton coil should also be used for additional safety and client comfort.

Rinsing the Neutralizer

Depending on the manufacturer's directions, neutralizers are rinsed from the hair in one of two ways:

- *Rinsing with the rods in place*

    - After a thorough rinsing with tepid water, followed by blotting, the rods are carefully removed in preparation for styling.
    - Some directions may require a second rinse after the removal of the rods.

- *Rinsing after the rods have been removed*

    - An alternative method is to carefully remove the rods, without stretching the hair, after neutralization has taken place.
    - Apply the balance of the neutralizing solution and allow it to remain on the hair for an additional minute.
    - Then rinse with tepid water and proceed with setting and/or styling the hair.

Post-permanent Wave Care

Most manufacturers recommend a 24- to 48-hour waiting period before shampooing freshly permed hair. Always follow the manufacturer's directions and be sure to educate your clients about the most appropriate shampoos and conditioners to use after a perm service. Unless there are signs of scalp irritation, deposit-only haircolor can also be applied sooner than three days after a permanent wave.

Reconditioning treatments can be used in the aftercare and between permanent waves. Effective post-perm care helps keep the hair in the best possible condition until the next chemical service. Suggest the following guidelines to your clients:

- Shampoo the hair as needed with an acid-balanced shampoo.

- Use a moisturizing hair conditioner.

- Schedule regular shop visits for trims and/or conditioning treatments to maintain the hairstyle.

figure 17-45
Partial perm style.

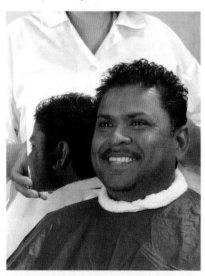

PARTIAL PERMANENT WAVES

Partial perming means that only a section of the hair is curled. In men's permanent waving, this is usually hair on the top and crest area of the head (**Figure 17-45**). Partial perms can be used to create volume and lift in these areas or to re-curl previously curled sections that have been trimmed due to normal hair growth and maintenance haircuts.

The same wrapping patterns and techniques used for a full permanent wave can be used for a partial perm with the following considerations:

- To make a smooth transition from the wrapped section to the non-wrapped section, wrap as far as the client wants, then before neutralizing, remove the bottom row and soften the curl. This will transition from permed to straight hair.

- After wrapping, place a coil of cotton around the wrapped rods as well as around the entire hairline.

- Before applying the waving lotion, apply a heavy conditioner or barrier cream to the sections that will not be permed to protect this hair from the effects of the waving lotion.

Many clients need the added texture and fullness that only a permanent wave can give. A permanent wave can help temporarily overcome common hair problems by redirecting a cowlick, making limp or unmanageable hair easier to style, or making sparse hair look fuller. Although men and women's hairstyles may be different, the techniques for permanent waving are essentially the same.

SPECIAL PROBLEMS

Dry, Damaged Hair

Dry, brittle, damaged, or overporous hair should be given reconditioning treatments before a permanent wave service. Avoid any treatment requiring massage or heat as this could create a sensitive scalp and irritation when the waving solution or neutralizer is applied. Special fillers that contain protein are available for reconditioning the hair and helping equalize its porosity. Some fillers also contain lanolin and cholesterol, which may help protect the hair against the harshness of the permanent waving solution.

Tinted or Lightened Hair

Hair that has been tinted or lightened should be shampooed with an extra-mild shampoo before waving. It may be advisable to use a pre-wrap or other leave-in conditioning product. While pre-wraps and leave-in conditioners may be sufficient for stronger hair types that have been previously tinted or lightened, extremely porous hair will probably not benefit from these applications. Extremely porous hair may absorb too much conditioner, which in turn may interfere with waving solution penetration and curl formation. Always select permanent waving solutions that are formulated for tinted and lightened hair conditions and always take the time to perform test curls.

Hair Tinted with Metallic Dye

Some over-the-counter haircoloring products still use metallic dyes in the formulations. Hair tinted with a metallic dye must first be treated with a dye remover to avoid hair discoloration or breakage. Do not chemically wave the hair if the test curls break or discolor. This type of haircoloring product is difficult to remove so the best option is to cut the color-treated hair in a series of shop visits until all the color is removed. Then proceed with the perm service on virgin hair, followed by the application of professional haircoloring products.

Curl Reduction

Sometimes a client is not pleased after a permanent wave because the hair seems too curly. If the hair is fine, do not suggest curl reduction before shampooing two or three times. This type of hair relaxes to a greater extent than does normal or coarse hair. Usually, after the second shampoo, the hair relaxes to a satisfactory level. If the hair has a normal or coarse texture, curl reduction may be done immediately following neutralization or

CAUTION
Do not attempt curl reduction on hair that has been overprocessed, as such treatment will only damage the hair further.

after a few days. Permanent waving solution may be used to relax the curl where required. Carefully comb it through the hair to widen and loosen the wave. When sufficiently relaxed, the hair is rinsed, towel-blotted, and neutralized.

Air-Conditioning and Heating Units

Because of its cooling effects, air-conditioning will usually slow the action of permanent waving solutions and additional processing time may be required. Make sure that clients are seated in an area of the shop away from drafts, vents, and fans to avoid slowing the processing time. Conversely, sitting too close to a heating vent or hood hair dryer can speed up the processing time.

SAFETY PRECAUTIONS FOR PERMANENT WAVING

- Always protect the client's clothing with the proper waterproof cape.
- Use two towels, one under the cape and one over the cape.
- Always examine the client's scalp before a perm service. Do not proceed if abrasions are present.
- Do not proceed with the perm if the client has ever experienced an allergic reaction to the products.
- Do not perm excessively damaged hair or hair that has been treated with hydroxide relaxers.
- Always apply a protective cream barrier around the client's hairline before applying the waving solution.
- Immediately replace cotton coils or towels that have become saturated with solution.
- Always protect the client's eyes when applying waving and neutralizing solutions by providing the client with a clean towel to hold over the eyes during the application. In case of accidental exposure, rinse thoroughly with cool water.
- Always follow the manufacturer's directions.
- Do not dilute or add anything to waving or neutralizing solutions unless specified in the manufacturer's directions.
- Wear gloves when applying solutions.
- Do not save opened or unused products, as the strength and effectiveness will change if not used promptly.
- Unless otherwise specified in the product instructions, apply waving and neutralizing solutions liberally to the top and underside of each rod.
- Start at the crown and progress systematically down each section. (Some barbers prefer to start at the top of the head.) Be sure that the surface area of the wound hair is wet with lotion so saturation is even.
- Follow the same application pattern for the neutralizer as used with the waving solution to avoid missing any rods.

- Sometimes it is necessary to resaturate the rods during processing. This may be due to evaporation of the solution, dryness of the hair, hair that was poorly saturated the first time, improper selection of solution strength, or failure to follow the manufacturer's directions. Reapplying the solution will hasten processing, so watch the wave development closely as negligence may result in hair damage.

- Make sure the hair stays evenly wet while wrapping on rods.

- Have client remove jewelry to avoid discoloration or skin reactions.

- Frequently change towels as they become soiled or saturated.

Know about Chemical Hair Relaxers

After reading this section, you will be able to:

LO⑧ Identify two types of chemical relaxers.

LO⑨ Explain the difference between *base* and *no-base* relaxers.

LO⑩ List three strand tests to be performed before a chemical relaxing process.

Chemical hair relaxing is the process of rearranging the basic structure of curly or wavy hair into a relaxed or straighter form. Like the permanent waving process, chemical relaxers change the shape of the hair by breaking and rearranging disulfide bonds in the hair. Relaxers can also soften coarse hair and make it more manageable.

The basic products used in the chemical relaxing process are:

- chemical relaxers (straighteners)

- neutralizers or neutralizing shampoos

- protective bases or creams

- conditioners

TYPES OF RELAXERS

The two most common types of relaxers are thio and hydroxide relaxers. Neither type of relaxer allows pre-shampooing unless there is an excessive buildup of dirt or styling products. In rare instances when the hair requires cleansing, the shampoo service should be performed gently to avoid scalp irritation and the hair should be thoroughly dried before the relaxer is applied.

Both types of relaxers are applied in the same manner, but thio relaxers require the application of a chemical neutralizing solution, whereas hydroxide relaxers are neutralized through the physical actions of rinsing and shampooing with a neutralizing shampoo product. Neutralizing shampoos or normalizing lotions are basically acid-balanced shampoos that neutralize any remaining hydroxide in the hair and help lower the pH of the hair and scalp.

Thio Relaxers

Thio (ATG) is the same reducing agent used in permanent waving, but thio relaxers usually have a pH above 10.0 and a higher concentration of ATG than permanent wave products. Thio relaxers are also thicker in consistency than permanent waving lotions for better adhesion and product control.

Hydroxide Relaxers

Hydroxide relaxers are ionic compounds formed by a metal combined with oxygen and hydrogen. Metal hydroxide relaxers include sodium hydroxide, potassium hydroxide, lithium hydroxide, and guanidine hydroxide.

Sodium Hydroxide Relaxers

These are known as *lye* relaxers. Sodium hydroxide is the oldest and most commonly used chemical relaxer. Sodium hydroxide content varies from 5 percent to 10 percent, with a pH range of 12.5 to 13.5. Generally speaking, the higher the percentage of sodium hydroxide, the faster the chemical reaction on the hair. The higher the pH factor, the greater the danger of hair damage or breakage.

Potassium and Lithium Hydroxide Relaxers

These are often sold as *no-mix/no-lye* relaxers. Although these two relaxers are not technically lye products, their chemistry is identical and there is little difference in their performance.

Guanidine Hydroxide Relaxers

These are usually advertised as no-lye relaxers. These relaxers contain two products, a relaxer cream and an activator, that must be mixed just prior to use and are recommended for sensitive scalps.

Calcium Hydroxide Relaxers

Many *calcium hydroxide* relaxers are often mistakenly referred to as *no-lye* relaxers. Obviously, this type of marketing statement can be misleading, so care must be taken when choosing the relaxer product. Calcium hydroxide relaxers require the addition of an activator. The strength of the relaxer is determined by the amount of activator used in the mixture. Although these relaxers are considered to be mild and tend to work more slowly on the hair, there are many professionals who feel that calcium hydroxide relaxers are more damaging to the cuticle layer of the hair than other hydroxide relaxers.

"Base" versus "No-Base" Relaxers

Hydroxide relaxers are usually sold in *base* and *no-base* formulas.

- **Base relaxers** require the application of a base cream to the entire scalp prior to relaxer application.

- **No-base relaxers** contain a base cream that is designed to melt at body temperature and do not require the application of a separate protective base.

RELAXER STRENGTHS

Most chemical relaxers are available in a variety of different strengths: mild, regular, and super. The strength of the relaxer reflects the concentration of hydroxide in its formulation.

- Mild strengths are recommended for fine, color-treated, or damaged hair.
- Regular-strength relaxers are intended for normal hair textures.
- Super strengths should be used for maximum straightening on extremely curly, coarse hair.
- Use Table 17-4 as a guide for selecting chemical relaxing products.

STRAND TESTS FOR CHEMICAL RELAXERS

Preliminary strand tests for chemical relaxer applications include:

- porosity test for determining the degree of porosity
- elasticity test for determining the degree of elasticity
- relaxer test for determining the hair's reaction to the chemical and processing time

table 17-4

SELECTING THE CORRECT RELAXER

Active Ingredient	pH	Marketed as	Advantages	Disadvantages
Sodium hydroxide	12.5 to 13.5	Lye relaxer	Very effective for extremely curly hair	May cause scalp irritation and damage the hair
Lithium hydroxide and potassium hydroxide	12.5 to 13.5	No-mix, lye relaxer	Very effective for extremely curly hair	May cause scalp irritation and damage the hair
Guanidine hydroxide	13 to 13.5	No-lye relaxer	Causes less skin irritation than other hydroxide relaxers	More drying to hair with repeated use
Ammonium thioglycolate	9.6 to 10.0	Thio relaxer, no-lye relaxer	Compatible with soft-curl permanent waves	Strong, unpleasant ammonia smell
Ammonium sulfite or ammonium bisulfite	6.5 to 8.5	Low-pH relaxer, no-lye relaxer	Less damaging to hair	Does not relax extremely curly hair sufficiently

Relaxer Strand Test Mini-Procedure

1. Thread a small section of hair through a hole cut into a piece of wax paper or paper towel; do not use foil. Do not use a base or cream. Apply relaxer to the hair section and smooth. Process according to the manufacturer's directions.

2. Thoroughly mist the hair section with water to remove product and blot.

3. Neutralize with neutralizer or neutralizing shampoo depending on the type of relaxing product used. Check results and note on the client record card.

4. If the hair has been satisfactorily straightened, apply conditioner or base cream to the strand, isolate it, and proceed with the relaxing treatment over the remainder of the hair.

SAFETY PRECAUTIONS FOR CHEMICAL RELAXERS

> ⚠️ **CAUTION**
> Hydroxide relaxers are incompatible with thio relaxers and products. *Never* use a hydroxide product on hair that has been previously relaxed with a thio product. *Never* use a thio product on hair that has been previously relaxed with a hydroxide product. Crossover of the products will result in hair breakage.

- Always protect the client's clothing with a proper waterproof cape.

- Use two towels, one under the drape and one over the cape.

- Always examine the client's scalp before a relaxer service. Do not proceed if abrasions are present.

- Do not proceed if the client has ever experienced an allergic reaction to the products.

- Do not relax excessively damaged hair.

- Do not use thio relaxers on hair that has been treated with hydroxide relaxers, or hydroxide relaxers on thio-treated hair.

- Always apply a protective cream barrier around the client's hairline before applying a relaxer.

- Base the scalp with a protective cream as directed by the product manufacturer.

- Always be careful of the client's eyes when applying relaxers and neutralizing solutions. In case of accidental exposure, rinse thoroughly with cool water.

- Always follow the manufacturer's directions.

- Do not dilute or add anything to relaxer creams unless specified in the manufacturer's directions.

- Wear gloves when applying relaxers.

- Do not save mixed products, as the strength and effectiveness will change if not used promptly.

- Apply relaxer cream to the most resistant area first.

- Follow the same pattern for smoothing the relaxer as was used during the application process.

- Frequently change towels as they become soiled or saturated.

Know about Chemical Curl Reformations

After reading this section, you will be able to:

LO⑪ Explain the three steps of a curl reformation process.

WHAT IS A CURL REFORMATION?

A curl reformation, also known as a *soft-curl permanent,* is a three-step process that is used to restructure very curly hair into looser and larger curls. First, naturally curly hair is relaxed into a straighter form using a thio-based rearranger. This step is similar to a thio-based relaxer application. After processing and rinsing, the hair is wrapped on perm rods using a thio-based curl booster, much like a lotion wrap permanent wave wrapping procedure. Finally, hair is neutralized, rehardening the bonds in the cortex into a new, wavy pattern. A curl reformation is a combination of a thio-based relaxer application followed by a permanent wave wrap and neutralizing process.

The products used in a curl reformation include:

- *Rearranger*
  - The thio relaxer product used for the partial relaxation of the hair in a curl reformation service is most commonly known as the *rearranger.*
  - The rearranger is an ATG product in a thick cream form that is applied to dry hair in the same way as a hydroxide relaxer.

- *Booster*
  - The waving solution is called the *booster* and is similar in composition to alkaline permanent waving solutions or lotions.
  - This chemical restructures the hair around perm rods.

- *Neutralizer*
  - The *neutralizer* is an oxidizing solution in a clear or milky liquid form and is part of the same product line as the rearranger and the booster.
  - This solution rebuilds the broken disulfide bonds.
  - The chemical reactions of the neutralizer are the same as those created by permanent waving neutralizers.

- *Additional products*
  - Styling products such as activators and moisturizers are often recommended as part of the finishing process.
  - These products, such as activators and moisturizers, serve as leave-in conditioners and styling products to promote curl retention, although excess application should be avoided to prevent drips and oversaturation.
  - Depending on the texture and condition of the hair, other professional products that retain moisture and promote manageability of the hair may be preferred.

> **⚠ CAUTION**
> Use only the manufacturer's recommended neutralizer with the waving lotion. Never mix brands or systems.

Ⓟ 17-7 **Curl Reforming** *pages 632–637*

Understand Texturizers and Chemical Blowouts

After reading this section, you will be able to:

LO⓬ Describe the intended outcomes of texturizer and chemical blowout services.

WHAT ARE THEY?

Overly curly hair has unique characteristics that may require special styling techniques. Relaxing products can be used to **texturize** the hair, to reduce it from an extremely curly state to a wave formation that makes haircutting and styling more versatile, or to perform a **chemical blowout** service that partially straightens the hair with the intent that it will be picked out and cut. Chemical blowouts were used for many of the semi-straightened "Afro" styles of the 1970s.

Using Thio

Texturizers and chemical blowouts are usually performed with a thio relaxer, although they may be performed with a sodium hydroxide relaxer. The primary consideration with either method is to not over-relax the hair to the point where the blowout process becomes impossible to perform. Consider the characteristics associated with using thio and hydroxide relaxers: Although thio relaxers may have a pH above 10, they are not as harsh as hydroxide relaxers. Depending on the strength of the thio relaxer, it may not straighten tightly curled hair textures to the desired degree. Since the objective of a chemical blowout is to remove some but not all of the curl, a thio relaxer may be used for most of its entire recommended application time. Check the curl pattern every few minutes until the desired amount of curl relaxation has been achieved.

> **CAUTION**
> Review the neutralization procedures for thio and hydroxide relaxers at the end of each procedure before proceeding.

Ⓟ 17-3 **Applying Thio Relaxer to Virgin Hair** *pages 619–622*

Ⓟ 17-4 **Thio Relaxer Retouch** *pages 623–625*

Using Hydroxide

Sodium hydroxide is an extremely alkaline product and may process the hair too quickly to the point where a blowout cannot be performed. When using sodium hydroxide, timing and controlling the amount of processing becomes very important. The chemical should not be kept on the hair for longer than 40 percent of the recommended processing time.

Ⓟ 17-5 **Applying Hydroxide Relaxer to Virgin Hair** *pages 626–628*

Ⓟ 17-6 **Hydroxide Relaxer Retouch** *pages 629–631*

Reminders

The important consideration to remember is to relax the hair only to the point where it has relaxed enough to achieve the desired style.

After the relaxer has been rinsed from the hair, apply:

- neutralizer conditioner if using a thio relaxer, or
- neutralizing (or stabilizing) shampoo and conditioner if using a sodium hydroxide product.

In both cases, the conditioner will help minimize possible damage or breakage and enable the hair to withstand combing, picking, and rearranging.

Procedural Reminders for a Chemical Blowout

While the degree of curl remaining after a texturizer service should leave the hair ready for cutting and styling, the chemical blowout requires an extra step before a haircut. After processing, perform the final steps of a chemical blowout service by:

1. Using a wide-tooth comb or pick, comb the hair upward and slightly forward. The hair closest to the scalp gives direction to the hair; therefore, it must be picked upward and outward. Start at the crown and continue until all of the hair has been combed out from the scalp and distributed evenly around the head.

2. Place the client under a hood hair dryer until the hair is dried.

3. Once dried, the hair is ready for shaping. Evenness is very important at this point. Check the hair length to make sure that the shortest hair is used as the guide for the balance of the head.

4. Begin cutting at the sides. The hair is evened out around the head with clippers or shears while picking the hair outward from the scalp. Cut the hair in the direction in which it is to be combed. The objective is to achieve a smooth, even cut that is properly contoured. The final cutting should be done with shears to even out loose or ragged ends.

5. Outline the hairstyle at the sides, around the ears, and in the nape area using either shears or an outliner. After the hair is cut to the desired style, apply the finishing touches. Fluff the hair slightly with the pick where required and spray lightly to hold the shape.

⚠ CAUTION

You may hear of keratin-based straightening treatments, also known as Brazilian keratin treatments. These advanced services are used to eliminate up to 95 percent of frizz and curl and last three to five months. If your state allows this service, educate yourself in order to protect you and your clients by following the requirements in Occupational Safety and Health Administration's (OSHA) formaldehyde and hazard communication standards. Potential health risks are involved if the formaldehyde released during the process exceeds the maximum concentration of 0.75 parts per million (ppm) allowed by OSHA over an 8-hour period. For more information, visit OSHA's website at http://www.osha.gov.

PRELIMINARY TEST CURL FOR A PERMANENT WAVE

MATERIALS, IMPLEMENTS, AND EQUIPMENT

You will need all of the following implements, materials, and supplies:

☐ Applicator bottles

☐ Clarifying and acid-balanced shampoo (optional)

☐ Conditioner (optional)

☐ Cotton coil or rope

☐ Disposable gloves

☐ End papers

☐ Neutralizer

☐ Neutralizing bib

☐ Perm rods

☐ Perm solution

☐ Plastic clips for sectioning

☐ Plastic tail comb

☐ Pre-neutralizing conditioner (optional)

☐ Protective barrier cream

☐ Roller picks

☐ Spray bottle

☐ Styling comb

☐ Timer

☐ Towels

☐ Waterproof cape

PREPARATION

1 Wash your hands.

2 Clean and disinfect all tools and implements.

3 Conduct client consultation.

4 Perform a hair and scalp analysis.

5 Select and arrange required materials.

PROCEDURE

1 Drape the client for shampoo.

2 Gently shampoo and towel-dry hair. Avoid irritating the client's scalp. Re-drape the client for a chemical service.

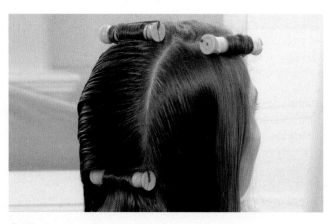

3 Wrap one rod in each different area of the head (top, side, and nape).

4 Wrap a coil of cotton around each rod.

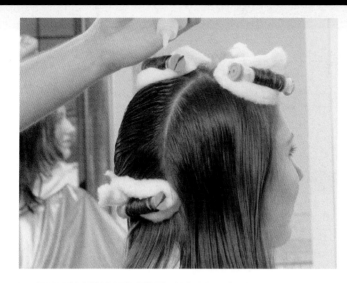

5 Apply perm solution to the wrapped curls. Do not allow perm solution to come into contact with unwrapped hair.

6 Set a timer, and process according to the manufacturer's directions.

7 Check each test curl frequently for proper curl development. Unfasten the rod and unwind the curl about one to two turns of the rod. Do not allow the hair to become loose or completely unwound. Gently move the rod toward the scalp to encourage the hair to fall loosely into the wave pattern.

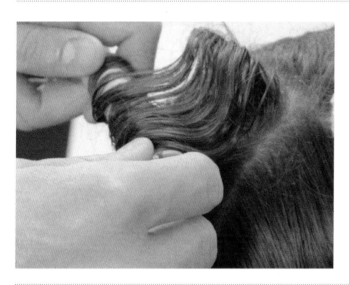

8 Curl development is complete when a firm S is formed that reflects the size of the rod used. Different hair textures will have slightly different S formations. The wave pattern for fine, thin hair may be weak, with little definition. The wave pattern for coarse, thick hair is usually stronger and better defined.

9 When the desired curl has been formed, rinse thoroughly with warm water for at least 5 minutes, blot thoroughly, apply neutralizer, and process according to the manufacturer's directions. Gently dry the hair and evaluate the results. Do not proceed with the permanent wave if the test curls are extremely damaged or overprocessed. If the test curl results are satisfactory, proceed with the perm, but do not re-perm these preliminary test curls. Rinse and process the test rods, but wait to remove them with the rest of the rods after the perm is completed.

CLEAN-UP AND DISINFECTION

☐ Clean and disinfect tools and implements.

☐ Clean and disinfect work area.

☐ Dispose of single-use items. Place all used linens, towels, and capes in the laundry.

☐ Wash your hands.

CHEMICAL (PERMANENT) WAVE AND PROCESSING USING A BASIC PERMANENT WRAP

MATERIALS, IMPLEMENTS, AND EQUIPMENT

You will need all of the following implements, materials, and supplies:

☐ Applicator bottles

☐ Clarifying and acid-balanced shampoo (optional)

☐ Conditioner (optional)

☐ Cotton coil or rope

☐ Disposable gloves

☐ End papers

☐ Neutralizer

☐ Neutralizing bib

☐ Perm rods

☐ Perm solution

☐ Plastic clips for sectioning

☐ Plastic tail comb

☐ Pre-neutralizing conditioner (optional)

☐ Protective barrier cream

☐ Roller picks

☐ Spray bottle

☐ Styling comb

☐ Timer

☐ Towels

☐ Waterproof cape

PREPARATION

1 Wash your hands.

2 Clean and disinfect all tools and implements.

3 Conduct client consultation.

4 Perform a hair and scalp analysis.

5 Select and arrange required materials.

PROCEDURE

1 After completing the pre-service procedure, seat the client. If the manufacturer's directions indicate a shampoo is necessary before the service, then drape the client for a shampoo and gently shampoo and towel-dry hair. Avoid irritating the client's scalp.

2 Re-drape the client for a chemical service.

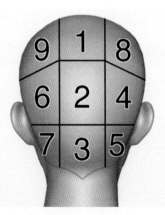

3 Divide the hair into nine panels. Use the length of the rod to measure the width of the panels. Remember to keep the hair evenly damp as you wrap.

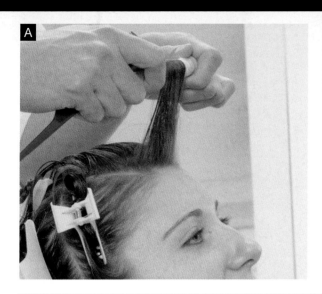

4A Begin wrapping at the front hairline or crown. Make a horizontal parting the same size as the rod. Using two end papers, roll the hair down to the scalp in the direction of hair growth, and position the rod half off-base.

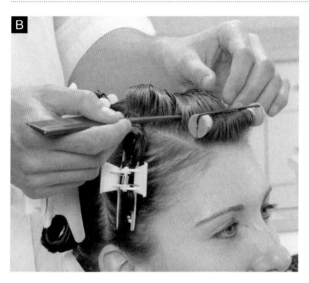

4B The band should be smooth, not twisted, and should be fastened straight across the top of the rod. Excessive tension may cause band marks or hair breakage.

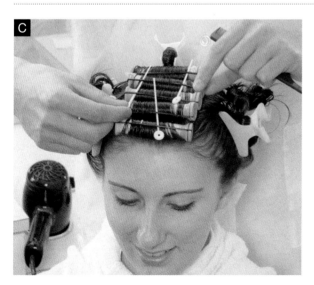

4C Continue wrapping the remainder of the first panel using the same technique. Option: Insert roller picks to stabilize the rods and eliminate any tension caused by the band.

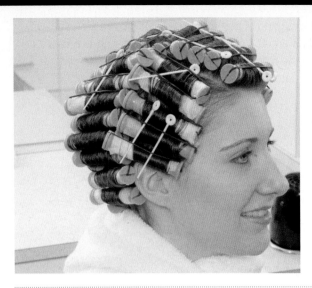

⑤ Continue wrapping the remaining eight panels in numerical order, holding the hair at a 90-degree angle.

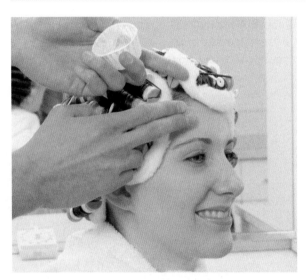

⑥ Apply protective barrier cream to the hairline and the ears. Apply a coil of cotton around the entire hairline and offer the client a towel to blot any drips. Put on gloves.

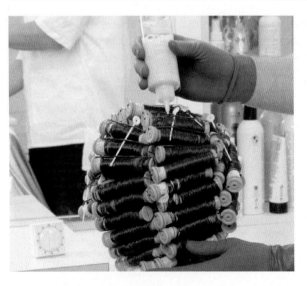

⑦ Slowly and carefully apply the perm solution to each rod. Ask the client to lean forward while you apply solution to the back area; ask the client to lean back as you apply solution to the front and sides. Avoid splashing and dripping. Continue to apply the solution slowly until each rod is completely saturated. Apply solution to the most resistant area first.

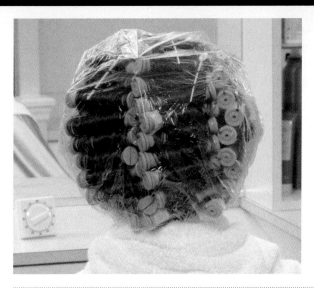

8 If a plastic cap is used, punch a few holes in the cap and cover all the hair completely. Do not allow the plastic cap to touch the client's skin.

9 Check cotton and towels. If they are saturated with solution, replace them.

10 Process according to the manufacturer's directions. Processing time varies according to the strength of the solution, hair type and condition, and desired results. As a general rule, processing usually takes less than 20 minutes at room temperature.

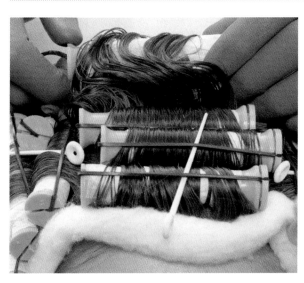

11 Check frequently for curl development. Unwind the rod and check the S pattern formation described in the preliminary test curl procedure. Check a different rod each time!

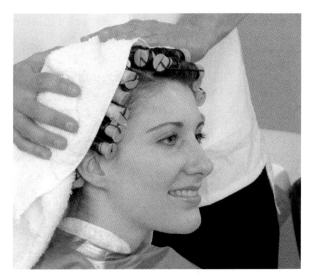

12 When processing is complete, rinse the hair thoroughly for at least 5 minutes. Then towel-blot each rod to remove excess moisture. Option: Some manufacturers recommend the application of a pre-neutralizing conditioner after rinsing and blotting and before applying the neutralizer. Always follow the manufacturer's directions and the procedures approved by your instructor.

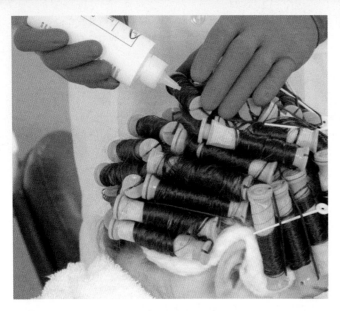

13 Apply the neutralizer slowly and carefully to the hair on each rod. Ask the client to lean forward while you apply solution to the back area, and then to lean back as you apply solution to the front and sides. Avoid splashing and dripping. Continue to apply the neutralizer until each rod is completely saturated.

14 Set a timer for the amount of time specified by the manufacturer.

15 Rinse thoroughly. Option: Shampoo and condition. Always follow the manufacturer's directions and the procedures approved by your instructor.

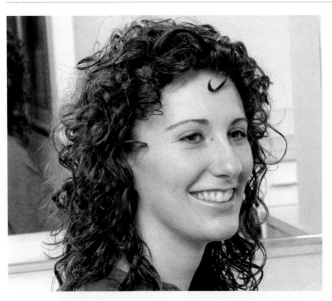

16 Style the hair as desired.

CLEAN-UP AND DISINFECTION

☐ Clean and disinfect tools and implements.

☐ Clean and disinfect work area.

☐ Dispose of single-use items. Place all used linens, towels, and capes in the laundry.

☐ Wash your hands.

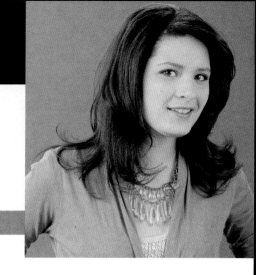

P 17-3

APPLYING THIO RELAXER TO VIRGIN HAIR

You will need all of the following implements, materials, and supplies:

- ☐ Acid-balanced shampoo
- ☐ Applicator brush or tail comb
- ☐ Conditioner
- ☐ Disposable gloves
- ☐ Hard rubber comb
- ☐ Plastic clips
- ☐ Plastic or glass bowl
- ☐ Pre-neutralizing conditioner
- ☐ Protective base cream
- ☐ Spray bottle
- ☐ Styling comb
- ☐ Thio neutralizer
- ☐ Thio relaxer
- ☐ Timer
- ☐ Towels
- ☐ Waterproof cape

PREPARATION

1. Wash your hands.
2. Clean and disinfect all tools and implements.
3. Conduct client consultation.

PROCEDURE

1. Perform an analysis of the hair and scalp. Perform tests for porosity and elasticity.

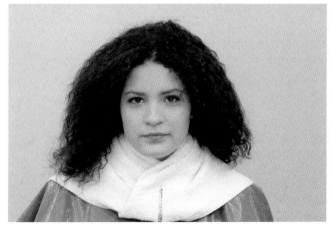

2. Drape the client for a chemical service. *The hair and scalp must be completely dry prior to the application of a thio relaxer.*

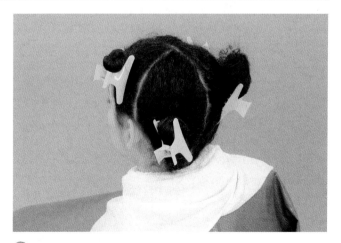

3. Part the hair into four sections, from the center of the front hairline to the center of the nape, and from ear to ear. Clip the sections up to keep them out of the way.

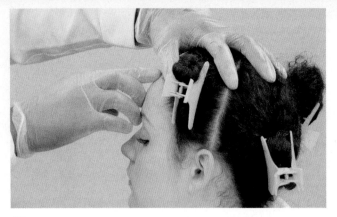

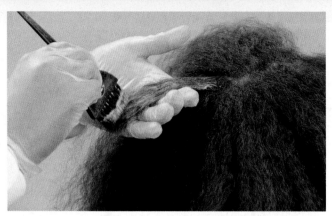

4 Apply protective base cream to the hairline and ears. Option: Take ¼-inch to ½-inch horizontal partings, and apply a protective base cream to the entire scalp. Always follow the manufacturer's directions and the procedures approved by your instructor.

5 Wear gloves on both hands. Begin application in the most resistant area, usually at the back of the head. Make ¼-inch to ½-inch horizontal partings, and apply the relaxer to the top of the strand first, and then to the underside. Apply the relaxer with an applicator brush, with the back of the comb, or with your fingers. Apply relaxer ¼-inch to ½-inch away from the scalp, and up to the porous ends. To avoid scalp irritation, do not allow the relaxer to touch the scalp until the last few minutes of processing.

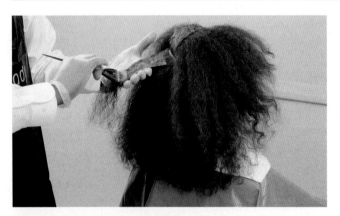

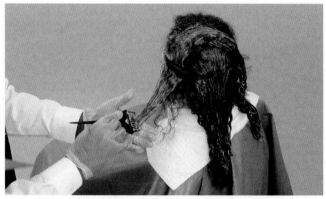

6 Continue applying the relaxer, working your way down the section toward the hairline.

7 Continue the same application procedure with the remaining sections. Finish the most resistant sections first.

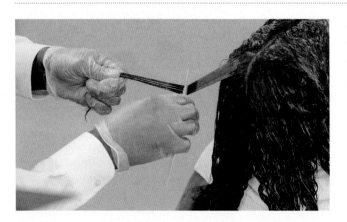

8 After the relaxer has been applied to all sections, use the back of the comb or your hands to smooth each section. Never comb the relaxer through the hair.

9 Process according to the manufacturer's directions. Perform periodic strand tests. Processing usually takes less than 20 minutes at room temperature. Always follow the manufacturer's processing directions.

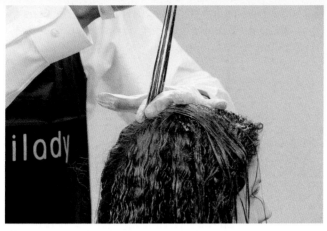

10 During the last few minutes of processing, work the relaxer down to the scalp and through the ends of the hair, using additional relaxer as needed. Carefully smooth all sections using an applicator brush, your fingers, or the back of the comb.

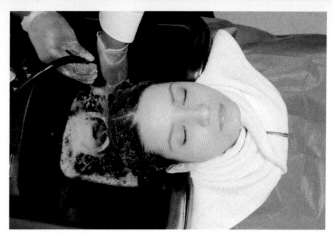

11 Rinse thoroughly with warm water to remove all traces of the relaxer.

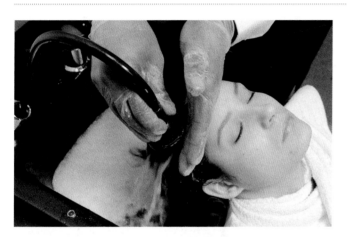

12 Shampoo at least three times with an acid-balanced shampoo. It is essential that all traces of the relaxer be removed from the hair. Optional: Apply the pre-neutralizing conditioner, and comb it through to the ends of the hair. Leave it on for approximately 5 minutes and then rinse. Always follow the manufacturer's directions and the procedures approved by your instructor.

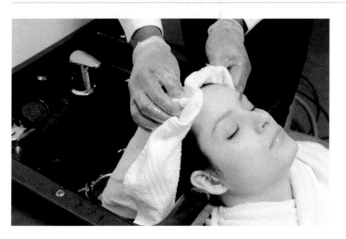

13 Blot excess water from the hair.

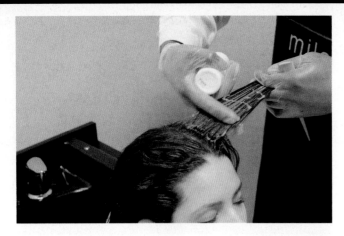

14 Apply thio neutralizer in ¼-inch to ½-inch sections throughout the hair and smooth with your hands or the back of the comb.

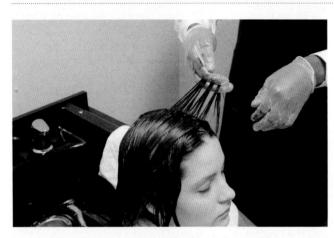

15 Process the neutralizer according to the manufacturer's directions.

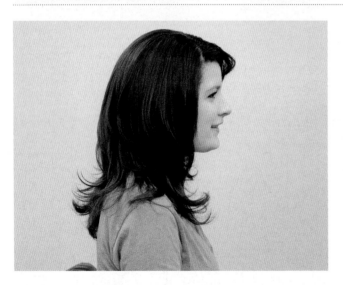

16 Rinse thoroughly. Shampoo, condition, and style.

CLEAN-UP AND DISINFECTION

☐ Clean and disinfect tools and implements.

☐ Clean and disinfect work area.

☐ Dispose of single-use items. Place all used linens, towels, and capes in the laundry.

☐ Wash your hands.

THIO RELAXER RETOUCH

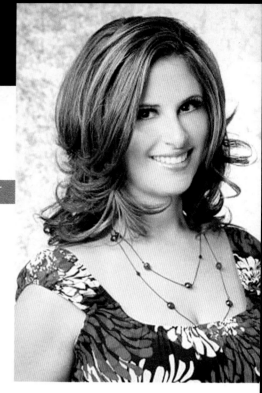

MATERIALS, IMPLEMENTS, AND EQUIPMENT

You will need all of the following implements, materials, and supplies:

- ☐ Acid-balanced shampoo
- ☐ Applicator brush or tail comb
- ☐ Conditioner
- ☐ Disposable gloves
- ☐ Hard rubber comb
- ☐ Plastic clips
- ☐ Plastic or glass bowl
- ☐ Pre-neutralizing conditioner
- ☐ Protective base cream
- ☐ Spray bottle
- ☐ Styling comb
- ☐ Thio neutralizer
- ☐ Thio relaxer
- ☐ Timer
- ☐ Towels
- ☐ Waterproof cape

Photography by Tom Carson.

PREPARATION

1. Wash your hands.
2. Clean and disinfect all tools and implements.
3. Conduct client consultation.
4. Perform a hair and scalp analysis.

PROCEDURE

1. Perform an analysis of the hair and scalp. Perform tests for porosity and elasticity.

2. Drape the client for a chemical service. To avoid scalp irritation, do not shampoo the hair prior to a thio relaxer. *The hair and scalp must be completely dry prior to the application of a thio relaxer retouch.*

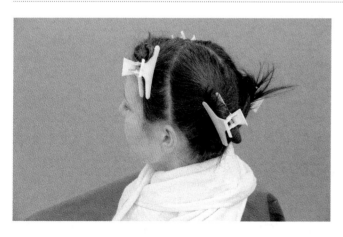

3. Divide the hair into four sections, from the center of the front hairline to the center of the nape, and from ear to ear. Clip sections up to keep them out of the way.

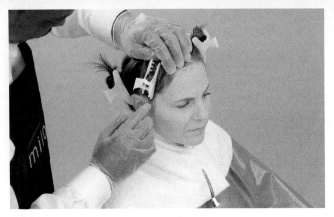

4 Wear gloves on both hands. Apply a protective base cream to the hairline and ears, unless you are using a no-base relaxing product. Option: Take ¼-inch to ½-inch horizontal partings, and apply protective base cream to the entire scalp.

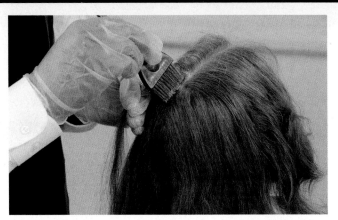

5 Begin application of the relaxer in the most resistant area, usually at the back of the head. Make ¼-inch to ½-inch horizontal partings, and apply the relaxer to the top of the strand. Apply the relaxer as close to the scalp as possible, but do not touch the scalp with the product. Only allow the relaxer to touch the scalp during the last few minutes of processing. To avoid overprocessing or breakage, do not overlap the relaxer onto the previously relaxed hair.

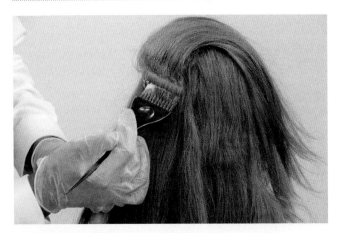

6 Continue applying the relaxer, using the same procedure and working your way down the section toward the hairline.

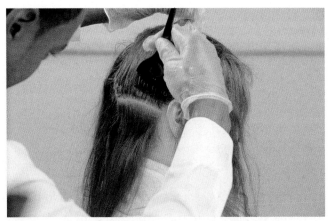

7 Continue the same application procedure with the remaining sections, finishing the most resistant sections first.

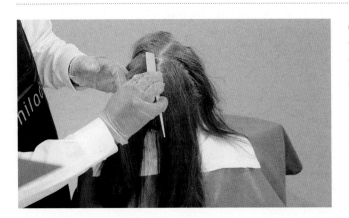

8 After the relaxer has been applied to all sections, use the back of the comb, the applicator brush, or your hands to smooth each section.

9 Process according to the manufacturer's directions. Perform periodic strand tests. Processing usually takes less than 20 minutes at room temperature. Always follow the manufacturer's processing directions.

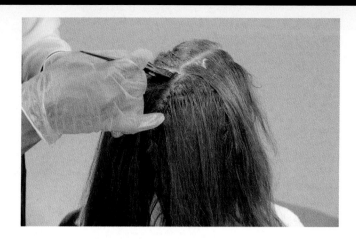

10 During the last few minutes of processing, gently work the relaxer down to the scalp.

> ⚠️ **CAUTION**
> Never intentionally overlap previously relaxed hair as this will result in damage and possible hair breakage!

11 Rinse thoroughly with warm water to remove all traces of the relaxer.

12 Shampoo at least three times with an acid-balanced shampoo (neutralizer). It is essential that all traces of the relaxer be removed from the hair. If the relaxer product recommends using a pre-neutralizing conditioner, comb it through the hair as per the recommendations of the manufacturer. Always follow the manufacturer's directions and the procedures approved by your instructor.

13 Blot excess water from hair.

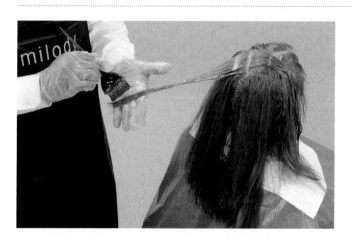

14 Apply thio neutralizer in ¼-inch to ½-inch sections throughout the hair and smooth with your hands or the back of the comb.

15 Process the neutralizer according to the manufacturer's directions.

16 Rinse thoroughly. Shampoo, condition, and style.

CLEAN-UP AND DISINFECTION

☐ Clean and disinfect tools and implements.

☐ Clean and disinfect work area.

☐ Dispose of single-use items. Place all used linens, towels, and capes in the laundry.

☐ Wash your hands.

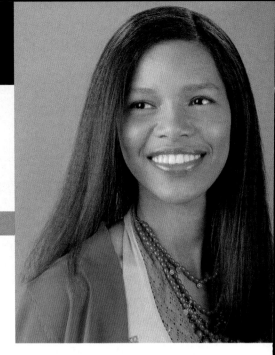

P 17-5

APPLYING HYDROXIDE RELAXER TO VIRGIN HAIR

MATERIALS, IMPLEMENTS, AND EQUIPMENT

You will need all of the following implements, materials, and supplies:

- ☐ Conditioner
- ☐ Disposable gloves
- ☐ Hydroxide relaxer
- ☐ Neutralizing acid-balanced shampoo
- ☐ Plastic clips
- ☐ Plastic or glass bowl
- ☐ Protective base cream
- ☐ Styling comb
- ☐ Tail comb or applicator brush
- ☐ Timer
- ☐ Towels
- ☐ Waterproof cape
- ☐ Wide-tooth hard rubber comb

PREPARATION

1. Wash your hands.
2. Clean and disinfect all tools and implements.
3. Conduct client consultation.
4. Perform a hair and scalp analysis.
5. Select and arrange required materials.
6. Drape client for a chemical service.

PROCEDURE

1. Perform an analysis of the hair and scalp by visually assessing the hair for breakage, sores on the scalp, or any visual signs of irritation. Feel the hair and perform an elasticity test. If hair fails the test for porosity and elasticity, do not perform the relaxer service.

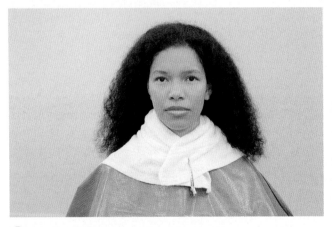

2. Drape the client for a chemical service.

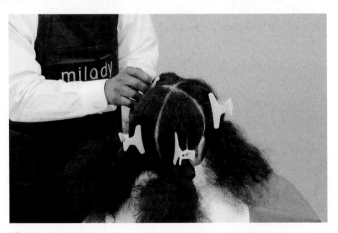

3. To avoid scalp irritation, do not shampoo the hair. *The hair and scalp must be completely dry prior to the application of a hydroxide relaxer.*

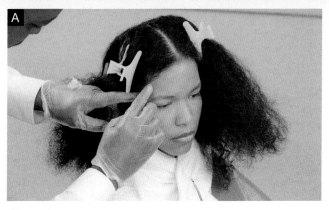

4A Part the hair into four sections, from the center of the front hairline to the center of the nape, and from ear to ear. Clip the sections up if necessary to keep hair out of the way.

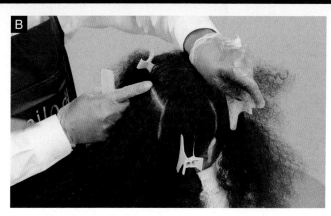

4B Apply protective base cream to the hairline and ears.

4C Optional: Take ¼-inch to ½-inch horizontal partings, and apply a protective base cream to the entire scalp. Always follow the manufacturer's directions and the procedures approved by your instructor. Set timer as indicated by the manufacturer and initial strand test.

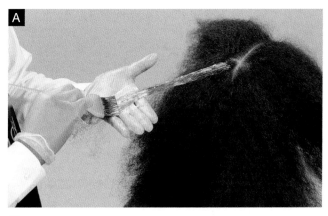

5A Put gloves on both hands. Begin the relaxer application in the most resistant area, usually at the back of the head or nape area. Make ¼-inch to ½-inch horizontal partings, and apply the relaxer to the top of the strand first. Do not apply to the scalp.

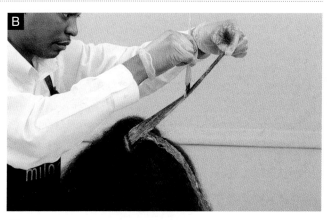

5B Apply relaxer to the underside of the first section using an applicator brush or the back of a tail comb. Apply relaxer ¼-inch to ½-inch away from the scalp, and up to the porous ends. To avoid scalp irritation, do not allow the relaxer to touch the scalp until the last few minutes of processing.

6 Continue applying relaxer to other sections, working your way down the section toward the hairline. Continue the same application procedure with the remaining sections.

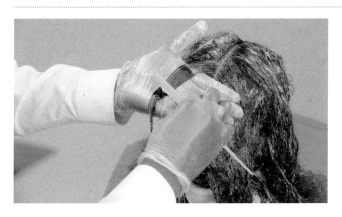

7 After the relaxer has been applied to all sections, use the back of the comb or your hands to smooth each section. Never comb the relaxer through the hair as this may break the hair.

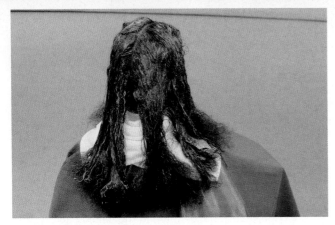

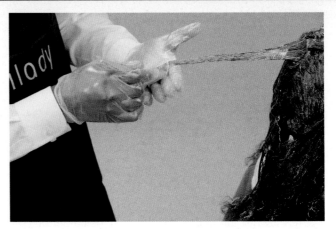

8 Process according to the manufacturer's directions and what your initial strand test indicated regarding timing. Perform periodic strand tests.

9 During the last few minutes of processing, work the relaxer down to the scalp and through the ends of the hair, using additional relaxer as needed. Carefully smooth all sections, using an applicator brush, your fingers, or the back of the tail comb.

10 Rinse thoroughly with warm water to remove all traces of the relaxer.

11 If the relaxer comes with a normalizing lotion or conditioner, comb it through the hair. Leave it on as indicated by the manufacturer. Rinse thoroughly. Always follow the manufacturer's directions and the procedures approved by your instructor.

12 Shampoo at least three times with an acid-balanced neutralizing shampoo. If you are using a neutralizing shampoo with a color indicator, usually the color will change from pink to white indicating that all traces of the relaxer are removed, and the natural pH of the hair and scalp has been restored.

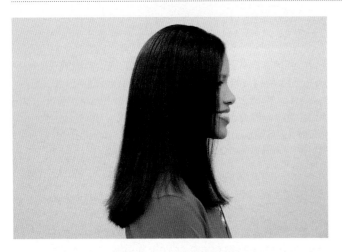

13 Rinse thoroughly, condition, and style as desired.

CLEAN-UP AND DISINFECTION

☐ Clean and disinfect tools and implements.

☐ Clean and disinfect work area.

☐ Dispose of any single use items, paper goods, and/or linens.

☐ Wash your hands.

HYDROXIDE RELAXER RETOUCH

MATERIALS, IMPLEMENTS, AND EQUIPMENT

You will need all of the following implements, materials, and supplies:

- ☐ Acid-balanced shampoo
- ☐ Conditioner
- ☐ Disposable gloves
- ☐ Hard rubber comb
- ☐ Hydroxide neutralizer
- ☐ Hydroxide relaxer
- ☐ Plastic clips
- ☐ Plastic or glass bowl
- ☐ Protective base cream
- ☐ Spray bottle
- ☐ Tail comb or applicator brush
- ☐ Timer
- ☐ Towels
- ☐ Waterproof cape

PREPARATION

1. Wash your hands.
2. Clean and disinfect all tools and implements.
3. Conduct client consultation.

PROCEDURE

1. Perform an analysis of the hair and scalp. Perform tests for porosity and elasticity.

2. Drape the client for a chemical service.

3. To avoid scalp irritation, do not shampoo the hair. *The hair and scalp must be completely dry prior to the application of a hydroxide relaxer retouch.*

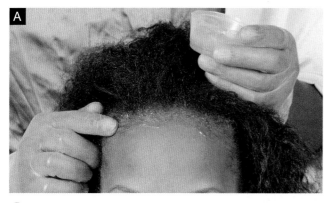

4A Divide the hair into four sections, from the center of the front hairline to the center of the nape, and from ear to ear. Clip sections up to keep hair out of the way if necessary.

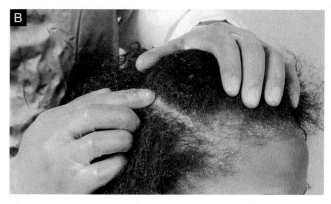

4B Apply a protective base cream to the hairline and ears. Put gloves on both hands.

4C Optional: Take ¼-inch to ½-inch horizontal partings and apply protective base cream to the entire scalp. Set timer as indicated by the manufacturer for retouch.

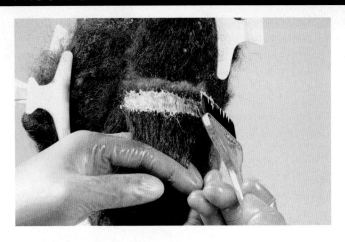

5 Begin application of the relaxer in the most resistant area, usually at the back of the head or nape area. Make ¼-inch to ½-inch horizontal partings, and apply the relaxer to the top of the strand. Apply the relaxer as close to the scalp as possible, but do not touch the scalp with the relaxer. Only allow the relaxer to touch the scalp during the last few minutes of processing. To avoid overprocessing or breakage, do not overlap the relaxer onto the previously relaxed hair.

6 Continue applying the relaxer, using the same procedure, and working your way down the section toward the hairline.

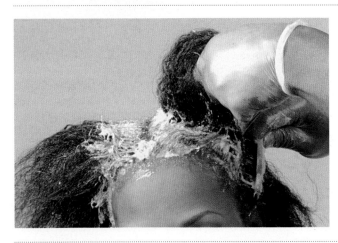

7 Continue the same application procedure with the remaining sections.

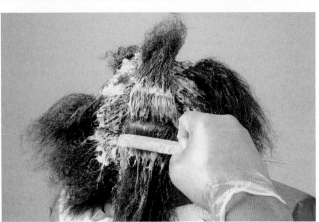

8 After the relaxer has been applied to all sections, use the back of the comb, the applicator brush, or your hands to smooth each section.

9 Process according to the manufacturer's directions. Perform periodic strand tests.

10 During the last few minutes of processing, gently work the relaxer down to the scalp.

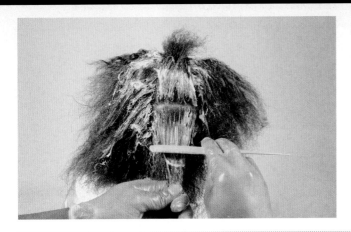

11 Do not relax mid-shaft or ends during the retouch service, as this will cause overprocessing. Option: Oil may be applied to previously relaxed ends to protect from overprocessing caused by overlapping.

12 Rinse thoroughly with warm water to remove all traces of the relaxer. If the relaxer comes with a normalizing lotion or conditioner, comb it through the hair. Leave it on as indicated by the manufacturer and rinse thoroughly. Always follow the manufacturer's directions and the procedures approved by your instructor.

13 Shampoo at least three times with an acid-balanced neutralizing shampoo. If you are using an acid-balanced neutralizing shampoo with a color indicator, usually the color change will go from pink to white indicating all traces of the relaxer have been removed and the natural pH of the hair and scalp has been restored. Apply conditioner as per manufacturer's recommendations. Rinse.

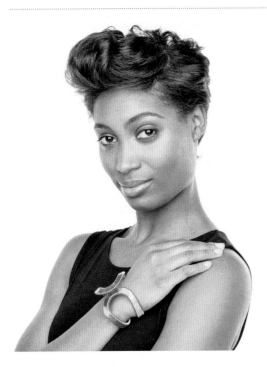

14 Style the hair as desired.

CLEAN-UP AND DISINFECTION

☐ Clean and disinfect tools and implements.

☐ Clean and disinfect work area.

☐ Dispose of single-use items. Place all used linens, towels, and capes in the laundry.

☐ Wash your hands.

CURL REFORMING (SOFT-CURL PERM)

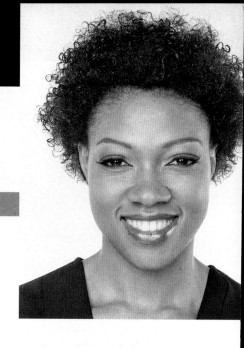

MATERIALS, IMPLEMENTS, AND EQUIPMENT

You will need all of the following implements, materials, and supplies:

- ☐ Applicator bottle
- ☐ Applicator brush
- ☐ Conditioner
- ☐ Disposable gloves
- ☐ End wraps
- ☐ Gentle clarifying shampoo
- ☐ Large-tooth comb
- ☐ Perm rods

- ☐ Plastic or glass bowl
- ☐ Plastic processing cap
- ☐ Protective base cream
- ☐ Tail comb
- ☐ Thio cream relaxer
- ☐ Thio neutralizing solution
- ☐ Thio waving lotion
- ☐ Waterproof cape

> ⚠️ **CAUTION**
> Hair that has been treated with hydroxide relaxers cannot be treated with thio products. The chemicals are not compatible!

PREPARATION

1. Wash your hands.
2. Clean and disinfect all tools and implements.
3. Conduct client consultation.

PROCEDURE

1. Perform an analysis of the hair and scalp. Perform tests for porosity and elasticity. Remember, this procedure requires that the hair and scalp be completely dry after completing the pre-service procedure. Most of the manufacturer's directions indicate a shampoo may be necessary before a soft-curl service; if so, drape the client for a shampoo and gently shampoo with a mild shampoo and towel-dry hair. Avoid irritating the client's scalp.

2. Re-drape the client for a chemical service.

3. Based on the manufacturer's recommendation for a preliminary strand test, conduct a strand test to determine proper timing and curl pattern prior to full-head application. Make note of the timing for the thio cream relaxer, strength used, and rod size.

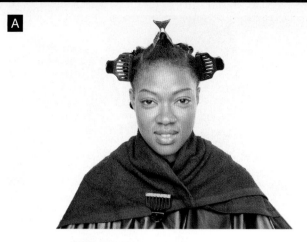

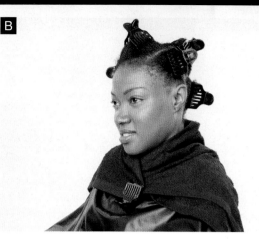

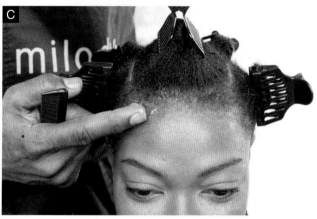

④ Divide the hair into four sections. Clip the sections up to keep them out of the way and for better application of product. Apply a protective base cream to the hairline and ears. It is best to make ¼-inch to ½-inch horizontal partings and apply protective base cream to the entire scalp.

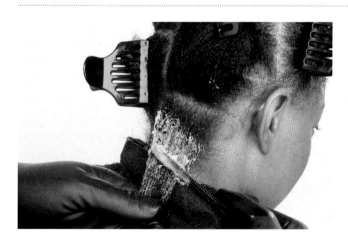

⑤ Wearing gloves on both hands, begin application of thio cream relaxer to the most resistant area, usually at the back of the head and nape area. Using an applicator brush or tail comb, apply cream ¼ inch away from the scalp and topside and underside of the strand. Do not apply the cream to the ends of hair during this step. To avoid possible scalp irritation, do not allow cream to touch the scalp until the last few minutes of processing.

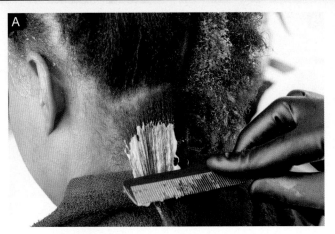

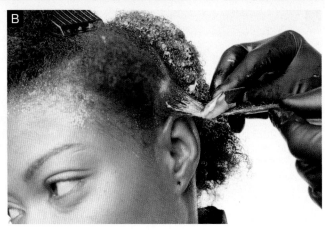

6 Repeat application in remaining sections. Apply thio cream to the hairline last, since hair is most fragile in this region.

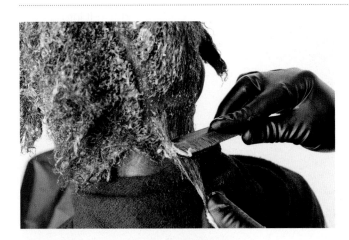

7 Review application of all four quadrants. If necessary apply more cream until all hair strands are covered. Apply cream to hairline and to ends of hair during this step.

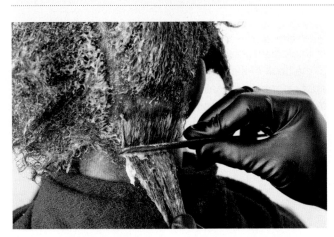

8 After the thio cream has been applied to all sections, using an applicator brush, the back of the comb, or your hands, begin to smooth each section, starting at the first section where thio cream was applied. Never comb the cream through the hair.

9 Process according to the manufacturer's directions and strand test results for timing. Perform periodic strand tests until time has elapsed.

10 During the final remaining minutes of processing, apply the thio cream down to the scalp and through the ends of the hair, using additional cream as needed. Carefully smooth all sections using an applicator brush, your fingers, or the back of the comb.

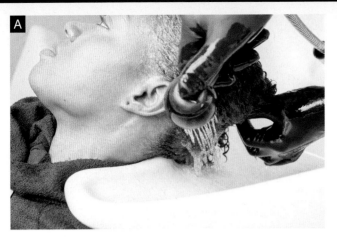

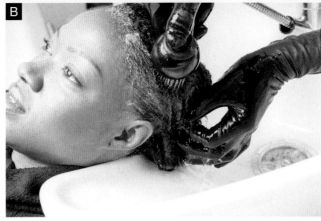

⑪ Rinse thoroughly with warm water to remove all traces of the thio cream.

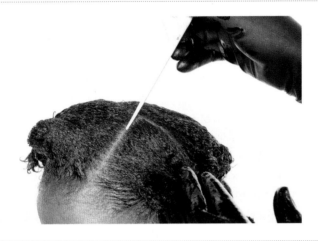

⑫ After rinsing the hair, towel-blot and part it into nine panels. Use the length of the rod to measure the width of the panels.

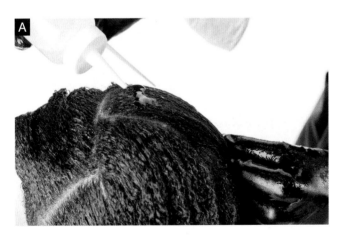

⑬Ⓐ Wearing disposable gloves, apply thio wrap lotion to each section, and roll hair on the appropriate-sized perm rods. Begin wrapping at the most resistant area, usually the nape.

B

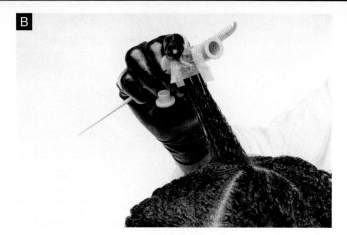

13B Make a horizontal parting the same size as the rod. Hold the hair at a 90-degree angle to the head. Using two end papers, roll the hair down to the scalp.

13B Position the rod half off-base. Option: Insert roller picks to stabilize the rods and eliminate any tension caused by the band.

C

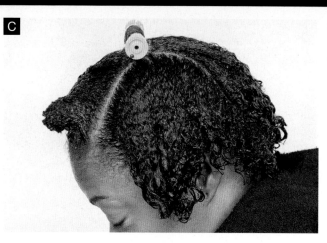

13C Continue wrapping the remaining eight panels in numerical order using the same technique.

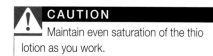

> **⚠ CAUTION**
> Maintain even saturation of the thio lotion as you work.

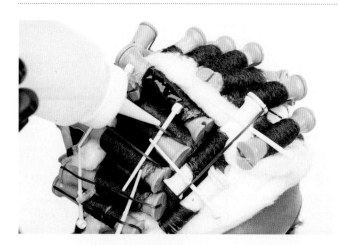

14 Place cotton strips around the hairline and neck to protect the client.

15 If the manufacturer or your instructor suggests using a plastic processing cap, cover all the hair completely. Do not allow the plastic cap to touch the client's skin.

16 Process according to the manufacturer's directions. Processing time will vary according to the strength of the product, hair type and condition, desired results, and strand test results. Check for proper curl development in 5-minute intervals.

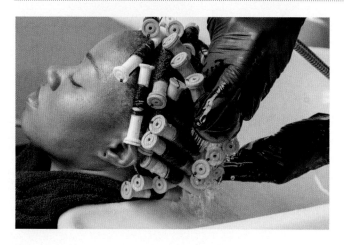

17 When processing is complete, rinse the hair thoroughly for at least 3 minutes. Gently towel-blot each rod to remove excess moisture. Do not rub.

18 Re-drape client with fresh strip cotton around hairline and neck.

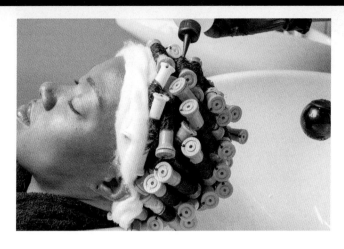

19 Measure approximately 6 to 8 ounces of the thio neutralizer in an applicator bottle, using more or less as needed. Slowly and carefully apply to each rod. Avoid splashing and dripping. Make sure each rod is completely saturated. Set a timer and neutralize according to the manufacturer's directions.

20 The average time to complete the neutralization process is 10 minutes without the use of a hair dryer.

21 After neutralizing is complete, thoroughly rinse hair with water for about 2 minutes with rods still in the hair. Do not remove rods during rinsing.

22 Gently blot to remove excess water.

23 Remove the rods from the hair, and rinse thoroughly for about 2 minutes.

24 Towel-dry and apply hydrating conditioner. Using a large-tooth comb, distribute the conditioner throughout the hair.

A

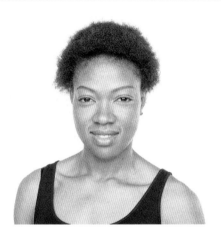

B

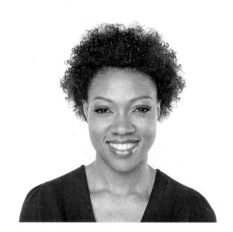

25 Rinse, towel-dry and style as desired.

CAUTION
Hair must not be shampooed for at least 48 hours, otherwise curls will be compromised!

CLEAN-UP AND DISINFECTION

☐ Clean and disinfect tools and implements.
☐ Clean and disinfect work area.
☐ Dispose of single-use items. Place all used linens, towels, and capes in the laundry.
☐ Wash your hands.

REVIEW QUESTIONS

1. Explain the physical and chemical changes that occur in the hair as a result of chemical texture services.

2. What characteristics or condition of the hair and scalp should be analyzed before performing chemical texture services?

3. List the similarities and differences between permanent wave, curl reformation, and hair relaxing processes.

4. List the chemical products used in permanent waving.

5. List at least five permanent waving safety precautions.

6. List the chemical products used with thio relaxers.

7. List the products used with hydroxide relaxers.

8. Explain the difference between base and no-base relaxers.

9. What chemical texture service requires a pre-service shampoo? Which services do not?

10. List the chemical products used in the curl reformation service.

11. Explain the difference between a texturizer and a chemical blowout.

12. List at least five chemical hair relaxing safety precautions.

CHAPTER GLOSSARY

acid-balanced waves	p. 597	permanent waves that have a 7.0 or neutral pH; do not require hair-dryer heat
alkaline or cold waves (AL-kuh-line WAYVZ)	p. 596	perms that process at room temperature without heat with a pH range between 9.0 and 9.6
ammonium thioglycolate (ATG) (uh-MOH-nee-um thy-oh-GLY-kuh-layt)	p. 596	main active ingredient or reducing agent in alkaline waves
base control	p. 593	the position of the perm rod in relation to its base section
base direction	p. 593	angle at which the perm rod is positioned on the head; also, the directional pattern in which the hair is wrapped
base relaxers	p. 606	relaxers that require the use of a base or protective cream
base sections	p. 592	subsections of panels into which the hair is divided for perm wrapping; one rod is normally placed on each base section
bookend wrap	p. 589	perm wrap in which an end paper is folded in half over the hair ends
chemical blowout	p. 610	partially straightens the hair with the intent that it will be picked out and cut
chemical hair relaxing	p. 579	the process of rearranging the basic structure of extremely curly hair into a straightened form

chemical texture services (KEM-uh-kul TEKS-chur SER-vicez)	p. 578	hair services that cause a chemical change that permanently alters the natural wave pattern of the hair
croquignole perm wrap (KROH-ken-yohl)	p. 594	rodding from the hair ends to the scalp
curl reformation	p. 579	a soft-curl permanent; combination of a thio relaxer and thio permanent, whereby the hair is wrapped on perm rods; used to make existing curl larger and looser
end wraps	p. 589	end paper; absorbent papers used to protect and control the ends of the hair during perming services
endothermic waves (en-duh-THUR-mik WAYVZ)	p. 596	perm activated by an outside heat source, usually a hood-type dryer
exothermic waves (ek-soh-THUR-mik WAYVZ)	p. 597	perms that create an exothermic chemical reaction that heats the solution and speeds up processing
glyceryl monothioglycolate (GMTG) (GLIS-ur-il mon-oh-THY-oh-GLY-kuh-layt)	p. 596	main active ingredient in true acid and acid-balanced waving lotions
hydroxide relaxers (hy-DRAHKS-yd re-LAX-uhrz)	p. 587	very strong alkalis with a pH over 13; the hydroxide ion is the active ingredient in all hydroxide relaxers
lanthionization (lan-THEE-ohn-iz-ay-shun)	p. 587	process by which hydroxide relaxers permanently straighten hair; lanthionization breaks the hair's disulfide bonds during processing and converts them to lanthionine bonds when the relaxer is rinsed from the hair
lotion wrap	p. 594	permanent waving wrapping technique in which the waving solution is applied to the section before rodding
neutralization (noo-truh-ly-ZAY-shun)	p. 601	process of stopping the action of a permanent wave solution and hardening the hair in its new form by the application of a chemical solution called the neutralizer
no-base relaxers	p. 607	relaxers that do not require application of a protective base
permanent or chemical waving	p. 578	a process used to chemically restructure natural hair into a different wave pattern
pre-wrap solution	p. 598	usually a type of leave-in conditioner that may be applied to the hair prior to permanent waving to equalize porosity
texturize	p. 610	a process used to semi-straighten extremely curly hair into a more manageable texture and wave pattern
thio relaxers (THY-oh re-LAX-uhrz)	p. 587	relaxers that usually have a pH above 10 and a higher concentration of ATG than is used in permanent waving
true acid waves (TROO AS-ud WAYVZ)	p. 596	perms that have a pH between 4.5 and 7.0 and require heat to speed processing; process more slowly than alkaline waves, and do not usually produce as firm a curl as alkaline waves

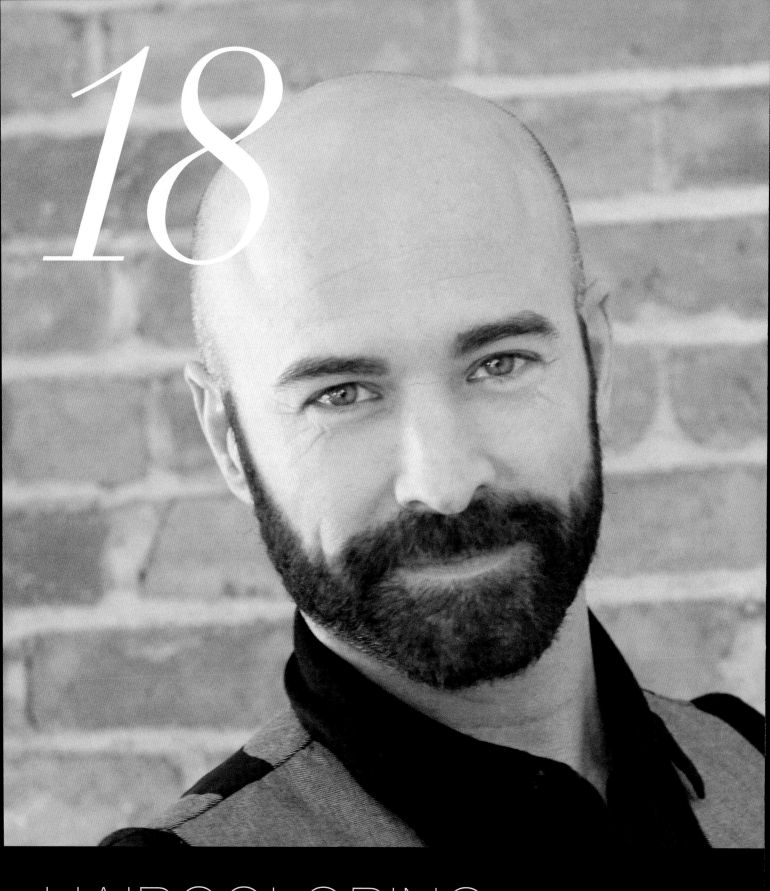

18

HAIRCOLORING
AND LIGHTENING

LEARNING OBJECTIVES

After completing this chapter, you should be able to:

LO❶
Identify six hair characteristics that are analyzed before performing haircoloring services.

LO❷
Explain color theory principles as they apply to hair color services.

LO❸
Identify haircolor products and explain their actions on hair.

LO❹
Explain the action of lighteners on hair.

LO❺
Explain procedure and application terms.

LO❻
Explain how haircolor products are selected and applied to hair.

LO❼
List haircoloring and lightening safety precautions.

figure 18-1a
Client before haircoloring service.

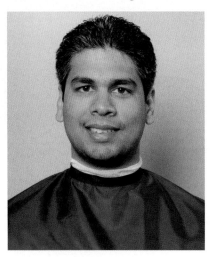

figure 18-1b
Client after haircoloring service.

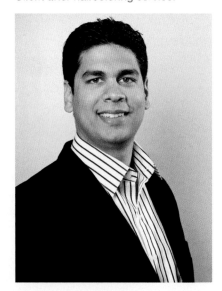

Introduction

Men and women have altered their hair color for thousands of years. Early cultures considered colors to be symbols of power and mysticism. This belief led to body painting and haircoloring from vegetable and mineral dyes, as evidenced by chemicals and tools found in Egyptian tombs. In the 1880s, American men had their beards and mustaches dyed in barbershops with coloring products that left the hair with strange iridescent tones or purple hues. These early formulations were made of silver nitrate, gold chloride, gum, and distilled water. Since the first synthetic dyes were developed in 1883, color technology and haircoloring processes have steadily improved in performance and safety.

Haircoloring (HAYR-KUL-ur-ing) is the art and science of changing the color of the hair. **Hair lightening** (HAYR LYT-un-ing) is the partial or total removal of natural pigment or artificial color from the hair. In today's barbershops, many clients expect barbers to be skilled in performing haircoloring and lightening services (**Figure 18-1a** and **18-1b**). Recently, there has been an increasing demand for beard and mustache coloring. As a barber, you need to be able to perform these services with knowledge and skill.

why study
HAIRCOLORING AND LIGHTENING?

You should study and have a thorough understanding of haircoloring and lightening because:

> Haircoloring and lightening services offer barbers an opportunity for building a reliable and lucrative clientele. The more knowledge and skill you have, the more services you can offer your clients.

> Knowing when to suggest a haircolor service will help build loyalty with your clients and confidence with your barbering skills.

> Barbers need to understand hair structure, the laws of color, and haircoloring procedures in order to be successful when performing haircoloring and lightening services.

> Haircoloring is a chemical service, and chemicals may cause damage and harm to clients and yourself if not used properly. To avoid these situations, it is important that you understand how to use these chemicals safely on clients.

Identify the Characteristics and Structure of Hair

After reading this section, you will be able to:

LO❶ Identify six hair characteristics that are analyzed before performing haircoloring services.

The client's hair structure and condition will affect the quality and success of the haircolor service. Six characteristics of the hair that are important considerations in determining haircoloring options and product selection are elasticity, texture, density, porosity, natural hair color, and contributing pigment.

ELASTICITY

Elasticity is an important factor to consider because it is an indication of the strength of the cortex, including cross-bonds and melanin molecules.

- *Normal* elasticity is indicated by wet hair that can stretch up to 50 percent of its original length and then return to that length without breaking.

- *Low* elasticity is indicated by wet hair that does not return to its original length when stretched.

TEXTURE

The diameter of the individual hair strand determines whether the hair texture is classified as fine, medium, or coarse. Melanin is distributed differently within the different textures:

- Fine hair has melanin granules grouped tightly, so the hair takes color faster and may appear darker.

- Medium-textured hair has an average response time to haircolor products.

- Coarse hair has a larger diameter with loosely grouped melanin granules and may take longer to process (Figure 18-2).

DENSITY

Density refers to the number of hairs per square inch on the scalp. It ranges from thin to thick and determines the subsection size to use to assure proper coverage of the haircolor or lightener. For example, you may need to part off subsections as thin as ⅛ inch on a client with very thick hair.

POROSITY

Porosity is the hair's ability to absorb moisture. The porosity level of the hair determines its ability to absorb haircolor products. Porous hair absorbs haircolor products faster and with more intensity and may appear darker than less porous hair. Degrees of porosity are:

- *High porosity:* Hair may not only absorb the color product quickly but also tend to fade quickly due to its inability to hold color pigments. The hair will feel very rough, dry, or may break during a porosity test.

- *Average porosity:* The cuticle is slightly raised and the hair tends to process normally. You should feel a slight roughness to the hair during a porosity test.

- *Low porosity:* The cuticle is tight, making the hair more resistant to chemical penetration, and may require a longer time to penetrate the hair shaft or a higher volume of developer for its strength. The hair will feel smooth and/or hard during a porosity test.

figure 18-2
Melanin distribution according to hair texture.

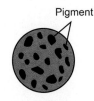

Pigment

Fine-textured hair

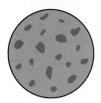

Medium-textured hair

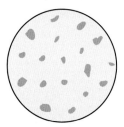

Coarse-textured hair

NATURAL HAIR COLOR

Natural hair color ranges from black to dark brown to red, and from dark blond to lightest blond. These natural color ranges are produced by two types of melanin:

- *Eumelanin* provides natural black and brown pigment (color) to hair.

- *Pheomelanin* provides yellow (blond) and red pigment (color) to hair.

  The three factors that determine what natural hair colors look like are the:

- thickness of the hair

- total number and size of pigment granules

- ratio of eumelanin to pheomelanin within the cortex layer

  Gray hair is the result of a reduction in the production of melanin pigments. White hair is actually the color of keratin without melanin and therefore does not contain either type of melanin.

CONTRIBUTING PIGMENT (OR "UNDERTONE")

Contributing pigment (kun-TRIB-yoot-ing PIG-ment) is the pigment that lies under the natural hair color. The foundation of haircoloring is based on modifying this pigment with haircoloring products to create new colors. When lightening a client's natural hair color, the darker the natural level, the more intense the contributing pigment.

Understand Color Theory

After reading this section, you will be able to:

LO❷ Explain color theory principles as they apply to haircolor services.

Color is a characteristic of visible light energy. Although the human eye sees only six basic colors, the brain is capable of visualizing combinations of different wavelengths relevant to the three primary and three secondary colors (see Chapter 8). The light rays that are absorbed or reflected by natural hair pigment or artificial pigment, added to the hair, create the colors we see.

THE LAWS OF COLOR

The **laws of color** is a system for understanding color relationships. The laws of color regulate the mixing of dyes and pigments to make other colors. Based in science and adapted to art, the laws of color serve as guidelines for harmonious color mixing. For example, equal parts of red and blue mixed together always make violet. A color wheel is a diagram that presents colors in a specific and sequential order to show the relationship of one color to another.

PRIMARY COLORS

Primary colors (PRY-mayr-ee KUL-urz) are basic or true colors that cannot be created by combining other colors. The three primary colors are yellow, red, and blue (**Figure 18-3**) and are found naturally in the world, such as yellow dandelions and red roses. All other colors are created by some combination of red, yellow, or blue. Colors with a predominance of blue are "cool-toned" colors and colors that are predominantly red are "warm-toned" colors.

- *Blue* is the strongest and the only cool primary color. Blue brings depth or darkness to any color to which it is added.

- *Red* is the medium primary color. Adding red to blue-based colors makes them appear lighter. Conversely, red added to a yellow color will cause it to appear darker.

- *Yellow* is the weakest of the primary colors and will lighten and brighten other colors.

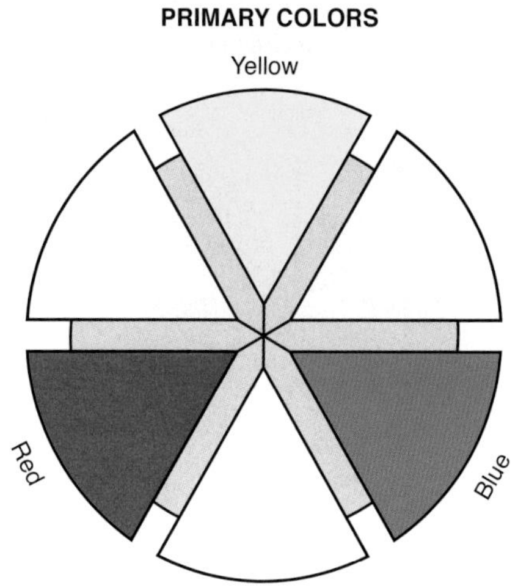

SECONDARY COLORS

Secondary colors (SEK-un-deh-ree KUL-urz) are created by mixing *equal* amounts of two primary colors. When mixed in equal parts:

- yellow and blue create green

- blue and red create violet

- red and yellow create orange (**Figure 18-4**)

TERTIARY COLORS

Tertiary colors, also called *quaternary colors*, are created by mixing equal amounts of one primary color with one of its adjacent secondary colors. Tertiary colors are:

- blue-green

- blue-violet

- red-violet

- red-orange

- yellow-green

- yellow-orange (**Figure 18-5**)

COMPLEMENTARY COLORS

Complementary colors (kahm-pluh-MEN-tur-ee KUL-urz) are primary and secondary colors positioned directly opposite each other on the color wheel. As seen in **Figure 18-6**, complementary colors include:

- blue and orange

- red and green

- yellow and violet

figure 18-3
Primary colors.

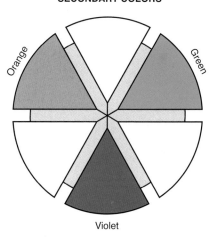

figure 18-4
Secondary colors.

figure 18-5
Tertiary colors.

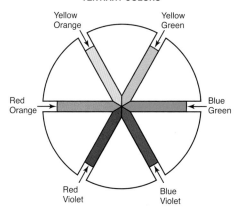

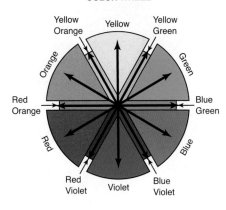

figure 18-6
Complementary colors neutralize each other.

COLOR WHEEL

When mixed together, complementary colors "neutralize" each other. For example, when mixed in equal amounts, red and green neutralize each other, creating brown, or a "neutral" tone.

Complementary colors are always composed of a primary and a secondary color, and complementary pairs always consist of all three primary colors. For example, the color wheel shows that the complement of red (a primary color) is green (a secondary color). Green is made up of blue and yellow (both primary colors). So, all three primary colors are represented to varying degrees in the complementary pair of red and green.

HUE AND TONE

- **Hue** (HYOO) is the basic name of a color, such as red, yellow, or violet. The color wheel is an arrangement of hues that makes the relationships among colors visible.

- **Tone** (TOHN) describes the warmth or coolness of a color (Figure 18-7). The warm colors, also known as *highlighting colors*, produce warmer tones because they reflect more light. Warm colors are red, orange, and yellow. The cool colors, also known as *ash or drab colors*, absorb more light and cast cool tones. Cool colors are blue, green, and violet.

LEVEL

Level (LEV-ul) is a unit of measurement used to identify the lightness or darkness of a color. Level is the saturation, density, or concentration of color:

- Colors lighten when mixed with white.

- Colors darken when mixed with black.

figure 18-7
The color wheel divided to represent both warm and cool colors.

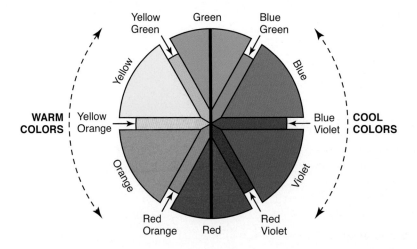

The **level system** (LEV-ul SIS-tum) is used to analyze the lightness or darkness of a hair color (Figure 18-8). The colors of hair and of haircolor products are arranged on a scale of 1 to 10:

- 1 is the darkest (black)
- 10 is the lightest (blond)

Although the names for the color levels may vary among manufacturers, the level system provides a guide to identify the lightness and darkness of each color level. This information is necessary to determine natural hair color levels and for formulating, matching, and correcting colors.

SATURATION

Saturation, or intensity, refers to the degree of concentration or amount of pigment in the color. It is the strength of a color. For example, a saturated red is very vivid. Any color can be more or less saturated. The more saturated the product, the more dramatic the change in hair color.

BASE COLOR

Artificial haircolors are developed from primary and secondary colors to form "base colors." The **base color** (BAYS KUL-ur) of a haircoloring product is the predominant tone of a color, which greatly influences the final color result. Examples of base colors used in a haircolor product are as follows:

- a violet base color produces cool results and helps minimize yellow tones
- a blue base color minimizes orange tones
- a red-orange base color creates warm, bright tones in the hair
- a neutral base color tends to soften and balance other colors

IDENTIFYING NATURAL LEVEL AND TONE

Haircoloring results depend on the combination of the:

- client's natural hair color
- artificial haircolor product that is added to it

Identifying the natural level and tone of the client's hair will determine which products to use and what the final results will look like. Identifying the natural level of the client's hair is accomplished by using a manufacturer's swatch or color ring to match the client's hair color (Figure 18-9).

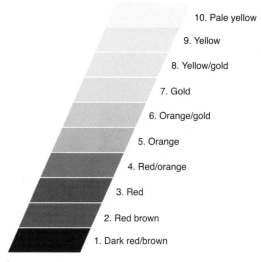

figure 18-8
The level system.

10. Pale yellow
9. Yellow
8. Yellow/gold
7. Gold
6. Orange/gold
5. Orange
4. Red/orange
3. Red
2. Red brown
1. Dark red/brown

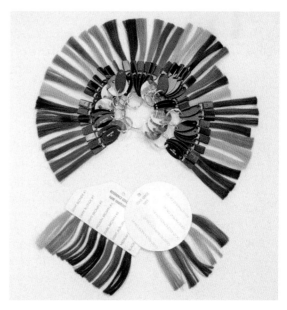

figure 18-9
Manufacturer's swatches are a useful tool.

Natural Level Mini-Procedure

figure 18-10
Take a ½-inch square section in the crown.

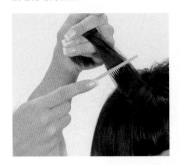

figure 18-11
Hold the color swatch against the hair strand.

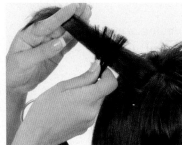

To determine a client's natural level:

1. Part off a ½-inch square section from just under the crown area, comb through, and hold the section so light will filter through (**Figure 18-10**).

2. Using the natural level swatch or color ring, select a swatch that best matches the hair color.

3. Move the swatch from the scalp along the entire strand (**Figure 18-11**).

4. Determine the natural hair color level.

> ⚠️ **CAUTION**
> If the hair has been previously colored, use the natural level swatch on the new growth and the manufacturer's color swatches on previously colored sections.

GRAY HAIR

Gray hair is normally associated with aging, although heredity is also a contributing factor. In most cases, the loss of pigment increases as a person ages, resulting in a range of gray tones from blended to solid. The amount of gray in an individual's hair is measured in percentages (**Table 18-1**) and requires special care when formulating haircolor applications.

table 18-1
DETERMINING THE PERCENTAGE OF GRAY HAIR

Percentage of Gray Hair	Characteristics	Level 5 Natural Hair	
30%	More pigmented, or colored, than gray hair		Level 5 natural hair with 30% gray
50%	Even mixture of gray and pigmented hair		Level 5 natural hair with 50% gray
70 to 90%	More gray than pigmented hair; most of remaining pigment is located at the back of the head		Level 5 natural hair with 75% gray
100%	Virtually no pigmented or colored hair; tends to look white		100% gray hair

© NinaMalyna/Shutterstock.com
© Budimir Jevtic/Shutterstock.com
© Oshchepkov Dmitry/Shutterstock.com

The challenges and solutions associated with coloring gray hair are discussed later in the chapter (**Figure 18-12a** and **18-12b**).

Identify Haircoloring Products

After reading this section, you will be able to:

LO❸ Identify haircolor products and explain their actions on hair.

Haircoloring products are categorized as nonoxidative and oxidative. The nonoxidizing haircolor products are:

- *temporary haircolor:* washes out with one shampoo
- *semipermanent haircolor:* washes out or fades within a few weeks

The oxidizing haircolor products are:

- *demipermanent:* lasts longer than a semipermanent, but not as long as a permanent haircolor
- *permanent:* stays in the hair until the hair grows out

Nonoxidizing versus oxidizing haircolor products determine a product's colorfastness, or its ability to remain on the hair, and that is determined by the chemical composition and molecular weight of the pigments and dyes within the products (**Tables 18-2** and **18-3**).

Ⓟ 18-1 **Patch Test** *pages 678–679*

Ⓟ 18-2 **Strand Test** *pages 680–681*

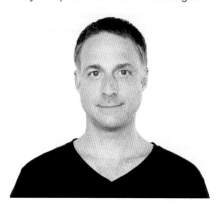
figure 18-12a
Gray hair presents certain challenges.

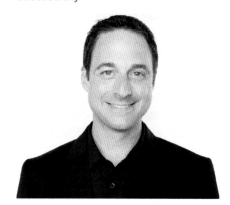
figure 18-12b
Many haircolor options cover gray successfully.

table 18-2

HAIRCOLOR CLASSIFICATIONS AND THEIR USES

Category	Uses
Temporary color	• Create fun, bold results that easily shampoo from the hair (e.g., haircolor sprays used at Halloween) • Neutralize yellow or other unwanted tones (e.g., a blue rinse used on gray hair)
Semipermanent color	• Introduces a client to haircolor services • Adds subtle color results
Demipermanent color	• Blends gray hair • Enhances natural color • Tones pre-lightened hair • Refreshes faded color • Can act as a filler in color correction
Permanent haircolor	• Changes existing haircolor permanently • Covers gray • Creates bright or natural-looking haircolor

table 18-3

CHARACTERISTICS OF HAIRCOLOR CLASSIFICATIONS

Characteristic	Temporary	Semipermanent	Demipermanent	Permanent
Size/weight of dye molecule	Large	Medium	Medium-small	Small
pH	Acid	Slightly alkaline	Moderately alkaline	Alkaline
Type of reaction or change	Physical	Chemical and physical	Chemical and physical	Chemical and physical
How long will it last?	Removed with shampooing	Fades gradually	Some fading, may leave a line of demarcation	Permanent
What does it do?	Deposits on outside of cuticle	Deposits and slightly penetrates cortex	No-lift, deposits and slightly penetrates cortex	Lifts (lightens) and deposits into the cortex
Is it mixed with hydrogen peroxide?	No	No	Yes	Yes
Is a predisposition test required?	One ingredient, **aniline derivative** (AN-ul-un DUR-ive-it-ive), requires that a predisposition test (also called a *patch test*) be performed. These tests are required by the Food and Drug Administration (FDA) before the application of any product that contains aniline derivative. Always read the manufacturer's instructions. If the manufacturer requires a predisposition test, it means that the product contains aniline derivative.			

TEMPORARY HAIRCOLOR (NON-OXIDATION COLOR)

Temporary colors (TEM-poh-rayr-ee KUL-urz) use color molecules that are the largest found in haircoloring products. The large size of the color molecule prevents penetration beyond the cuticle layer, producing only a coating on the outside of the hair. This coating usually lasts only until the next shampoo (**Figure 18-13**). The chemical composition of a temporary color is acidic, creating a physical change rather than a chemical change in the hair shaft. Temporary rinses have a pH range of 2.0 to 4.5. If a temporary haircolor has aniline derivative as an ingredient, a predisposition test is required. Be sure to read the manufacturer's instructions.

Different types of temporary haircolors include:

- *Color rinses* highlight the existing color or add color to the hair and remain on the hair until the next shampoo.

- *Color-enhancing shampoos* are a combination of a color rinse with a shampoo and produce highlights and impart slight color tones to the hair.

- *Crayons* are sticks of coloring compounded with soaps or synthetic waxes and sometimes used to color gray or white hair between hair tint retouches. They can also be used as temporary coloring for mustaches, beards, or sideburns. They are available in several standard colors:

figure 18-13
Action of temporary haircolor.

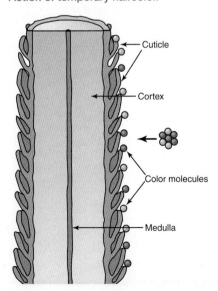

Cuticle

Cortex

Color molecules

Medulla

- blond
- light, medium, and dark brown
- black
- auburn

- *Haircolor sprays* are applied to dry hair from aerosol containers. They are usually available in vibrant colors and generally used for special effects.

- *Haircolor mousses and gels* are a combination of a little bit of color and styling mousse or gel in one product.

 18-3 **Temporary Color Rinse** *pages 682–683*

SEMIPERMANENT HAIRCOLOR (NON-OXIDATION COLOR)

Semipermanent colors are no-lift, deposit-only haircolor products. Semipermanent pigment molecules are of a lesser molecular weight and size than those of temporary colors. The pigment molecules are small enough to partially penetrate the hair shaft and stain the cuticle layer. However, these molecules are also small enough to leave the hair during shampooing and to fade with each shampoo. Traditional semipermanent colors usually last from six to eight shampoos as the color molecules are shampooed from the hair (Figure 18-14). The chemical composition of semipermanent color is mildly alkaline, causes the cortex to swell, and raises the cuticle to allow some penetration. This chemical composition combines small color molecules, solvents, alkaline swelling agents (mild oxidizer), and surfactants to create a type of color that is known as self-penetrating. Self-penetrating colors tend to make a mild chemical change as well as a physical change. Most semipermanent colors do not contain ammonia and may be used right out of the bottle. Although normally gentle on the hair, semipermanent colors require a patch test (predisposition test) prior to application to prevent the occurrence of product sensitivity or allergic reaction. These tests are required by FDA before the application of any product that contains aniline derivative. Semipermanent haircolor typically falls within the 7.0 to 9.0 pH range. Due to the slight alkalinity of semipermanent color, haircolor services should be followed with a mild, acid-balanced shampoo and conditioning. This process neutralizes any residual alkalinity and helps restore the hair to normal pH levels.

Semipermanent haircolor may be used to:

- cover or blend partially gray hair without affecting its natural color when the hair color and product color are matched correctly

- cover gray hair on a client who has up to 25 percent gray

- enhance or deepen color tones in the hair

- serve as a non-peroxide toner for pre-lightened hair

DEMIPERMANENT HAIRCOLOR (OXIDATION COLOR)

Demipermanent haircolors (DEM-ih PUR-muh-nent HAYR-KUL-urz), also known as *no-lift, deposit-only haircolors*, are longer lasting than semipermanent colors. They are designed to deposit color without lifting (lightening)

figure 18-14
Action of semipermanent haircolor.

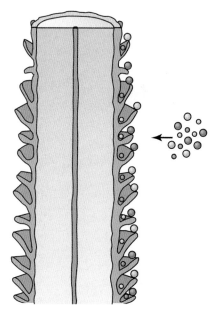

> **DID YOU KNOW?**
> During the past several decades, some manufacturers labeled their tube color products as semipermanent color, even though a mild developer was required. Since then, most now call these products *demipermanent*.

figure 18-15
Action of demipermanent color.

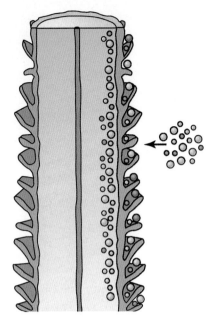

natural or artificial color in the hair and are a type of oxidation color. They are not used directly out of the bottle but must be mixed with a low-volume developer or activator immediately before use. The agent in the developer causes "oxidation" to occur, which develops the color (**Figure 18-15**). Demipermanents darken the natural hair color when applied. They are available in gel, cream, or liquid forms. Because they contain aniline derivative, a patch test is required before application.

Demipermanent haircolor may be used to:

- get vivid color results
- introduce a client to a color service
- blend or cover up to 50 percent gray
- refresh faded permanent color
- deposit color changes without lightening the hair
- reverse highlights
- perform corrective coloring

Ⓟ 18-4 **Demipermanent Color Applications** *pages 684–685*

PERMANENT HAIRCOLOR (OXIDATION COLOR)

Permanent haircolors (PUR-muh-nent HAYR-KUL-urz) are mixed with developers (hydrogen peroxide) and remain in the hair permanently. When the hair grows, a touch-up or retouch application is required to blend the new growth with the previously colored hair. A permanent haircolor is also called a *tint*.

Permanent haircolor products usually contain all of the following:

- ammonia
- oxidative tints (color molecules; aniline derivative)
- hydrogen peroxide (developer)

Permanent haircolor products contain aniline derivative, so they require a patch or predisposition test. They can lighten and deposit color in one process. They can lighten natural hair color because they are more alkaline than demipermanent oxidation colors and are usually mixed with a higher-volume developer. The amount of lift is controlled by the pH and concentration of peroxide in the developer. The amount of deposit depends on the amount of color in the product.

Permanent haircolor products are usually mixed with an equal amount of 20-volume peroxide and are capable of lifting one or two levels. When mixed with higher volumes of peroxide, permanent colors can lift up to four levels. Since some manufacturers recommend a 2:1 ratio of developer to haircolor, always read the manufacturer's directions.

When a permanent haircolor is mixed with a developer and applied to the hair, the cuticle layers will swell and begin to open allowing the undeveloped, small color molecules to enter the cortex. This process usually takes place in the first 10 to 15 minutes after the color is mixed. The molecule (aniline derivative) will then oxidize and grow in size in the remaining processing time, trapping the molecule in the cortex. They are then too big to get out of the cortex (**Figure 18-16**).

figure 18-16
Action of permanent haircolor.

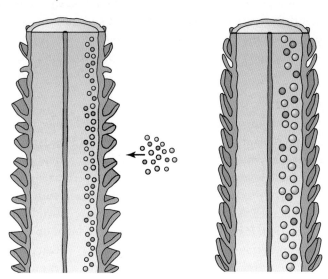

Permanent haircolor products are alkaline and generally range between 9.0 and 10.5 on the pH scale. After processing, the hair is shampooed and as it dries it begins to return to its normal pH. This process causes the cortex to shrink and the cuticle to close, which tends to further trap the color molecules. Except for residual color, permanent haircolor does not wash out during the shampoo process. Eventually the color may fade and may require refreshing.

When new growth occurs, a **line of demarcation** (LYN UV dee-mar-KAY-shun) develops between the new growth and the previously colored hair. This stage requires an application of permanent haircolor to the new growth, known as a *retouch application.*

Permanent haircoloring products are regarded as the best products for covering gray hair. They diffuse natural pigment through the action of lifting and add artificial color to the hair as the color molecules are trapped in the cortex. The gray and non-gray areas blend uniformly with full coverage.

TYPES OF PERMANENT HAIRCOLOR

There are four types of permanent haircolors.

Oxidation Tints

Oxidation tints are also known as aniline derivative tints, penetrating tints, synthetic-organic tints, and amino tints. They can lighten and deposit color in a single process and are available in a wide variety of colors. *Toners* also fall into the category of permanent color and are aniline derivative products of pale, delicate shades designed for use on pre-lightened hair. Most oxidation tints contain aniline derivatives and require a predisposition (patch) test before the service is performed. As long as the hair is of normal strength and in good condition, oxidation tints are compatible with other professional chemical services, such as chemical waves and relaxers. Oxidation tints are sold in bottles, canisters, and tubes, in either a semiliquid or cream form. Tints must be mixed with hydrogen peroxide, which activates the chemical reaction known as *oxidation.* This reaction begins as soon as the two products are combined, so the mixed tint must be used immediately. Any leftover tint must be discarded since it deteriorates quickly. Timing the application of the tint depends upon the product and the volume of peroxide selected. Consult the manufacturer's directions and your instructor for assistance. A strand test should always be performed to ensure satisfactory results.

Vegetable Tints

Vegetable tints, also known as *natural haircolors*, are haircoloring products made from various plants, such as herbs and flowers. In the past, indigo, chamomile, sage, Egyptian henna, and other plants were used to color the hair. Even though vegetable tints are considered permanent, they are non-oxidation color products because they are not mixed with a developer.

Henna is still used as a professional haircoloring product, but should be used with caution. It has a coating action that can build up with overuse and prevent the penetration of other chemicals. It may penetrate the cortex and attach to the salt bonds, leaving the hair unfit for other professional treatments.

Metallic or Mineral Dyes

Metallic dyes are not professional haircoloring products. Metallic dyes are advertised as *color restorers* or **progressive colors** (pruh-GRES-iv KUL-urz). The metallic ingredients, such as lead acetate or silver nitrate, react with the keratin in the hair, turning it brown. This reaction creates a colored film coating that produces a dull metallic appearance. If a product has silver nitrate in it, it oxidizes over time with oxygen in the air and tarnishes, turning the hair to blackish-gray (much like silverware made of silver does over time if it is not kept polished). Repeated treatments of metallic dyes can damage the hair and can react adversely with many professional chemical services, such as relaxers and chemical waves.

Compound Dyes

Like metallic dyes, compound dyes are not used professionally. Compound dyes are metallic or mineral dyes combined with a vegetable tint. Metallic salts are added to vegetable tints, such as henna, to give the product more staying power and to create different colors. Like metallic dyes, these products can change color, coat the hair, and make hair unfit for other chemical services.

HYDROGEN PEROXIDE DEVELOPERS

A hydrogen peroxide **developer** (dee-VEL-up-ur) is an oxidizing agent that supplies oxygen gas for the development of color molecules when mixed with an oxidative haircolor product. When diluted with water and other substances for use in haircoloring, hydrogen peroxide has a mildly acidic pH of 3.5 to 4.0.

Hydrogen peroxide alone produces a relatively mild lightening of the natural hair color and causes little damage to the hair shaft. A color change occurs in the hair when the oxygen combines with the melanin in the hair. As the oxygen and melanin combine, the peroxide solution begins to diffuse and lighten the melanin within the cortex. The smaller structure and spread-out distribution of the diffused melanin gives the hair a lighter appearance. This diffused melanin is called *oxymelanin*. When very pale, light shades are desired, however, chemical lighteners must be used.

Hydrogen peroxide (H_2O_2) serves as the main oxidizing agent used in haircoloring. The chemical action of the oxygen with the artificial haircolor molecules in the haircoloring product is called *oxidation*. The small, artificial color molecules (aniline derivative) expand into a larger form because of this chemical action.

In haircoloring, the term *volume* is used to denote the different strengths of hydrogen peroxide (**Table 18-4**). **Volume** (VAHL-yoom) measures the concentration and strength of hydrogen peroxide:

- The lower the volume, the lesser the lift or lightening achieved.
- The higher the volume, the greater the lifting or lightening action.

Hydrogen peroxide is distributed for use under a variety of names that include:

- developer
- oxidizer
- generator
- catalyst

Regardless of the name used, hydrogen peroxide is available in three forms:

- *Cream peroxides* contain additives such as thickeners, drabbers, conditioners, and acids for stabilization. The thickeners help create a product that tends to stay moist on the hair longer than liquid peroxide, is easy to control, and does not drip during the brush-and-bowl method of application.
- *Liquid hydrogen peroxides* contain a stabilizing acid that brings the pH to between 3.5 and 4.0. They are convenient because they can be used with most of today's bleach and tint formulas.

table 18-4

VOLUMES AND USES OF HYDROGEN PEROXIDE

Volume	Uses
10-Volume	• Used with demipermanent products to deposit color or when less lift/lightening is desired. • Recommended when less lightening is desired.
20-Volume	• The standard volume used with many permanent color products. • Used with permanent color products to cover gray. • Produces up to one or two levels of lift/lightening in one step.
30-Volume	Used with permanent haircolor to achieve up to three levels of lift/lightening in one step.
40-Volume	Used with permanent and high-lift haircolor to achieve up to four levels of lift/lightening in one step.

- *Dry peroxides* are available in either tablet or powder form and are dissolved in liquid hydrogen peroxide to boost the volume. The availability of liquid and cream peroxides in a variety of volumes has made this product somewhat obsolete.

The safety precautions for using hydrogen peroxide include the following:

- Use clean implements when measuring, using, and storing hydrogen peroxide. Even a small amount of dirt or impurities can cause hydrogen peroxide to deteriorate.

- Never measure the needed amount of hydrogen peroxide by pouring it into the lid of another product. The residue will cause the product in the container to oxidize as it sits on the shelf and render it unusable.

- Do not allow hydrogen peroxide formulations to come in contact with metal. Metal causes the oxidation process to occur too quickly to allow proper color development.

- Avoid breathing in vapors caused by mixing hydrogen peroxide and haircolor products.

- A hydrogen peroxide volume of 20 or more can cause skin irritations, chemical burns, and hair damage.

- Keep the cap closed securely on the hydrogen peroxide at all times when not in use. Overexposure to the air will affect the strength.

ACTIVATORS

An **activator** (AK-tih-vay-ter) is an oxidizer, consisting of powdered persulfate salts, that is added to haircolors, lighteners, or hydrogen peroxide to increase the chemical action of the product. This addition results in an increased lifting power, which is controlled by the number of activators that are added to the product. Generally, up to three activators can be used for on-the-scalp applications and up to four for off-the-scalp processes; however, since formulas and strengths will vary from brand to brand, always refer to the manufacturer's directions for mixing instructions. Activators are also known as boosters, protinators, and accelerators.

P 18-5   **Single-Process Permanent Color Applications: Virgin and Retouch** *pages 686–688*

Understand Hair Lighteners

After reading this section, you will be able to:

LO❹   Explain the action of lighteners on hair.

Lighteners (LYT-un-urz) are chemical compounds that lighten hair by dispersing, dissolving, and decolorizing the natural hair pigment (melanin) (**Figure 18-17**), which is accomplished by a mixture of bleach

figure 18-17
Hair lighteners diffuse pigment.

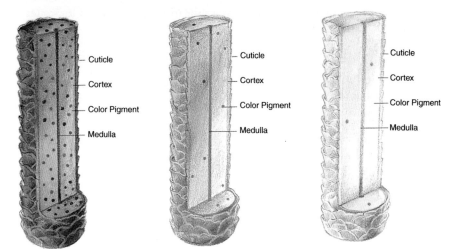

and hydrogen peroxide. When mixed, the pH of lighteners is around 10.0. As soon as hydrogen peroxide is mixed into the lightener formula, it begins to release oxygen.

The hair pigment goes through different stages of color as it lightens. The amount of change depends on:

- how much natural pigment, or melanin, the hair has
- the strength of the lightener
- the length of time the lightener is on the hair

During this decolorization process, natural hair may go through many stages of lightening from the darkest to the lightest: natural black hair can lighten through the brown and/or red stages to orange, gold, yellow, and finally to pale yellow (**Figure 18-18**). Hair lighteners are used to:

- create blond shades that are not possible with permanent haircolor
- pre-lighten the hair to prepare it for the application of a toner or tint (double-process application)
- lighten the hair to a particular shade or stage
- brighten and lighten an existing shade
- lighten only certain areas of the hair
- lighten naturally dark hair
- lighten hair without depositing color

TYPES OF LIGHTENERS

Lighteners are available in three forms: cream, powder, and oil. Cream and oil lighteners are considered **on-the-scalp light-eners** (AWN-THE-SKALP LYT-un-urz) and powder lighteners are

figure 18-18
Ten degrees of decolorization.

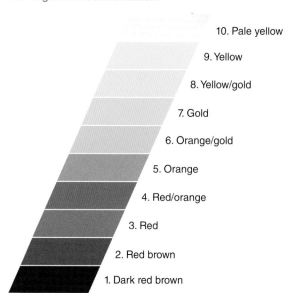

10. Pale yellow

9. Yellow

8. Yellow/gold

7. Gold

6. Orange/gold

5. Orange

4. Red/orange

3. Red

2. Red brown

1. Dark red brown

off-the-scalp lighteners (AWF-THE-SKALP LY-Tun-urz). That said, some newer powder lighteners may be used on the scalp, so always refer to the manufacturer's directions before purchase or application. Each type of lightener has unique abilities, chemical compositions, and formulation procedures.

- *Cream lighteners* are the most popular type of on-the-scalp lightener. They contain conditioning agents, bluing agents, and thickeners, which makes them easy to apply, and will not run, drip, or dry out. Cream lighteners provide the following benefits:
  - The conditioning agents give some protection to the hair.
  - The bluing agent helps drab undesirable red and gold tones.
  - The thickener provides control during application and prevents overlap.

- *Powder lighteners,* also called *paste, speed,* or *quick lighteners* contain oxygen-releasing boosters and substances for quick and strong lightening. These lighteners will stay in place and not run or drip, but do not contain conditioning agents and tend to dry out quickly. Because they are stronger than oil or cream lighteners, they may also be too strong to use directly on the scalp. Be sure to read the directions to see if it is safe to use powder lightener for a virgin lightener or lightener retouch.

- *Oil lighteners* are not as popular as cream or powder lighteners nowadays. They are usually mixtures of hydrogen peroxide with sulfonated oil. As on-the-scalp lighteners, they are the mildest form of lightener and may be used when only one or two levels of lift are desired. There are two types of oil lighteners:
  - *Color oil lighteners* add temporary color as they lighten:
    - *Gold:* lightens and adds golden to reddish tones depending on the base color of the hair
    - *Silver:* lightens and adds silvery highlights to gray or white hair and minimizes red and gold tones in other shades
    - *Red:* lightens and adds red highlights
    - *Drab:* lightens and adds ash highlights, and tones down or reduces red and gold tones
  - *Neutral oil lighteners* remove pigment without adding color tone and may be used to pre-soften hair for a tint application.

CONTRIBUTION OF UNDERLYING PIGMENT

It is essential to lighten the hair to the correct stage of lightness needed, because the pigment that remains in the hair will impact the final result of the hair lightening and coloring process. For example, let's say you need to lighten to the pale yellow stage, but only lighten to the yellow or gold stage. The tint or toner you have selected has a blue base. If you were to apply this blue-based tint to the yellow/gold hair, the hair will turn green because you only lightened to the yellow/gold stage, and blue added to yellow (think color theory) makes green. Use Figure 18-19 as a guide to determine the contributing pigment or undertones of color at various hair color levels.

figure 18-19
Contributing pigment (undertones).

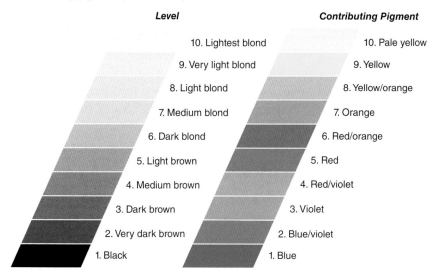

Level	Contributing Pigment
10. Lightest blond	10. Pale yellow
9. Very light blond	9. Yellow
8. Light blond	8. Yellow/orange
7. Medium blond	7. Orange
6. Dark blond	6. Red/orange
5. Light brown	5. Red
4. Medium brown	4. Red/violet
3. Dark brown	3. Violet
2. Very dark brown	2. Blue/violet
1. Black	1. Blue

TONERS

A toner is a permanent haircoloring product that is applied to pre-lightened hair for the purpose of achieving the desired color or tones in the hair or to neutralize unwanted undertones (contributing pigment). For example, brassy red tones that remain in the hair after lightening can be "neutralized" with a green-based toner if they are at the same level of lightness. Toners only add or deposit pigment into the hair shaft; they do not lighten the hair. Because toners are applied only to pre-lightened hair, they typically come in pale, delicate, blond shades. Aniline derivative is an ingredient in toners, so a patch test is required 24 to 48 hours before application. Toners usually have a very different color in the bottle than the final shade they produce. They may appear to be purple, blue, orange, or pink in the bottle. As toner color oxidizes, it goes through several visual color changes; therefore, a preliminary strand test should be done to determine the processing time required for a desired shade. Toners are used in double-process applications:

1. the lightener application is the first process

2. the toner application is the second process

After the hair goes through the desired stages of lightening, the color left in the hair is known as its *contributing color*, which is usually the darkest degree of contributing pigment that remains after the lightening process. Achieving the correct lightening stage is necessary for proper toner development and to achieve even color. Toner manufacturers provide recommendations about the contributing color needed to achieve various color results. As a general rule, the lighter the desired color, the lighter the foundation must be. It is important to follow the guide closely.

Overlightened hair will absorb or *grab* the base color of the toner, while underlightened hair will appear to have more red, yellow, or orange than the intended color. While color manufacturers produce toners to complement their color lines, toning is also a process that can be performed using a semipermanent, demipermanent, or permanent haircolor as a "toner" to achieve the desired result. Read the manufacturer's directions carefully for appropriate color selection, mixing, and application instructions. Toner formulations and color ranges vary with each manufacturer. Using products from the same product line is recommended.

TINT OR DYE REMOVERS

The removal of artificial haircoloring products, such as a tint, is sometimes desired if:

* the client wants to change to a lighter shade
* a coloring mistake has been made
* the hair has processed too dark due to an overporous condition

Dye removers (DYE ree-MOOV-urz) are also known as *color or tint removers*. There are two basic types of products available to remove artificial pigment, such as tints and toners, from the hair:

* *Oil-base dye removers* lift trapped color pigments, stain, or buildup from cuticle layers, do not create structural changes in the hair shaft or pigment (natural or artificial) of the hair, and will not make drastic changes in the level of color.
* *Tint or dye solvents* produce strong lightening effects on melanin and diffuse artificial pigment within the cortex, are nonallergenic, and do not require a predisposition test because they do not contain aniline derivative. As these are strong and fast-acting, follow the manufacturer's directions carefully.

FILLERS

Fillers (FIL-urz) are designed to correct excessive porosity and/or to create a color base in the hair by penetrating the cuticle and filling in empty, small holes or pockets in the cortex. They help even out porosity in the hair shaft that can cause uneven color deposit or lightening. There are two types of fillers:

* Conditioner fillers are available in protein and nonprotein and in gel, cream, and liquid forms.
* **Color fillers** (KUL-ur FIL-urz) are dual-purpose haircoloring products that are able to create a color base and equalize excessive porosity in one application. They are available in clear, neutral, and a variety of colors:
  * A clear filler is designed to correct porosity without affecting color and does not deposit a color base.

- Neutral fillers (a balance of all three primary colors) have minimal saturation and color correction abilities, but have power to equalize porosity.

Hair with uneven color distribution or pre-lightened hair may benefit from a color filler application before applying a toner or tint. Color fillers can be used to:

- deposit color to faded hair shafts and ends
- help hair hold color
- help ensure a uniform color from the scalp to the hair ends
- prevent color streaking
- prevent off-color results
- prevent dullness
- facilitate more uniform color in tinting the hair back to its natural shade

Color fillers use certified colors as pigments and are safe to use without a predisposition test if they contain no aniline derivative, may be used directly from the container and applied to the hair before tinting, and should match the same basic shade as the toner or tint to be used.

SKIN STAIN REMOVERS

Generally, soap and water will remove most tint stains from the skin. Stain removers are commercially prepared solutions that are designed for this purpose. When soap and water is not capable of removing haircolor from the skin, use one of the following methods:

1. Dampen a piece of cotton with the leftover tint. Use a rotary movement to cover the stained areas and follow with a damp towel. Apply a small amount of face cream and wipe clean.

2. Use a prepared stain remover.

Understand Procedure and Application Terms

After reading this section, you will be able to:

LO**5** Explain procedure and application terms.

Successful haircoloring usually requires a series of steps to accomplish the desired end result. Due to the wide range of haircoloring products, application methods, and procedures, it is important to have a clear understanding of the terms used in haircoloring processes. Review the following section to become familiar with procedure and application terms used in haircoloring and lightening services (see Table 18-5).

table 18-5

PROCEDURE AND APPLICATION TERMS

Patch or predisposition test	An individual's reaction to aniline derivative tints can be unpredictable. Some clients may show an immediate sensitivity, while others may suddenly develop an allergy to the product after years of use. To identify a client who has a sensitivity to aniline derivatives, the U.S. Federal Food, Drug, and Cosmetic Act prescribes that a **patch test** (PACH TEST), also known as a *predisposition test*, be given 24 to 48 hours prior to each application of an aniline derivative tint or toner (refer to Procedure 18-1).
Strand test	A **strand test** (STRAND TEST) is performed for color applications to determine: • how the hair will react to the haircolor product • how long it will take to process • what the final outcome will look like After the results of the patch test, the strand test is the next step in performing a haircolor service (refer to Procedure 18-2). A strand test is a smart and safe thing to do, but, unlike patch tests, it is not required by law.
Soap cap	A **soap cap** (SOHP KAP) is a combination of equal parts of a permanent haircolor, hydrogen peroxide, and shampoo that is applied like a regular shampoo. An example of a soap cap mixture is 1 ounce of permanent haircolor, 1 ounce of developer, and 1 ounce of shampoo. Soap caps can be used to: • brighten existing color • reduce unwanted yellow tones in gray hair • blend lines of demarcation when a retouch application does not quite match the former color application
Tint back	*Tint back* is the term used to describe the process of coloring hair back to its natural color (or close to its natural color). It is important to keep in mind that previously processed hair will be more porous and, therefore, may process darker than intended. In some cases, a filler is required to even out the hair's porosity or to achieve accurate color correction. A demipermanent haircoloring product is usually an effective choice because it is a deposit-only color with minimal oxidation.
Virgin application	A **virgin application** (VUR-jin ap-lih-KAY-shun) is the application of haircolor to hair that has not been previously colored. Hair that is in a "virgin" state is usually healthy hair that does not have any chemical damage. A virgin application also indicates that the haircoloring product will be applied to the entire hair strand versus the new growth only.
Retouch application	When permanent haircolor or lighteners are used, new hair growth will become obvious after a few weeks. The new growth, or regrowth, is that section of the hair shaft between the scalp and the hair that has been previously colored or lightened. This growth creates a *line of demarcation* between the natural color of the hair and the previously colored or lightened hair that requires blending by applying color or lightener to the new hair growth. The term **retouch application** (ree-TUCH ap-lih-KAY-shun) is used to describe this blending process.
Single-process haircoloring	**Single-process haircoloring** (SING-gul-PRAH-ses HAYR KUL-ur-ing) is a process that lightens (or lifts) and deposits color, or only deposits color in the hair in one, single application. Examples of single-process coloring are: • virgin tint applications • tint retouch applications Single-process haircoloring is also known as: • single-application coloring • one-step coloring • one-step tinting • single-application tinting

Double-process haircoloring	**Double-process haircoloring** (DUB-ul PRAH-ses HAYR-KUL-ur-ing) requires two separate and distinct applications to achieve the desired lighter hair color: 1. The hair is lightened. 2. A depositing color is applied. This process allows the practitioner to independently control the lightening and coloring actions. Double-process haircoloring is also known as: • double-application coloring • two-step coloring • two-step tinting • double-application tinting Double-process haircoloring may include the use of: • lighteners and toners • lighteners and tints • pre-softeners and tints • fillers and tints
Pre-softening	**Pre-softening** (pree-SOF-en-ing) is the process of treating gray or other resistant hair to facilitate better color penetration. Pre-softening swells and opens the cuticle. It can be accomplished with a mixture of 1 ounce of 20-volume peroxide and 8 drops of 28 percent ammonia water or with an oil or cream bleach product.
Highlighting	**Highlighting** (HY-lyt-ing) is the process of coloring some of the hair strands lighter than the natural or artificial color to add an illusion of sheen and depth. Forms of highlighting include: • cap frost • foil frost • tipping • streaking • painting/free-form
Lowlighting	**Lowlighting** or *reverse highlighting* is the process of coloring strands or sections of the hair darker than the natural or artificial color. Contrasting dark areas appear to recede and make detail less visible to the eye. Forms of lowlighting include: • cap frost • foil frost • tipping • streaking • painting/free-form
Cap technique	The **cap technique** involves pulling strands of hair through the holes of a perforated cap with a hook. A lightener, haircolor, or both (lightener and haircolor) are applied to only these hair strands, giving a natural, streaked look. The number of strands pulled through the cap determines the degree of highlighting or lowlighting that is achieved.
Foil technique	The **foil technique** (FOYL tek-NEEK) involves slicing or weaving out sections of hair to be placed on a piece of foil. The color or lightening product is usually brushed onto the hair section within the foil, after which the foil is folded and sealed for processing.
Free-form technique	The **free-form technique** (FREE-form tek-NEEK), or *balyage* (also spelled baliage), is the process of painting a lightener or color directly onto clean, styled hair. The effects can be subtle or dramatic, depending on the type of product (color or lightener) and the amount of hair that it is applied to.

RECORD KEEPING

Before performing a haircoloring service, a client record card should be completed for each client (Figure 18-20). The client record card is used to log all information pertaining to the haircoloring service. In addition to the

figure 18-20
Haircolor record card.

HAIRCOLOR RECORD

Name _____ Tel. _____

Address _____ City _____

Patch Test: ☐ Negative ☐ Positive   Date _____

Eye Color _____ Skin Tone _____

DESCRIPTION OF HAIR

Form	Length	Texture	Density	Porosity	
☐ straight	☐ short	☐ coarse	☐ sparse	☐ very porous	☐ resistant
☐ wavy	☐ medium	☐ medium	☐ moderate	☐ porous	☐ very resistant
☐ curly	☐ long	☐ fine	☐ thick	☐ normal	☐ perm. waved

Natural hair color _____

level	Tone	Intensity
(1-10)	(Warm, Cool, etc.)	(Mild, Medium, Strong)

Scalp Condition
☐ normal   ☐ dry   ☐ oily   ☐ sensitive

Condition
☐ normal   ☐ dry   ☐ oily   ☐ faded   ☐ streaked (uneven)

% unpigmented _____ Distribution of unpigmented _____

Previously lightened with _____ for _____ (time)

Previously tinted with _____ for _____ (time)

☐ original hair sample enclosed   ☐ original hair sample not enclosed

Desired hair color _____

level	Tone	Intensity
(1-10)	(Warm, Cool, etc.)	(Mild, Medium, Strong)

CORRECTIVE TREATMENTS

Color filler used _____ Conditioning treatments with _____

HAIR TINTING PROCESS

whole head _____ retouch inches (cm) _____ shade desired _____

formula: (color/lightener) _____ application technique _____

Results: ☐ good   ☐ poor   ☐ too light   ☐ too dark   ☐ streaked

Comments: _____
_____
_____
_____
_____

Date	Operator	Price	Date	Operator	Price

---

client's contact information, the record card should be descriptive enough that it provides pre-service and post-service data about the client's hair. For example, key information items should include:

- characteristics of the hair's condition
- scalp condition
- haircolor history
- any corrective treatments
- results of the haircoloring process

This information can be used for future visits as a basis for other services and should be maintained from one visit to the next.

A release statement form should be used when the client's hair is in a questionable condition that may not withstand chemical processes and treatments. See **Figure 18-21** for a sample barber school release form. To some degree, the release statement is designed to protect the school or shop owner from responsibility for accidents and damages and is a requirement of most malpractice insurance. It should be noted, however, that a release statement is not a legally binding contract and will not fully protect the barber or the shop from liability.

figure 18-21
Sample school release form.

RELEASE FORM

I, the undersigned, _____
(name)

residing at _____
(street, address)

_____
(city, state and zip)

about to receive services in the Clinical Department of
_____

and having been advised that the services shall be performed by either students, graduate students, and/or instructors of the school, in consideration of the nominal charge for such services, hereby release the school, its students, graduate students, instructors, agents, representatives, and/or employees, from any and all claims arising out of and in any way connected with the performance of these services.

The Proprietor Is Not Responsible for Personal Property

Signed _____

Date _____

Witnessed _____

THIS RELEASE FORM MUST BE SIGNED BY THE PARENT OR GUARDIAN IF THE CLIENT BEING SERVED IS UNDER 18 YEARS OF AGE.

CLIENT CONSULTATION

A thorough client consultation is the first step in a haircoloring service. Consultations should be held in a well-lit room that provides either a strong natural light or incandescent lighting. Fluorescent lighting is not suitable for judging existing hair colors.

Use the following as a guide to perform a haircoloring service consultation:

1. Drape the client.

2. Have the client fill out a client record card.

3. Perform a hair and scalp analysis and write the results on the record card. Use color swatches to determine client's natural level (**Figure 18-22**).

4. Ask the client leading questions about the desired end result to determine the:
   a. preferred color
   b. product (temporary, permanent, etc.)
   c. method (all-over color, retouch, highlights, etc.)

5. Show examples of appropriate colors and make a determination with the client (**Figure 18-23**). Ask if they have any pictures of a hair color they like or don't like.

6. Review with the client:
   a. the procedure
   b. application technique
   c. maintenance needed
   d. cost of the service

7. Perform a patch test if the haircolor product requires it.

8. Gain the client's approval and begin the service.

9. Record end results on the client record card.

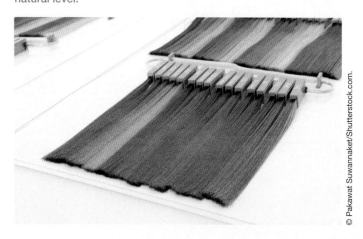

figure 18-22
Use color swatches to determine the natural level.

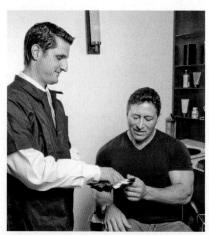

© Pakawat Suwannaket/Shutterstock.com.

figure 18-23
Discuss appropriate colors with the client.

Understand Product Selection and Application

After reading this section, you will be able to:

LO⑥ Explain how haircolor products are selected and applied to hair.

Given the many choices in haircoloring formulations and applications, it is important that you provide the client with the appropriate product and follow the correct application method. Use the following as a guide for haircoloring product selection and application.

TEMPORARY COLOR RINSES

Temporary color rinses may be used to give clients a preview of how a color change will look. They are also an option for clients who want to highlight the color of their hair or add slight color to gray hair. These rinses wash out when shampooed and are available in a variety of color shades. Temporary rinses are easily and quickly applied at the shampoo bowl and can serve as an introduction to other, longer lasting color services. Temporary color rinses can be used to:

- bring out highlights
- temporarily restore faded hair color to its natural shade
- neutralize yellow tones in white or gray hair
- tone down overlightened hair

Perform a preliminary strand test to determine proper color selection.

SEMIPERMANENT HAIRCOLOR

Semipermanent haircolor (sem-ee-PUR-muh-nent HAYR-KUL-ur) products are appropriate for the client who may want more color change than is available with a temporary rinse, but who is hesitant about a permanent color change and its related maintenance. A semipermanent color fills the gap between temporary color rinses and permanent haircolor without replacing either of them.

Since semipermanent products are deposit-only colors, the final outcome will depend on the:

- hair's original color and texture
- color that is applied
- length of development time

These haircoloring products are available in liquid and cream forms in a variety of colors. Some formulations are specifically designed in blue-gray or silver-gray hues to brighten or blend gray color tones.

Characteristics of Semipermanent Colors

The basic characteristics of semipermanent haircolors that influence the decision to choose this color product over another are:

- Semipermanent tints do not require the use of hydrogen peroxide.

- The color is self-penetrating to the extent that it stains the cuticle and deposits color molecules into the cortex.

- The color is applied the same way for each application.

- Hair will usually return to its natural color after six to eight shampoos, provided a mild, non-stripping shampoo is used.

- Retouching is eliminated.

- Semipermanent colors contain aniline derivative, so a patch test is required.

- Some semipermanent haircolors require pre-shampooing; others do not. Always follow the manufacturer's instructions.

Selecting Semipermanent Color

The addition of artificial color to the natural pigment in the hair shafts creates a darker color. When using a color chart to determine the level and shade of semipermanent color to use, consider the natural color to represent half of the formula. Use the following to select the correct color to perform the strand test:

- The use of ash or cool shades will create a color that appears darker than if a warm shade is applied.

- Warm colors appear shinier due to the reflection of light.

- For clients with up to 25 percent gray, select a shade that matches the client's natural hair color.

Special Problems

Some semipermanent haircolor products have a tendency to build up on the hair shaft with repeated applications. If this happens:

1. apply the semipermanent color to the new growth only
2. process until the desired color shade develops
3. wet the hair with warm water
4. blend the color through the hair for a few minutes
5. rinse or shampoo the color from the hair, following the manufacturer's instructions

DEMIPERMANENT HAIRCOLOR

Since demipermanent color is considered to be deposit-only color, the same procedures used for the application of a semipermanent haircolor product can be used. The difference between a semipermanent and a demipermanent color is that you mix demipermanent color with a low-volume developer or an activator immediately before applying it to the client's hair. Follow the manufacturer's guidelines for application, color selection, and processing time.

PERMANENT HAIRCOLOR

Professional permanent haircolor products contain aniline derivative color molecules and are mixed with developer. These penetrating tints are available in liquid, cream, and gel forms and are used as either single-process or double-process tints.

Single-Process Tints

Single-process tints provide a simple method of haircoloring. In one application, the hair can be permanently colored without pre-shampooing, pre-softening, or **pre-lightening** (pree-LYT-tin-ing). A single-application tint is applied on dry hair. If the hair is extremely oily or dirty and a shampoo is necessary, it must be dried before applying the tint. Single-process tints contain aniline derivative molecules and an alkaline agent and are formulated for use with 20-volume hydrogen peroxide. When other volumes of peroxide are used, the color results change. The choice of colors available vary from deepest black to lightest blond. Some characteristics of single-process tints are that they:

- save time by eliminating pre-lightening
- color the hair lighter or darker than the client's natural color
- blend in gray or white hair to match the client's natural hair color
- tone down streaks, off-shades, discoloration, and faded hair ends

Color Selection of Single-Process Tints

The porosity of the hair is one of the most important characteristics to consider when choosing haircolor tint shades. Use the following guide for choosing the level of color when tinting darker:

- *Normal porosity:* half level lighter than desired color
- *Slightly porous:* one level lighter than desired color
- *Very porous:* one to two levels lighter than desired color

  General rules for single-process color selection for gray hair:

- To match the natural color of hair and to cover gray, select the color closest to the natural shade.

- To brighten or lighten hair color and to cover gray, select a shade lighter than the natural color. The selected tint must contain enough color to produce the desired shade on gray hair.

- To darken the hair and cover gray, select a color darker than the natural hair color.

- Study the manufacturer's color chart for correct color selections.

- If a vibrant color is desired, add a natural shade to it in order to ensure better coverage.

DOUBLE-PROCESS HAIRCOLORING

Double-process haircoloring begins with hair lightening, followed by either a tint or a toner.

> **? DID YOU KNOW?**
> Skin tones change with age. The natural color of the client's hair, which harmonized with the skin coloring at the age of 20 or 30, may seem harsh and unbecoming at the age of 40 or 50. For clients in this age group, keep to the lighter shades of color.

This double process requires two separate steps as discussed in this section and demonstrated in Procedure 18-6.

P 18-6   **Double-Process Haircoloring** *pages 689–693*

LIGHTENERS

Lightening creates a new color foundation that is lighter than the client's natural hair color. This new color foundation may be the finished result or it may be the first step of a double-process application.

To achieve the desired shade of lightness, consideration must be given to the:

- existing hair color
- processing and development time
- resulting porosity
- color selection

Depending on the manufacturer's directions, hair lighteners can be used to:

- lighten the entire head of hair
- lighten the hair to a particular shade or stage
- brighten and lighten the existing shade
- paint, streak, or frost certain sections of the hair
- remove undesirable casts and off-shades
- correct dark streaks or spots in hair that has already been lightened

Selection of Lighteners

Together with the manufacturer's directions, be guided by the following general rules when choosing a lightening product:

- *Cream lighteners* can be used on the scalp when performing virgin or retouch lightening services. They offer some protection to the hair, are controllable during application, and can be used to drab undesirable red and gold tones. For increased strength, up to three activators can be added for on-the-scalp applications and up to four activators for off-the-scalp processes.
- *Powder lighteners* are strong enough to lighten the hair through several stages of lightening and may be too strong to use directly on the scalp— read and follow the manufacturer's directions carefully.
- *Oil lighteners* are the mildest form of lighteners and may be used when only one or two levels of lift are desired.

Lightener Retouch

Lightener retouch is the term used when a lightener is applied only to the new hair growth to match the rest of the lightened hair. The client's record card should be used as a guide to determine the:

- lightener that was previously used
- processing time required for the desired stage of lightness to develop

Cream lightener is often used for a lightener retouch because it helps prevent overlapping on the previously lightened hair. Powdered lighteners may be used if the manufacturer's directions state that it is safe to use on the scalp. When retouching, the lightener is applied to the new growth only. If a lighter or different level is desired overall, wait until the new growth is almost light enough or has developed fully. Then distribute the remainder of the lightener through the hair shaft. One to five minutes should be ample time to create a lighter-level effect.

TONERS

Toners (TOHN-urz) have the same chemical ingredients as permanent hair-color tints, except they contain less amounts of color, which gives toners pale, delicate shades of color for depositing in pre-lightened hair.

Color Selection of Toners

Pastel colors, such as silver, platinum blond, and beige-blond, are popular toners for lighter blond colors. Gray hair and skin tone changes that accompany advancing years may benefit from light, silver tones. When extremely pale toner shades such as very light silver, platinum, or beige are desired, the hair must be pre-lightened to pale yellow or almost white.

Toner Retouch

A toner retouch must be given the same careful consideration as you would give a double-process tint retouch application. The new growth must be pre-lightened to the same degree of lightness achieved in the previous application. The lightener is applied to the new growth only. To avoid damage to the hair, be careful not to overlap the lightener on previously lightened hair. After the lightening process has been completed, follow the manufacturer's instructions for toner application:

- Some toners are applied to the entire length of the hair at one time.

- Some toners are first applied to the new growth area to process, and then applied briefly to the length of the remaining hair.

Toner Suggestions and Reminders

Toners are completely dependent on the proper preliminary lightening treatment, which must leave the hair light and porous enough to receive the pale toner shades. Semipermanent and demipermanent color can be used after lighteners to achieve specific tones and colors. Strand tests are vital in double-process applications. A complete explanation of the possible outcome should be discussed with the client. It is always possible that the hair cannot be decolorized sufficiently for the color choice without resulting in serious damage to the hair. Gold or red pigments remaining in the hair after lightening indicate underlightening. Ash tones indicate overlightening—when this happens, the shade of toner should be chosen to neutralize the unwanted tones.

SPECIAL-EFFECTS HAIRCOLORING AND LIGHTENING

Special-effects haircoloring refers to any technique that involves the partial lightening or coloring of the hair. One way of creating special effects is to strategically place light and dark colors in the hair. Highlighting is the process of lightening or coloring some of the hair strands lighter than the natural color. Lowlighting, or reverse highlighting, is the process of coloring strands or sections of the hair darker than the natural color. Both of these techniques can be used to create special-effects haircoloring and may consist of an overall dramatic dimensional change or something more subtle. Consult your client about where they would like to see the change in color. The three most frequently used techniques for creating highlights or lowlights are:

- cap frost
- foil frost
- balyage, free-form, or painting

Ⓟ 18-7 **Special Effects** *pages 694–698*

SPECIAL PROBLEMS AND CORRECTIVE HAIRCOLOR

Each haircoloring or lightening service has the potential to create unique problems. Some problems can be avoided by performing preliminary strand tests, but others can be the result of unique properties within the client's hair structure that are unforeseen. Most haircoloring and lightening problems can be resolved with:

- a calm approach
- an accurate assessment of the problem
- knowledge to correct the situation

GRAY HAIR CHALLENGES

Gray, white, or salt-and-pepper hair shades have characteristics that can present unique color challenges (**Figure 18-24**). Since both gray and white hair contain little melanin within the cortex, a large number of coloring services are performed with the intent to cover or enhance the color. Depending on the amount of gray, the hair may have a yellowish cast or process differently from one strand to another. Some gray hair also tend to be resistant to chemical processes and may require pre-softening before a service.

Gray Hair with a Yellowish Cast

Gray, white, and salt-and-pepper hair with a yellowish cast can be treated with violet-based colors that range from highlighting shampoos and temporary rinses to lighteners. The longevity of the product used will depend on the client's desired result and the options offered

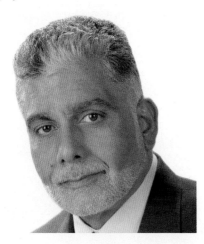

figure 18-24
Many people choose to cover or blend gray hair.

by the barber. If lightening and coloring services are not typically offered in the barbershop, it is highly recommended that, at a minimum, highlighting shampoos or temporary rinses with violet bases be available to clients.

Determining the Percentage of Gray

Since most people retain some dark hair as they turn gray, the hair must be analyzed for level, hue, and percentage of gray before the appropriate product selection can be made. Gray hair may be evenly distributed or isolated in various sections of the head, such as the temple areas.

Formulating Haircolor for Naturally Gray Hair

Gray hair will usually accept the level of the color applied. Because there is no melanin in the hair, gray hair may appear lighter after haircolor is applied.

When a client has 80 to 100 percent gray, lighter haircolors are usually more flattering than darker shades. The client's skin tone, eye color, and personal preference will determine whether warm or cool tones are used (**Figure 18-25**). Many color product lines have a specific gray coverage series that provides greater saturation of the color.

Occasionally, gray hair is so resistant that pre-softening is necessary for better color penetration. It is always a good idea to mix a small amount of the haircolor product and perform a strand test. A strand test indicates:

- if the hair is resistant to the product
- how long it takes for the product to be absorbed by the hair
- what the color results will be

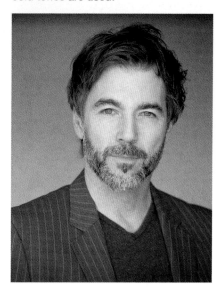

figure 18-25
Skin tone, eye color, and personal preference will determine if warm or cold tones are used.

RECONDITIONING DAMAGED HAIR

Hair that is damaged due to careless chemical applications, excessive heat, or misused styling products must be reconditioned before it can be tinted or lightened successfully. Sometimes hair is naturally brittle, thin, and lifeless. Both neglect and the client's physical condition may contribute to these conditions. Hair is considered damaged when it exhibits one or more of the following characteristics:

- overporous
- brittle and dry
- breaks easily
- little to no elasticity
- rough and harsh to the touch
- spongy and mats easily when wet
- resists color or absorbs too much color during a tinting process

Any of these conditions may create undesirable results during a tinting or lightening service. Therefore, damaged hair should receive reconditioning treatments before and after haircolor applications.

Reconditioning Treatment

To restore damaged hair to a healthier condition, hair conditioners containing lanolin or protein substances should be used. The conditioning product is applied to the hair according to the manufacturer's directions. If heat is applied, use a heating cap, a steamer, or a heating lamp. Be guided by your instructor as to the frequency and length of time for each treatment.

TINT BACK TO NATURAL COLOR

Clients who have been tinting or lightening their hair may want to return to their natural shade, which is known as a *tint back*. Each tint back must be handled as an individual situation. The determining factors in the selection of the tint shade are the:

- present condition of the hair
- present color of the hair
- final result desired
- original color

To determine the client's natural hair color, check the natural shade of the hair next to the scalp. Next, select an appropriate shade of filler to correspond with the tint to be used; otherwise, it will be difficult to obtain a uniform color from the scalp to hair ends, due to uneven porosity levels. Perform strand tests as needed to determine the expected final outcome.

COLORING MUSTACHES AND BEARDS

- *Aniline derivative tints* should *never* be used for coloring mustaches. Doing so may cause serious irritation or damage to the lips or the delicate membranes of the nostrils.

- *Metallic or progressive dyes* have been known to cause severe allergic reactions when applied to facial hair or around freshly cut hairlines.

- *Hair color crayons* are waxy sticks that are available in several colors: blond, medium, dark brown, black, and auburn. They are applied by rubbing it directly on the facial hair.

- *Pomades* are formulated specifically for coloring mustaches and beards. These products are available in a variety of shades, including black, brown, blond, chestnut, and white (neutral). The pomade is applied with a small brush and is stroked from the nostrils downward. Liquid pomades are also available and may be preferred for use on beards. Some pomades contain heavy waxing ingredients that can be used to style mustaches with rolled or twisted ends for dramatic looks.

- *Liquid eyebrow and eyelash tints* are available in brown and black for coloring facial hair.

Ⓟ 18-8   **Coloring Mustaches and Beards** *pages 699–701*

COATING DYES

Many clients buy and use over-the-counter haircoloring products at home. Some of these products are actually progressive dyes and must be removed prior to any other chemical service. Hair treated with a compound, metallic, or other coating dye looks dry and dull, and may feel harsh and brittle to the touch. These colors usually fade to unnatural tones, such as:

- silver dyes have a green or gray cast
- lead dyes leave a purple color
- those containing copper turn red

If you are unsure as to whether the client has used a progressive dye, a test for metallic salts and dyes should be performed on the hair.

Test for Metallic Salts and Coating Dyes

In a glass container, mix 1 ounce of 20-volume (6 percent) peroxide and 20 drops of 28 percent ammonia water. Cut a few strands of the client's hair, bind it with tape, and immerse it in the solution for 30 minutes. Remove, towel-dry, and observe the strand. Refer to the following for analysis of the hair:

- Hair dyed with lead will lighten immediately.
- Hair treated with silver will show no reaction at all, which indicates that other chemicals will not be successful because they will not be able to penetrate the coating.
- Hair treated with copper will start to boil and will pull apart easily. This hair would be severely damaged or destroyed if other chemicals such as those found in permanent colors or perm solutions were applied to it.
- Hair treated with a coating dye either will not change color or will lighten in spots. Hair in this condition will not receive chemical services easily and the length of time necessary for penetration may result in further damage to the hair.

Removing Coatings from the Hair Mini-Procedure

The removal of metallic dyes from the hair shaft may not always be effective the first time. Performing a strand test after the treatment will indicate whether the metallic deposits have been removed. If not, the entire application must be repeated until the hair is sufficiently free of metal salts to perform other chemical services.

Supplies

- ☐ 70 percent alcohol
- ☐ Concentrated shampoo for oily hair
- ☐ Mineral, castor, vegetable, or commercially prepared color-removing oil

Procedure

1. Apply 70 percent alcohol to dry hair.

2. Allow alcohol to stand for 5 minutes.

3. Apply the oil to the hair thoroughly.

4. Cover the hair completely with a plastic cap.

5. Place under a hot dryer for 30 minutes.

6. To remove the oil, saturate with concentrated shampoo.

7. Work the shampoo into the oil for 3 minutes, and then rinse with warm water.

8. Repeat the shampoo steps until the oil is removed completely.

REMINDER
Keep up to date! Manufacturers are constantly improving and developing new haircoloring products. Be sure to attend seminars and trade shows as often as possible to stay current in your profession.

Discuss Haircoloring and Lightening Safety Precautions

After reading this section, you will be able to:

LO⑦ List haircoloring and lightening safety precautions.

HAIRCOLORING SAFETY PRECAUTIONS

- Perform a 24- to 48-hour patch test before the application of a haircolor product containing aniline derivative.
- Examine the scalp before applying a tint.
- Do not apply tint if abrasions are present on the scalp.
- Use only clean swabs, brushes, applicator bottles, combs, and linens.
- Always wash your hands before and after each client.
- Do not brush the hair prior to a tint.
- Do not apply a tint without reading the manufacturer's directions.
- Perform a strand test for color and processing results.
- Choose a shade of tint that harmonizes with the client's complexion.
- Use an applicator bottle or bowl (plastic or glass) for mixing tint.
- Do not mix tint before ready for use; discard leftover tint.
- If required, use the correct shade of color filler.
- Make frequent strand tests until the desired shade is reached.
- Suggest a reconditioning treatment for tinted hair.
- Do not apply tint if metallic or compound dye is present.
- Do not apply tint if a patch test is positive.

- Perform a strand test for the correct color shade before applying tint.
- Do not use an alkaline or harsh shampoo for tint removal.
- Do not use water that is too hot for removing tint. Use lukewarm or tepid water.
- Protect the client's clothing by proper draping.
- Do not permit tint to come in contact with the client's eyes.
- Do not overlap during a tint retouch.
- Cap all bottles of developer and tint to avoid loss of strength.
- Fill out a tint record card.
- Do not apply hydrogen peroxide or any material containing hydrogen peroxide directly over dyes known or believed to contain a metallic salt. Breakage or complete disintegration of the hair may result.
- Wear protective gloves.

HAIR LIGHTENING SAFETY PRECAUTIONS

- Analyze the condition of the hair and suggest reconditioning treatments, if required.
- When working with a cream or paste lightener, it must be the thickness of whipped cream to avoid dripping or running and overlapping.
- Do not use off-the-scalp lightener for virgin or retouch lightener applications.
- Apply lightener to resistant areas first. Use ⅛-inch sections when applying lightener to ensure complete coverage.
- Check strands frequently until the desired lightness is reached.
- Immediately after completing the lightener application, check the client's skin (face, neck, hairline, etc.) and remove any lightener to avoid skin irritation.
- Check the towel around the client's neck. Lightener on the towel that is allowed to come in contact with the skin will cause irritation.
- Lightened hair is fragile and requires special care. Use only a very mild shampoo and only cool water for rinsing.
- If a preliminary shampoo is necessary, comb and shampoo the hair carefully. Avoid irritating the scalp during the shampoo or when combing the hair.
- Work as rapidly as possible when applying the lightener to produce a uniform shade without streaking.
- Never allow lightener to stand; use it immediately.
- Cap all bottles of developer and lightener to avoid loss of strength.
- Keep a completed record card of all lightening treatments.

PATCH TEST

MATERIALS, IMPLEMENTS, AND EQUIPMENT

- ☐ Cotton swab
- ☐ Developer
- ☐ Glass or plastic mixing bowl
- ☐ Haircolor product
- ☐ Mild soap
- ☐ Towels

PREPARATION

1. Wash your hands.
2. Conduct client consultation and select a haircolor product.
3. Perform hair and scalp analysis.
4. Select and arrange required materials.
5. Drape client for a chemical service.

PROCEDURE

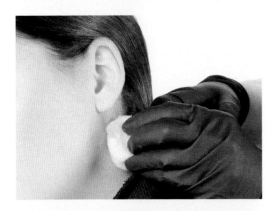

1. Select a test area; behind the ear or on the inside of the elbow are good choices.
2. Using a mild soap, clean and dry an area about the size of a quarter.

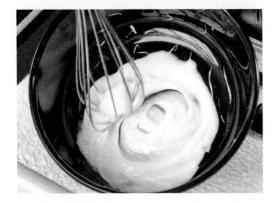

3. Mix a small amount of the same product you plan on using for the service according to the manufacturer's directions.

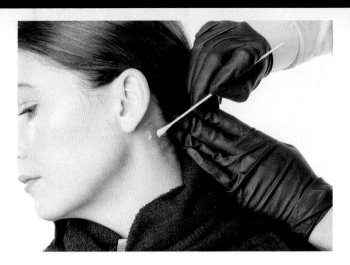

4 Apply a small amount of the haircolor mixture to the test area with a sterile cotton swab.

5 Leave the mixture undisturbed for 24 to 48 hours.

6 Examine the test area. If there are no signs of redness or irritation, the test result is negative, and you can proceed with the color service.

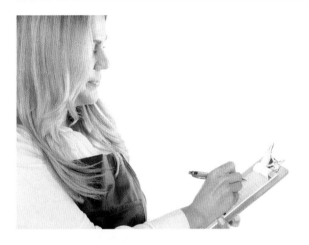

7 Record the results on the haircolor service record card.

CLEAN-UP AND DISINFECTION

☐ Wash and disinfect tools and implements.

☐ Clean and disinfect work area.

☐ Dispose of single-use items. Place all used linens, towels, and capes in the laundry.

☐ Wash your hands.

STRAND TEST

- ☐ Bowl and brush
- ☐ Chemical cape
- ☐ Color brushes
- ☐ Developer
- ☐ Glass or plastic mixing bowl
- ☐ Protective gloves
- ☐ Selected haircolor

- ☐ Service record card
- ☐ Shampoo
- ☐ Sheet of foil or plastic wrap
- ☐ Spray bottle containing water
- ☐ Timer
- ☐ Towels

PREPARATION

1. Wash your hands.
2. Conduct client consultation and select a haircoloring product.
3. Perform hair and scalp analysis.
4. Select and arrange required materials.
5. Drape client for a chemical service.

PROCEDURE

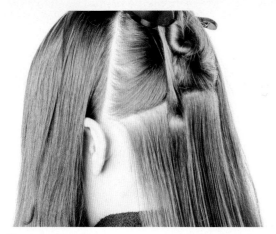

1. Apply gloves. Part off a ½-inch square section of hair in the interior nape area, so it is not visible from the hairline. Using plastic clips, fasten other hair out of the way.

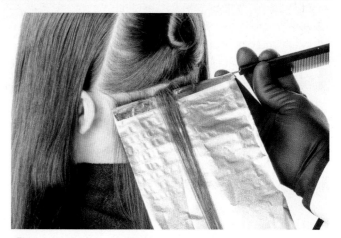

2. Place the hair strand over the foil or plastic wrap and apply the color mixture you plan on using for the service.

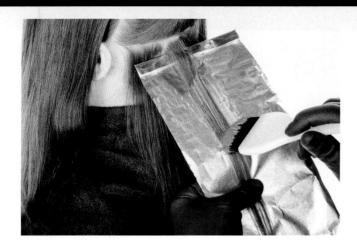

3 Follow the application method for the color you will be using to apply the color mixture.

4 Check the development at 5-minute intervals until the desired color has been achieved. Note the timing on the service record card.

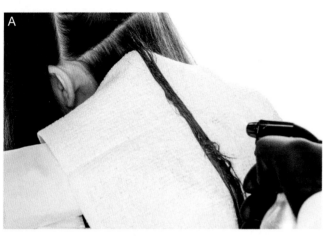

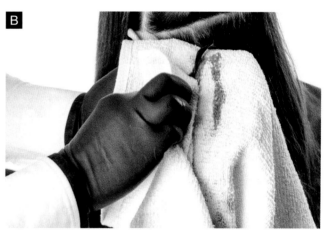

5 When satisfactory color has developed, remove the protective foil or plastic wrap. Place a towel under the strand, mist it thoroughly with water, add shampoo, and massage through. Rinse by spraying with water. Dry the hair strand with the towel and observe the results.

6 Adjust the timing, haircolor formulation, or application method as necessary and proceed with the color service.

CLEAN-UP AND DISINFECTION

☐ Discard disposable items.

☐ Clean and disinfect the chair and workstation.

☐ Dispose of single-use items. Place all used linens, towels, and capes in the laundry.

☐ Store products, materials, and service record card.

☐ Wash your hands.

TEMPORARY COLOR RINSE

MATERIALS, IMPLEMENTS, AND EQUIPMENT

☐ Applicator bottle

☐ Comb

☐ Protective gloves

☐ Service record card

☐ Shampoo

☐ Shampoo cape

☐ Temporary haircolor product

☐ Timer

☐ Towels

⚠ CAUTION
If the client is to receive a haircut, perform the cut before applying a color rinse.

PREPARATION

1. Assemble all necessary supplies.

2. Prepare the client and drape with towels and waterproof cape.

3. Examine the client's scalp and hair.

4. Select the desired shade of color rinse.

5. Perform a strand test.

PROCEDURE

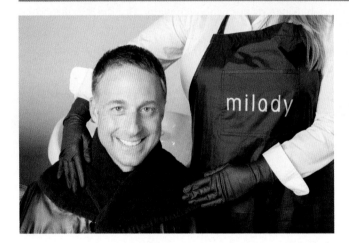

1. Drape the client for a haircoloring service. Slide a towel down from the back of the client's head and place lengthwise across the client's shoulders. Cross the ends of the towel beneath the chin and place the cape over the towel. Fasten the cape in the back. Fold the towel over the top of the cape and secure in front.

2. Shampoo and towel-dry the hair.

3. Make sure the client is comfortably reclined at the shampoo bowl.

4. Put on gloves.

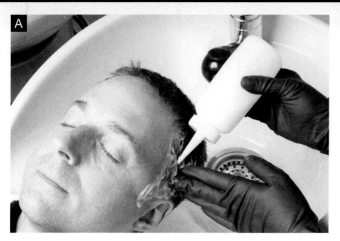

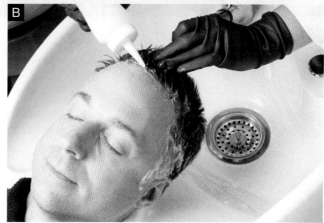

5 Put the color into the applicator bottle and apply as directed by the manufacturer's instructions.

6 Apply the color and work around the entire head.

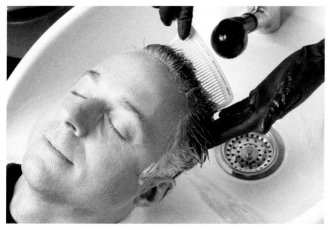

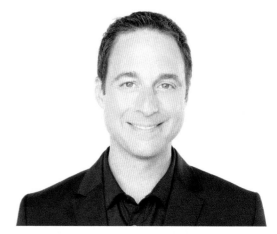

7 Blend the color with your gloved hands or comb it through the hair, applying more color as necessary.

8 Do not rinse the hair. Towel-blot excess product.

9 Proceed with styling and finish.

CLEAN-UP AND DISINFECTION

☐ Wash and disinfect tools and implements.

☐ Clean and disinfect the work area.

☐ Sweep up hair and deposit in closed receptacle.

☐ Dispose of single-use items. Place all used linens, towels, and capes in the laundry.

☐ Wash your hands.

☐ Record the results on the service record card.

DEMIPERMANENT COLOR APPLICATION

MATERIALS, IMPLEMENTS, AND EQUIPMENT

☐ Chemical cape

☐ Color brushes

☐ Color chart

☐ Comb

☐ Conditioner

☐ Cotton

☐ Glass or plastic bowl

☐ Plastic cap (optional)

☐ Plastic clips

☐ Protective cream

☐ Protective gloves

☐ Selected color

☐ Service record card

☐ Shampoo

☐ Timer

☐ Towels

PREPARATION

1 Perform a preliminary patch test with any haircolor product containing aniline derivative 24 to 48 hours before the service. Proceed only if the test is negative.

2 Perform client consultation, select a haircolor product, and record results on client record card.

3 Drape client and apply protective cream.

4 Perform a strand test and record the results.

PROCEDURE

1 Shampoo the client's hair with mild shampoo, and towel-dry.

2 Put on gloves.

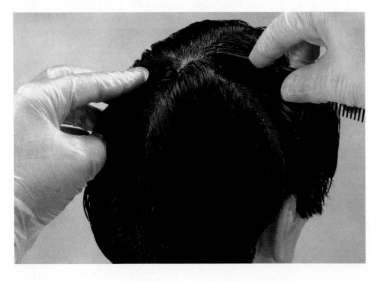

3 Part the hair into four sections—from ear to ear and from front center of forehead to center nape—and apply protective cream around the hairline and over the ears.

4 Outline the partings with color product.

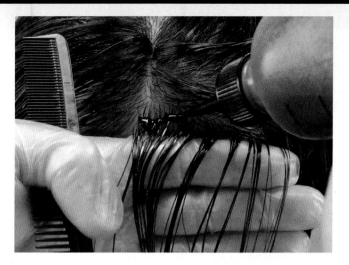

5 Take ¼- to ½-inch partings, and apply the color to the new growth or scalp area in all four sections. Take horizontal subsections, starting in the nape of a rear quadrant, repeat on other rear quadrant. When you reach the front, you will take vertical sections applying product so the hair lays away from the face.

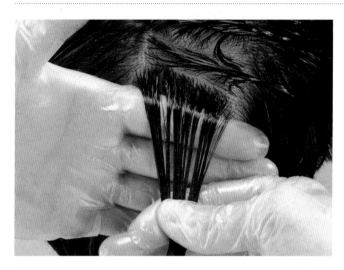

6 After all four sections are completed, work the color through the rest of the hair shaft to the ends until the hair is fully saturated.

7 Set timer to process. In addition to following the manufacturer's directions, check the haircolor every 5 minutes as it is processing to ensure you are not overdepositing color on porous hair. Some colors require the use of a plastic cap. To prevent the elastic of the plastic cap from leaving a mark on client's face, place cotton under cap elastic on face and hairline.

8 When processing is complete, massage color into a lather and rinse thoroughly with warm water.

9 Remove any stains from around the hairline with shampoo or stain remover.

10 Shampoo the hair. Condition as needed.

CLEAN-UP AND DISINFECTION

☐ Wash and disinfect tools and implements.

☐ Clean and disinfect the work area.

☐ Dispose of single-use items. Place all used linens, towels, and capes in the laundry.

☐ Wash your hands.

☐ Record the results on the service record card.

SINGLE-PROCESS PERMANENT COLOR APPLICATIONS: VIRGIN AND RETOUCH

MATERIALS, IMPLEMENTS, AND EQUIPMENT

☐ Applicator bottle or brush and bowl

☐ Color chart

☐ Comb

☐ Conditioner

☐ Cotton

☐ Hydrogen peroxide (developer)

☐ Measuring cup or beaker

☐ Plastic cap (optional, depending on the manufacturer's directions)

☐ Plastic clips (optional, depending on length of hair)

☐ Protective cream

☐ Protective gloves

☐ Service Record card

☐ Shampoo

☐ Shampoo cape

☐ Single-process permanent color product

☐ Timer

☐ Towels

PREPARATION

1 Perform a preliminary patch test with any hair-color product containing aniline derivative 24 to 48 hours before the service. Proceed only if the test is negative.

2 Perform client consultation, select haircolor product, and record results on client record card.

3 Drape client and apply protective cream.

4 Perform a strand test and record the results.

VIRGIN APPLICATION PROCEDURE

1 Follow the manufacturer's directions.

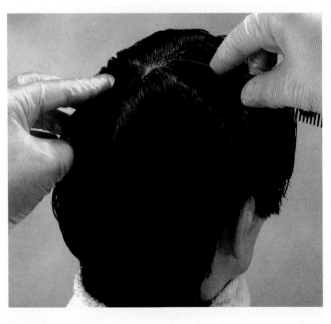

2 Put on gloves and part dry hair into four sections. Most permanent haircolors do not require shampooing before the application of color.

3 Prepare color formula for either bottle or brush application method.

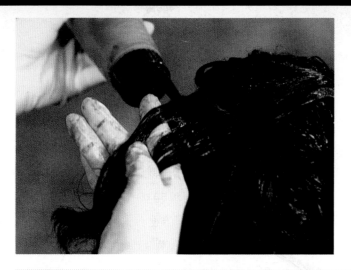

4 Begin in the section where the hair is most resistant or where there will be the most color change, usually in the back of the head.

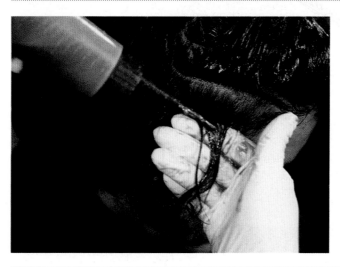

5 Part off ¼-inch subsections and apply color to the mid-shaft area. Stay at least ½ inch from the scalp and do not apply to the porous ends at this time.

6 Process according to the strand test results and the manufacturer's directions.

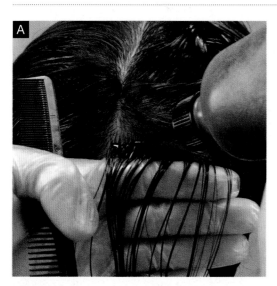

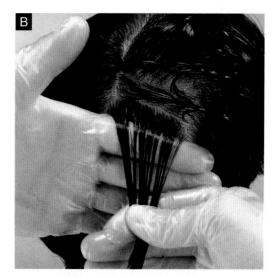

7 Check color development. When the hair is halfway to the desired color, apply remaining product to hair at the scalp, then pull the color through to the hair ends.

8 Lightly wet client's hair with warm water and lather. Massage lather through the hair.

9 Rinse thoroughly using lukewarm or tepid water, shampoo, and condition. Remove skin stains as necessary.

10 Rinse, towel-blot, and style.

11 Record results.

TINT RETOUCH PROCEDURE

To retouch new hair growth, use the same preparation steps as for coloring virgin hair. Then proceed as follows:

12 Refer to the client record card for correct color selection and other information.

13 Section the hair into four quadrants and apply the tint to dry hair, starting in the areas where hair is most resistant.

14 Apply the tint to the new growth using ¼-inch partings. Do not overlap onto previously tinted hair. Check frequently for color development.

15 When color has almost developed, dilute the remaining tint by adding a mild shampoo or warm water. Apply and gently work the mixture through the hair with the fingertips. Blend the color from the scalp through the hair ends for even distribution.

16 Process for the required time, following the manufacturer's directions.

17 Rinse with warm water to remove excess color.

18 Use an acid-balanced shampoo, condition, and rinse thoroughly. Remove skin stains, if necessary.

19 Style the hair as desired.

CLEAN-UP AND DISINFECTION

☐ Wash and disinfect tools and implements.

☐ Clean and disinfect the work area.

☐ Dispose of single-use items. Place all used linens, towels, and capes in the laundry.

☐ Wash your hands.

☐ Record the results on the service record card.

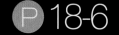

DOUBLE-PROCESS HAIRCOLORING

STEP 1: LIGHTENING VIRGIN HAIR

MATERIALS, IMPLEMENTS, AND EQUIPMENT

- ☐ Chemical cape
- ☐ Color brushes
- ☐ Comb
- ☐ Conditioner
- ☐ Cotton

- ☐ Glass or plastic mixing bowl
- ☐ Hydrogen peroxide developer
- ☐ Lightener
- ☐ Plastic clips
- ☐ Protective cream

- ☐ Protective gloves
- ☐ Service record card
- ☐ Shampoo
- ☐ Timer
- ☐ Towels

PREPARATION

1 Perform a preliminary patch test with any haircolor product containing aniline derivative 24 to 48 hours before the service. Proceed only if the test is negative.

2 Perform client consultation, select haircoloring and lightening products, and record on client record card.

3 Drape client and apply protective cream.

4 Perform a strand test and record the results.

PROCEDURE FOR LIGHTENING VIRGIN HAIR

1 Section dry hair into four quadrants.

2 Apply protective cream around hairline. Put on gloves.

3 Prepare the lightening formula and use it immediately.

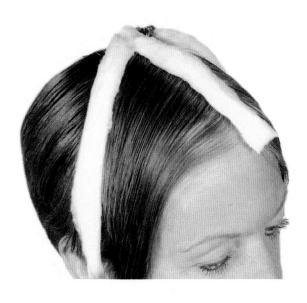

4 An option for a clean and comfortable application is to place cotton around and through all four sections to protect the scalp. Continue by placing strips of cotton at the scalp area along the partings for each subsection. This process will prevent the lightener from touching the base of the hair.

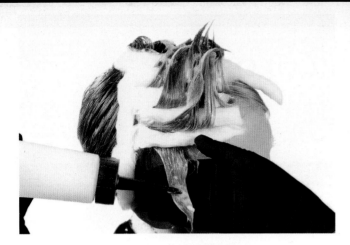

5 Part off ⅛-inch subsection and apply the lightener ½ inch away from the scalp, working the lightener through the mid-strands and up to the porous ends.

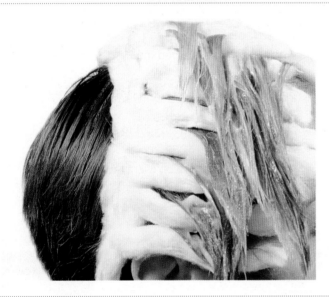

6 Continue to apply the lightener. Double check the application, adding more lightener if necessary. Do not comb the lightener through the hair. The lightener will stop processing if it dries out. Keep the lightener moist during development by reapplying if the mixture dries on the hair.

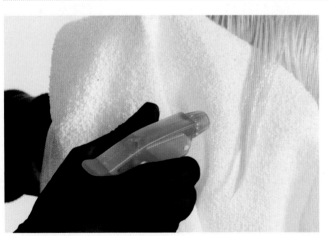

7 Check for lightening action about 15 minutes before the time indicated by the preliminary strand test. Spray a hair strand with a water bottle and remove the lightener with a damp towel. Examine the strand. If the strand is not light enough, reapply the mixture and continue testing frequently until the desired level is reached.

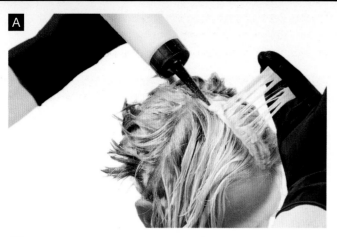
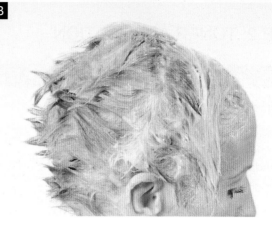

8 Remove the cotton from the scalp area. Apply the lightener to the hair near the scalp with ½-inch partings.

9 Apply lightener to the porous ends and process until the entire hair strand has reached the desired stage.

10 Rinse the hair thoroughly with warm water. Shampoo gently and condition as needed, keeping your hands under the hair to avoid tangling.

11 Neutralize the alkalinity of the hair with an acidic conditioner. Recondition if necessary.

12 Towel-dry the hair, or dry it completely under a cool dryer if required by the manufacturer.

13 Examine the scalp for any abrasions. Analyze the condition of the hair.

14 Proceed with a toner application if desired. If no toner is needed, dry and style the hair.

CLEAN-UP AND DISINFECTION

☐ Wash and disinfect tools and implements.

☐ Clean and disinfect work area.

☐ Dispose of single-use items. Place all used linens, towels, and capes in the laundry.

☐ Wash your hands.

☐ Record the results on the service record card.

STEP 2: TONER APPLICATION

MATERIALS, IMPLEMENTS, AND EQUIPMENT

- ☐ Applicator bottle
- ☐ Bowl
- ☐ Chemical cape
- ☐ Conditioner
- ☐ Cotton
- ☐ Glass or plastic mixing bowl
- ☐ Hydrogen peroxide developer
- ☐ Plastic clips
- ☐ Protective cream
- ☐ Protective gloves
- ☐ Selected toner
- ☐ Service record card
- ☐ Shampoo
- ☐ Tail comb
- ☐ Timer
- ☐ Tint brush
- ☐ Towels

PREPARATION

1. Perform a preliminary patch test with any haircolor product containing aniline derivative 24 to 48 hours before the service. Proceed only if the test is negative.
2. Perform client consultation.
3. Drape client.
4. Pre-lighten the hair to the desired level.
5. Shampoo with cool or tepid water, rinse, condition, and towel-dry the hair.

PROCEDURE FOR TONER APPLICATION

1. Put on gloves.
2. Select the desired toner shade.
3. Apply protective cream around the hairline and over the ears.
4. Take a strand test and record the results on the client's service record card.
5. If using a toner with developer, mix the toner and the developer in a nonmetallic bowl or bottle, following the manufacturer's directions.

6 Part the hair into four equal sections, using the end of the tail comb or applicator brush. Avoid scratching the scalp.

7 Take a strand test. At the crown of one of the back sections, part off ¼-inch partings and apply the toner from the scalp up to, but not including, the porous ends. If it indicates proper color development, start application in the back at the nape and work application forward.

8 Gently work the toner through the ends of the hair, using an applicator brush or your fingers.

9 If necessary for coverage, apply additional toner to the hair and distribute evenly. Leave the hair loose or cover with a plastic cap if required.

10 Time the procedure according to your strand test. Check frequently until the desired color has been reached evenly throughout the entire hair shaft and ends.

11 Remove the toner by wetting the hair and massaging the toner into a lather.

12 Rinse with warm water, shampoo gently, and thoroughly rinse again.

13 Apply an acidic conditioner to close the cuticle, lower the pH, and help prevent fading.

14 Remove any stains from the skin, hairline, and neck.

15 Style as desired. Use caution to avoid stretching the hair.

CLEAN-UP AND DISINFECTION

☐ Wash and disinfect tools and implements.

☐ Clean and disinfect the work area.

☐ Dispose of single-use items. Place all used linens, towels, and capes in the laundry.

☐ Wash your hands.

☐ Record the results on the service record card.

SPECIAL EFFECTS

MATERIALS, IMPLEMENTS, AND EQUIPMENT

- ☐ Applicator bottle
- ☐ Chemical cape
- ☐ Color brushes
- ☐ Conditioner
- ☐ Foil
- ☐ Glass or plastic mixing bowl
- ☐ Gloves

- ☐ Lightener
- ☐ Plastic clips
- ☐ Service record card
- ☐ Shampoo
- ☐ Tail comb
- ☐ Timer
- ☐ Towels

PREPARATION FOIL TECHNIQUES

1. Perform a preliminary patch test 24 to 48 hours before the service with any product containing aniline derivative. Proceed only if the test is negative.
2. Perform client consultation and record on client record card.
3. Drape client.
4. Perform a strand test and record the results.

PROCEDURE FOR FOIL TECHNIQUE

1. Part hair into six sections. Start by dividing the hair into four quadrants, from front hairline to nape, and ear to ear. In the front, you will then subdivide your right and left quadrants into a top and side section at the parietal ridge above the ear.

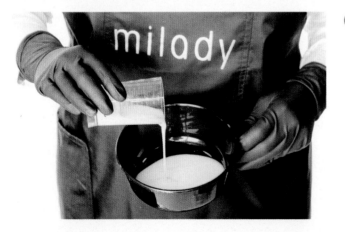

2. Prepare the lightening formula, and use it immediately.

> **FOCUS ON**
> When performing the foil technique over the entire head, the sequence of application should be back, lower crown, sides, top, and front.

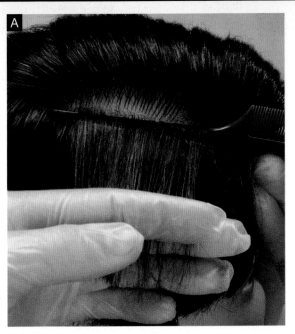

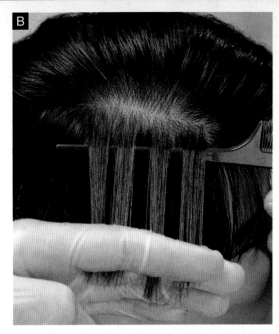

3 Starting in the right back section, with a tail comb, take a thin diagonal slice or weave out the strands, following the shape of the hairline. From this slice you will then take a fine weave of hair and place a piece of foil under it.

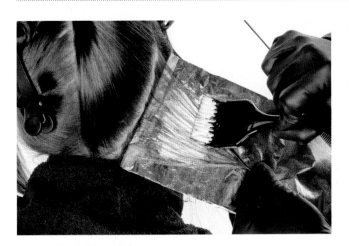

4 Holding the hair taut, brush lightener starting from 2 inches from the top of the foil to the ends, using only enough product to secure the foil in place. Work the product up to ¼ inch from the edge of the foil.

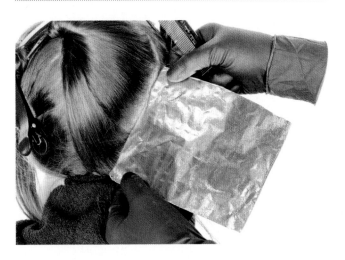

5 Fold the foil in half until the ends meet.

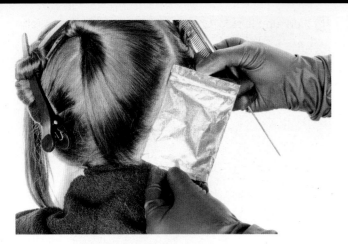

6 Fold the foil in half again, using the comb to crease it.

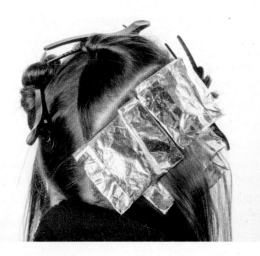

7 Take a ¼-inch subsection in between foils. Clip this hair up and out of the way. Note the contrast in size between the foiled and unfoiled subsections.

8 Continue working up the back right side of the head until the section is complete.

9 Repeat this procedure on the back left side of the head.

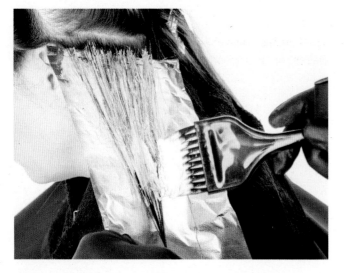

10 Work around the head to the left side.

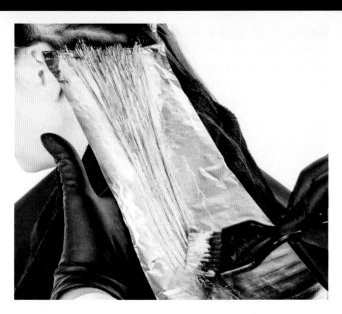

11 Work up the side, bring fine slices of hair into the foil, and apply lightener to the hair.

12 Move to the other side of the head and complete the matching sections.

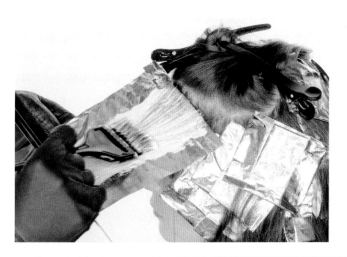

13 Move to the top right side of the head. Take a fine slice of hair, from the top of the side section to the center part, following the shape of the hairline. Place it on the foil, and apply lightener.

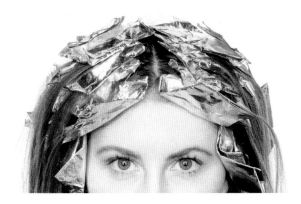

14 Continue toward the top until the last foil is placed. Repeat on the top left side of the head.

15 Allow the lightener to process according to the strand test.

16 Check the foils for the desired lightness.

17 Remove the foils one at a time at the shampoo area. Rinse the hair immediately to prevent the color from affecting the untreated hair.

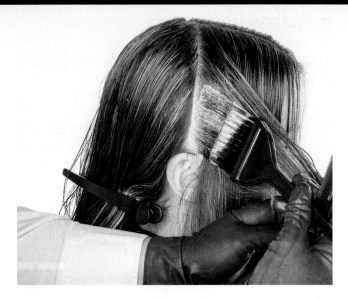

18 A haircolor glaze is an optional service added onto a highlighting to add shine to the finished result. If desired, apply a haircolor glaze to the hair from the scalp to the ends. Skip to step 20 if you do not use a haircolor glaze.

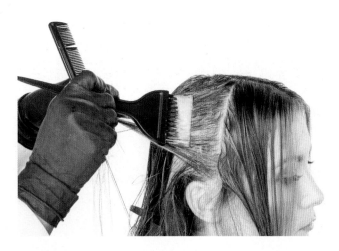

19 Work the glaze into the hair to make sure it is completely saturated, and process per the manufacturer's directions.

20 Rinse the hair, shampoo, condition, and style the hair as desired.

CLEAN-UP AND DISINFECTION

☐ Wash and disinfect tools and implements.

☐ Clean and disinfect the work area.

☐ Dispose of single-use items. Place all used linens, towels, and capes in the laundry.

☐ Wash your hands.

☐ Record the results on the service record card.

COLORING MUSTACHES AND BEARDS

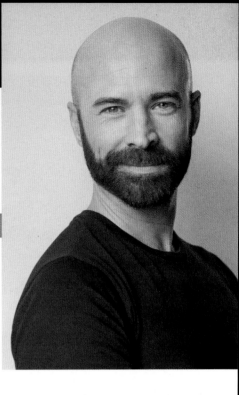

- ☐ Chemical cape
- ☐ Coloring solutions (nos. 1 and 2)
- ☐ Cotton-tipped applicators
- ☐ Petroleum jelly
- ☐ Soap
- ☐ Stain remover
- ☐ Towels

PROCEDURE

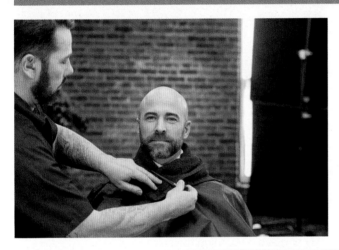

1 Seat the client in a comfortable position and drape for a chemical service.

2 Apply clean headrest cover.

3 Recline chair slightly about 45 degrees to access hair under the chin.

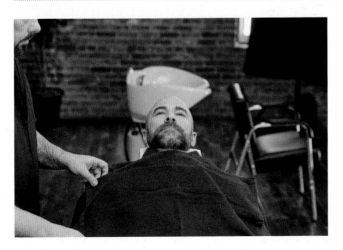

4 Place a clean towel across the chest and shoulders.

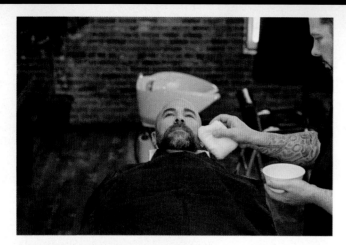

5 Cleanse the facial hair with warm, soapy water and pat dry with a cloth towel.

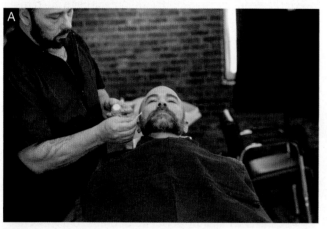

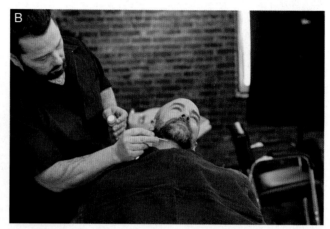

6 Apply petroleum jelly around the facial hairline.

7 Remove the cap on solution no. 1. Moisten a cotton-tipped applicator in the solution. Replace the cap on bottle no. 1.

8 Remove any excess solution by touching the tip of the applicator to a towel.

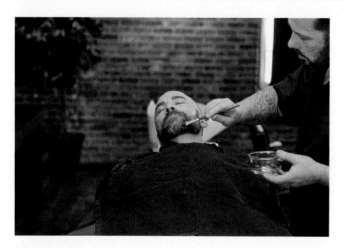

9 Apply the solution to the mustache and/or beard hair only and avoid touching the skin.

10 Set timer according to the manufacturer's direction.

11 Following the manufacturer's instructions, solution no. 1 may be reapplied two more times, using a new cotton-tipped applicator for each application.

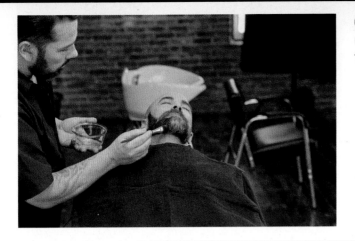

12 Use a small square-tipped brush to apply solution no. 2, taking care to apply the solution from the hairline in the direction of hair growth.

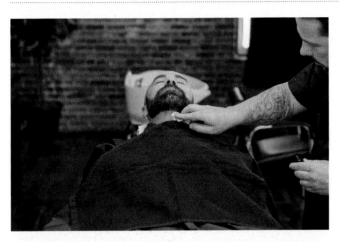

13 Remove any stains with the manufacturer's stain remover. Do not rub.

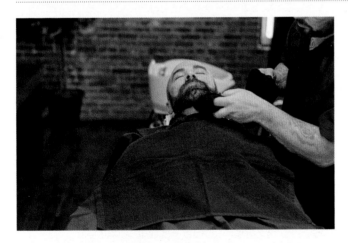

14 Wash the mustache or beard gently with soap and cool water.

15 Repeat the process if a deeper color is desired.

16 Style the mustache and/or beard as desired.

⚠ **CAUTION**
Do not use an aniline derivative tint with facial coloring. Using this may cause serious irritation and damage.

CLEAN-UP AND DISINFECTION

☐ Wash and disinfect tools and implements.

☐ Clean and disinfect work area.

☐ Dispose of single-use items. Place all used linens, towels, and capes in the laundry.

☐ Wash your hands.

☐ Record the results on the service record card.

REVIEW QUESTIONS

1. Define haircoloring and lightening.

2. List the colors of the color wheel. Identify primary, secondary, and complementary colors.

3. List four types of haircoloring products.

4. Identify the types of non-oxidation and oxidation haircolors.

5. Explain the difference between semipermanent and demipermanent haircolor products.

6. List the one haircolor ingredient that requires a patch or predisposition test.

7. List the volumes of hydrogen peroxide used in haircoloring.

8. Explain how to test for sensitivities or allergies to haircolor products.

9. What is a strand test?

10. What professional products use a single-process application? Double-process application?

11. Explain the lightening process.

12. List the products used to color beards and mustaches.

CHAPTER GLOSSARY

activator (AK-tih-vay-ter)	p. 656	an oxidizer, consisting of powdered persulfate salts, that is added to haircolors, lighteners, or hydrogen peroxide to increase the chemical action of the product
aniline derivatives (AN-ul-un DUR-ive-it-ivez)	p. 650	uncolored dye precursors that combine with hydrogen peroxide to form larger, permanent color molecules in the cortex; the ingredient that requires a patch test
base color (BAYS KUL-ur)	p. 647	the predominant tone of an existing color
cap technique	p. 663	coloring or lightening technique that involves pulling strands of hair through a perforated cap with a plastic or metal hook
color fillers (KUL-ur FIL-urz)	p. 660	equalize porosity and deposit color in one application to provide a uniform contributing pigment on pre-lightened hair
complementary colors (kahm-pluh-MEN-tur-ee KUL-urz)	p. 645	a primary and secondary color positioned opposite each other on the color wheel
contributing pigment (kun-TRIB-yoot-ing PIG-ment)	p. 644	pigment that lies under the natural hair color that is exposed when the natural color is lightened
demipermanent haircolor (DEM-ih PUR-muh-nent HAYR-KUL-ur)	p. 651	deposit-only haircolor product similar to semipermanent but longer lasting
developer (dee-VEL-up-ur)	p. 654	also known as *oxidizing agents* or *catalysts*; when mixed with an oxidation haircolor, supplies the necessary oxygen gas to develop color molecules and create a change in hair color
double-process haircoloring (DUB-ul PRAH-ses HAYR-KUL-ur-ing)	p. 663	a two-step combination of lightening and haircoloring
dye removers (DYE ree-MOOV-urz)	p. 660	products used to strip built-up color from the hair
fillers (FIL-urz)	p. 660	preparations designed to equalize porosity and/or deposit a base color in one application
foil technique (FOYL FRAWST)	p. 663	coloring or highlighting technique using foil to apply product to specific hair sections
free-form technique (FREE-form tek-NEEK)	p. 663	also known as *balyage* or baliage; the painting of a lightener on clean, styled hair
haircoloring (HAYR-KUL-ur-ing)	p. 642	industry-coined term referring to artificial haircolor products and services; the addition of color on or into the hair shaft

hair lightening (HAYR LYT-un-ing)	p. 642	the chemical process of diffusing natural or artificial pigment from the hair
highlighting (HY-lyt-ing)	p. 663	coloring or lightening some strands of hair lighter than the natural color
hue (HYOO)	p. 646	the basic name of a color
laws of color	p. 644	a system for understanding color relationships
level (LEV-ul)	p. 646	unit of measurement to identify the lightness or darkness of a color
level system (LEV-ul SIS-tum)	p. 647	system used to analyze the lightness or darkness of a hair color or color product
lighteners (LYT-un-urz)	p. 656	chemical compounds that lighten hair by dispersing and diffusing natural pigment
line of demarcation (LYN UV dee-mar-KAY-shun)	p. 653	a visible line separating colored hair from new growth
lowlighting	p. 663	coloring some strands of hair darker than the natural hair color
off-the-scalp lighteners (AWF-THE-SKALP LYT-un-urz)	p. 658	lighteners that cannot be used directly on the scalp
on-the-scalp lighteners (AWN-THE-SKALP LYT-un-urz)	p. 657	lighteners that can be used directly on the scalp
patch test (PACH TEST)	p. 662	test for identifying a possible allergy to aniline derivative products; required by the FDA 24 to 48 hours before the application of the product
permanent haircolor (PUR-muh-nent HAYR-KUL-ur)	p. 652	lighten and deposit color at the same time and in a single process because they are more alkaline than no-lift, deposit-only colors and are usually mixed with a higher-volume developer
pre-lightening (pree-LYT-tin-ing)	p. 669	the first step of a double-process haircoloring; used to lighten natural pigment
pre-softening (pree-SOF-en-ing)	p. 663	process of treating resistant hair for better color penetration
primary colors (PRY-mayr-ee KUL-urz)	p. 645	red, blue, and yellow; colors that cannot be achieved from a mixture of other colors
progressive colors (pruh-GRES-iv KUL-urz)	p. 654	haircolor products that contain compound or metallic dyes, which build up on the hair; not used professionally
retouch application (ree-TUCH ap-lih-KAY-shun)	p. 662	application of the product to new growth only
secondary colors (SEK-un-deh-ree KUL-urz)	p. 645	colors obtained by mixing equal parts of two primary colors
semipermanent haircolor (sem-ee-PUR-muh-nent HAYR-KUL-ur)	p. 667	deposit-only haircolor product formulated to last through several shampoos
single-process haircoloring SING-gul-PRAH-ses HAYR-KUL-ur-ing	p. 662	process that lightens and colors the hair in a single application
soap cap (SOHP KAP)	p. 662	equal parts of tint and a shampoo
strand test (STRAND TEST)	p. 662	the application of a coloring or lightening product to determine how the hair will react to the formula and the amount of time it will take to process
temporary colors (TEM-poh-rayr-ee KUL-urz)	p. 650	color products that last only from shampoo to shampoo
tone (TOHN)	p. 646	term used to describe the warmth or coolness of a color.
toners (TOHN-urz)	p. 671	semipermanent, demipermanent, or permanent haircolor products used primarily on pre-lightened hair to achieve pale and delicate colors
virgin application (VUR-jin ap-lih-KAY-shun)	p. 662	the first time the hair is tinted or lightened
volume (VAHL-yoom)	p. 655	the measure of the potential oxidation of varying strengths of hydrogen peroxide

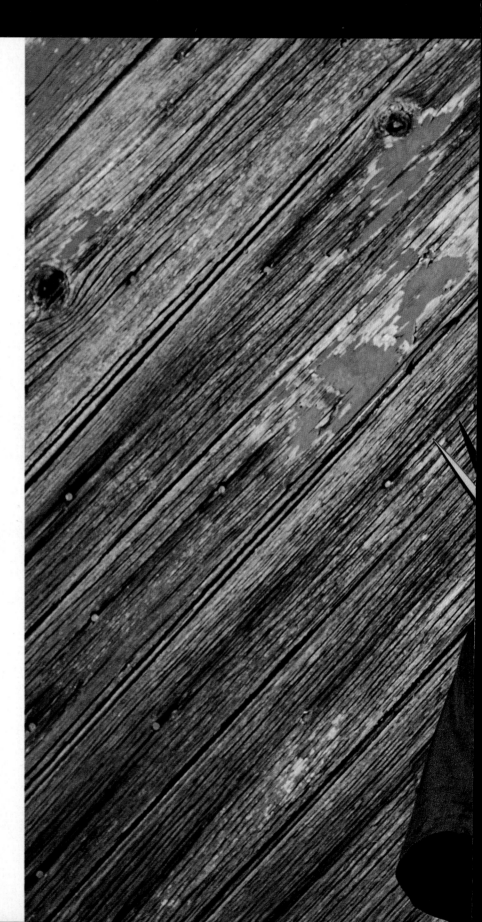

PART **5** BUSINESS SKILLS

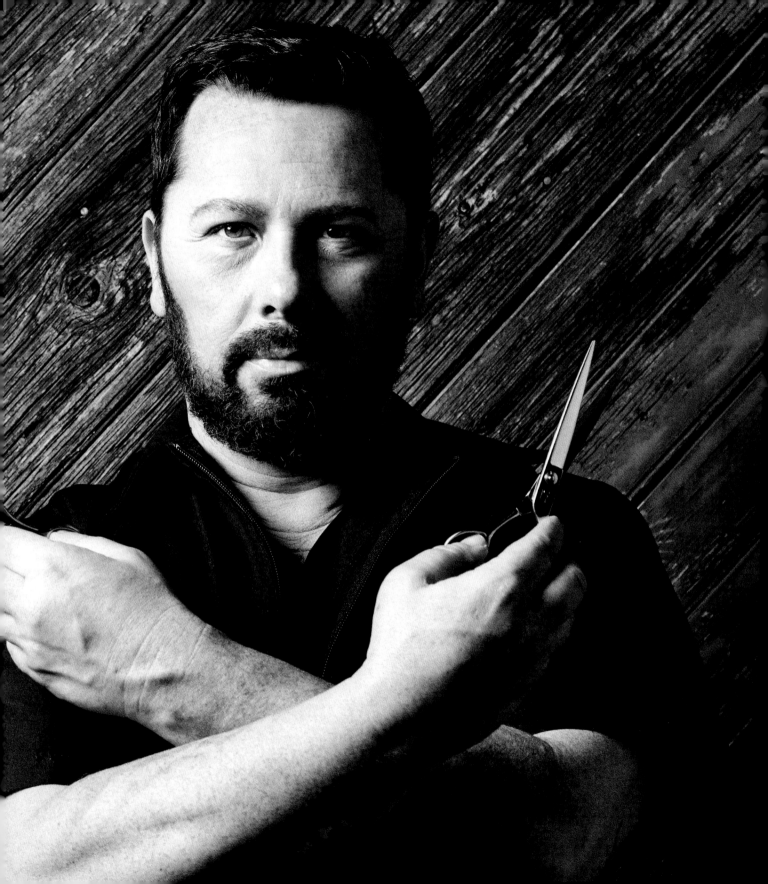

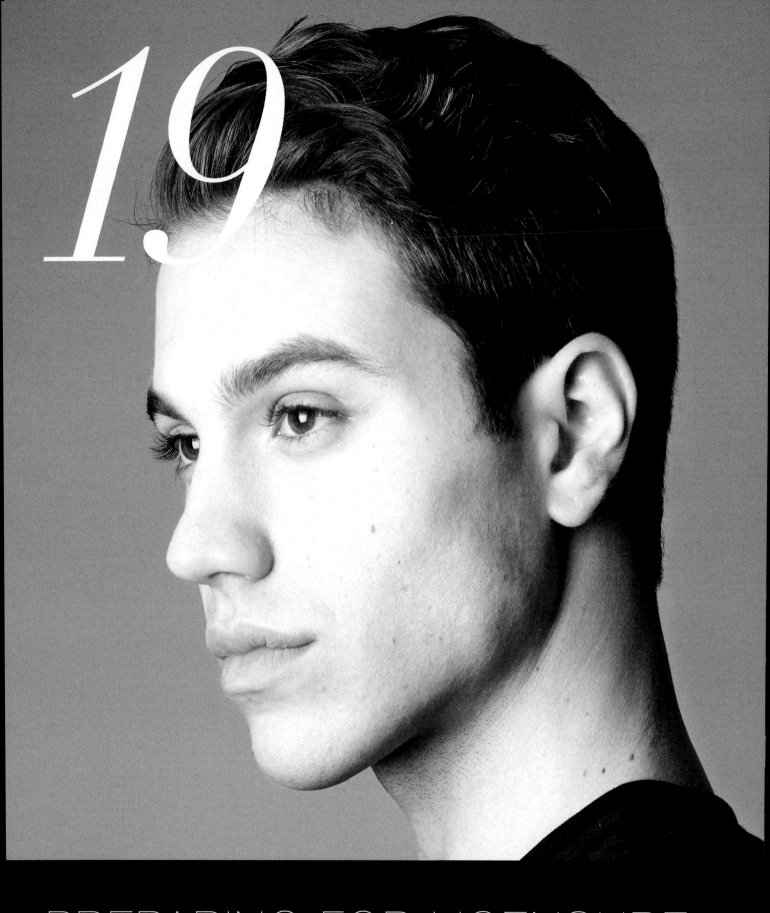

19

PREPARING FOR LICENSURE
AND EMPLOYMENT

LEARNING OBJECTIVES

After completing this chapter, you will be able to:

LO❶
Describe the process of taking and passing your state licensing examinations.

LO❷
Develop a resume and employment portfolio.

LO❸
Know how to explore the job market, research potential employers, and operate within the legal aspects of employment.

Introduction

There are plenty of great jobs out there for energetic, hardworking, and talented people. If you look at the top professionals in the barbering field, you will find they were not born successful; they achieved success through self-motivation, energy, and persistence. Like you, these barbers began their careers by enrolling in barbering school, while others may have taken the apprenticeship route. In either case, they were the ones who used their time wisely, planned for the future, went the extra mile, and drew on a reservoir of self-confidence to meet challenges. They owe their success to no one but themselves, because they created it. If you want to enjoy similar success, you must prepare for the opportunities that await you.

No matter what changes occur in the economy, there are often more jobs available for entry-level barbers than there are people to fill them. This is a tremendous advantage for you, but you must still thoroughly research the job market in your geographical area before committing to your first job (Figure 19-1). If you make the right choice, your career will be on the road to success. If you make the wrong choice, your career will not be a tragedy, but there will be unnecessary delay.

figure 19-1
Many barbering jobs are available.

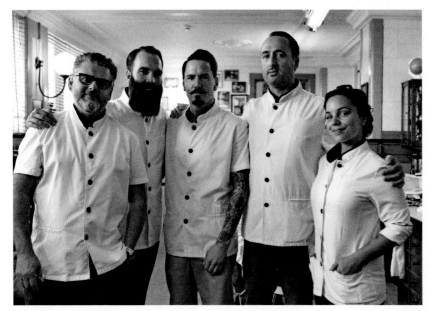

why study
PREPARING FOR LICENSURE AND EMPLOYMENT?

Barbers should study and have a thorough understanding of preparing for licensure and employment because:

> You must pass your state board exam to be licensed, and you must be licensed to be hired; therefore, preparing for licensure and passing your exam is your first step to employment success.

> A successful employment search is a job in itself, and there are many tools that can give you the edge—as well as mistakes that can cost you an interview or a job.

> The ability to pinpoint the right barbershop for you and target it as a potential employer is vital for your career success.

> Proactively preparing the right materials, such as a great resume, and practicing for interviewing give you the confidence that is needed to secure a job in a barbershop you love.

Prepare for Licensure

After reading this section, you will be able to:

LO ❶ Describe the process of taking and passing your state licensing examinations.

Before you can obtain the career position you are hoping for, you must pass your state licensing examinations (usually a written and a practical exam) and secure the required credentials from your state's licensing board by filling out an application and paying a fee. For details on fees, testing dates, requirements, and more, visit the website of your state barber board or your state's department of licensing.

Many factors affect how well you perform during that licensing examination and on tests in general. They include your physical and psychological state; your memory; your time management skills; and your academic skills, such as reading, writing, note taking, test taking, and general learning.

Of all the factors that affect your test performance, the most important is your mastery of course content. However, even if you feel that you have truly learned the material, it is still very beneficial to have strong test-taking skills. Being **test-wise** (TEST-whys) means understanding the strategies for successfully taking tests.

PREPARING FOR THE WRITTEN EXAM

A test-wise student begins to prepare for a test by practicing good study habits and time management. These habits include the following:

- Have a planned, realistic study schedule (**Figure 19-2**).
- Read content carefully and become an active studier.
- Keep well-organized notes.
- Develop a detailed vocabulary list.
- Take effective notes during class.
- Organize and review handouts.
- Review past quizzes and tests.
- Listen carefully in class for cues and clues about what could be expected on the test.

More holistic hints to keep in mind include the following:

- Make yourself mentally ready and develop a positive attitude toward taking the test.
- Get plenty of rest the night before the test.
- Dress comfortably and professionally.
- Anticipate some anxiety (feeling concerned about the test results may actually help you do better).
- Avoid cramming the night before an examination.
- Find out if your state uses computers for the written portion of the test. If so, make certain you are comfortable with computerized test taking.

figure 19-2
Studying for your exam.

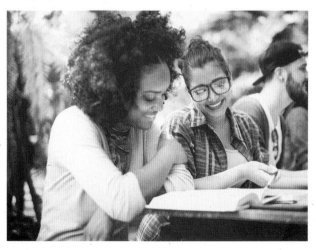

ON TEST DAY

After you have taken all the necessary steps to prepare for your test, you can adopt a number of strategies on the day of the exam that may be helpful.

- Relax and try to slow down physically.

- Review the material lightly on the day of the exam.

- If possible, do a "test drive" to the site before test day if you are unsure of the location. Some exams may be administered at your school, and some may be given in alternate locations.

- Arrive early with a self-confident attitude; be alert, calm, and ready for the challenge.

- Read all written directions and listen carefully to all verbal directions before beginning.

- If there are things you do not understand, do not hesitate to ask the examiner questions.

- Scan the entire test before beginning.

- Budget your time to ensure that you have plenty of opportunity to complete the test; do not spend too much time on any one question.

- Wear a watch so that you can monitor the time.

- Begin work as soon as possible, and mark the answers in the test carefully but quickly.

- Answer the easiest questions first to save time for the more difficult ones. Quickly scanning all the questions first may clue you in to the more difficult questions.

- Make a note of the questions you skip so that you can find them again later. If the test is administered online, you may not be given this option. Some software prevents you from moving forward without first answering all the questions on the page. Discuss this with your instructor or the testing facility before taking the exam.

- Read each question carefully to make sure that you know exactly what the question is asking and that you understand all parts of the question.

- Answer as many questions as possible. For questions that cause uncertainty, guess or estimate.

- Look over the test when you are done to ensure that you have read all questions correctly and that you have answered as many as possible.

- Make changes to answers only if there is a good reason to do so.

- Check the test carefully before turning it in. (For instance, you might have forgotten to put your name on it!)

DEDUCTIVE REASONING

Deductive reasoning (DEE-duck-tiv REAS-on-ing) is the process of reaching logical conclusions by employing logical reasoning. *Deductive reasoning* is a technique that students should learn to use for better test results. Some strategies associated with deductive reasoning include the following:

- Eliminate options that are known to be incorrect. The more incorrect answers you can eliminate, the better your chances of identifying the correct answer.

- Watch for key words or terms. Look for any qualifying conditions or statements. Keep an eye out for phrases and words such as *usually, commonly, in most instances, never,* and *always.*

- Study the **stem** (STEM), which is the basic question or problem. It often provides a clue to the correct answer. Look for a match between the stem and one of the choices.

- Watch for grammatical clues. For instance, if the last word in a stem is *an,* the answer must begin with a vowel sound rather than a consonant.

- Look at similar or related questions. They may provide clues.

- When answering essay questions, watch for words such as *compare, contrast, discuss, evaluate, analyze, define,* or *describe,* and develop your answer accordingly.

- When questions include paragraphs to read and questions to answer, read the questions first. This helps you identify the important information as you read the paragraph.

UNDERSTANDING TEST FORMATS

There are a few additional tips that all test-wise learners should know, especially with respect to the state licensing examination. Keep in mind, of course, that the most important strategy of test taking is to know your material. Beyond that, consider the following tips on the various types of question formats.

True/False

Watch for qualifying words (*all, most, some, none, always, usually, sometimes, never, little, no, equal, less, good, bad*). Absolutes (*all, none, always, never*) are generally not true (**Figure 19-3**).

- For a statement to be true, the *entire* statement must be true.

- Long statements are more likely to be true than short statements. It takes more detail to provide truthful, factual information.

Multiple Choice

- Read the entire question carefully, including all the choices.

- Look for the best answer; more than one choice may be true.

- Eliminate incorrect answers by crossing them out (if taking the test on the test form).

- When two choices are close or similar, one of them is probably right.

- When two choices are identical, both must be wrong.

- When two choices are opposites, one is probably wrong and one is probably correct, depending on the number of other choices.

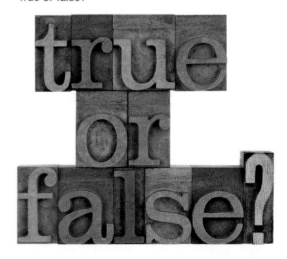

figure 19-3
True or false?

- "All of the above" and similar responses are often the correct choice.
- Pay special attention to words such as *not*, *except*, and *but*.
- Guess if you do not know the answer (provided that there is no penalty).
- The answer to one question may be in the stem of another.

Matching

- Read all items in each list before beginning.
- Check off items from the brief response list to eliminate choices.

Essays

- Organize your answer according to the cue words in the question.
- Think carefully and outline your answer before you begin writing.
- Make sure that what you write is complete, accurate, relevant to the question, well organized, and clear.

Remember that understanding test formats and effective test-taking strategies still does not take the place of having a complete understanding of the material on which you are being tested. To be successful at taking tests, you must follow the rules of effective studying and be thoroughly knowledgeable of the exam content for both the written and the practical examination.

BARBER LAW

In addition to testing basic theory concepts, the written exam often contains questions about your state's barber laws and rules. The basic concept and functions of state barber boards remain the same: to protect the health, safety, and welfare of the public as it relates to the practice of barbering. However, when it comes to studying for your exam, it is important to be aware of the specific rules and regulations of your state. For example, there may be a test question that asks, "How many members of the barber board must be licensed barbers?" The answer to this question varies from state to state, so you need to know what the configuration of the barber board is in *your* state. Other questions relating to barber laws and regulations that may vary from state to state include, but are not limited to, the following:

- Chapter or administrative code number
- Number of board members
- Configuration of the board (barbers, public members, etc.)
- Terms of office
- Definitions
- Exemptions and exceptions
- Examination prerequisites (school hours, age, service requirements, etc.)
- Reexamination requirements
- Types of licenses
- License display

- License renewal dates

- Fees and penalties

- Minimum square footage for a barbershop

- Continuing education requirements

- Prohibited acts

- Qualifications for endorsement

Obtain copies of the barber board rules and regulations and candidate information literature for your state. Review these documents thoroughly and be guided by your instructor when preparing for written exams.

THE PRACTICAL EXAM

After completing the barber school curriculum, examination candidates should be competent in their technical skills and ready for state board **practical exams** (prac-ti-cal x-amz). Although performance criteria for practical examinations vary from state to state, the basic skills or procedures that are usually evaluated are haircutting, shaving, shampooing, infection control, and possibly blowdrying or a chemical service. A fairly standard testing protocol requires candidates to demonstrate competence with the comb, shears, razor, and clippers. Safety precautions, proper draping procedures, and the safe handling of tools are also important performance standards. Review barber board rules and candidate information literature for details about what you will be tested on at the practical exam.

Practical exam preparation requires a different approach than written exams. After all, performing services is what barbering is all about, and practical exams are the best way to evaluate a person's competency in barbering techniques and safety.

Basic preparation for practical exams should always include practice on the model that you will be taking to the examination. To feel confident about your performance, you must be familiar with the model's hair texture and the haircut that you will be performing. For example, many states require a taper haircut—knowing the characteristics of your model's hair and the best techniques for cutting it will help to eliminate some nervousness and stress during the practical exam.

To be better prepared for the practical portion of the examination, follow these tips:

- Practice the correct skills required for the test as often as you can.

- Participate in mock licensing examinations, complete with timed sections.

- Familiarize yourself with the content in the examination bulletin.

- Make a list of equipment and implements you are expected to bring to the examination.

- Make certain that all equipment and implements are clean and in good working order prior to the exam.

- If allowed by the regulatory or licensing agency, observe other practical examinations prior to taking yours.

? DID YOU KNOW?

Although the extent of information made available to exam candidates varies from state to state, many states now maintain candidate information online for easy access, so be sure to review these valuable test-taking tools. In most cases, candidate information booklets or materials contain the following:

- Introduction to written and practical exams

- Examination rules

- Location and contact information for exams

- Manner of testing (computer-based, paper and pencil, etc.)

- Requirements, procedures, and reservation information for computer-based testing, if applicable

- Content overview—written (number of questions, subject areas, sample questions, etc.)

- Content overview—practical (specific procedures to be tested, possible points, etc.)

- Model requirements (practical)

- Tool and equipment requirements (practical)

- What to bring and what not to bring (written and practical)

- References used to write or develop the examinations

- Grading and scoring policies (reexamination information, notification of results, etc.)

- Administrative policies (late arrivals, cancellations, exam review process, etc.)

- As with any exam, listen carefully to the examiner's instructions, and follow them explicitly.

- Focus on your own knowledge and do not allow yourself to be concerned with what other test candidates are doing.

- Follow all infection control and safety procedures throughout the entire examination.

- Look the part. Every little bit helps; make certain your appearance is neat, clean, and professional.

Prepare for Employment

After reading this section, you will be able to:

 LO❷   Develop a resume and employment portfolio.

When you chose to enter the field of barbering, your primary goal was to find a good job after being licensed. Now you need to reaffirm that goal by reviewing a number of important questions.

- What do you really want out of a career in barbering?

- What particular areas within barbering are most interesting to you?

- What are your strongest practical skills? In what ways do you wish to use these skills?

- What personal qualities will help you have a successful career?

One way that you can answer these questions is to copy and complete the Inventory of Personal Characteristics and Technical Skills (**Figure 19-4**). After you have completed this inventory and identified the areas that need further attention, you can determine where to focus the remainder of your training. In addition, you should have a better idea of what type of establishment would best suit you for your eventual employment.

During your training, you may have the opportunity to network with various industry professionals who are invited to the school as guest speakers. Be prepared to ask them questions about what they like most and least in their current positions. Ask them for any tips they might have that will assist you in your search for the right barbershop. In addition, be sure to take advantage of your institution's in-house placement assistance program, if available, when you begin your employment search.

Your willingness to work hard is a key ingredient to your success. The commitment you make now in terms of time and effort will pay off later in the workplace, where your energy will be appreciated and rewarded. Having enthusiasm for getting the job done can be contagious, and when everyone works hard, everyone benefits. You can begin to develop this enthusiasm by establishing good work habits as a student.

figure 19-4
Inventory of personal characteristics and technical skills.

INVENTORY OF PERSONAL CHARACTERISTICS

PERSONAL CHARACTERISTIC	Exc.	Good	Avg.	Poor	Plan for improvement
Posture, Deportment, Poise					
Grooming, Personal hygiene					
Manners, Courtesy					
Communication skills					
Attitude					
Self-motivation					
Personal habits					
Responsibility					
Self-esteem, Self-confidence					
Honesty, Integrity					
Dependability					

INVENTORY OF TECHNICAL SKILLS

TECHNICAL SKILL	Exc.	Good	Avg.	Poor	Plan for improvement
Hair shaping/cutting					
Hairstyling					
Haircoloring					
Texture services, Perming					
Texture services, Relaxing					
Shaving					
Razor cutting					
Hair replacement					
Other					

After analyzing the above responses, would you hire yourself as an employee in your business? Why or why not?

State the short-term goals that you hope to accomplish in 6 to 12 months:

State the long-term goals that you hope to accomplish in 1 to 5 years:

Ask yourself: Do you want to work in a big city or small town? Would you feel more comfortable in a traditional barbershop or a trendy, upscale shop? Which clientele are you able to communicate with more effectively? Do you want to start out slowly and carefully, or do you want to jump in and throw everything into your career from the starting gate? Will you be in this industry throughout your working career, or is this just a stopover? Will you only work a 30- or 40-hour week, or will you go the extra mile when opportunities are available? How ambitious are you, and how many risks are you willing to take?

HOW TO GET THE JOB YOU WANT

There are several key personal characteristics that will not only help you get the position you want, but will also help you keep it. These characteristics include the following points:

- **Motivation.** This means having the drive to take the necessary action to achieve a goal. Although motivation can come from external sources—parental or peer pressure, for instance—the best kind of motivation is internal.

- **Integrity.** When you have integrity, you are committed to a strong code of moral and artistic values. Integrity is the compass that keeps you on course over the long haul of your career.

- **Good technical and communication skills.** While you may be better in either technical or communication skills, you must develop both to reach the level of success you desire.

- **Strong work ethic.** In the barbering business, having a strong **work ethic** (WOHRK ETH-IK) means taking pride in your work and committing yourself to consistently doing a good job for your clients, employer, and barbershop team.

- **Enthusiasm.** Try never to lose your eagerness to learn, grow, and expand your skills and knowledge.

WHERE TO WORK?

As you research employment opportunities, do not limit yourself to searching for barbershop positions alone. While the vast majority of barbers do work in barbershops, some perform services in either beauty or unisex salons—and increasing numbers find employment in hotels, resorts, and spas. Barbershops can vary significantly, not just in style, culture, and target market, but also in their organization. Many are small, independent shops in close contact with their owners and their personal tastes, while others are part of independent local chains or are regional franchise shops. All of these situations offer different opportunities that may or may not fit your needs and interests as a new barbering professional.

Another form of employment for barbers is renting a booth or chair, often within one of the locations mentioned earlier—indeed, almost half of all barbers and cosmetologists are booth renters. Booth renting is possibly the least expensive way of owning your own business, but this type of business is regulated by complex laws. The following two chapters will discuss booth rental in detail.

RESUME DEVELOPMENT

A **resume** (res-oo-MAY) is a written summary of a person's education and work experience. It tells potential employers at a glance what your achievements and accomplishments are. If you are a new graduate, you may have little or no work experience, in which case your resume should focus on skills and accomplishments. Here are some basic guidelines to follow when preparing your professional resume.

ACTIVITY

For 1 week, keep a daily record of your performance in the following areas, and ask a few of your fellow students to provide feedback as well.

- Positive attitude
- Punctuality
- Diligent practice of newly learned techniques
- Teamwork
- Professional appearance
- Regular class and clinic attendance
- Interpersonal skills
- Helping others

- Keep it simple; limit it to one page.

- Print a hard copy from your electronic version, using good-quality paper.

- Include your name, address, phone number, and e-mail address on both the resume and your cover letter.

- List recent, relevant work experience.

- List relevant education and the name of the institution from which you graduated, as well as relevant courses attended.

- List your professional skills and accomplishments.

- Focus on information that is relevant to the position you are seeking.

The average time that a potential employer will spend scanning your resume before deciding whether to grant you an interview is about 20 seconds. That means you must market yourself in such a manner that the reader will want to meet you. If your work experience has been in an unrelated field, show how the position helped you develop transferable skills. Restaurant work, for example, helps employees develop customer-service skills and learn to deal with a wide variety of clientele.

As you list former and current positions on your resume, focus on achievements instead of detailing duties and responsibilities. Accomplishment statements enlarge your basic duties and responsibilities. The best way to show concrete accomplishment is to include numbers or percentages, whenever possible. As you describe former and current positions on your resume, ask yourself the following questions:

- How many regular clients did I serve?

- How many clients did I serve weekly?

- What was my service ticket average?

- What was my client retention rate?

- What percentage of my client revenue came from retailing?

- What percentage of my client revenue came from color or texture services?

If you cannot express your accomplishment numerically, can you address which problems you solved or other results you achieved? For instance, did your office job help you develop excellent organizational skills?

This type of questioning can help you develop accomplishment statements that will interest a potential employer. There is no better time for you to achieve significant accomplishments than while you are in school. Even though your experience may be minimal, you must still present evidence of your skills and accomplishments. This may seem a difficult task at this early stage in your working career, but by closely examining your training and school clinic performance, extracurricular activities, and the full- or part-time jobs you have held, you should be able to create a good, attention-getting resume.

For example, consider the following questions:

- Did you receive any honors during your course of training?

- Were you ever selected "student of the month"?

- Did you receive special recognition for your attendance or academic progress?

- Did you win any barbering-related competitions while in school?
- What was your attendance average while in school?
- Did you work with the student body to organize any fundraisers? What were the results?

Answers to these types of questions may indicate your people skills, personal work habits, and personal commitment to success.

Since you have not yet completed your training, you have the opportunity to make some of the examples a reality before you graduate. Positive developments of this nature while you are still in school can do much to improve your resume.

The Dos and Don'ts of Resumes

You will save yourself from many problems and a lot of disappointment right from the beginning of your job search if you keep a clear idea in your mind of what to do and what not to do when it comes to creating a resume. Here are some of the dos:

- **Always put your complete contact information on your resume.** If your cell phone is your primary phone, list its number first, and add a landline if you have one.
- **Make your resume easy to read.** Use concise, clear sentences and avoid overwriting or flowery language.
- **Know your audience.** Use vocabulary and language that will be understood by your potential employer.
- **Keep your resume short.** One page is preferable.
- **Stress accomplishments.** Emphasize past accomplishments and the skills you used to achieve them.
- **Focus on career goals.** Highlight information that is relevant to your career goals and the position you are seeking.
- **Emphasize transferable skills.** The skills mastered at other jobs that can be put to use in a new position are **transferable skills** (TRANZ-fur-able SKILLZ).
- **Use action verbs.** Begin accomplishment statements with action verbs such as *achieved, coordinated, developed, increased, maintained,* and *strengthened.*
- **Make your resume neat.** A poorly structured, badly typed resume does not reflect well on you.
- **Include professional references.** Use only professional references on your resume, and make sure you give potential employers the person's title, place of employment, and telephone number.
- **Be realistic.** Remember that you are just starting out in a field that you hope will be a wonderful and fulfilling experience. Be realistic about what employers may offer to beginners.
- **Include a cover letter.** A cover letter is used to introduce yourself to the employer and to identify the position you are seeking.
- **Note any skills with new technologies.** Include software programs, web development tools, and computerized barbershop management systems.

Here are some of the don'ts for resume writing:

- **Avoid salary references.** Do not state your salary history.
- **Avoid information about why you left former positions.**
- **Do not stretch the truth.** Misinformation or untruthful statements usually catch up with you.

If you do not feel comfortable writing your own resume, consider seeking a professional resume writer or a job coach. There may be employment agencies that can help you as well; many online job search websites offer easy-to-use resume templates.

Review **Figure 19-5** that represents an achievement-oriented resume for a recent graduate of a barbering course. Remember that you are a total package, not just a resume. With determination, you will find the right position to begin your barbering career. Utilize all available resources during your resume development and job search process. For example, there is an abundance of best practice information available on the Internet, or you can communicate with an individual you may already know who has gone through the hiring process and can provide recommendations. Milady also has fantastic resources that can provide you with additional assistance when you begin your job search.

? DID YOU KNOW?

Use your creativity and artistic abilities as a barber to create a resume that represents your style and sets you apart from the competition. Do a search for contemporary resumes on Pinterest, for instance, for ideas to get started on color options, new styles, and formatting to create a unique resume.

EMPLOYMENT PORTFOLIO

As you prepare to work in the field of barbering, an employment portfolio can be extremely useful. An **employment portfolio** (EM-ploy-ment PORT-fo-lee-oh) is a collection of photos and documents that reflect your skills, accomplishments, and abilities in your chosen career field. You may choose to have a printed or an online portfolio.

While the actual contents of the portfolio vary from graduate to graduate, there are certain items that have a place in any portfolio. A powerful online or printed portfolio includes the following elements:

- Diplomas, including high school and barbering school
- Awards and achievements received while being a barbering student
- Current resume, focusing on accomplishments
- Letters of reference from former employers
- Summary of continuing education and/or copies of training certificates
- Statement of membership in industry and other professional organizations
- Statement of relevant civic affiliations and/or community activities
- Before-and-after photographs of services that you have performed on clients or models
- Brief statement about why you have chosen a career in barbering
- Any other information that you regard as relevant

When you write the statement about why you chose a career in barbering, you might include the following elements:

- A statement that explains what you love about your new career
- A description about the importance of teamwork and how you see yourself as a contributing team member

John Styles

143 Fern Circle • Anytown, USA, 12345 • 123.555.1234 • Johnstyles@barberstyles.net • StyledToTheNines.blogspot.com

Objective

My objective is to obtain an apprentice position in an upscale barbershop focusing on straight razor shaving and education so I may become a seasoned hair designer.

Education

ABC Barbering Academy, Chicago, IL, May 2016
Oak Park River Forest High School, Oak Park, IL, May 2012
Overall GPA: 3.0
Clubs: Paint/Sketch Club, Theater Club, Yearbook Committee

Qualifications

- Creative, energetic, and devoted to the barbering industry
- Hold a current Illinois barber license and have a strong knowledge of trends
- Proven ability to retain clients and was booked solid with requests during my final 4 months of training
- Served as mentor to new students of the ABC Barbering Academy

Professional Experience

Creative

- Won Regional Barber Battle: Best Fade Design
- Developed an outstanding digital portfolio of photos showing cuts, color, and beards designs
- Received Award for Best Student Fade: IBS 2014

Sales and Client Retention

- Increased chemical services to 30 percent of my clinic volume by graduation
- Named *Student of the Month* for best attendance, best attitude, highest retail, and most services delivered
- Developed and retained a school-clinic client base of over 75 individuals, both male and female

Team Spirit

- Peer resource and mentor for new students' during their first 3 months of training
- Volunteered as the "go-to person" for other students to consult regarding formal hairstyles
- Created the official Academy Facebook page, where I regularly shared new industry information

Administration

- Supervised a student "shop team" that developed a business plan for opening a 12-chair, full-service barbershop. This project earned an "A" and was recognized for thoroughness, accuracy, and creativity
- Led the reorganization of the school dispensary, allowing for increased inventory control, and the streamlining of clinic operations
- Internet savvy with abilities in Microsoft Word, Excel, and PowerPoint

References

Please see the attached page for references.

- A description of methods and ideas you would use to increase service and retail revenue (**Figure 19-6**)

figure 19-6
How will you increase retail revenue?

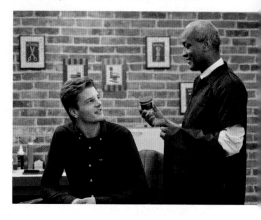

Once you have assembled your portfolio, ask yourself whether it accurately portrays you and your career skills. If it does not, identify what needs to be changed. If you are not sure, run it by a neutral party for feedback about how to make it more interesting and accurate. This kind of feedback is also useful when creating a resume. The portfolio, like the resume, should be prepared in a way that projects professionalism.

- For ease of use, you may want to separate sections of a printed portfolio with tabs.

- A bound portfolio should be easy to carry and show to potential employers and clients.

- If you are showing your online portfolio, be sure your electronic device is fully charged and the web page is bookmarked for easy retrieval.

- The photos should all have the same dimensions.

Online Portfolios

If you are technologically savvy or can hire someone to assist you, create a digital portfolio or an online showcase of your work. However, do not expect potential employers to take the extra time to visit a website or view a DVD. Bring along a printed copy of everything you want the employer to see.

Make it a habit to take photos of your work for your portfolio. Bring in models and practice the latest haircut, styling, or coloring techniques. Take compelling before-and-after photos to show your ability to transform your clients. For ideas, browse the Internet by doing a Google image search for *barbering portfolios*. Showcase your versatility by providing photos of various haircuts so your potential employer will gain a sense of your abilities.

There are many options you can use to create an online or electronic version of your portfolio. You can simply save your photos and scanned documents on a DVD, or you can easily create an online portfolio for free by utilizing a blog. Websites such as blogger.com or wordpress.com offer free blog sites that can easily serve as your online portfolio.

Do your homework, research carefully, and think long term. You, your portfolio, and web address want to be around for years to come. If creating a website is currently not in your budget, then create a "Fan Page" on Facebook to showcase your work. Remember: Your fan page is your business page and a representation of your professional image.

TARGETING THE ESTABLISHMENT

One of the most important steps in the process of job hunting is narrowing your search. Listed here are some points to keep in mind when targeting potential employers.

- Accept that your first job will probably not be your dream job. Few people are so fortunate.

- Do not wait until graduation to begin your search. If you do, you may be tempted to take the first offer you receive instead of carefully investigating all possibilities before making a decision.

figure 19-7
What type of shop do you see yourself working in?

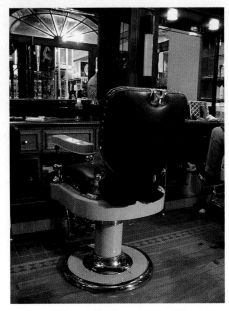

- Locate a barbershop that serves the type of clients you wish to serve. Finding a good fit with the clients and staff is critical from the outset of your career (**Figure 19-7**).

- Make a list of your area barbershops. The Internet will be your best source for this. If you are considering relocating to another area, go to anywho.com for a complete listing of businesses in every state, or find top barbershops in any region or city at citysearch.com. You may also want to do a Google search for your area of interest and city, using key words such as *barbershop Austin.*

- Watch for barbershops that advertise locally, to get a feel for the market each barbershop is targeting. Then check the barbershop's website or see if it is part of a social network, such as Facebook.

- Check out websites and social networking sites for various types of barbershops. If you contact them, do not waste their time. Get right to the point that you are a student, and ask specific questions about the profession.

- Keep the barbershop's culture in mind. Do the barbers dress like you? Are the clients in different age groups or just one? Look for the barbershop that will be best for you and your goals.

FIELD RESEARCH

A great way to find out about potential jobs is to network. Actually get out there; visit barbershops; and talk to shop owners, managers, educators, and barbers. Whether your first contact is online, in person, or on the phone, sooner or later you will want to arrange a face-to-face meeting or an exploratory visit to the barbershop. To set up a shop visit, consider the following:

- If you call, use your best telephone manner; speak with confidence and self-assurance. If you e-mail, be brief, and check spelling and punctuation. Do not text message barbershop owners or managers, unless they request that you do so.

- Explain that you are preparing to graduate from school in barbering, that you are researching the market for potential positions, and that you have a few quick questions.

- If the person is receptive, ask whether the barbershop is in need of any new barbers, and how many the barbershop currently employs.

- Ask if you can make an appointment to visit the barbershop to observe sometime during the next few weeks. If the shop representative is agreeable, be on time! When timing allows, confirm the appointment the day before, via e-mail.

Remember that a rejection is not a negative reflection on you. Many professionals are too busy to make time for this kind of networking. The good news is that you are bound to discover many genuinely kind people who remember what it was like when they started out and who are willing to devote a bit of their time to help others who are beginning their careers.

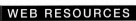

WEB RESOURCES

To start looking for a barbering job, begin at these websites:

Industry specific:
- barber-license.com

General:
- careerbuilder.com
- resumeedge.com
- craigslist.org
- jobbank.com
- jobs.net
- monster.com
- snagajob.com

© iStock.com/CraigPJ.

THE BARBERSHOP VISIT

When you visit the barbershop, take along a checklist to ensure that you observe all the key areas that might ultimately affect your decision making. The checklist will be similar to the one used for field trips that you probably have taken to area barbershops while in school. Keep the checklist on file for future reference so that you can make informed comparisons among establishments (Figure 19-8).

After your visit, always remember to follow up with a handwritten note or e-mail, thanking the barbershop representative for his time (Figure 19-10). Do this even if you did not like the barbershop and would never consider working there (Figure 19-10).

Never burn your bridges. Instead, build a network of contacts who have a favorable opinion of you.

figure 19-8
Barbershop visit checklist.

BARBERSHOP VISIT CHECKLIST

When you visit a barbershop, observe the following areas and rate them from 1 to 5, with 5 considered being the best.

_____ **BARBERSHOP IMAGE:** Is the barbershop's image consistent and appropriate for your interests? Is the image pleasing and inviting? What is the decor and arrangement? If you are not comfortable or if you find it unattractive, mark the barbershop off your list of employment possibilities.

_____ **PROFESSIONALISM:** Do the employees present the appropriate professional appearance and behavior? Do they give their clients the appropriate levels of attention and personal service, or do they act as if work is their time to socialize?

_____ **MANAGEMENT:** Does the barbershop show signs of being well managed? Is the phone answered promptly with professional telephone skills? Is the mood of the barbershop positive? Does everyone appear to work as a team?

_____ **CLIENT SERVICE:** Are clients greeted promptly and warmly when they enter the barbershop? Are they kept informed of the status of their appointment? Are they offered a magazine or beverage while they wait? Is there a comfortable reception area?

_____ **PRICES:** Compare price for value. Are clients getting their money's worth? Do they pay the same price in one barbershop but get better service and attention in another? If possible, take home barbershop brochures and price lists.

_____ **RETAIL:** Is there a well-stocked retail display offering clients a variety of product lines and a range of prices? Do the barbers and receptionist (if applicable) promote retail sales?

_____ **IN-SHOP MARKETING:** Are there posters or promotions throughout the barbershop? If so, are they professionally made, and do they reflect contemporary styles?

_____ **SERVICES:** Make a list of all services offered by each barbershop and the product lines they carry. This will help you decide what earning potential the barbers have in each barbershop.

BARBERSHOP NAME: _____

BARBERSHOP MANAGER: _____

figure 19-9
Sample thank-you note.

Dear Ms. (or Mr.) _____,

I appreciate having had the opportunity to observe your barbershop in operation last Friday. Thank you for the time you and your staff gave me. I was impressed by the efficient and courteous manner in which your barbers served their clients. The atmosphere was pleasant, and the mood was positive. Should you ever have an opening for a professional with my skills and training, I would welcome the opportunity to apply. You can contact me at the e-mail address and phone number listed below. I hope we will meet again soon.

Sincerely,

(your name, address, telephone, e-mail address)

figure 19-10
Sample thank-you note to a barbershop where you do not expect to seek employment.

Dear Ms. (or Mr.) _____,

I appreciate having had the opportunity to observe your barbershop in operation last Friday. I know how busy you and all your staff are, and I want to thank you for the time that you gave me. I hope my presence didn't interfere with the flow of your operations too much. I certainly appreciate the courtesies that were extended to me by you and your staff. I wish you and your barbershop continued success.

Sincerely,

(your name)

Arrange for a Job Interview

After reading this section, you will be able to:

LO③ Know how to explore the job market, research potential employers, and operate within the legal aspects of employment.

After you have graduated and completed the first two steps in the process of securing employment—targeting and observing barbershops—you are ready to pursue employment in earnest. The next step is to contact the establishments that you are most interested in by sending them a resume and requesting an interview. Choosing a barbershop that is the best match to your skills will increase your chances of success.

figure 19-11
Sample cover letter.

Your Name
Your Address
Your Phone Number

Ms. (or Mr.) _____
Barbershop Name
Barbershop Address

Dear Ms. (or Mr.) _____,

We met in August when you allowed me to observe your barbershop and staff while I was still in training. Since that time, I have graduated and have received my license. I have enclosed my resume for your review and consideration.

I would appreciate the opportunity to meet with you and discuss either current or future career opportunities at your barbershop. I was extremely impressed with your staff and business, and I would like to share with you how my skills and training might add to your barbershop success.

I look forward to meeting with you again soon.

Sincerely,
(your name)

Many barbershops have websites with special employment areas; others post position openings on barbering- or job-related websites. Follow instructions exactly for filling out forms or sending resumes (some barbershops do not want attachments, such as letters of recommendation or digital portfolios sent with the resumes). In rare instances, you may need to send a resume and cover letter by traditional snail mail (**Figure 19-11**). Comply with the barbershop's guidelines.

Mark your calendar to remind yourself to make a follow-up contact. A week after submitting your resume is generally sufficient. When you call or e-mail, try to schedule an interview appointment. Keep in mind that some barbershops may not have openings and may not be granting interviews. When this is the case, send a resume, if you have not already, and ask the barbershop to keep it on file should an opening arise in the future. Be sure to thank your contacts for their time and consideration.

INTERVIEW PREPARATION

When preparing for an interview, make sure that you have all the necessary information and materials in place, including the following items.

Identification

- Social Security number
- Driver's license number

- Names, mailing addresses, e-mail addresses, and phone numbers of former employers
- Name, phone number, and e-mail address of the nearest relative not living with you

Interview Wardrobe

Your appearance is crucial, especially since you are applying for a position in the barbering industry. It is recommended that you obtain one or two interview outfits. You may be requested to return for a second interview, hence the need for the second outfit. Consider the following points:

- Is the outfit appropriate for the position?

- Is it both fashionable and flattering, and similar to what the barbershop's current barbers wear? (If you have not visited the barbershop, walk by or check out its website to gauge its style culture so that you can dress accordingly.)

- Are your accessories both fashionable and functional (e.g., not noisy or so large that they would interfere with performing services)?

- Are your nails well groomed?

- Is your hairstyle current? Does it flatter your face and your overall style?

- Is your makeup current? Does it flatter your face and your overall style?

- Are you clean shaven? If not, is your beard properly trimmed?

- Is your perfume or cologne subtle (or nonexistent)?

- Are you carrying either a handbag or a briefcase, but not both?

Supporting Materials

- **Resume.** Even if you have already sent a resume, take another copy with you.

- **Facts and figures.** Have ready a list of names and dates of former employment, education, and references.

- **Employment portfolio.** Even if you have just two photos in your portfolio and they are pictures of haircuts you did for friends, bring them along.

Review and Prepare for Anticipated Interview Questions

Certain questions are typically asked during an interview. Being familiar with these questions allows you to reflect on your answers ahead of time. You might even consider role-playing an interview situation with friends, family, or fellow students. Typical questions include the following:

- Why do you want to work here?

- What did you like best about your training?

- Are you punctual and regular in attendance?

- Will your school director or instructor confirm this?

- What skills do you feel are your strongest?

HERE'S A TIP

When you contact a barbershop to make an appointment for an interview, you may be told that they are not currently hiring but would be happy to conduct an interview for future reference. Never think that this would be a waste of time.

Take advantage of the opportunity. Not only will it give you valuable interview experience, but it may also provide opportunities that you would otherwise miss.

- In which areas do you consider yourself to be less strong?

- Are you a team player? Please explain.

- Do you consider yourself flexible? Please explain.

- What are your career goals?

- What days and hours are you available for work?

- Are there any obstacles that would prevent you from keeping your commitment to full-time employment? Please explain.

- What assets do you believe that you would bring to this barbershop and this position?

- What computer skills do you have?

- How would you handle a problem client?

- How do you feel about retailing?

- Would you be willing to attend our company's training program?

- Would you please describe ways that you provide excellent customer service?

- What consultation questions might you ask a client?

- Are you prepared to train for a year before you have your own clients?

Be Prepared to Perform a Service

Some barbershops require applicants to perform a service in their chosen discipline as part of the interview, and many of these barbershops require that you bring your own model. Be sure to confirm whether this is a requirement. If it is, make sure that your model is appropriately dressed and properly prepared for the experience and that you bring the necessary supplies, products, and tools to demonstrate your skills.

THE INTERVIEW

On the day of the interview, try to make sure that nothing occurs that will keep you from completing the interview successfully. You should practice the following behaviors in connection with the interview itself.

- Always be on time or, better yet, early. If you are unsure of the location, find it the day before, so there will be no reason for delays.

- Turn off your cell phone! Do not arrive with earbuds or a hands-free cell phone device in your ear.

- Project a warm, friendly smile. Smiling is the universal language.

- Walk, sit, and stand with good posture.

- Be polite and courteous.

- Do not sit until you are asked to do so or until it is obvious that you are expected to do so.

- Never smoke or chew gum, even if one or the other is offered to you.

- Do not come to an interview with a cup of coffee, a soft drink, snacks, or anything else to eat or drink.

<table>
<tr><td>? DID YOU KNOW?</td></tr>
<tr><td>It can be difficult for new graduates to afford the two or three outfits necessary to project a confident and professional image when going out into the workplace. Fortunately, several nonprofit organizations have been formed to address this need. These organizations receive donations of clean clothes in good repair from individuals and manufacturers. The items are then passed along to people who need them. For more information, visit Wardrobe for Opportunity at wardrobe.org and Dress for Success at dressfor-success.org.</td></tr>
</table>

ACTIVITY

Find a partner among your fellow students and role-play the employment interview. Each of you can take turns as the applicant and the employer. After each session, conduct a brief discussion regarding how it went; that is, what worked and what did not work. Discuss how your performance could be improved. Bear in mind that a role-playing activity will never predict exactly what will occur in a real interview. However, the process will help prepare you for the interview and boost your confidence.

- Never lean on or touch the interviewer's desk. Some people do not like their personal space broached without an invitation.

- Try to project a positive first impression by appearing as confident and relaxed as you can be.

- Speak clearly. The interviewer must be able to hear and understand you.

- Answer questions honestly. Think about the question and answer carefully. Do not speak before you are ready, and not for more than 2 minutes at a time.

- Never criticize former employers.

- Always remember to thank the interviewer at the end of the interview.

Another critical part of the interview comes when you are invited to ask the interviewer questions of your own. You should think about those questions ahead of time and bring a list if necessary. Doing so will show that you are organized and prepared. Some questions that you might consider include the following:

- What are you looking for in a barber?

- Is there a job description? May I review it?

- Is there a shop manual? May I review it?

- How does the barbershop promote itself?

- How long do barbers typically work here?

- Are employees encouraged to grow in skills and responsibility? How so?

- Does the barbershop offer continuing education opportunities?

- What does your training program involve?

- Is there room for advancement? If so, what are the requirements for promotion?

- What key benefits does the barbershop offer, such as advanced training and medical insurance?

- What outside and community activities is the barbershop involved in?

- What is the form of compensation?

- When will the position be filled?

- May I contact you in a week regarding your decision?

- May I have a tour of the barbershop?

Do not feel that you have to ask all of your questions. The point is to create as much of a dialogue as possible. Be aware of the interviewer's reactions and make note of when you have asked enough questions. By obtaining the answers to at least some of your questions, you can compare the information you have gathered about other barbershops and choose the one that offers the best package of income and career development.

Remember to follow up the interview with a thank-you note or e-mail. It should simply thank the interviewer for the time she spent with you.

Close with a positive statement that you want the job (if you do). If the interviewer's decision comes down to two or three possibilities, the one expressing the most desire may be offered the position. Also, if the interviewer suggests that you call to learn about the employment decision, then by all means do so.

LEGAL ASPECTS OF THE EMPLOYMENT INTERVIEW

Over the years, a number of legal issues have arisen about questions that may or may not be included in an employment application or interview, including ones that involve race/ethnicity, religion, and national origin; marital status; sexual orientation; and if you have children. Generally, there should be no questions in any of these categories. Additional categories of appropriate and inappropriate questions are listed here.

- **Age or date of birth.** It is permissible to ask the age if the applicant is younger than 18. Otherwise, age should not be relevant in most hiring decisions; therefore, date-of-birth questions prior to employment are improper.

- **Disabilities or physical traits.** The Americans with Disabilities Act prohibits general inquiries about health problems, disabilities, and medical conditions.

- **Drug use or smoking.** Questions regarding drug or tobacco use are permitted. In fact, the employer may obtain the applicant's agreement to be bound by the employer's drug and smoking policies and to submit to drug testing.

- **Citizenship.** Employers are not allowed to discriminate because an applicant is not a U.S. citizen. However, employers can request to see a Green Card or work permit.

It is important to recognize that not all potential employers understand that they may be asking improper or illegal questions. If you are asked such questions, you might politely respond that you believe the question is irrelevant to the position you are seeking and that you would like to focus on your qualities and skills that are suited to the job and the mission of the establishment.

EMPLOYEE CONTRACTS

Employers can legally require you to sign contracts as a condition of employment. In the barbering business, the most common ones are noncompete and confidentiality agreements. Barbershop owners often invest a great deal in training, and they do not want you taking all that education to a competing barbershop across the street once your apprenticeship or initial training is complete. Noncompete agreements address this issue, prohibiting you from seeking employment within a given time period and

> **? DID YOU KNOW?**
> These are examples of illegal questions as compared to legal questions.
>
> **Illegal Questions**
> - How old are you?
> - Please describe your medical history.
> - Are you a U.S. citizen?
> - What is your native language?
>
> **Legal Questions**
> - Are you over the age of 18?
> - Are you physically able to perform this job?
> - Are you authorized to work in the United States?
> - In which languages are you fluent?

geographic area after you leave employment with them. Often, noncompete agreements also forbid employees from gathering and keeping client records, including client phone numbers. A contract cannot interfere with your right to work, and as a result, these contracts must be very specific and are sometimes controversial. If you are presented with any contract, take it home, read it, and make certain you completely understand it. If you do not completely understand any part of it, consult with a labor-law attorney before signing it.

THE EMPLOYMENT APPLICATION

Any time that you are applying for any position, you will be required to complete an application, even if your resume already contains much of the requested information. Your resume and the list you have prepared prior to the interview will assist you in completing the application quickly and accurately.

DOING IT RIGHT

You are ready to set out on your exciting new career as a professional barber. The right way to proceed is by learning important study and test-taking skills early and applying them consistently.

Think ahead to your employment opportunities and use your time in school to develop a record of interesting, noteworthy activities that will make your resume more exciting. When you compile a history that shows how you have achieved your goals, your confidence will grow.

- Always take one step at a time. Be sure to take the helpful preliminary steps that we have discussed when preparing for employment.

- Develop a dynamic portfolio. Keep your materials, information, and questions organized to ensure a high-impact interview.

Once you are employed, take the necessary steps to learn all that you can about your new position and the establishment you will be serving. Read all you can about the industry. Attend trade shows and take advantage of as much continuing education as you can manage. Become an active participant in efforts to make the barbering industry even better.

As you transition into your new career as a barbering professional, let us at Milady continue the journey with you. Be sure to visit the MiladyPro.com website. In addition to helping you prepare for your State Board Exam, MiladyPro.com offers access to materials designed to help you hit the ground running and grow your skill set, assuring long-term success no matter where you may take your career.

REVIEW QUESTIONS

1 What are three habits of test-wise students?

2 What is *deductive reasoning*?

3 What are the four most common testing formats?

4 What basic skills or procedures are usually evaluated during the practical examination?

5 Where can a barber expect to work?

6 What is a *resume*?

7 What are the skills mastered at other jobs that can be put to use in a new position?

8 What items should be included in an employment portfolio?

9 What are the three things you should bring to an interview?

10 What are the three questions that are illegal to be asked when interviewing for a job?

CHAPTER GLOSSARY

deductive reasoning (DEE-duck-tiv REAS-on-ing)	p. 710	the process of reaching logical conclusions by employing logical reasoning
employment portfolio (EM-ploy-ment PORT-fo-lee-oh)	p. 719	a collection, usually bound, of photos and documents that reflect your skills, accomplishments, and abilities in your chosen career field
practical exams (prac-ti-cal x-amz)	p. 713	hands-on testing on a live model or mannequin
resume (res-oo-MAY)	p. 716	written summary of a person's education and work experience
stem (STEM)	p. 711	the basic question or problem
test-wise (TEST-whys)	p. 709	understanding the strategies for successful test taking
transferable skills (TRANZ-fur-able SKILLZ)	p. 718	skills mastered at other jobs that can be put to use in a new position
work ethic (WOHRK ETH-IK)	p. 716	taking pride in your work and committing yourself to consistently doing a good job for your clients, employer, and barbershop team

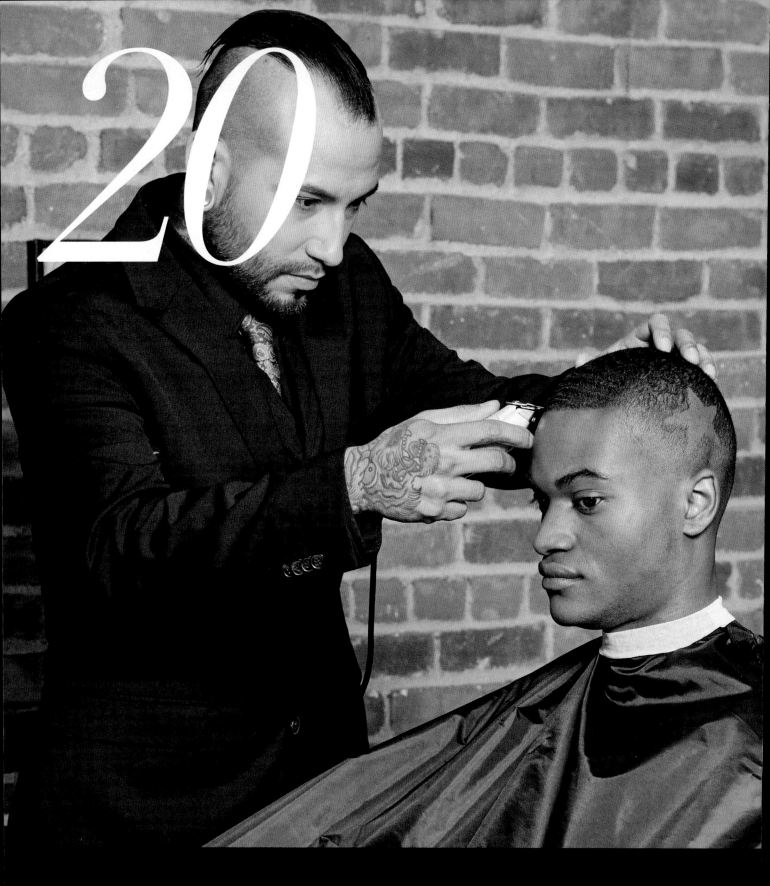

20

WORKING BEHIND
THE CHAIR

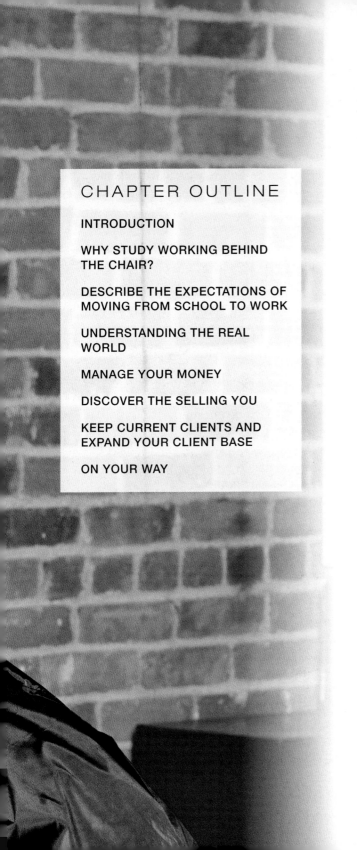

LEARNING OBJECTIVES

After completing this chapter, you will be able to:

LO❶
Describe what is expected of a new employee and what this means in terms of your everyday behavior.

LO❷
List the habits of a good barbershop team player.

LO❸
Describe three different ways in which barbers are compensated.

LO❹
Determine the best way to record your tips and make additional income.

LO❺
Explain the principles of selling products and services in the barbershop.

LO❻
List the most effective ways to build a client base.

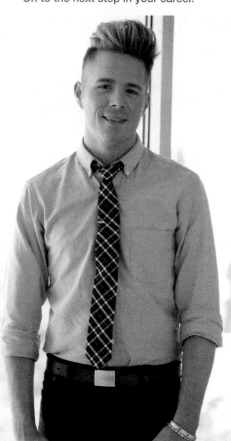

figure 20-1
On to the next step in your career.

Introduction

Congratulations! You have worked hard in barbering school, passed your state's licensing exam, and been offered your first job in the field. Now, more than ever, you need to prioritize your goals and commit to personal rules of conduct and behavior. These goals and rules should guide you throughout your career. If you let them do so, you can expect to always have work and to enjoy all the freedom that your chosen profession can offer (**Figure 20-1**).

why study
WORKING BEHIND THE CHAIR?

Barbers should study and have a thorough understanding of working behind the chair because:

> Working in a barbershop requires each staff member to belong to and work as a team member of the shop. Learning to do so is an important aspect of being successful in the barbershop environment.

> There are a variety of ways that a barbershop may compensate employees. Being familiar with each way and knowing how it works will help you determine if the compensation system at a particular shop can work for you and what to expect from it.

> Once you are working as a barbering professional, you will have financial obligations and responsibilities, so learning the basics of financial management while you are building your clientele and business is invaluable.

> As you build your clientele and settle into your professional life, there will be opportunities for you to use a variety of techniques for increasing your income, such as retailing and upselling services. Knowing and using these techniques will help you promote yourself, build a loyal client base, and create a sound financial future for yourself.

Describe the Expectations of Moving from School to Work

After reading this section, you will be able to:

 LO ❶ Describe what is expected of a new employee and what this means in terms of your everyday behavior.

Making the transition from school to work can be difficult. While you may be thrilled to have a job, working for a paycheck brings with it a number of duties and responsibilities that you may not have considered.

Barbering school is a forgiving environment. You are given the chance to do a certain procedure over and over again until you get it right. Making and fixing mistakes is an accepted part of the process, and your instructors

figure 20-2
(a) Time to transition from your school life (b) to your life behind the chair.

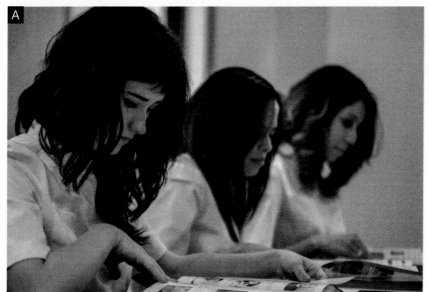

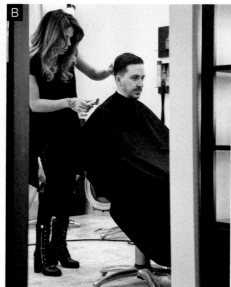

and mentors are there to help you. Schedules may be adjusted if necessary, and you are given some leeway in the matter of juggling your personal life with the demands of your schooling (**Figure 20-2a** and **20-2b**).

When you work in a barbershop, however, you will be expected to put the needs of the barbershop and its clients ahead of your own. This means that you must be on time for every scheduled shift and be prepared to perform whatever services or functions are required of you, regardless of what is happening in your personal life. For example, if someone comes to you with tickets for a concert on a day when you are scheduled to work, you cannot just take the day off. To do so would definitely inconvenience your clients, who might even decide not to return to the barbershop. It could also burden your coworkers, who might feel resentful if they are asked to take on your appointments.

Understanding the Real World

After reading this section, you will be able to:

LO❷ List the habits of a good barbershop team player.

LO❸ Describe three different ways in which barbers are compensated.

Many barbering graduates believe they should be rewarded with a high-paying job, performing only the kinds of services they wish to do, as soon as they graduate from school. It does not work out that way for most people. In a job, you may be asked to do work or perform services that are not your first choice. The good news is that when you are really working in the trenches, you are learning every moment, and there is no substitute for that kind of experience.

What is important is to determine which type of position is right for you by being honest with yourself as you evaluate your skills. If you need help and direction in sorting out the issues around the various workplaces you are considering, ask your instructor for advice. If you choose a barbershop carefully, based on its culture and the type of shop and benefits you prefer, you will be off to a great start.

THRIVING IN A SERVICE PROFESSION

The first reality when you are in a service business is that your career revolves around serving your clients. There will always be some people who do not treat others with respect; however, the majority of people you encounter will truly appreciate the work you perform for them. They will look forward to seeing you, and they will show their appreciation for your hard work with their loyalty.

Here are some points that will help guide you as you meet your clients' needs:

- **Put others first.** You will have to quickly get used to putting your own feelings or desires aside and putting the needs of the barbershop and the client first. This means performing what is expected of you, unless you are physically unable to do so.

- **Be true to your word.** Choose your words carefully and honestly. Be someone who can be counted on to tell the truth and to do what you say you will do.

- **Be punctual.** Scheduling is central to the barbering business. Getting to work on time shows respect not only for your clients but also for your coworkers who will have to handle your clients if you are late.

- **Be a problem solver.** No job or situation comes without its share of problems. Be someone who recognizes problems promptly and finds ways to resolve them constructively.

- **Be a lifelong learner.** Valued employees continue to learn throughout their careers. Thinking that you are done learning once you are out of school is immature and limiting. Your career might go in all kinds of interesting directions, depending on what new things you learn. This applies to every aspect of your life. Besides learning new technical skills, you should continue gaining more insight into your own behavior and better ways to deal with people, problems, and issues.

BARBERSHOP TEAMWORK

Working in a barbershop requires that you practice and perfect your people skills. A barbershop is very much a team environment (**Figure 20-3**).

figure 20-3
The barbering team.

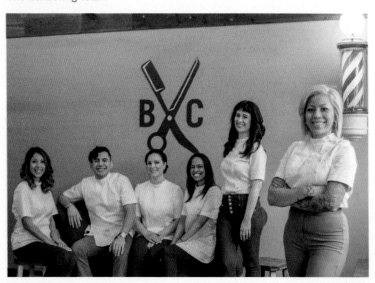

Photography by Jason Lott. Lilly Benitez, Founder of Blade Craft Barber Academy.

To become a good team player, you should do your best to practice the following workplace principles:

- **Strive to help.** Be concerned not only with your own success, but also with the success of others. Be willing to help a teammate by staying a little later or coming in a little earlier.

- **Pitch in.** Be willing to help with whatever needs to be done in the barbershop—from folding towels to making appointments—when you are not busy servicing clients.

- **Share your knowledge.** Be willing to share what you know. This will make you a respected member of any team. At the same time, be willing to learn from your coworkers by listening to their perspectives and techniques.

- **Remain positive.** Resist the temptation to give in to maliciousness and gossip.

- **Become a relationship builder.** Just as there are different kinds of people in the world, there are different types of relationships within the barbering world. You do not have to be someone's best friend to build a good working relationship with that person.

- **Be willing to resolve conflicts.** The most difficult part of being in a relationship is when conflict arises. A real teammate is someone who knows that conflict and tension are bad for the people who are in it, those who are around it, and the barbershop as a whole. Nevertheless, conflict is a natural part of life. If you can work constructively toward resolving conflict, you will always be a valued member of the team. If you do have a conflict, discuss it with the individual, not with others in the shop.

- **Be willing to be subordinate.** No one starts at the top. Keep in mind that beginners almost always start out lower down in the pecking order.

- **Be sincerely loyal.** Loyalty is vital to the workings of a barbershop. Barbers need to be loyal to the shop and its management. Management needs to be loyal to the staff and clients. Ideally, clients will be loyal to the employee and the barbershop. As you work on all the team-building characteristics, you will start to feel a strong sense of loyalty to your shop (**Figure 20-4**).

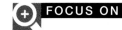

FOCUS ON

Being a Good Teammate

While each individual may be concerned with getting ahead and being successful, a good teammate knows that no one can be successful alone. You will be truly successful if your entire barbershop is successful!

THE JOB DESCRIPTION

When you take a job, you will be expected to behave appropriately, perform services asked of you, and conduct your business professionally. To do this to the best of your abilities, you should be given a **job description** (JOHB des-CRIP-shun), a document that outlines all the duties and responsibilities of a particular position in a barbershop. Many shops have a preprinted job description available. If you find yourself at a shop that does

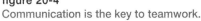

figure 20-4
Communication is the key to teamwork.

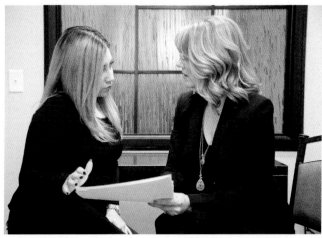

not use job descriptions, you may want to write one for yourself. You can then present it to your shop manager for review, to ensure that you both have a good understanding of what is expected of you.

Once you have your job description, be sure you understand it. While reading it over, make notes and jot down questions you want to ask your manager. When you assume your new position, you are agreeing to do everything as it is written down in the job description. If you are unclear about something or need more information, it is your responsibility to ask.

Remember, you will be expected to fulfill all of the functions listed in the job description. How well you fulfill these duties will influence your future at the barbershop, as well as your financial rewards.

In crafting a job description, the best barbershops cover all the bases. They outline not only the employees' duties and responsibilities but also the attitudes that they expect their employees to have and the opportunities that are available to them. Like the shops that generate them, job descriptions come in all sizes and shapes, and they feature a variety of requirements, benefits, and incentives.

EMPLOYMENT CLASSIFICATIONS

When you assess a job offer, your first concern will probably be the compensation for your work. The way you will be paid for services performed in the barbershop will depend primarily on your employment status as an employee, independent contractor, or booth renter. Most barbers work as independent contractors or booth renters, although employee positions are available in some shops and salons. The U.S. Internal Revenue Service (IRS) categorizes independent contractors and booth renters as self-employed workers; these worker categories have certain required criteria and restrictions that are used to separate them from being designated as an employee for tax liability purposes.

Employee Status

As an **employee** (EM-ploy-ee), you might work on a salary, commission, or salary-plus-commission basis. You can expect to be told when and where to work in the form of required work hours, how to perform the job, and whether or not a uniform is required. Your clients will more than likely be booked for you, and you probably will not handle any money for services other than your tips. Training may be offered or required, depending on the needs of the business, and some establishments may provide insurance or vacation benefits.

As an employee, your employer is responsible for withholding income and Medicare taxes, paying a portion of your Social Security tax, paying unemployment taxes, and providing you with a Form W-2, Wage and Tax Statement. Your responsibilities as an employee include reporting all wages, tips of $20.00 or more per month, commissions for product sales, and filing your personal income tax statement.

Independent Contractor Status

As an **independent contractor** (IN-dee-pen-dant CON-tract-uhr), you may rent a chair or work for a percentage of the proceeds of services you perform, but you must apply for a tax identification number and provide your own business insurance coverage. You are also responsible for your own income and self-employment taxes and should receive a Form 1099-MISC from the shop owner when you earn over $600.00 a year. Although business expenses may be deducted, all income and tips are to be reported and estimated quarterly tax payments may be required. To prove that you are working as an independent contractor for tax purposes, there must be a written agreement or contract between you and the shop owner. This agreement must include how you will be compensated, your responsibilities, what is included in the chair rental, and an end date for your work, along with additional stipulations as required. When set up properly, independent contractor agreements may be renewable. You are recommended to seek the guidance of an accountant to ensure the agreement conforms to current federal tax laws.

Booth Renter Status

In a **booth rental** (BOO-th ren-tal) arrangement, you are actually setting up a small business. This requires a contract with the shop owner, appropriate business licenses, insurance, a tax ID number, and tax designation as a booth renter or independent businessperson. As a booth renter, you lease space from the shop owner and are solely responsible for your own clientele, supplies, record keeping, workstation maintenance, and accounting. You handle all money transactions and are responsible for booking your own appointments. Usually, the only obligation to the shop owner is the weekly or monthly rent. You should be given a key to the establishment and be able to set your own hours and schedule.

One of the main advantages of booth rental is that you can become self-employed for a relatively small investment. The initial expenses are fairly low and usually limited to the costs incurred for rent, supplies, products, and personal promotion or advertising. For some booth renters, a very low overhead may balance equitably with the income generated as a beginning barber with a small clientele. However, a good rule to follow is to make sure your clientele is large enough to cover all overhead costs *and* pay you a salary.

Chair or booth rental may also be ideal for those individuals who are interested in part-time employment, want to supplement another income, or prefer to take a stepping-stone approach to shop ownership. Regardless of the motivation, a booth rental arrangement provides the means for an individual to retain most of the control and decision making as it applies to work schedules and professional goals.

Position availability, personal choice, convenience, and the level of responsibility you care to assume will influence the capacity in which you work. Be sure to familiarize yourself with applicable state and federal tax laws. Working as an independent contractor and working as a booth renter are forms of self-employment, meaning that paid holidays or vacation benefits are nonexistent. Instead, you will have to plan ahead and set aside savings for times when you are not working or an emergency arises.

WAGE STRUCTURES

As discussed previously, booth rental involves paying the shop owner a fixed amount of rent for the space. All the fees brought in from the performance of services are basically yours after paying for the rent and supplies. For the employee or independent contractor, however, compensation may be structured in one of several different ways.

Straight or hourly salaries are most often seen in chain or franchise shops or salons but can provide you with a chance to earn a fixed income while building a clientele. Some shops offer an hourly wage that is slightly higher than the minimum wage to encourage new barbers to take the job and stick with it. With experience in the field and increased clientele, the fixed salary arrangement may evolve into a commission-based form of compensation.

In a **commission** (KAHM-ish-un) compensation structure, the employer pays you a percentage of the gross service sales you generate. Commission is usually offered once an employee has built up a loyal clientele. A commission payment structure is very different from an hourly wage, because any money you are paid is a direct result of the total amount of service dollars you generate for the shop. Commission percentages for barbers can vary greatly, anywhere from 40 to 70 percent, and depend on a variety of factors that may include your level of experience or the number of clients the shop services on a regular basis. Keep in mind that it may take you up to 2 years of performing services and building your clientele to make a living on straight commission compensation. Additionally, many states do not allow straight commission payments unless they average out to at least minimum wage.

A salary-plus-commission (sometimes called a *guarantee*) compensation arrangement usually guarantees a minimum base salary with a percentage of the amount over the base added to it for a total wage. This kind of structure is often used to motivate employees to perform more services, thereby increasing their productivity. As with salaried compensation, salary-plus-commission may also evolve into a commission-only wage status.

Commission wages are usually paid as a straight percentage of the total fees taken in for services; however, sometimes a fee is taken "off the top" for the shop, and the commission percentage is based on the remainder. Both employees and independent contractors may be paid on a commission basis. Table 20-1 provides a summary of the differences involved when working as an employee, independent contractor, or booth renter.

Tips

When you receive satisfactory service at a hotel or restaurant, you are likely to leave your server a tip. It has become customary for clients to acknowledge their barbers in this way, too. Some barbershops have a tipping policy; others have a no-tipping policy. This is determined by what the shop feels is appropriate for its clientele.

Tips are income in addition to your regular compensation and must be tracked and reported on your income tax return. Reporting tips will be beneficial to you if you wish to take out a mortgage or another type of loan and want your income to appear as strong as it really is.

As you can see, there are a number of ways to structure compensation for a barbershop professional. You will probably have the opportunity to try each of these methods at different points in your career. When deciding whether a certain compensation method is right for you, it is important to be aware of what your monthly expenses are and to have a personal financial budget in place. Budget issues are addressed later in this chapter.

table 20-1

EMPLOYMENT CLASSIFICATION OVERVIEW

Employee	Independent Contractor	Booth Renter
Work instructions are provided; job performance is evaluated	No instruction, training, or evaluation is provided	No instruction, training, or evaluation is provided
Training may be provided or required	May require personal investment in advanced training	Requires personal investment in advanced training
Operating hours are set or scheduled	Sets own hours and schedule with agreement	Sets own hours and work schedule
Appointments are scheduled by business	May schedule own appointments	Schedules own appointments
Services revenue most often collected at front desk	Services revenue may be collected at front desk	Services revenue is collected by booth renter
Equipment and facilities are provided	May pay for certain equipment or arrange an agreement; opportunity for profit and loss exists	Certain equipment included in lease; opportunity for profit and loss
Benefits may be provided	No benefits are provided	No benefits are provided
No rental agreement exists	Independent contractor agreement required. Requires agreement with an end date, wage payment information, responsibilities, etc.	Booth rental agreement is required. Requires lease with dates, fee, booth renter responsibilities, etc.
Expenses may be reimbursed	Expenses are not usually reimbursed	Expenses are not reimbursed
May be paid on hourly, salaried, commission, or salary-plus-commission basis	May work on percentage, commission, or flat fee; and agreements may be renewed. May work in more than one location	Responsible for collecting all service revenues
Uniforms may be required	Attire may be discussed in agreement	Generally the renter's decision
Income tax, portion of social security tax, Medicare tax, and unemployment tax are paid by employer	Is responsible for all taxes, licenses, and insurance	Is responsible for all taxes, licenses, insurance, and advertising
Amount of tips are recorded by employer	Responsible for own tips and taxes	Responsible for own tips and taxes
Employer is required to provide Form W-2, Wage and Tax Statement	May work within confines of shop hours. Owner is required to provide 1099 form	Requires submitting 1099 form to owner for rent paid

Photography by Jason Lott. Lilly Benitez, Founder of Blade Craft Barber Academy.

figure 20-5
A good role model can provide guidance as you start out.

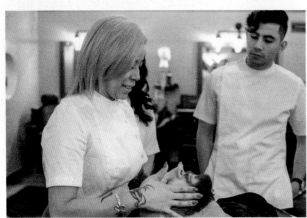

Barbers can increase their chances of building a solid and loyal clientele more quickly if they:

- live in a large city or choose areas within their cities that have a large number of potential clients
- select a location where the competition for clients is less saturated
- have advanced training, skills, and certifications
- have and use their artistic abilities
- employ marketing and publicity strategies
- concentrate on an unusual niche within the beauty business (e.g., teens)

EMPLOYEE EVALUATION

The best way to keep tabs on your progress is to ask for feedback from your shop manager and key coworkers. Most likely, the barbershop will have a structure in place for evaluation purposes. Commonly, evaluations are scheduled 90 days after hiring, and then once a year after that. But you should feel free to ask for help and feedback any time you need it. This feedback can help you improve your technical abilities as well as your customer service skills.

Ask a senior barber to sit in on one of your client consultations and to make note of areas where you can improve. Ask your manager to observe your technical skills and to point out ways you can perform your work more quickly and efficiently. Have a trusted coworker watch and evaluate your skills when it comes to selling retail products. All of these evaluations will benefit your learning process enormously.

Find a Role Model

One of the best ways to improve your performance is to model your behavior after someone who is having the kind of success that you wish to have (Figure 20-5).

Watch other barbers in your shop. You will easily be able to identify who is really good and who is just coasting along. Focus on the skills of the ones who are really good. What do they do? How do they treat their clients? How do they treat the shop staff and manager? How do they book their appointments? How do they handle their continuing education? What process do they use when formulating color or selecting a product? What is their attitude toward their work? How do they handle a crisis or conflict?

Go to these professionals for advice. Ask for a few minutes of their time, but be willing to wait for it, because it may not be easy to find time to talk during a busy barbershop workday. If you are having a problem, explain your situation and ask if the mentor can help you see things differently. Be prepared to listen and not argue your points. Remember that you asked for help, even when what your coworker is saying is not what you want to hear. Thank your coworker for their help, and reflect on the advice you have been given.

A little help and direction from skilled, experienced coworkers will go a long way toward helping you achieve your goals.

Manage Your Money

After reading this section, you will be able to:

LO④ Determine the best way to record your tips and make additional income.

Although a career in the barbering industry is very artistic and creative, it is also a career that requires financial understanding and planning. Too many barbers live for the moment and do not plan for the future. They may end up feeling cheated out of the benefits that their friends and family in other careers are enjoying.

In a corporate structure, the human resources department of the corporation handles a great deal of the employees' financial planning for them. For example, health and dental insurance, retirement accounts, savings accounts, and many other items may be automatically deducted and paid out of the employees' salary. Most barbering professionals, however, must research and plan for all of those expenses on their own. This may seem difficult, but in fact it is a small price to pay for the kind of freedom, financial reward, and job satisfaction that a career in barbering can offer. And the good news is that managing money is something everyone can learn to do.

REPAYMENT OF YOUR DEBTS

In addition to making money, responsible adults are concerned with paying back their debts. Throughout your life and your career, you will undoubtedly incur debt in the form of car loans, home mortgages, or student loans. While it is easy for some people to merely ignore their responsibility in repaying these loans, it is extremely irresponsible and immature to accept a loan and then shrug off the debt. Not paying back your loans is called *defaulting*, and it can have serious consequences regarding your personal and professional credit. Legal action can be taken against you if you fail to repay your loans. The best way to meet all of your financial responsibilities is to know precisely what you owe and what you earn so that you can make informed decisions regarding your finances. Before committing to a loan, make sure you understand the payment terms, interest rate, and what you realistically can afford.

REPORTING YOUR INCOME

As you enter your new career and work to become established, you most likely will be in a commissioned or salaried structure. When you receive your paycheck, taxes and other deductions will already be taken according to your state. When you complete your yearly taxes, it is critical that you report cash tips and other income that is not shown on your paycheck. Other income may be from performing work outside of the barbershop, such as performing services on location for weddings, parties, or in a private residence. There are serious legal consequences for not reporting such income including:

- fines and even potential jail time

- decreasing your borrowing power as it is based on your reported income

- reducing the amount of Social Security benefits for retirement

- lowering the Bureau of Labor's endorsement as a sustainable industry, leading to lower federal loans and grants available

The best way to record your tips and additional income is to keep a daily log. At the end of each week, add the total amount of your additional income. Next, add the total for the month and keep it on a single page in the front of your log book. At the end of the year, you will be able to easily report your total cash income for your taxes. Ethical barbers take the responsibility to comply with tax laws seriously and report their income accurately at the end of each year.

WEB RESOURCES

Optional info on budget topics and tutorials can be found at MiladyPro.com Keyword: *FutureBarberPro*

FOCUS ON

Barbershop Technology

Today, it is common for most barbershops to utilize computer technology to support their shop. The increase in the number of computerized barbershops could be advantageous for technology-savvy students. You may be able to master barbershop software programs more easily than other barbers. These programs now handle cash flow management, inventory tracking, payroll automation, client appointment books, performance evaluation tracking, and more. Just remember, these client records are usually considered the barbershop's property. Additionally, cost-effective, online continuing education is increasingly popular.

If you are accustomed to working with technology, you may be able to help a barbershop set up e-mail access, a website, social networking pages, and more. With many clients enjoying the freedom of online booking and text-message appointment reminders, and with shops benefiting from e-mail or even electronic marketing programs, it is important for you to understand technology. Today, hair care manufacturers even have special educational programs you can access on your mobile phone and social networking pages where you can share inspiration or ask for instant help.

Go through the budget worksheet and fill in the amounts that apply to your current living and financial situation. If you are unsure of the amount of an expense, put in the amount you have averaged over the past 3 months or give it your best guess. You may need to have 3 or 4 months of employment history to complete the income item, but fill in what you can. If the balance is a minus number, start listing ways you can decrease expenses or increase income.

Personal Budget

It is amazing how many people work hard and earn very good salaries but never take the time to create a personal budget. Many people are afraid of the word *budget*, because they think that it will be too restrictive on their spending or that they will have to be mathematical geniuses to work with a budget. Thankfully, neither of these fears is rooted in reality.

Personal budgets range from being extremely simple to extremely complex. The right one for you depends on your needs. At the beginning of your career, a simple budget should be sufficient. To get started, take a look at the Personal Monthly Budget Worksheet (**Figure 20-6**). It lists the standard monthly expenses that most people have to budget. It also includes school loan repayment, savings, and payments into an individual retirement account (IRA).

figure 20-6
A budget worksheet.

Personal Monthly Budget Worksheet

A. Expenses

1. Monthly rent (or share of the rent) $_____
2. Car payment   _____
3. Car insurance   _____
4. Auto fuel/upkeep and maintenance   _____
5. Electricity   _____
6. Gas   _____
7. Health insurance   _____
8. Entertainment (movies, dining, etc.)   _____
9. Groceries   _____
10. Dry cleaning   _____
11. Personal grooming   _____
12. Prescriptions/medical   _____
13. Cell phone   _____
14. Internet/television/home phone   _____
15. Student loan   _____
16. IRA   _____
17. Savings deposit   _____
18. Other expenses   _____

TOTAL EXPENSES $_____

B. Income

1. Monthly take-home pay   _____
2. Tips   _____
3. Other income   _____

TOTAL INCOME $_____

C. Balance

Total Income (B)   _____
Minus Total Expenses (A)   _____

BALANCE $_____

Keeping track of where your money goes is one step toward making sure that you always have enough. It also helps you to plan ahead and save for bigger expenses such as a vacation, your own home, or even your own business. All in all, sticking to a budget is a good practice to follow faithfully for the rest of your life.

Giving Yourself a Raise

Once you have taken some time to create, use, and work with your personal budget, you may want to look at ways in which you can have more money left over after paying bills. You might automatically jump to the most obvious sources, such as asking your employer for a raise or asking for a higher percentage of commission. While these tactics are certainly valid, you will also want to think about other ways to increase your income. Here are a few tips:

- **Spend less money.** Although it may be difficult to reduce your spending, it is certainly one way to increase the amount of money that is left over at the end of the month. These dollars can be used to invest, save, or pay down debt.

- **Work more hours.** If possible, choose times when the shop is busiest, which are the most convenient for clients. Come early and stay late to accommodate clients' booking needs. Saturday is a peak workday in most barbershops.

- **Increase service prices.** It will probably take some time before you are in a position to increase your service prices. For one thing, to do so, you need a loyal **client base** (KLY-ent baze), customers who are loyal to a particular barber, which in this instance is you. Also, you must have fully mastered all the services that you are performing. But if you have a loyal client base and service mastery, there is nothing wrong with increasing your prices every year or two, as long as you do so by a reasonable amount. Do a little research to determine what your competitors are charging for similar services, and increase your fees accordingly.

- **Retail more.** Most barbershops pay a commission on every product you recommend and sell to your clients. If you sell more products, you make more money!

Seek Professional Advice

Just as you will want your clients to seek out your advice and services for their hair care needs, sometimes it is important for you to seek out the advice of experts, especially when it comes to your finances. You can research and interview financial planners who will be able to give you advice on reducing your credit card debt, on how to invest your money, and on retirement options. You can speak to the officers at your local bank, who may be able to suggest bank accounts that offer you greater returns or flexibility with your money, depending on what you need.

When seeking out advice from other professionals, be sure not to take anyone's advice without carefully considering whether the advice makes sense for your particular situation and needs. Before you buy into anything, be an informed consumer about other people's goods and services. Ask yourself these questions as you begin to think about going on a budget:

- How do your expenses compare to your income?
- What is your balance after all your expenses are paid?
- Were there any surprises for you in this exercise?
- Do you think that keeping a budget is a good way to manage money?
- Do you know of any other methods people use to manage money?

Discover the Selling You

After reading this section, you will be able to:

LO**5** Explain the principles of selling products and services in the barbershop.

Another area that touches on the issue of you and money is selling. As a barber, you will have enormous opportunities to sell retail products and upgrade service tickets. **Ticket upgrading** (TIK-it UP-grayd-ing), also known as *upselling services*, is the practice of recommending and selling additional services to your clients. These services may be performed by you or other professionals licensed in a different field. **Retailing** (REE-tail-ing) is the act of recommending and selling products to your clients for at-home use (**Figure 20-7**). These two activities can make all the difference in your economic picture. The following dialogue is an example of ticket upgrading. In this scene, Joey, the stylist, suggests an additional service to Mr. King, his client, who has just had his hair trimmed for a wedding he will be attending that evening.

figure 20-7
Retailing is vital to increasing revenue.

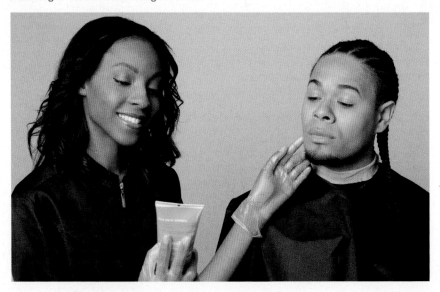

Read the script yourself and change the words to make them fit your personality. Then try it the next time you feel that an additional service could help one of your clients.

Joey: I'm really glad you like your haircut. I think it will be perfect with the new suit you described.

Mr. King: I don't know. To tell you the truth, I don't get dressed up all that often.

Joey: Yes, I know what you mean, but you're going to look great! We could even cover your grays to add more dimension to the cut, if you like.

Mr. King: Well, actually, I was sort of wondering about that.

Joey: I have an opening, if you want to do it now. How does that sound to you?

Mr. King: Definitely. That sounds terrific!

PRINCIPLES OF SELLING

Some barbers shy away from sales. They think that selling is being pushy. A close look at how selling works can set your mind at ease. Not only can you become very good at selling once you understand the principles behind it, but you can also feel good about providing your clients with a valuable service.

To be successful in sales, you need ambition, determination, and a pleasing personality. The first step in selling is to sell yourself. Clients must like and trust you before they will purchase services, skin care items, shampoos and conditioners, or other merchandise.

Remember, every client who enters the shop is a potential purchaser of additional services or merchandise. Recognizing the client's needs and preferences lays the foundation for successful selling (Figure 20-8).

To become a proficient salesperson, you must be able to apply the following principles of selling barbering products and services:

- Be familiar with the features and benefits of the various services and products that you are trying to sell, and recommend only those that the client really needs. You should try and test all the products in the barbershop yourself.

- Adapt your approach and technique to meet the needs and personality of each client. Some clients may prefer a soft sell that involves informing them about the product, without stressing that they purchase it. Others are comfortable with a hard-sell approach that focuses emphatically on why a client should buy the product.

figure 20-8
Every client is a potential purchaser of additional services and products.

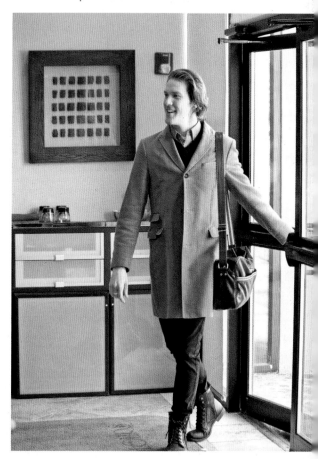

figure 20-9
Demonstrate the product if possible.

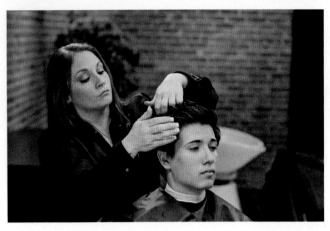

- Be self-confident when recommending products for sale. You become confident by knowing about the products you are selling and by believing that they are as good as you say.

- Generate interest and desire in the customer by asking questions that determine a need.

- Never misrepresent your services or products. Making unrealistic claims will only lead to your client's disappointment, making it unlikely that you will ever again make a sale to that client.

- Do not underestimate the client's intelligence or their knowledge of their own home care regimen or particular needs.

- To sell a product or service, deliver your sales talk in a relaxed, friendly manner. If possible, demonstrate the use of the product (**Figure 20-9**).

- Recognize the right psychological moment to close any sale. Once the client has offered to buy, quit selling. Do not oversell; simply praise the client for making the purchase and assure the client that they will be happy with it.

THE PSYCHOLOGY OF SELLING

Most people have reasons for doing what they do, and when you are selling something, it is your job to figure out the reasons that will motivate a person to buy. When dealing with barbershop clients, you will find that their motives for buying barbering products vary widely. Some may be concerned with issues of vanity. (They want to look better.) Some are seeking personal satisfaction. (They want to feel better about themselves.) Others need to solve a problem that is bothersome. (They want to spend less time maintaining their hair.)

 FOCUS ON

Overcoming Objections

Making sales won't always be easy. For example, sometimes a client is stuck on a haircolor that is not flattering. Other times, the client may not feel convinced a product is any better than a drugstore brand or the client may have a genuine price objection.

To overcome an objection, reword the objection in a way that addresses the client's need. For instance, let's say you recommend a shampoo based on the fact that your client has dry hair and he just had it colored. In response, he says he already has a shampoo for color-treated hair.

First, acknowledge what he said. Then reword his objection that he already has the right shampoo in a different way, which gets him thinking. For example:

"I know, but not all shampoos for color-treated hair are alike. This shampoo not only protects your color from fading, it will definitely moisturize it more, which is what adds the shine you told me you wanted. I can leave it at the front desk, so you can think about it."

If the objection is a price objection, base your reaction on the client's. For strong objections, acknowledge the price and offer a free sample, if you can. If the objection is moderate, acknowledge it and reiterate the product's benefits.

"It is a little more expensive, but if you really want your color to last and your hair to feel good and look shiny, this is the best product I've ever found. We used it on you today. See what you think, and let me know."

Always state things in terms of the client's benefit, based on the information you gathered during the consultation.

Sometimes a client may inquire about a product or service but still be undecided or doubtful. In this type of situation, you can help the client by offering honest and sincere advice. When you explain a barbering service to a client, address the results and benefits of that service. Always keep in mind that the best interests of the client should be your first consideration. You will need to know exactly what your client's needs are, and you need to have a clear idea as to how those needs can be fulfilled.

Here are a few tips on how to get the conversation started on retailing products:

- Ask all your clients what products they are using for home maintenance of their hair, skin, and nails.

- Discuss the products you are using as you use them. For instance, tell the client why you are using the particular mousse or spray gel and what it will do for them. Also explain how the client should use the product at home.

- Place the product in the client's hands whenever possible or have the product in view.

- Advise the client about how the recommended service will provide personal benefit (more manageable hairstyling or longer-lasting haircolor, for instance).

- Keep retail areas clean, well lit, and appealing.

- Inform clients of any promotions and sales that are going on in the barbershop.

- Be informed about the merits of using a professional product, as opposed to generic store brands.

- If you have time, offer a quick styling lesson. If your client has difficulty home styling, they will appreciate your guidance. After demonstrating, watch as the client mimics the recommended styling technique, so you can guide them.

While you realize that retailing products is a service to your clients, you may not be sure how to go about it. Imagine the following scenes and see how Louis highlights the benefits and features of a product to his client, Mr. Steiner. Notice that price is not necessarily the most important factor.

Scenario: Meet a Need

Mr. Steiner: I really like my new haircut. When should I be back for a trim?

Louis: You should come back in 3 to 4 weeks to maintain the style. By then, you'll have had time to work with the styling product I suggested.

Mr. Steiner: Is that what you used on me today? It seemed easy enough to use and doesn't look greasy.

Louis: Absolutely. Just dispense a little into your palms and distribute it through your hair. It's just that easy.

Mr. Steiner: Great!

FOCUS ON

Retailing

For quick reference, keep these five points in mind when selling:

1. Establish rapport with the client.
2. Determine the client's needs.
3. Recommend products/services based on these needs.
4. Emphasize benefits.
5. Close the sale.

ACTIVITY

Pick a partner from class and role-play the dynamics of a sales situation. Take turns being the customer and the barber. Evaluate each other on how you did, with suggestions about where you can improve. Then try this exercise with someone else because no two customers are the same.

Keep Current Clients and Expand Your Client Base

After reading this section, you will be able to:

LO**6** List the most effective ways to build a client base.

Once you have mastered the basics of good service, take a look at some marketing techniques that will expand your client base—the customers who keep coming back to you for services.

The following are only a few suggestions; there are many others that may work for you. The best way to decide which techniques are most effective is to try several!

- **Send birthday cards.** Ask clients for their birthday information (just the month and day, not the year) on the client consultation card, and then use it as a tool to get them into the shop again. About 1 month prior to the client's birthday, send a card with a special offer. Make it valid only for the month of their birthday. This form of advertisement is not expensive, and it is always greatly appreciated.

- **Provide consistently good service.** It seems basic enough, but it is amazing how many professionals work hard to get clients, and lose them because they rush through a service, leaving clients feeling dissatisfied. Providing good-quality service must always be your first concern (**Figure 20-10**).

- **Be reliable.** Always be courteous, thoughtful, and professional. Be at the barbershop when you say you will be there, and do not keep clients waiting. Give your clients the style they ask for, not something else. Recommend a retail product only when you have tried it yourself and know what it can and cannot do.

- **Be respectful.** When you treat others with respect, you become worthy of respect yourself. Being respectful means that you do not gossip or make fun of anyone or anything related to the barbershop. Negative energy brings everyone down, especially you.

- **Be positive.** Be one of those people who always sees the glass as half full. Look for the positive in every situation. No one enjoys being around a person who is always unhappy.

- **Be professional.** Sometimes a client may try to make your relationship more personal than it ought to be. It is in your best interest, and your client's best interest, not to cross that line.

- **Ask for your clients' e-mail addresses.** E-mail is now the preferred mode of

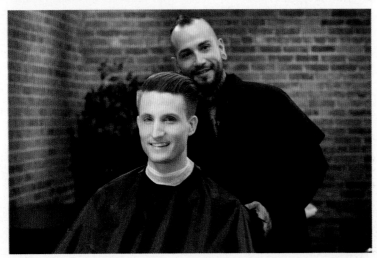

figure 20-10
Quality service must always come first.

communication for many people. In fact, many clients now prefer to book appointments using e-mail.

- **Utilize social media.** The Internet is a powerful medium to build your reputation and attract new clients. Utilize social media tools such as Facebook and Yelp to establish your credibility, showcase your work, and provide a space for satisfied clients to recommend you. Create a Facebook page dedicated to your business, and make it a place to share barbering tips, trends, and shop information and promotions. Post before-and-after photos to illustrate your skills (but always gain approval from your clients before sharing their photos). Yelp is a powerful tool to build your brand. If the barbershop has a Yelp listing, be sure to utilize it as a way to strengthen your business. Satisfied clients are able to post a review of your services and provide a rating of their overall experience. It is always a good practice to casually invite your clients to provide a review; however, it is not ethical to pressure anyone to do so.

- **Business card referrals.** Make up a special business card with your information on it, but leave room for a client to put his name on it as well. If your client is clearly pleased with your work, give him several cards. Ask him to put his name on them and to refer his friends and associates to you. For every card you receive from a new customer with the client's name on it, give him 10 percent off his next barbering service or a complimentary added service to his next appointment. This gives the client lots of motivation to recommend you to others, which in turn helps build up your clientele.

- **Local business referrals.** Another terrific way to build business is to work with local businesses to get referrals. Look for gyms, tailors, diners, cigar shops, tattoo parlors, and other small businesses near your barbershop. Offer to have a card swap and commit to referring your clients to them when they are in the market for goods or services that your neighbors can provide, if they will do the same for you. This is a great way to build a feeling of community among local vendors and to reach new clients you may not be able to otherwise.

- **Public speaking.** Make yourself available for public speaking at local groups, the PTA, organizations for young men and women, and anywhere else that will put you in front of people in your community who are all potential clients. Put together a short program (20 to 30 minutes) in which, for example, you might discuss professional appearance with emphasis in your chosen field and other grooming tips for people looking for jobs or who are already employed.

REBOOKING CLIENTS

The best time to think about getting your clients back into the shop is while they are still in your shop. It may seem a little difficult to assure your clients that you are concerned with their satisfaction on this visit while you are talking about their next visit, but the two go together. The best way to encourage your clients to book another appointment before they leave is to simply talk with them, ask questions, and listen carefully to their answers.

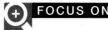
FOCUS ON

Building Your Efficiency

Some professionals believe that the more time they spend with their clients performing services, the better the service will be. Not so! Unless your shop has a lounge, your client should be in the barbershop only as long as is necessary for you to adequately complete a service.

Be aware of how much time it takes you to perform your various services, and then schedule accordingly. As you become more and more experienced, you should see a reduction in the amount of time it takes you to perform these services. That means clients wait less, and you can increase the number of services you perform each day. The increase in services naturally increases your income.

When you are working on a client's hair, for instance, talk about the condition of their hair, their hairstyling habits at home, and the benefits of regular or special shop maintenance. You will want to listen carefully to what your clients tell you during their visit, because they will often give the careful listener many good clues as to what is happening in their lives. Those clues will open the door to a discussion about their next appointment.

On Your Way

Your first job in this industry will most likely be the most difficult. Getting started in this business means spending some time on a steep learning curve. Be patient with yourself as you transition from the "school you" to the "professional you." Always remember that in your work life, as in everything else you do, practice makes perfect. You will not know everything you need to know right at the start, but be confident in the fact that you are graduating from barbering school with a solid knowledge base. Make use of the many generous and experienced professionals you will encounter, and let them teach you the tricks of the trade. Make the commitment to perfecting your technical and customer service skills.

Above all, always be willing to learn. If you let the concepts that you have learned in this book be your guide, you will enjoy your life and reap the amazing benefits of a career in barbering (**Figure 20-11**).

figure 20-11
Welcome to your career in barbering!

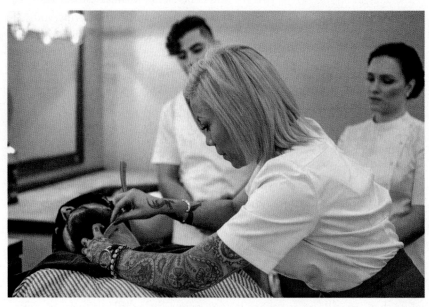

Photography by Jason Lott. Lilly Benitez, Founder of Blade Craft Barber Academy.

REVIEW QUESTIONS

1 What are the workplace principles to practice to become a good team player?

2 If your employer does not provide a job description, what should you do?

3 What are the three common employment statuses for barbers?

4 What are the three most common methods of compensation you're likely to encounter?

5 What are six ways to build a solid and loyal clientele more quickly?

6 What are four serious legal consequences for not reporting income, including tips?

7 What are four tips for increasing your income?

8 What is ticket upgrading?

9 What are the principles of selling barbering products and services?

10 What are three possible marketing techniques for maintaining and expanding your client base?

CHAPTER GLOSSARY

booth rental (BOO-th ren-tal)	p. 739	also known as *chair rental*; a form of self-employment, business ownership, and tax designation, distinguished by renting a booth or station in a barbershop
client base (KLY-ent baze)	p. 745	customers who are loyal to a particular barber
commission (KAHM-ish-un)	p. 740	a percentage of the revenue that the barbershop takes in from services performed by an employee, usually offered to that employee once the individual has built up a loyal clientele
employee (EM-ploy-ee)	p. 738	employment classification in which the employer withholds certain taxes and has a high level of control
independent contractor (IN-dee-pen-dant CON-tract-uhr)	p. 738	a form of self-employment and tax designation with specific responsibilities for bookkeeping, taxes, insurances, and so on
job description (JOHB des-CRIP-shun)	p. 737	document that outlines all the duties and responsibilities of a particular position in a barbershop
retailing (REE-tail-ing)	p. 746	the act of recommending and selling products to your clients for at-home use
ticket upgrading (TIK-it UP-grayd-ing)	p. 746	also known as *upselling services*; the practice of recommending and selling additional services to your clients

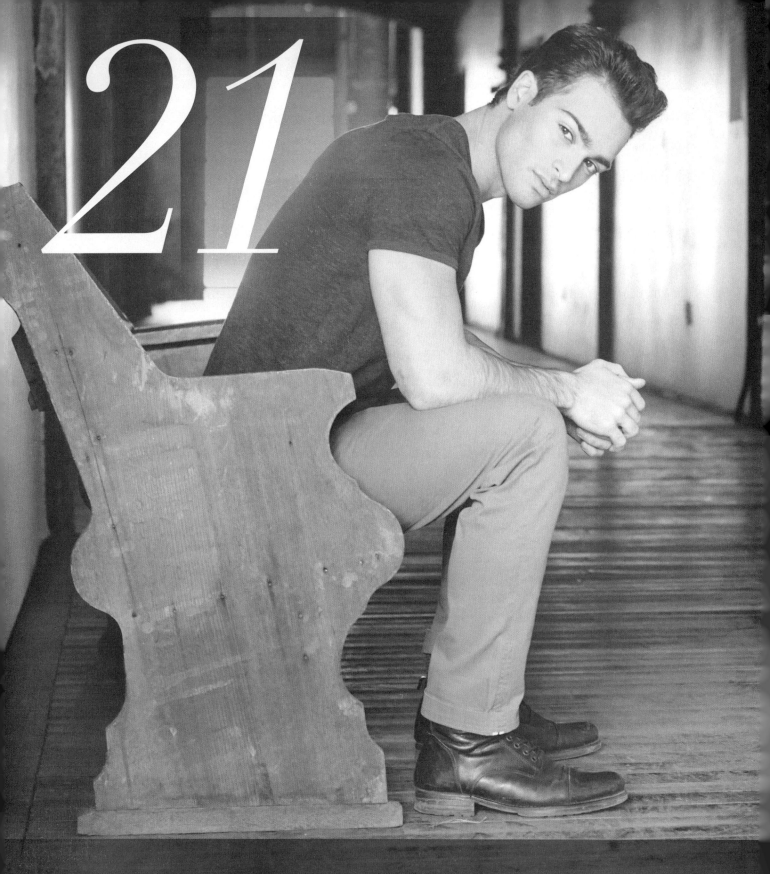

21

THE BUSINESS OF
BARBERING

LEARNING OBJECTIVES

After completing this chapter, you will be able to:

LO❶
Identify two options for going into business for yourself.

LO❷
List the basic factors to be considered when opening a barbershop.

LO❸
Compare types of barbershop ownership.

LO❹
Recognize the information that should be included in a business plan.

LO❺
Explain the importance of record keeping.

LO❻
Examine the responsibilities of a booth renter.

LO❼
Distinguish the elements of successful barbershop operations.

LO❽
Validate why advertising is a vital aspect of a barbershop's success.

figure 21-1
Be successful.

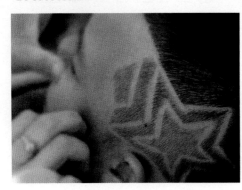

Introduction

The better prepared you are to be both a great artist and a successful businessperson, the greater your chances of success (**Figure 21-1**).

Entire books have been written on each of the topics touched on in this chapter, so be prepared to read and research your business idea extensively before making any final decisions about opening a business. The following information is only meant to be a general overview.

why study
THE BUSINESS OF BARBERING?

Barbers should study and have a thorough understanding of the business of barbering because:

> As you become more proficient in your craft and your ability to manage yourself and others, you may decide to become an independent booth renter or even a barbershop owner. In fact, most owners are barbers.

> Even if you spend your entire career as an employee of someone else's barbershop, you should be familiar with the rules of business that affect the shop. It is also important to look at your career behind the chair as your own business.

> To become a successful entrepreneur, you will need to attract employees and clients to your business and maintain their loyalty over long periods of time.

> Business knowledge will serve you well in managing your career and professional finances, as well as your business practices.

Review Types of Business Options

After reading this section, you will be able to:

LO**❶** Identify two options for going into business for yourself.

LO**❷** List the basic factors to be considered when opening a barbershop.

LO**❸** Compare types of barbershop ownership.

LO**❹** Recognize the information that should be included in a business plan.

LO**❺** Explain the importance of record keeping.

If you reach a point in your life when you feel that you are ready to become your own boss, you will have two main options to consider: (1) owning your own barbershop or (2) renting a booth in an existing shop or salon.

Both options are extremely serious undertakings that require significant financial investment and a strong line of credit. Barbershop owners have a very different job than barbers because typically, they continue to work behind the chair while they manage the business. This is extremely time consuming, and there is no guarantee of profits, which is why barbershop ownership is definitely not for everyone. Owning your own shop and renting a booth have different pros and cons.

OPENING YOUR OWN BARBERSHOP

Opening your own barbershop is a huge undertaking—financially, physically, creatively, and mentally—because you will face challenges that are complex and unfamiliar to you. Before you can open your doors, you need to decide what products to use and carry, what types of marketing and promotions you will employ, the best method and philosophy for running the business and creating a culture, and whom to hire if you need additional staff.

Regardless of the type of barbershop you hope to open, you should carefully consider basic issues and perform basic tasks, as outlined in the following section.

Create Your Brand Identity

Creating your brand identity at the start is essential for building a unique, successful business. To create your brand, start by identifying a few simple concepts to use as building blocks for your brand identity.

- What is your point of difference? What is going to make a client want to visit your business versus the one across the street?

- What are you selling? Every barbershop sells haircuts; think beyond the obvious. Are you selling a luxury experience, a family-friendly environment, or a cost-conscious express service?

- What is your aesthetic? Will there be a consistent color, theme, or uniform for your staff?

Identifying the answers to these three main questions solidifies your concepts and serves as reference. Refer to them frequently for inspiration, guidance, and a reminder of what your business is built upon.

Create a Vision and Mission Statement for the Business with Goals

A **vision statement** (VIZ-uhn state-ment) is a sweeping picture of the long-term goals for the business, what it is to become, and what it will look like when it gets there. A mission statement is a guide to the actions of the organization: It spells out the overall goals, provides a path, and contains the core values to help guide decision making. The mission statement lays the foundation for how your company's strategies are created. **Goals** (GOHLZ) are an essential set of benchmarks that, once achieved, help you to realize your mission and your vision. It is important to set realistic goals for both the short term and long term.

Create a Business Timeline

While initially you will be concerned with the first two aspects of the timeline, once your business is successful you will need to think about the others as well.

- **Year 1.** It could take a year or more to determine and complete all of the aspects of starting the business.

- **Years 2 to 5.** This time period is for tending to the business, its clientele, and its employees and for growing and expanding the business so that it is profitable.

- **Years 5 to 10.** This time period, if successfully achieved, can be for adding more locations, expanding the scope of the business, constructing a larger space, or anything else you or your clients need and want.

- **Years 11 to 20.** In this time period, you may want to move from being a working barber into a full-time manager of the overall business and to begin planning for your eventual retirement.

- **Year 20 Onward.** This may be the perfect time to consider selling your successful business or changing it in some way, such as taking on a junior partner and training him to take over the day-to-day operations of the business so you can have time away from the business to explore your interests or hobbies.

Determine Business Feasibility

Determining whether or not the business you envision is feasible means addressing certain practical issues. For example, do you have a special skill or talent that can help you set your business apart from other barbershops in your area? Does the town or area where you are planning to locate the business offer you the appropriate type of clientele for the products and services you want to offer? Based on what you envision for the business, how much money will you need to open the business? Is this funding available to you?

Choose a Business Name

The name you select for your business explains what it is and can also identify characteristics that set your business apart from competitors in the marketplace. The name you select for your business will also influence how clients and potential clients perceive the business. The name will create a picture of your business in clients' minds, and once that picture is imagined, it can be very difficult to change the perception. In addition, once your business is named, it is complicated to make all of the legal, banking, and tax changes if you change your mind.

Choose a Location

You will want to base your business location on your primary clientele and their needs. Select a location that has good visibility, high traffic, easy access, sufficient parking, and handicap access (**Figure 21-2**).

Written Agreements

Many **written agreements** (RIT-en UH-gree-mentz) and documents govern the opening of a barbershop, including leases, vendor contracts, and employee contracts. All of these written agreements detail, usually for legal purposes, who does what and what is given in return. You must be able to read and understand them. Additionally, before you open a barbershop, you must

figure 21-2
Scout the best location for your shop.

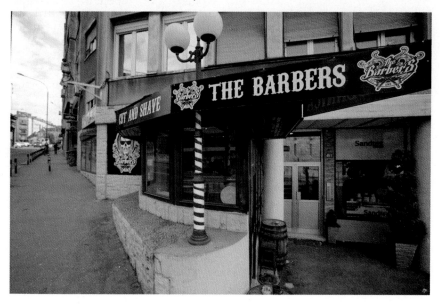

© Zoran Milich/Moment Mobile/Getty Images.

develop a **business plan** (BIZ-nez plahn), a written description of your business as you see it today and as you foresee it in the next 5 years (detailed by year). A business plan is more of an agreement with yourself, and it is not legally binding. However, if you wish to obtain financing, it is essential that you have a business plan in place first. The plan should include a general description of the business and the services that it will provide; area **demographics** (dem-oh-graf-iks), which consist of information about a specific population, including data on race, age, income, and educational attainment; expected salaries and cost of related benefits; an operations plan that includes pricing structure and expenses, such as equipment, supplies, repairs, advertising, taxes, and insurance; and projected income and overhead expenses for up to 5 years. A certified public accountant (CPA) can be invaluable in helping you gather accurate financial information. The Chamber of Commerce in your proposed area typically has information on area demographics.

Business Regulations and Laws

Business regulations and laws (BIZ-nez reg-U-lay-shuns AND LAWZ) are any and all local, state, and federal regulations and laws that you must comply with when you decide to open your barbershop or rent a booth. Since the laws change from year to year and vary from state to state and from city to city, it is important that you contact your local authorities regarding business licenses, permits, and other regulations, such as zoning and business inspections. Additionally, you must know and comply with all federal Occupational Safety and Health Administration (OSHA) guidelines, including those requiring that information about the ingredients of cosmetic preparations be available to employees. OSHA requires Safety Data Sheets (SDSs) for this purpose. There are also many federal laws that apply to hiring and firing, payment of benefits, contributions to employee entitlements (e.g., Social Security and unemployment), and workplace behavior.

Understanding the laws and rules of owning a barbershop is imperative to running a successful business. The laws and rules not only lay the foundation of acceptable guidelines regarding hiring and firing but also build a framework for day-to-day policies and procedures and safety. Not following the laws and rules can result in costly fines and heavy penalties. It is important to become very familiar with the local, state, and federal laws and rules before you open your business.

When you open your business, you need to purchase **insurance** (in-SHUR-ens) that guarantees protection against financial loss from malpractice, property liability, fire, burglary and theft, and business interruption. You need to have disability policies as well. Make sure that your policies cover you for all the monetary demands you have to meet on your lease.

Barbershop Operation

Business or **barbershop operation** refers to the ongoing, recurring processes or activities involved in the running of a business for the purpose of producing income and value.

Record Keeping

Record keeping (REK-urd KEEP-ing) is the act of maintaining accurate and complete records of all financial activities in your business.

Barbershop Policies

Barbershop policies are the rules and regulations adopted by a barbershop to ensure that all clients and associates are being treated fairly and consistently. Even small shops and booth renters should have barbershop policies in place.

TYPES OF BARBERSHOP OWNERSHIP

A barbershop can be owned and operated by an individual, a partnership, or a corporation or franchise. Before deciding which type of ownership is most desirable for your situation, research each option thoroughly. There are excellent reference tools available, and you can also consult a small business attorney for advice.

Individual Ownership

If you like to make your own rules and are responsible enough to meet all the duties and obligations of running a business, individual ownership may be the best arrangement for you.

The **sole proprietor** (SOHL PRHO-pry-eh-tohr) is the individual owner and, most often, the manager of the business who:

- determines policies and has the last say in decision making
- assumes expenses, receives profits, and bears all losses

Partnership

Partnerships may mean more opportunity for increased investment and growth. They can be fantastic if the right chemistry exists, or they can be disastrous if you find yourself linked with someone you wish you had known better in the first place. Your partner can incur losses or debts that you may not even be aware of unless you use a third-party accountant. Trust is just one of the requirements for this arrangement (**Figure 21-3**).

In a **partnership** (PART-nur-ship) business structure, two or more people share ownership—although not necessarily equally.

- One reason for going into a partnership arrangement is to have more **capital** (KAP-uh-tal), or money to invest in a business; another is to have help running your operation.

- Partners also pool their skills and talents, making it easier to share work, responsibilities, and decision making.

- Keep in mind that partners must assume one another's liability for debts.

Corporation

A **corporation** (KOR-pour-aye-shun) is an ownership structure controlled by one or more stockholders. Incorporating is one of the best ways that a business owner can protect their personal assets. Most people choose to incorporate solely for this reason, but there are other advantages as well. For example, the corporate business structure saves you money in taxes, provides greater business flexibility, and makes raising capital easier. It also limits your personal financial liability if your business accrues unmanageable debts or otherwise runs into financial trouble.

Characteristics of corporations are generally as follows:

- Corporations raise capital by issuing stock certificates or shares.

- Stockholders (people or companies that purchase shares) have an ownership interest in the company. The more stock they own, the bigger that interest becomes.

- You can be the sole stockholder (or shareholder), or you can have many stockholders.

- Corporate formalities, such as director and stockholder meetings, are required to maintain a corporate status.

- Income tax is limited to the salary that you draw and not the total profits of the business.

- Corporations cost more to set up and run than a sole proprietorship or partnership. For example, there are the initial formation fees, filing fees, and annual state fees.

- A stockholder of a corporation is required to pay unemployment insurance taxes on their salary, whereas a sole proprietor or partner is not.

Your accountant may suggest that your business become an S Corporation (Small Business Corporation), which is a business elected for S Corporation status through the IRS. This status allows the taxation of the company to be similar to a partnership or sole proprietor as opposed to paying taxes based on a corporate tax structure. Or your accountant may suggest that your business become registered as an LLC (Limited Liability Company), which is a type of business ownership combining several features of corporation and partnership structures. Owners of an LLC also have the liability protection of a corporation. An LLC exists as a separate entity, much like a corporation. Members cannot be held personally liable for debts unless they have signed a personal guarantee.

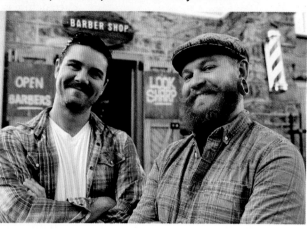

figure 21-3
Business partnerships can have many benefits.

© Monkey Business Images/Shutterstock.com.

? DID YOU KNOW?

When you open your own business, you should consult with an attorney and an accountant before filing any documents to legalize your business. It is helpful to find these kinds of professionals who have previous experience in the barbering business. Your attorney will advise you of the legal documents and obligations that you will take on as a business owner, and your accountant can inform you of the ways in which your business may be registered for tax purposes.

Franchise Ownership

A franchise is a form of business organization in which a firm that is already successful (the franchisor) enters into a continuing contractual relationship with other businesses (franchisees) operating under the franchisor's trade name in exchange for a fee. When you operate a franchise shop, you usually operate under the franchisor's guidance and must adhere to a contract with many stipulations. These stipulations ensure that all locations in the franchise are run in a similar manner, look the same way, use the same logos, and, sometimes, even train the same way or carry the same retail products.

Franchises offer the advantage of a known name and brand recognition, and the franchisor does most of the marketing for you. Also, many have protected territories, meaning another franchise barbershop with the same name cannot open up within your fixed geographic area. However, franchise agreements vary widely in what you can and cannot do on your own. Owning a franchise is no guarantee of making a profit, and you should always research the franchise, talk to other owners of the franchise's shops, and have an attorney read the contract and explain anything you do not understand, including your precise obligations and arrangements for paying the franchise fee. In most cases, whether or not you are profitable, you must pay the fee.

BUSINESS PLAN

Regardless of the type of barbershop you plan to own, it is imperative that you have a thorough and well-researched business plan. Remember, the business plan is a written plan of a business as it is seen in the present and envisioned in the future, and it follows your business throughout the entire process from start-up through many years in the future. Many books, classes, DVDs, and websites offer much more detailed information than can be provided here, but the following is a sampling of the kinds of information and materials that a business plan should include (**Figure 21-4**).

figure 21-4
Create a solid business plan.

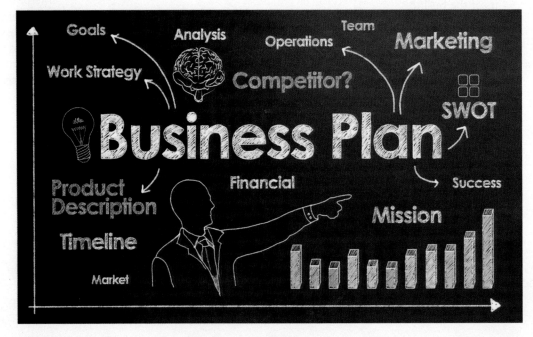

© T. L. Furrer/Shutterstock.com.

- **Executive summary.** Summarizes your plan and states your objectives.
- **Vision statement.** A long-term picture of what the business is to become and what it will look like when it gets there.
- **Mission statement.** A description of the key strategic influences of the business, such as the market it will serve, the kinds of services it will offer, and the quality of those services.
- **Organizational plan.** Outlines employees and management levels and also describes how the business will run administratively.
- **Marketing plan.** Outlines all of the research obtained regarding the clients your business will target and their needs, wants, and habits.
- **Financial documents.** Includes the projected financial statements, actual (historical) statements, and financial statement analysis.
- **Supporting documents.** Includes the owner's resume, personal financial information, legal contracts, and any other agreements.
- **Barbershop policies.** Even small shops and booth renters should have policies that they adhere to. These policies ensure that all clients and employees are treated fairly and consistently.

PURCHASING AN ESTABLISHED BARBERSHOP

Purchasing an existing barbershop could be an excellent opportunity, but, as with anything else, you have to look at all sides of the picture. If you choose to buy an established shop, seek professional assistance from an accountant and a business lawyer. You can purchase all the assets of a shop or some or all of its stock. It is important to know, if you purchase an established barbershop, you are not purchasing the staff or clientele. There is no guarantee that with new ownership the staff will be retained or that the clients will continue to return. In general, any agreement to buy an established barbershop should include the following items:

- A financial audit to determine the actual value of the business once the current owner's bookings are taken out of the equation. Often, the barbershop owner brings in the bulk of the business income, and it is unlikely you will retain all the former owner's clients without a lot of support and encouragement from that former owner. Any existing financial statements should also be audited.
- Written purchase and sale agreement to avoid any misunderstandings between the contracting parties.
- Complete and signed statement of inventory (goods, fixtures, etc.) indicating the value of each article.
- If there is a transfer of a note, mortgage, lease, or bill of sale, the buyer should initiate an investigation to determine whether there are defaults in the payment of debts.
- Confirmed identity of the owner.
- Use of the barbershop's name and reputation for a definite period of time.

- Disclosure of any and all information regarding the barbershop's clientele and its purchasing and service habits.

- Disclosure of the conditions of the facility. If you are buying the actual building, a full inspection is in order, and many other legalities apply. Be guided by your realtor and attorney.

- Noncompete agreement stating that the seller will not work in or establish a new barbershop within a specified distance from the present location.

- An employee agreement, either formal or informal, that lets you know if the employees will stay with the business under its new ownership. Existing employee contracts should be transferable.

DRAWING UP A LEASE

In most cases, owning your business does not mean that you own the building that houses your business. When renting or leasing space, you must have an agreement between you and the building's owner that has been well thought out and well written. The lease should specify clearly who owns what and who is responsible for which repairs and expenses. You should also secure the following:

- Exemption of fixtures or appliances that might be attached to the barbershop so that they can be removed without violating the lease.

- Agreement about necessary renovations and repairs, such as painting, plumbing, fixtures, and electrical installation.

- Option from the landlord that allows you to assign the lease to another person. In this way, obligations for the payment of rent are kept separate from the responsibilities of operating the business, should you decide to bring in another person or owner.

PROTECTION AGAINST FIRE, THEFT, AND LAWSUITS

As a business owner, you must protect the business, clients, and shop staff on several levels. Some of the ways you can reduce risk and ensure this protection include:

- Ensure that your business has adequate locks, fire alarm system, burglar alarm system, and surveillance system.

- Purchase liability, fire, malpractice, and burglary insurance, and do not allow these policies to lapse while you are in business.

- Be thoroughly familiar with all laws governing barbering and with the safety and infection control codes of your city and state.

- Keep accurate records of the number of employees, their salaries, lengths of employment, and Social Security numbers as required by various state and federal laws that monitor the social welfare of workers.

- Ignorance of the law is no excuse for violating it. Always check with your regulatory agency if you have any questions about a law or regulation.

BUSINESS OPERATIONS

Whether you are an owner or a manager, there are certain skills that you must develop to successfully run a barbershop. To run a people-oriented business, you need:

- an excellent business sense, aptitude, good judgment, and diplomacy

- knowledge of sound business principles

Because it takes time to develop these skills, it would be wise of you to establish a circle of contacts—business owners, including some barbershop owners—who can give you advice along the way. Consider joining a local entrepreneurs' group or your city's Chamber of Commerce to extend the reach of your networking. The Chamber of Commerce is a local organization of businesses and business owners whose goal is to promote, protect, and further the interests of businesses in a community. Smooth business management depends on the following factors:

- Sufficient investment capital

- Efficiency of management

- Good business procedures

- Strong computer skills

- Cooperation between management and employees

- Trained and experienced barbershop personnel

- Excellent customer service delivery

- Proper pricing of services

Allocation of Money

As a business operator, you must always know where your money is being spent. A good accountant and an accounting system are indispensable. Table 21-1 serves as a guideline, but the figures may vary depending on the locality.

THE IMPORTANCE OF RECORD KEEPING

Good business operations require a simple and efficient record system. Proper business records are necessary to meet the requirements of local, state, and federal laws regarding taxes and employees. Records are of value only if they are correct, concise, and complete. Proper bookkeeping methods include keeping an accurate record of all income and expenses. Income is usually classified as receipts from services and retail sales. Expenses include rent, utilities, insurance, salaries, advertising, equipment, and repairs. Retain all check stubs, cancelled checks, receipts, and invoices. A professional accountant or a full-charge bookkeeper is recommended to help keep records accurate. Table 21-1 is a generalization, and percentages can vary from city to city. For example, rent in New York City may be a different percentage of sales than in Duluth, Minnesota.

table 21-1

FINANCIAL BENCHMARKS FOR BARBERSHOPS IN THE UNITED STATES

Expenses	Percent of Total Gross Income
Salaries and Commissions (Including Payroll Taxes)	53.5
Rent	13.0
Supplies	5.0
Advertising	3.0
Depreciation	3.0
Laundry	1.0
Cleaning	1.0
Light and Power	1.0
Repairs	1.5
Insurance	0.75
Telephone	0.75
Miscellaneous	1.5
Total Expenses	85.0
Net Profit	15.0
Total	100.0

Courtesy Kopsa Otte CPAs & Advisors in York, NE, nationally known as the only accounting firm that specializes in salons and spas.

The term *full-charge bookkeeper* refers to someone who is trained to do everything from recording sales and payroll to generating a profit-and-loss statement. The most important part of record keeping is having the ability to defend your business in the case of an audit by the federal or state government and to have accurate proof of all sales made and taxes paid.

Purchase and Inventory Records

The purchase of inventory and supplies should be closely monitored. Purchase records help you maintain a perpetual inventory, which prevents overstocking or a shortage of needed supplies, and they alert you to any incidents of theft. Purchase records also help establish the net worth of the business at the end of the year.

Keep a running inventory of all supplies, and classify them according to their use and retail value. Those to be used in the daily business operation are **consumption supplies** (KON-sump-shun sup-LYZ). Those to be sold to clients are **retail supplies** (REE-tail sup-LYZ). Both categories have different tax responsibilities, so be sure to check with your accountant that you are charging the proper taxes.

Service Records

Always keep service records or client cards that describe treatments given and merchandise sold to each client. Using a barbershop-specific software program for this purpose is highly recommended. All service records should include the name and address of the client, the date of each purchase or service, the amount charged, the products used, and the results obtained. Clients' preferences and tastes should also be noted.

Understand Booth Rental

After reading this section, you will be able to:

LO⑥ Examine the responsibilities of a booth renter.

Booth rental involves renting a booth or a station in a barbershop or salon. This practice is popular in shops all over the United States. Many people see booth rental or renting a station as a more desirable alternative to owning a barbershop.

In a booth rental arrangement, a professional generally rents a station or work space in a barbershop or salon for a weekly fee paid to the shop owner. Booth renters are solely responsible for their own clientele, supplies, record keeping, and accounting and have the ability to be their own boss with very little capital investment.

Booth rental is a desirable situation for many barbers who have large, steady clientele and who do not have to rely on the shop's general clientele to keep busy. Unless you are at least 70 percent booked all the time, however, it may not be advantageous to rent a booth.

Although it may sound like a good option, booth renting has its share of obligations, such as the following:

- Keeping records for income tax purposes and other legal reasons.

- Paying all taxes, including higher Social Security (double that of an employee).

- Carrying adequate malpractice insurance and health insurance.

- Complying with all IRS obligations for independent contractors. Go to irs.gov and search for independent contractors.

- Using your own telephone and booking systems.

- Collecting all service fees, whether they are paid in cash or via a credit card.

- Creating all professional materials, including business cards and a service menu.

- Purchasing of all supplies, including back bar and retail supplies and products.

- Tracking and maintaining inventory.

- Managing the purchase of products and supplies.

- Budgeting for advertising or offering incentives to ensure a steady flow of new clients.

> **? DID YOU KNOW?**
> Some state do not recognize booth rental as an acceptable method of doing business. Check with your state to be aware of all the latest laws and regulations.

- Paying for all continuing education.

- Working in an independent atmosphere where teamwork usually does not exist and where barbershop standards are interpreted on an individual basis.

- Adhering to state laws and regulations. To date, TWO STATES (Pennsylvania and New Jersey) do not allow booth rental at all; others may require that each renter in an establishment hold his own establishment license and carry individual liability insurance. Always check with your state regulatory agency.

As a booth renter, you will not enjoy the same benefits as an employee of a barbershop would, such as paid days off or vacation time when they are provided. Remember, as a booth renter, when you do not work, you do not get paid. Perhaps, most important, you must continually attract new clients and maintain the ones you have, which means working the hours your clients need you to be available. For more information on booth rental as a business option, reference Milady's: *Booth Renting 101: A Guide for the Independent Stylist.*

Understand the Elements of a Successful Barbershop

After reading this section, you will be able to:

 Distinguish the elements of successful barbershop operations.

The only way to guarantee that you will stay in business and have a prosperous barbershop is to take excellent care of your clients. Clients visiting your shop should feel that they are being well taken care of, and they should always have reason to look forward to their next visit. To accomplish this, your barbershop must be physically attractive, well organized, smoothly run, and, above all, sparkly clean.

PLANNING THE BARBERSHOP'S LAYOUT

One of the most exciting opportunities ahead of you is planning and constructing the best physical layout for the type of barbershop you envision. Maximum efficiency should be the primary concern. For example, if you are opening a low-budget barbershop offering quick service, you will need several stations and a small- to medium-sized reception area because clients will be moving in and out of the shop fairly quickly. Retail sales are essential to a profitable barbering business. Make sure the products you carry and the space you design reflect the importance of high retail sales (**Figure 21-5**).

However, if you are opening a high-end barbershop where clients expect the quality of the service to be matched by the environment, you may want to plan for more room in the waiting area. In fact, you might choose to have several areas where clients can lounge and enjoy light snacks or

figure 21-5
Barbershop floor plans.

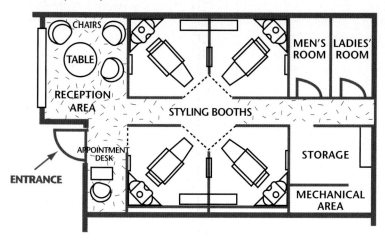

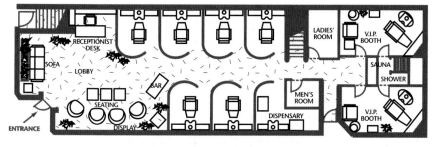

beverages—from soda and coffee to alcoholic beverages. Most shops also provide complimentary Wi-Fi access to their guests.

Layout is crucial to the smooth operation of a barbershop. Once you have decided the type of shop that you wish to run, seek the advice of an architect with plenty of experience in designing barbershops. Ideally, the shop design you develop should include:

- ample aisle space

- space for each piece of equipment

- quality mirrors

- fixtures, furniture, and equipment chosen on the basis of cost, durability, utility, and appearance

- decoration and paint that is thematic and pleasing to the eye

- restrooms for clients and employees

- handicap-accessible facilities and doors

- good plumbing and lighting for services

- ventilation, air-conditioning, and heating

- sufficient electrical outlets and current adequate to service all equipment

- storage areas

- display areas

- an attractive, furnished, and comfortable reception or waiting area

Costs to create even a small barbershop in an existing space can range from $75 to $125 per square foot. Renovating existing space requires familiarity with building codes and the landlord's restrictions before you do anything. All the plumbing should be in the same area, and electrical wiring must be up to code. If they are not, you will pay thousands extra. Before you begin, get everything in writing from contractors, design firms, equipment manufacturers, and architects. It is a good idea to get three quotes on everything from contractors and cleaning services to barber stations and equipment. Do not be afraid to negotiate whenever you can.

Try to estimate how much each area in the barbershop will earn, so you can use space efficiently. An inviting retail display in your reception area is a good investment; on the other hand, an employee break area produces no income. In addition to start-up costs for creating your barbershop, you will need financing for operational expenses. Realistically, you should plan to have at least several months and up to 1 year of expenses available to help get you up and running. It takes most new shops about 6 months to begin operating at full capacity.

PERSONNEL

Your **personnel** (PER-son-elle) is your staff or employees. The size of your barbershop will determine the size of your staff. Large shops may require receptionists, barbers, colorists, manicurists, assistants, and housekeepers (Figure 21-6).

Smaller barbershops have some combination of these personnel who perform more than one type of service. For example, a barber might also be the colorist. Ultimately, whether your barbershop is large or small, high end or economical, the success of a shop depends on the attitude and quality of work done by the staff.

figure 21-6
Your barber personnel.

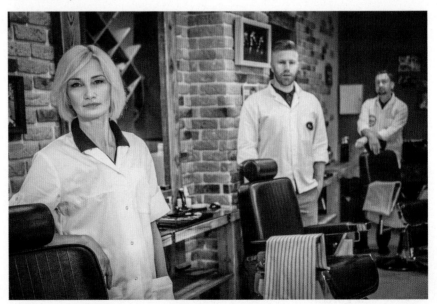

When interviewing potential employees, consider the following:

- **Level of skill.** What is their educational background? When was the last time they attended an educational event? How long have they been in the industry? What can they bring to the organization beyond barbering?

- **Personal grooming.** Do they look like professionals you would consult for personal grooming advice?

- **Image as it relates to the barbershop.** Are they too progressive or too conservative for your environment? Does their image reflect the image of your business?

- **Overall attitude.** Are they mostly positive or mostly negative in their responses to your questions? Do they seem self-motivated and self-directed?

- **Communication skills.** Are they able to understand your questions? Can you understand their responses?

- **Work history.** Have they been at a previous barbershop for many years, or do they hop from shop to shop? Are they bringing a clientele, or do they expect you to build one for them?

Making good hiring decisions is crucial. Undoing bad hiring decisions is painful for all involved, and it can be more complicated than one might expect.

Payroll and Employee Benefits

To have a successful business, one in which everyone feels appreciated and is happy to work hard to service clients well, you must be willing to share your success with your staff whenever it is financially feasible to do so. You can do this in a number of ways:

- Make it your top priority to meet your payroll obligations. In the allotment of funds, this comes first. It will also be your largest expense.

- Whenever possible, offer hardworking and loyal employees as many benefits as possible. Either cover the cost of these benefits, or simply make them available to employees, who can decide if they can cover the cost themselves.

- Provide staff members with a schedule of employee evaluations. Make it clear what is expected of them if they are to receive pay increases.

- Create and stay with a tipping policy. It is a good idea for both your employees and your clients to know exactly what is expected. It is also important to be familiar with the tax laws around tipping.

- Put your entire pay plan in writing.

- Create incentives by giving your staff opportunities to earn more money, prizes, or tickets to educational events and trade shows; when a reward is involved, it can inspire employees to achieve more.

- Create barbershop policies and stick to them. Everyone in the shop should be governed by the same rules, including you!

ACTIVITY

What would your dream barbershop look like? Try your hand at designing a shop that would attract the kinds of clients you want; offer the services you would like to specialize in; and provide an efficient, comfortable working environment for barbers.

Draw pictures, use word pictures, or try a combination of both. Pay attention to practical requirements, but feel free to dream a little, too. Skylights? A mechanical bull? You name it. It's your dream!

Managing Personnel

As a new barbershop owner, one of your most challenging tasks will be managing your staff. At the same time, leading your team can also be very rewarding. If you are good at managing others, you can make a positive impact on their lives and their ability to earn a living. If managing people does not come naturally, do not despair. People can learn how to manage other people, just as they learn how to drive a car or perform hair services. Keep in mind that managing others is a serious job. Whether it comes naturally to you or not, it takes time to become comfortable with the role.

Human resources, or HR, is an entire specialty in its own right. It covers not only how you manage employees but also what you can and cannot say when hiring, managing, or firing them. All employers must be familiar with various civil rights laws, including Equal Employment Opportunity Commission (EEOC) regulations, and the Americans with Disabilities Act (ADA), which pertains to hiring and firing, as well as business design for accessibility. Every business should have a written personnel policies and procedures manual, and every employee must read and sign it. If you choose to use a payroll company, it can provide HR services and employee manuals for a nominal fee. The more documented systems you have for managing human resources, the better.

There are many excellent books, both within and outside the professional barbering industry, that you can use as resources for learning about managing employees and staff. Spend an afternoon online or at your local bookstore researching the topic and purchasing materials or registering for classes that will educate and inform you. Once you have a broad base of information, you will be able to select a technique or style that best suits your personality and that of your barbershop.

THE FRONT DESK

Most shop owners believe that the quality and pricing of services are the most important elements of running a successful barbershop. Certainly these are crucial, but too often the front desk—the operations center—is overlooked. The best barbershops employ professional receptionists to handle the job of answering phones, scheduling appointments, greeting clients, and attending to the clients' needs.

The Reception Area

First impressions count, and since the reception area is the first area clients see, it needs to be attractive, appealing, and comfortable. This is your barbershop's nerve center, where retail merchandise is on display, the phone system is centered, financial transactions are carried out, and your receptionist stands, should you employ one.

Make sure that the reception area is stocked with business cards and there is a prominently displayed price list that shows at a glance what your clients should expect to pay for various services.

The Receptionist

When it comes to staffing, your receptionist is second in importance only to your licensed professionals. A well-trained receptionist is crucial because the receptionist is the first and last person the client contacts. The receptionist should have an image that reflects your brand, should be pleasant and patient, should greet each client with a smile, and should address each client by name. Efficient, friendly, and consistent service fosters goodwill, confidence, and satisfaction.

In addition to filling the crucial role of greeter, the receptionist handles other important functions, including answering the phone, booking appointments, informing barbers that a client has arrived, preparing daily appointment information for the staff, and recommending additional services and products to clients. The receptionist should have a thorough knowledge of all retail products carried by the shop so that they or he can also serve as a salesperson and information source for clients.

During slow periods, it is customary for the receptionist to perform certain other duties and activities, such as straightening up the reception area and maintaining inventory and daily reports. Personal calls or personal projects are done on personal time, not at work.

Booking Appointments

The key duty of the receptionist is booking appointments. This must be done with care because services are sold in terms of time on the appointment page. Appointments must be scheduled to make the most efficient use of everyone's time—both the client and the barber. Under ideal circumstances, a client should not have to wait for a service, and a barber should not have to wait for the next client.

Booking appointments is primarily the receptionist's job, but when they are not available, the barbershop owner or manager, or one of the other professionals in small barbershops, can help with scheduling. It is important for each person involved in working the reception area to understand how to book an appointment and how much time is needed for each service. Regardless of who actually makes the appointment, anyone who answers the phone or deals with clients must have a pleasing voice and personality.

Appointment Book

The appointment book helps barbers arrange time to suit their clients' needs. It should accurately reflect what is taking place in the shop at any given time. In larger barbershops, the receptionist prepares the appointment schedule for staff members; in smaller shops, each person may prepare their own schedule (Figure 21-7).

Increasingly, the appointment book is a computerized book that is easily accessed through the barbershop's computer system. It may also be an actual hard copy book that is located on the reception desk. Some shops have websites with online booking systems, which tie into barbershop management software.

figure 21-7
Schedule appointments.

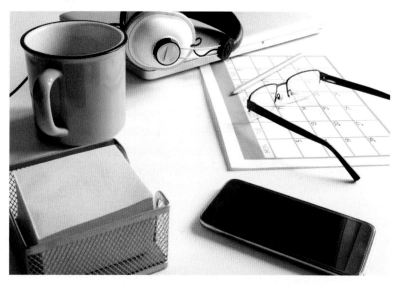

USE OF TELEPHONE IN THE BARBERSHOP

A majority of barbershop business is handled over the telephone. Good telephone habits and techniques make it possible for the barbershop owner and employees to increase business and improve relationships with clients and suppliers. With each call, a gracious, appropriate response helps build the shop's reputation. For example, "Thank you for calling Milady Barbers, Shannon speaking. How may I help you?"

Good Planning

Because it can be noisy, business calls to clients and suppliers should be made at a quiet time of the day or from a quiet area of the shop. When using the telephone, you should:

- have a pleasant telephone voice, speak clearly, and use correct grammar. A smile on your face should reflect in your voice and counts a lot.

- show interest and concern when talking with a client or a supplier.

- be polite, respectful, and courteous to all, even though some people may test the limits of your patience.

- be tactful. Do not say anything to irritate the person on the other end of the line.

Incoming Telephone Calls

An incoming call is often your client's first impression of your business. Clients usually call ahead for appointments with a preferred barber, or they might call to cancel or reschedule an appointment. The person answering the phone should have the necessary telephone skills to handle these calls.

When you answer the phone, say, "Good morning (afternoon or evening), thank you for calling Milady Barbers. How may I help you?" or "Thank you for calling Milady Barbers. This is Jonathan speaking. How may I help you?" Some barbershops require that you give your name to the caller. The first words you say tell the caller something about your personality. Let callers know that you are glad to hear from them.

Answer the phone promptly. A good rule of thumb is to not let the phone ring more than three times. On a system with more than one line, if a call comes in while you are talking on another line, ask to put the first person on hold, answer the second call, and ask that person to hold while you complete the first call. Take calls in the order in which they are received.

If you do not have the information requested by a caller, either put the caller on hold and get the information or offer to call the person back with the information as soon as you have it.

Do not talk with a client standing nearby while you are speaking with someone on the phone. Have one conversation at a time to avoid doing a disservice to both clients.

Booking Appointments by Phone

When booking appointments, take down the client's first and last name, their phone number, their e-mail address, and the service booked. Many barbershops call the client to confirm the appointment 1 or 2 days before it is scheduled. Automated systems can send an e-mail or even a text message confirmation.

You should be familiar with all the services and products available in the barbershop and their costs, as well as which barbers or specialists perform specific services, such as color correction. Be fair when making assignments. Do not schedule six appointments for one professional and only two for another, unless it is necessary because you are working with specialists.

However, if someone calls to ask for an appointment with a particular barber on a particular day and time, make every effort to accommodate the client's request. If the barber is not available, handle the situation in one of the following ways:

- Suggest other times that the barber is available.

- If the barber cannot come in at any of those times, suggest another professional.

- If the client is unwilling to try another barber, offer to call the client if there is a cancellation at the desired time.

Handling Complaints by Telephone

Handling complaints, particularly over the phone, is a difficult task. The caller is probably upset and possibly short tempered. Respond with self-control, tact, and courtesy, no matter how trying the circumstances. Only then will the caller feel that they have been treated fairly.

The tone of your voice must be sympathetic and reassuring. Your manner of speaking should convince the caller that you are really concerned about the complaint. Do not interrupt the caller. After hearing the complaint in full, try to resolve the situation quickly and effectively.

Know How to Build Your Business

After reading this section, you will be able to:

LO⑧   Validate why advertising is a vital aspect of a barbershop's success.

A new barbershop owner will want to get the business up and running as soon as possible to start earning some revenue and to begin paying off debts. The first area of opportunity for building your business is through social media.

SOCIAL MEDIA

The term **social media** refers to a platform used to engage and communicate with groups of people by way of online communities, networks, websites, or blogs, for personal or professional means. Social media platforms such as Facebook, Twitter, YouTube, and Instagram are free to use and a great way to build awareness about your business and at the same time engage your audience in an interactive format. Some barbershops have one person in charge of their social media to control the content and ensure certain standards are met. Other shops allow the staff to post on their behalf.

Some guidelines to effectively using social media are listed here:

- Have the same username for all accounts.
- Get permission from clients if you use their image in your posting.
- Post regularly so your followers pay attention.
- Respond to questions, comments, or "likes."

Another, more costly option the new shop owner should consider is advertising the barbershop. It is important to understand the many aspects of advertising.

ADVERTISING

The term *advertising* encompasses promotional efforts that are paid for and are directly intended to increase business.

Advertising includes all activities that promote the barbershop favorably, from newspaper ads to radio spots to charity events that the shop participates in, such as fashion shows. To create a desire for a service or product, advertising must attract and hold the attention of readers, listeners, or viewers.

Satisfied clients are the very best form of advertising because they will refer your barbershop to friends and family. So make your clients happy (**Figure 21-8**)! Then, have your clients work for you. Develop a referral program and a loyalty program in which the referring client reaps a reward.

If you have some experience developing ads, you may decide to do your own advertising. On the other hand, if you need help, you can hire an agency or ask a local newspaper or radio station to help you produce the ad. As a general rule, an advertising budget should not exceed 3 percent of your gross income. Make sure you plan well in advance for holidays and special yearly events, such as proms, New Year's Eve, or the wedding season.

figure 21-8
Keep your clients happy.

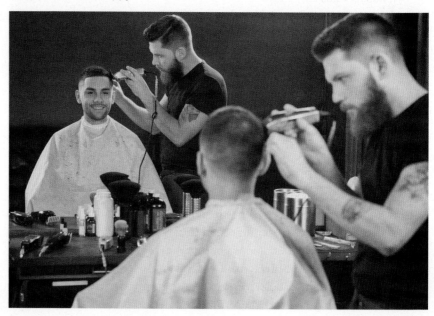

© Nestor Rizhniak/Shutterstock.com.

Make certain you know what you are paying for. Get everything in writing. No form of advertising can promise that you will get business. Sometimes, local circulars can work well. You must know your clientele, which types of media they use, and what kinds of messages attract them.

Here are some tools you may choose to attract customers to the barbershop:

- Newspaper ads and coupons.

- Build a website. If you don't have a large budget now, buy your domain name and keep that ownership current. You can set up a site very inexpensively, and as your business grows, you can build it to have many pages and features. Building a website is an easy way for new clients to find you through Internet searches or friends sharing links.

- E-mail newsletters and discount offers to all clients who have agreed to receive such mailings. (Always include an *Unsubscribe* link.) You can also purchase e-mail lists targeted to your demographic to help you build your subscriber list.

- Website offerings, including those on your own website, social networking websites, and blogs.

- Direct mail to mailing lists and your current barbering client list.

- Classified advertising.

- Giveaway promotional items, such as branded combs, or retail packages, like shampoos and colognes.

ACTIVITY

All the planning in the world cannot guarantee success as much as a happy client can. Great customer service and a fabulous customer experience are the most important aspects of barbershop success. What will your customer service look like? Imagine you are calling or walking into your dream shop. Write down everything about your ideal experience as a customer, from the way you are greeted, to the actual service, to checkout at the desk when you leave. Include all five senses.

- Window displays that attract attention and feature the barbershop and your retail products.
- Radio advertising.
- Television advertising.
- Community outreach by volunteering at men's and women's clubs, church functions, political gatherings, and charitable affairs and on TV and radio talk shows.
- Make donations of services for local organizations like school fundraisers.
- Client referrals.
- In-shop videos that promote your services and products.
- Create an on-hold message featuring your shop's best attributes.

Many of these vehicles can help you attract new clients, but the first goal of every business should be to maintain current clients. It takes at least three shop visits for a new client to become a loyal current client. Encourage your staff to have their guests prebook their appointments: Just because a client has visited the barbershop 100 times does not mean they will come again. By having a prebooking system in place, you are guaranteeing future business. Once you have a loyal client base, it is far less expensive to market to that base. That is why you should follow up every visit to determine the client's satisfaction and why you should personally contact any client who has not been in the shop for more than 8 weeks.

SELLING IN THE BARBERSHOP

An important aspect of the barbershop's financial success revolves around upselling (adding on additional services), cross promoting (encouraging a client who is booked for a haircut to also get a manicure or facial), and retailing (selling take-home or maintenance products). No matter the size or style of your business, adding services and retail sales to your service ticket means additional revenue. Remember: your clients will spend money during their visit. It is your job to encourage your clients to invest in retail and services that will keep them coming back for more, while also helping to maintain the look you just gave them!

It is important that we as professionals feel confident in selling services and retail. Remove any negative feelings or stereotypes you have toward sales or sales people and start fresh. Helpful and knowledgeable professionals make customer care their top priority. These people play a major role in the lives of their customers and are very valuable to clients because they offer good advice. In fact, the successful barbershop owner, like the successful barber, makes their living by giving complete image advice every day (**Figure 21-9**).

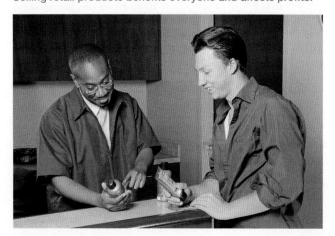

figure 21-9
Selling retail products benefits everyone and affects profits.

REVIEW QUESTIONS

1. What are the two most common options for going into business for yourself?

2. List at least three of the basic factors that potential barbershop owners should consider before opening their doors.

3. How many types of barbershop ownership are there? What are they?

4. List the categories of information that should be included in a business plan.

5. Why is it important to keep good records? What types of records should be kept?

6. When interviewing potential employees, what are the six factors to keep in mind?

7. What responsibilities does a booth renter assume?

8. List the four elements of a successful barbershop.

9. Name five advertising tools you might use to attract customers to your barbershop.

10. Why is selling services and products such a vital aspect of a barbershop's success?

CHAPTER GLOSSARY

barbershop operation	p. 760	the ongoing, recurring processes or activities involved in the running of a barbershop for the purpose of producing income and value
barbershop policies	p. 760	the rules or regulations adopted by a barbershop to ensure that all clients and associates are being treated fairly and consistently
business plan (BIZ-nez plahn)	p. 759	a written description of your business as you see it today and as you foresee it in the next 5 years (detailed by year)
business regulations and laws (BIZ-nez reg-U-lay-shuns AND LAWZ)	p. 759	any and all local, state, and federal regulations and laws that you must comply with when you decide to open your barbershop or rent a booth
capital (KAP-uh-tal)	p. 761	money needed to invest in a business
consumption supplies (KON-sump-shun sup-LYZ)	p. 766	supplies used in the daily business operation
corporation (KOR-pour-aye-shun)	p. 761	an ownership structure controlled by one or more stockholders
demographics (dem-oh-graf-iks)	p. 759	information about a specific population including data on race, age, income, and educational attainment
goals (GOHLZ)	p. 757	a set of benchmarks that, once achieved, help you to realize your mission and your vision
insurance (in-SHUR-ens)	p. 760	guarantees protection against financial loss from malpractice, property liability, fire, burglary and theft, and business interruption
partnership (PART-nur-ship)	p. 760	business structure in which two or more people share ownership, although not necessarily equally
personnel (PER-son-elle)	p. 770	your staff or employees
record keeping (REK-urd KEEP-ing)	p. 760	maintaining accurate and complete records of all financial activities in your business
retail supplies (REE-tail sup-LYZ)	p. 766	supplies sold to clients
social media	p. 775	a platform used to engage and communicate with groups of people through online communities, networks, websites, or blogs, for personal or professional means
sole proprietor (SOHL PRHO-pry-eh-tohr)	p. 760	individual owner and, most often, the manager of a business
vision statement (VIZ-uhn state-ment)	p. 757	a long-term picture of what the business is to become and what it will look like when it gets there
written agreements (RIT-en UH-gree-mentz)	p. 758	documents that govern the opening of a barbershop, including leases, vendor contracts, and employee contracts; all of these detail, usually for legal purposes, who does what and what is given in return

APPENDIX

FORMERLY CHAPTER 20, NAILS AND MANICURING IS PRESENTED HERE TO MEET THE INSTRUCTIONAL NEEDS OF THE FEW STATES THAT INCLUDE THIS SUBJECT IN THEIR BARBERING CURRICULUM.

NAIL CARE

LEARNING OBJECTIVES

After reading through the Appendix, you will be able to:

LO❶
Describe the composition of the nail.

LO❷
Identify common nail disorders and diseases.

LO❸
Identify nail care equipment, implements, materials, and products.

LO❹
Recognize the five general shapes of nails.

LO❺
Understand table setup, hand massage, and manicure procedures.

APPENDIX OUTLINE

Introduction

Barbershops of the first half of the twentieth century routinely provided manicures as part of the traditional shave, haircut, and shoeshine service. Today's barbershops can offer the service through a licensed manicurist, nail technician, or in a few states, by a licensed barber. Always refer to your state board rules and regulations to confirm the services you are licensed to perform.

why study
NAIL CARE?

Barbers should study and have a thorough understanding of nail care because:

> They need to know the procedures for performing a manicure or to oversee a manicure that is performed by others.

> They need to recognize conditions that may benefit from a manicure service.

> They need to recognize conditions that prohibit a manicure service.

Describe the Nail Unit

After reading this section, you will be able to:

LO **1** Describe the composition of the nail.

The **nail** (NAYL) is a horny, translucent plate of hard keratin that serves to protect the tips of the fingers and toes. Nails are part of the integumentary system and are considered to be appendages of the skin. The technical term for nail is **onyx** (AHN-iks).

The condition of the nail, like that of the skin, reflects the general health of the body. The normal, healthy nail is firm, flexible, and translucent with the pinkish color of the nail bed below showing through. Its surface should be smooth, curved, and unspotted, without any hollows or wavy **ridges** (RIJ-ez). No nerves or blood vessels are contained within the horny nail plate. The nail unit consists of the nail plate, nail bed, matrix, cuticle, eponychium, perionychium, hyponychium, specialized ligaments, and nail folds (**Figure A-1**).

* The **nail plate** (NAYL PLAYT) is a hardened keratin plate, constructed of layers of matrix cells, that sits on and covers the nail bed. The nail plate slowly slides upon the nail bed as it grows and extends to the **free edge** (FREE EJ) of the nail.

* The **nail bed** (NAYL BED) is the portion of living skin that supports the nail plate as it grows toward the free edge. It is supplied with blood vessels that provide the pinkish tone from the lunula almost to the free edge and nerves that are attached to the nail plate. The nail bed is attached to the nail plate by a thin layer of tissue called the **bed epithelium** (BED ep-ih-TH-EE-lee-um), which helps guide the nail plate along the nail bed as it grows.

figure A-1
Structure of the natural nail.

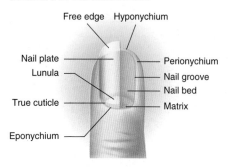

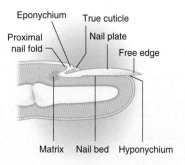

- The **matrix** (MAY-triks) is where the nail plate cells are formed. The cells are nourished by nerves, lymph, and blood vessels, and continue to grow as long as the matrix receives nutrition and remains healthy. The visible portion of the matrix is called the **lunula** (LOO-nuh-luh) or half-moon. It is located at the base of the nail where the matrix and the connective tissue of the nail bed join.

- The **cuticle** (KYOO-tih-kul) is the crescent of *dead*, colorless tissue attached to the nail plate around the base of the nail that forms a seal between the eponychium and the nail plate to help prevent injury and infection.

- The **eponychium** (ep-oh-NIK-ee-um) is the *living* skin at the base of the nail plate covering the matrix area and should not be confused with the cuticle.

- The **perionychium** (payr-ee-uh-NIK-ee-um) is the living skin bordering the root and sides of a nail.

- The **hyponychium** (hy-poh-NIK-ee-um) is the slightly thickened layer of skin between the fingertip and the free edge of the nail plate that forms a protective barrier against microorganisms and infection of the nail bed.

- The **specialized ligaments** form bands of fibrous tissue that attach the nail bed and matrix to the underlying bone that are located at the base of the matrix and around the edges of the nail bed.

- The **nail folds** (NAYL FOHLDZ) are folds of normal skin that surround the nail plate. These folds form the **nail grooves** (NAYL GROOVZ) on the sides of the nail that permit the nail to move as it grows.

NAIL GROWTH

Nail growth is influenced by nutrition, health, and disease. A normal, healthy nail grows forward, starting at the matrix and extending over the fingertip. The average rate of growth in the normal adult is about $\frac{1}{10}$ inch per month. Typically, nails grow faster in summer than they do in winter. Children's nails grow more rapidly, whereas those of elderly persons grow more slowly. The nail of the middle finger grows the fastest and the thumbnail the most slowly. Although toenails grow more slowly than fingernails, they are thicker and harder (**Figure A-2**).

figure A-2
Various shapes of nails.

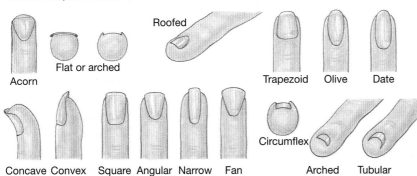

Acorn
Flat or arched
Roofed
Trapezoid Olive Date

Concave Convex Square Angular Narrow Fan Circumflex Arched Tubular

NAIL MALFORMATION

If the nail is separated from the nail bed through injury, it becomes distorted or **discolored** (dis-KUL-urd). Should the nail bed be injured after the loss of a nail, a badly formed new nail will result.

Nails are not shed in the same way that hair is shed. If a nail is torn off accidentally or lost through infection or disease, it will be replaced only if the matrix remains in good condition. In some cases, the replacement nails are shaped abnormally, due to interference at the base of the nail. Replacement of the nail takes about four to six months.

Recognize Nail Disorders and Diseases

After reading this section, you will be able to:

LO❷ Identify common nail disorders and diseases.

A *nail disorder* is a condition caused by injury to the nail, disease, or a chemical or nutritional imbalance. Most clients will have experienced a common nail disorder at some time in their lives. If a client has a nail disorder, you may be able to help them in one of two ways: either cosmetically improve the condition or appearance of the nail plate or refer them to a physician. Be observant and if the nail or the skin surrounding it looks infected or inflamed, do not perform the manicure and recommend the client seek medical attention. Review **Tables A-1** and **A-2** to be able to recognize common nail disorders.

table A-1

OVERVIEW OF NAIL DISORDERS

Disorder	Signs or Symptoms
Beau's Lines (BOWZ LYNZ)	Visible depressions running across the width of the natural nail plate; usually a result of major illness or injury that has traumatized the body.
Blue Fingernails	Blue or purple nail bed, usually from poor circulation.
Bruised Nail Beds	Dark purplish spots, usually due to physical injury.
Discolored Nails	Nails turn a variety of colors; may indicate surface staining, a systemic disorder, or poor blood circulation.
Eggshell Nails	Noticeably thin, white nail plates that are more flexible than normal and can curve over the free edge; usually caused by improper diet, hereditary factors, internal disease, or medication.
Hangnails (HANG-NAYLZ)	Living skin around the nail plate (often the eponychium) that becomes split or torn.
Koilonychia (koyal-oh-NICK-ee-uh)	Also known as *spoon nails*; inverted or concave nails.

Leukonychia Spots (loo-koh-NIK-ee-ah SPATZ)	Also known as *white spots*; whitish discolorations of the nail usually caused by minor injury to the nail matrix. Not related to the body's health or vitamin deficiencies.
Melanonychia (mel-uh-nuh-NIK-ee-uh)	Darkening of the fingernails or toenails; may be seen as a black band within the nail plate extending from the base to the free edge.
Nail Pterygium (NAYL teh-RIJ-ee-um)	Abnormal stretching of skin around the nail plate; usually caused by serious injury, such as burns, or an adverse skin reaction to chemical nail enhancement products or an allergic skin reaction.
Onychauxis (ahn-ih-KAHK-sis)	Thickening of the fingernails or toenails.
Onychogryposis (ahn-ih-koh-gry-POH-sis	Also known as *ram's horn* or *claw nails*; an enlargement of the fingernails or toenails accompanied by increased thickening and curvature.
Onychophagy (ahn-ih-koh-FAY-jee)	Also known as *bitten nails*; chewed nails or chewed hardened skin surrounding the nail plate.
Onychorrhexis (ahn-ih-koh-REK-sis)	Split or brittle nails that have a series of lengthwise ridges giving a rough appearance to the surface of the nail plate.
Pincer Nail (PIN-sir NAYL)	Also known as *trumpet nail*; increased crosswise curvature throughout the nail plate caused by an increased curvature of the matrix; the edges of the nail plate may curl around to form the shape of a trumpet or sharp cone at the free edge.
Plicatured Nail (plik-a-CHOORD NAYL)	Also known as *folded nail*; a type of highly curved nail plate, usually caused by injury to the matrix, but it may be inherited.
Ridges	Vertical lines running the length of the natural nail plate that are caused by uneven growth of the nails, usually the result of normal aging.
Splinter Hemorrhage (SPLIN-tohr HEM-err-aje)	Physical trauma or injury to the nail bed that damages the capillaries and allows a small amount of blood flow.

table A-2

OVERVIEW OF NAIL DISEASES

Disease	Signs or Symptoms
Nail Psoriasis (NAYL suh-RY-uh-sis)	Tiny pits or severe roughness on the surface of the nail plate.
Onychia (uh-NIK-ee-uh)	Inflammation of the nail matrix followed by shedding of the nail.
Onychocryptosis (ahn-ih-koh-krip-TOH-sis)	Also known as *ingrown nails*; nail grows into the sides of the tissue around the nail.
Onycholysis (ahn-ih-KAHL-ih-sis)	Lifting of the nail plate from the nail bed, without shedding, usually beginning at the free edge and continuing toward the lunula area.
Onychomadesis (ahn-ih-koh-muh-DEE-sis)	Separation and falling off of a nail plate from the nail bed; can affect fingernails and toenails.

(Continues)

Onychomycosis (ahn-ih-koh-my-KOH-sis)	Fungal infection of the natural nail plate.
Paronychia (payr-uh-NIK-ee-uh)	Bacterial inflammation of the tissues surrounding the nail. Redness, pus, and swelling are usually seen in the skin fold adjacent to the nail plate.
Pseudomonas Aeruginosa (SUE-duh-MOAN-us aye-ru-jin-oh-sa)	Common bacteria that can lead to a bacterial infection that appears as a green, yellow, or black discoloration on the nail bed.
Pyogenic Granuloma (py-oh-JEN-ik gran-yoo-LOH-muh)	Severe inflammation of the nail in which a lump of red tissue grows up from the nail bed to the nail plate.
Tinea Pedis (TIN-ee-uh PED-us)	Also known as *athlete's foot*; red, itchy rash on the skin on the bottom of feet and/or between the toes, usually between the fourth and fifth toe.

Learn about Manicuring

After reading this section, you will be able to:

LO③ Identify nail care equipment, implements, materials, and products.

LO④ Recognize the five general shapes of nails.

LO⑤ Understand table setup, hand massage, and manicure procedures.

The ancients regarded long, polished, and colored fingernails as a mark of distinction between aristocrats and common laborers. The word *manicure* is derived from the Latin *manus* (meaning "hand") and *cura* (meaning "care"), which means the care of the hands and nails.

To perform professional manicures, it is important to develop competence when working with nail care tools. Nail care tools include equipment, implements, materials, and products.

IDENTIFY MANICURE EQUIPMENT, IMPLEMENTS, MATERIALS, AND PRODUCTS

Equipment

Equipment used to perform nail services do not require replacement until they are no longer in good repair.

- *Manicure table with adjustable lamp:* Most standard manicuring tables include drawers for storage and an attached, adjustable lamp (**Figure A-3**). The lamp should have a 40- to 60-watt bulb. Heat from a higher-wattage bulb will interfere with manicuring and sculptured nail procedures. A lower-wattage bulb will not warm a client's nails in a room that is highly air-conditioned. The warmth from the bulb will help maintain product consistency.

- *Client's chair and technician's chair or stool.*

figure A-3
Manicure table.

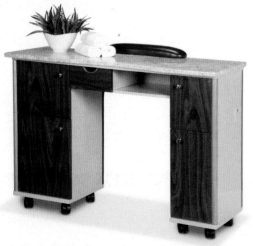

- *Finger bowl:* A plastic, china, metal, or glass bowl is used for soaking the client's fingers in warm water and antibacterial soap (**Figure A-4**).

- *Disinfection container:* This receptacle must be large enough to hold the disinfectant solution in which to immerse implements for sanitizing purposes. A cover is provided with most containers to prevent contamination of the solution when it is not in use.

- *Client's arm cushion:* The cushion is usually 8 to 12-inches long and especially made for manicuring (a towel that is folded to cushion size can also be used). The cushion or folded towel should be covered with a clean towel before each appointment.

- *Gauze and cotton container:* This container holds clean, absorbent cotton, lint-free wipes, or gauze squares.

- *Supply tray:* The tray holds cosmetics such as polishers, polish removers, and creams. It should be sturdy and easy to clean.

- *Electric nail dryer:* A nail dryer is an optional item used to shorten the length of time necessary for drying the client's nails.

- *Metal trash can:* The trash can should have a foot pedal and lid and be lined with a plastic bag.

- *Approved solution for jar sanitizer:* Depending on state laws, *disinfected* metal implements may be placed in a small jar containing a disinfectant to maintain sanitary standards during the manicure. Always follow-up with thorough washing and disinfection of the implements and jar after each use. Check your state rules and regulations for further information.

Implements

Implements are tools that must be cleaned and disinfected or discarded after use with each client.

- *Wooden pusher:* Use a wooden pusher, also known as an *orangewood stick*, to loosen the cuticle around the base of a nail or clean under the free edge. Hold the stick similarly to a pencil (**Figure A-5**).

- *Metal pusher:* The metal pusher is used to push back excess cuticle growth. Hold the pusher in the same way as the wooden pusher. The spoon end is used to loosen and push back the cuticle. If the pusher has rough or sharp edges, use an abrasive board to dull them. This prevents digging into the nail plate.

- *Abrasive nail file:* An abrasive nail file is used to shape the free edge of natural or sculptured nails (**Figure A-6**). Abrasive files are available in different grits; the lower the grit number, the more aggressive its action. Most professional nail technicians use 7- or 8-inch nail files because some states do not allow shorter files to be used. When using a nail file, hold it with the thumb on one side of the handle and four fingers on the other side at an angle to the free edge. Emery boards are another type of abrasive file.

- *Nipper:* A nipper is used to trim away dead skin at the base of the nail (**Figure A-7**). To use the nipper, hold it in the palm of the hand with the blades facing the cuticle. Place the thumb on one handle and three fingers on the other handle, with the index finger on the screw to help guide the blade around the cuticle.

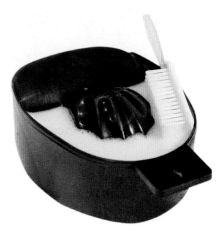

figure A-4
Finger bowl for manicures.

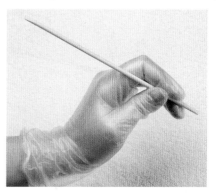

figure A-5
Wooden pusher.

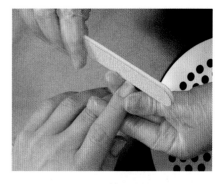

figure A-6
Typical abrasive nail file.

> ⚠ **CAUTION**
> Always prep abrasive boards by rubbing a clean board across the sharp edges before use.

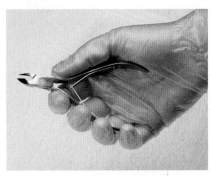

figure A-7
Nail nipper.

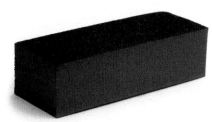

figure A-8
Abrasive nail block buffer.

- *Tweezers:* Tweezers can be used to lift small particles from the nail.
- *Nail brush:* A nail brush is used to clean fingernails and remove bits of cuticle with warm, soapy water. Hold the nail brush with the bristles turned down and away from you. Place the thumb on the handle side of the brush facing you and the fingers on the other side.
- *Nail buffer:* Buffers used to be made with a chamois cover, but new disposable materials have replaced them. Two- or three-way buffers are used to add shine to the nail and to smooth out corrugations or wavy ridges (**Figure A-8**).
- *Fingernail clippers:* Fingernail clippers are used to shorten nails. For very long nails, clipping reduces filing time.
- *Plastic or metal spatula:* The spatula is used to remove nail cosmetics from their containers. Never use your fingers because you will transfer bacteria into the container and contaminate the product.

Materials

Materials are supplies that need to be replaced for each client.

- *Disposable towels or terry cloth towels:* A fresh, sanitized terry towel is used to cover the client's cushion before each manicure. Another fresh towel should be used to dry the client's hands after soaking in the finger bowl. Other terry or lint-free disposable towels are used to wipe spills that may occur around the finger bowl.
- *Cotton or cotton balls:* Cotton is used to remove polish, wrap the end of the wooden pusher, and apply nail cosmetics. Some nail technicians prefer to use small, fiber-free squares to remove polish because they do not leave cotton fibers on the nails that might interfere with polish application.
- *Gloves:* Use gloves when disinfecting implements and surfaces. Check with state board laws regarding required use during a manicure. Gloves are personal protective equipment (PPE) worn to protect the barber from exposure to microbes during services.
- *Plastic bags:* Tape or clip a bag to the side of the manicuring table to hold materials used during a service. Line all trash cans with plastic bags. Be sure to have a generous supply of bags so that they can be changed regularly during the day.

Products

This section describes some basic nail cosmetics that are often used during a manicure.

- *Antibacterial soap:* This soap is mixed with warm water and used in the finger bowl to clean.
- *Buffing powder or cream:* Buffing powder is used with a chamois buffer or three-way buffer to polish and add shine to the surface of the nail plate. The dry version may also be known as *pumice powder*.
- *Polish remover:* Polish remover is used to dissolve and remove nail polish; use non-acetone polish remover for clients who have artificial nails, since acetone will weaken or dissolve the tips, wrap glues, and sculptured nail compound.

- *Cuticle cream:* Cuticle cream is used to lubricate and soften dry cuticles and brittle nails.
- *Cuticle oil:* Cuticle oil keeps the cuticle soft and helps prevent hangnails or rough cuticles.
- *Cuticle solvent or cuticle remover:* Cuticle solvent makes cuticles easier to remove and minimizes nipper work.
- *Nail bleach:* Nail bleach is applied to the nail plate and under the free edge to remove yellow stains.
- *Nail whitener:* Nail whiteners are applied under the free edge of a nail to make the nail appear white.
- *Nail strengthener/hardener:* Nail strengthener is applied to the nail before the base coat to prevent splitting and peeling of the nail. Two types of nail strengtheners are protein hardeners and nylon fiber hardeners.
- *Base coat:* The base coat is colorless and is applied to the nail before the application of colored polish or a clear top coat unless a nail strengthener is being used.
- *Colored polish, liquid enamel, or lacquer:* Colored polish is used to add color and gloss to the nail and is usually applied in two coats.
- *Top coat or sealer:* The top coat, a colorless polish, is applied over colored polish to prevent chipping and to add a shine to the finished nail.
- *Liquid nail dry:* Liquid nail dry promotes rapid drying and is available in brush-on or spray form.
- *Hand cream and hand lotion:* Hand lotion and hand cream add a finishing touch to a manicure and help replace lost moisture to the skin.
- *Nail conditioner:* Nail conditioner contains moisturizers and helps prevent brittle nails and dry cuticles.

TYPES OF POLISH APPLICATIONS

When men choose to wear polish, it is usually a clear polish that is applied to the entire nail plate (full coverage). Women, on the other hand, may request one of the following coverage options instead of full coverage:

- *Free edge:* The free edge of the nail is unpolished. This helps prevent the polish from chipping.
- *Hairline tip:* The nail plate is *polished* and a $\frac{1}{16}$ inch is removed from the free edge. This prevents the polish from chipping.
- *Slim-line or free walls:* Leave a $\frac{1}{16}$-inch margin on each side of the nail plate. This makes a wide nail appear narrower.
- *Half-moon or lunula:* The lunula at the base of the nail is left unpolished.

APPLYING POLISH

When applying polish, the base coat is applied first, followed by two coats of color and one or two applications of top coat. Roll the polish bottle in the palms of the hands to mix. Never shake polish. Shaking causes air bubbles to form, which can be transferred to the nail plate during application and cause marks in the finish. Apply all coats of polish in the following manner:

1. Remove the brush from the bottle and wipe one side on the bottleneck so that a bead of polish remains on the end of the brush.

2. Start in the center of the nail, position the brush $\frac{1}{16}$ inch away from the cuticle, and brush toward the free edge.

3. Using the same technique, do the left side of nail, then the right side. There should be enough polish on the brush to complete three strokes without having to dip it back into the bottle; however, the amount will need to be adjusted according to the size of the nail. The more strokes used, the more lines or lumps will show on the client's nail. Small areas missed with the first color coat can be covered with the second coat.

4. Apply two coats of colored polish using the same technique used for the base coat. Complete the first color coat on both hands before starting the second coat. Polish on the cuticle should be removed with a cotton-tipped orangewood stick saturated in polish remover.

5. Apply one or two coats of top coat to prevent chipping and to give nails a glossy look. The use of an instant nail dry spray is optional, but it is effective in preventing smudging and dulling.

CHAIR-SIDE MANICURE

In some barbershops, the manicurist performs the manicure at the barber's workstation. This procedure is called a *chair-side* or *booth manicure* and requires the manicurist to either balance the supply tray on their lap or to have a small table at hand. If manicures are to be performed chair-side, the styling chair should have a small, recessed hole at the end of the armrest to hold the finger bowl. The manicurist must then move around the client, depending on which hand is being manicured.

When performing a chair-side manicure, always be considerate of the barber's position during the haircutting and styling process. Try to anticipate the turn of the barber chair or a change in the client's position in order to prevent client discomfort and any interference with the barber's procedures.

Ⓟ A-1   **Pre-service Procedure** *pages 792–797*

Ⓟ A-2   **Post-service Procedure** *pages 798–799*

CLIENT CONSULTATION

Before performing a service on a client, take time to talk with that client. During the client consultation, discuss issues of general health, the health of nails and skin, and the client's lifestyle and needs. You will use your knowledge of skin, nails, and each type of nail service to help the client select the most appropriate service. If the client has a nail or skin disorder that prevents you from performing a service, refer that client to a physician and offer to perform a service as soon as the disorder has been treated. A good client consultation can make a difference between being a professional and just doing nails.

Finish the consultation with a determination of the desired shape and polish color of the nails. Consider the shape of the hands, the length of the fingers, the shape of the cuticles, and the type of work the client does. The five standard nail shapes are square, squoval, round, oval, and pointed (see **Table A-3**).

Most men prefer short nails. The square or round shapes can be accomplished on shorter nail lengths and usually look the most appropriate on male hands. Generally, tapering the nail ends to a point or oval shape should be reserved for use on female hands and nails.

Generally speaking, a woman's manicure is performed using the same steps as a man's manicure with the exception of Step 14 in Procedure A-4, which usually requires the application of a base coat, two coats of colored polish, and one or two coats of top coat.

Ⓟ **A-3A** Hand Massage Techniques *pages 800–801*

Ⓟ **A-3B** Arm Massage Techniques *pages 801–802*

Ⓟ **A-4** Men's Manicure *pages 803–806*

table A-3
BASIC NAIL SHAPES

Shape	Definition
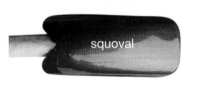	The **square nail** is completely straight across the free edge with no rounding at the outside edges.
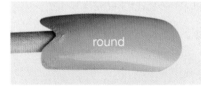	The **squoval nail** has a square free edge that is rounded off at the corner edges. If the nail extends only slightly past the fingertip, this shape will be sturdy because there is no square edge to break off, and any pressure on the tip will be reflected directly back to the nail plate, its strongest area. Clients who work with their hands—nurses, computer technicians, landscapers, or office workers—will need shorter, squoval nails.
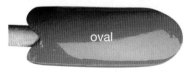	The **round nail** should be slightly tapered and usually should extend just a bit past the fingertip.
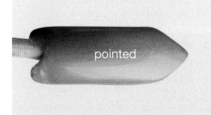	The **oval nail** is a conservative nail shape that is thought to be attractive on most women's hands. It is similar to a squoval nail with even more rounded corners. Professional clients who have their hands on display (e.g., businesspeople, teachers, or salespeople) may want longer oval nails.
	The **pointed nail** is suited to thin hands with long fingers and narrow nail beds. The nail is tapered and longer than usual to emphasize and enhance the slender appearance of the hand. Know, however, that this nail shape may be weaker, may break more easily, and is more difficult to maintain than other nail shapes. Rarely are natural nails successful with this nail shape, so they are usually enhancements. They are for fashion-conscious people who do not need the strongest, most durable shape of nail enhancements.

PRE-SERVICE PROCEDURE

MATERIALS, IMPLEMENTS, AND EQUIPMENT

- ☐ Buffing cream
- ☐ Cotton or pledgets
- ☐ Disinfecting container with disinfectant solution
- ☐ Disposable implements (abrasive file, wooden pusher, buffers)
- ☐ Finger bowl and brush
- ☐ Gloves
- ☐ Hand soap or sanitizer

- ☐ Linen or paper towels
- ☐ Manicure table and chairs
- ☐ Massage cream or lotion
- ☐ Metal implements (fingernail clippers, nippers, file, metal pusher)
- ☐ Metal trash receptacle with self-closing lid or small plastic bags and tape
- ☐ Polishes

PRE-SERVICE PROCEDURE

1. Apply gloves. Clean and disinfect reusable tools and implements and store in clean dry container until needed.
2. Clean and disinfect manicure table and drawer with an EPA-approved disinfectant.
3. Remove gloves and wash your hands.
4. Conduct client consultation.

PROCEDURES

A. CLEANING AND DISINFECTING

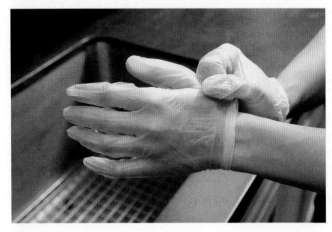

1. It is important to wear gloves while performing this pre-service procedure to prevent possible contamination of the implements by your hands and to protect your hands from the powerful chemicals in the disinfectant solution.

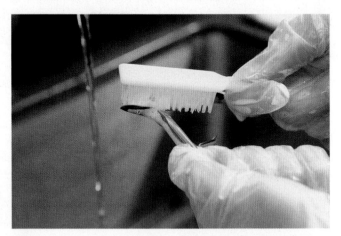

2. Rinse all implements with warm running water, and then thoroughly wash them with soap, a nail brush, and warm water. Brush grooved items, if necessary, and open hinged implements to scrub the area.

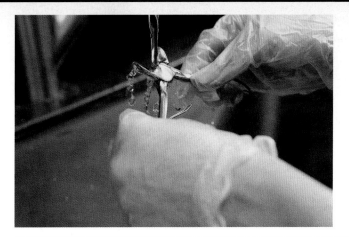

3 Rinse away all traces of soap with warm running water. The presence of soap in most disinfectants can cause the disinfectant to become inactive. Soap is most easily rinsed off in warm, but not hot, water. Dry implements thoroughly with a clean cloth towel or a disposable towel. Your implements are now properly cleaned and ready to be disinfected.

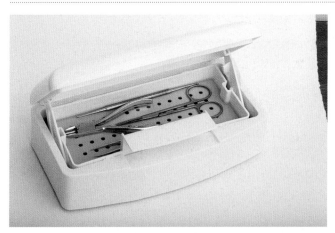

4 It is extremely important that your implements be cleaned before placing them in the disinfectant solution. Otherwise, your disinfectant may become contaminated. Before immersing the cleaned implements, bring any hinged implements to the open position. Immerse cleaned implements in a disinfection container holding an EPA-registered disinfectant for the required time (usually 10 minutes). Change the disinfectant solution daily or sooner if the disinfectant becomes visibly dirty during the course of the day. Avoid skin contact with all disinfectants by using tongs or by wearing disposable gloves.

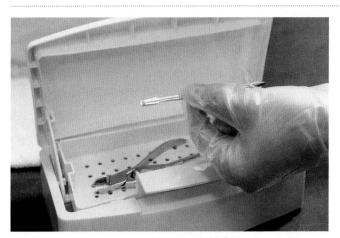

5 Remove implements, avoiding skin contact, and rinse and dry tools thoroughly.

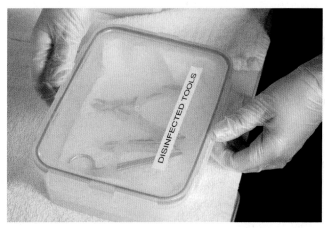

6 Store disinfected implements in a clean, dry container until needed.

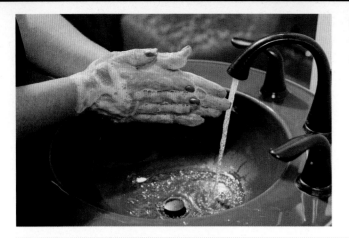

7 Remove gloves and thoroughly wash your hands with liquid soap. Rinse and dry with a clean fabric or disposable towel.

B. BASIC TABLE SETUP

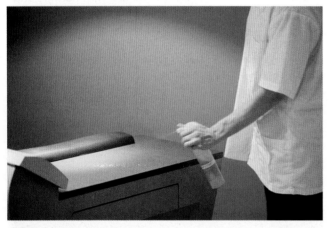

8 Following the directions on the product label, clean and then disinfect the manicure table and drawer with an EPA-approved disinfectant.

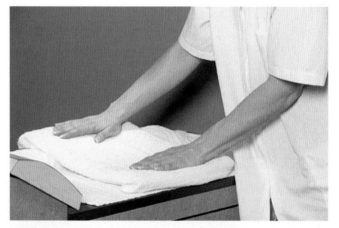

9 Wrap your client's arm cushion, if you are using one, with a clean cloth or disposable towel. Place the cushion in the middle of the table so that one end of the towel extends toward the client and the other end extends toward you.

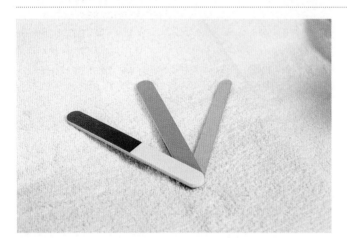

10 Place the abrasives and buffers of your choice on the table to your right (or to the left if you are left-handed). Many technicians wrap them neatly in a towel to ward off dust and potential contaminants.

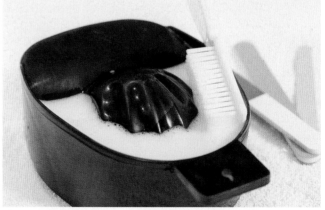

11 Place the finger bowl filled with warm water and the manicure brush in the middle of the table. The finger bowl should not be moved from one side to the other of the manicure table. It should stay in place for the duration of your manicure.

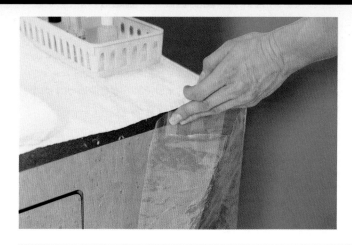

12 Tape or clip a plastic bag that can be closed securely to the side of the table if a metal trash receptacle with a self-closing lid is not available. This is used for depositing used materials during your manicure. These bags must be sealed and thrown away after each client to prevent product vapors from escaping into the shop air.

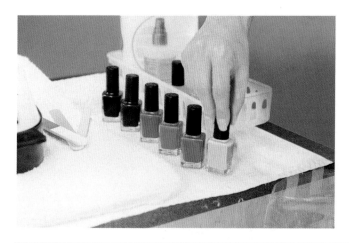

13 Place polishes to the right if you are right-handed and to the left if you are left-handed.

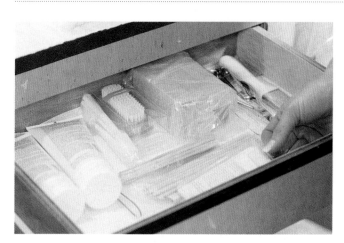

14 The drawer can be used to store the following items in clean, covered containers for immediate use: extra cotton or cotton balls, abrasives, buffers, nail polish dryer, and other supplies. Never place used materials in your drawer. Only completely cleaned and disinfected implements in a clean, covered container (to protect them from dust and recontamination) are stored in the drawer; extra materials or professional products are also placed in a clean, covered container in the drawer. Your drawer should always be organized and clean.

C. GREET THE CLIENT

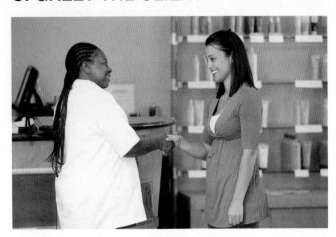

15 Greet your client with a smile, introduce yourself if you have never met, and shake hands. If the client is new, ask for the consultation card or sheet they filled out in the reception area.

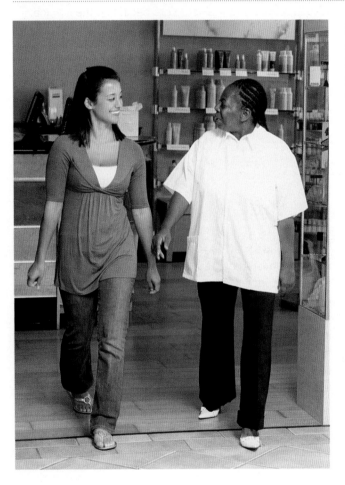

16 Escort your client to the hand-washing area and demonstrate the hand-washing procedure on your own hands. Once you have completed the demonstration, hand your client a fresh nail brush to use and ask them to wash their hands.

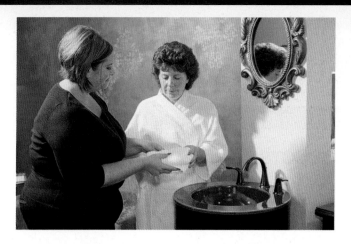

17 Hand your client a fresh towel for drying their hands. Be sure that your towels are clean and are not worn. A dirty towel can cause a client to not come back or to report the shop to the state board.

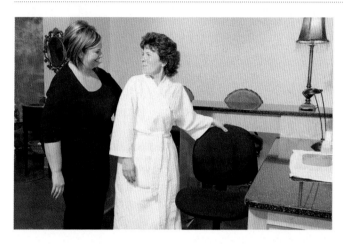

18 Show your client to your manicure table and make sure they are comfortable before beginning the service.

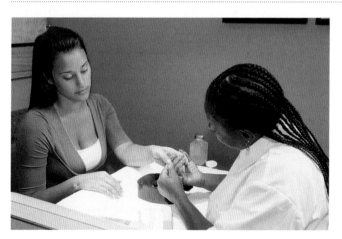

19 Discuss the information on the consultation card and determine a course of action for the service.

POST-SERVICE PROCEDURE

PROCEDURES

A. ADVISE CLIENTS AND PROMOTE PRODUCTS

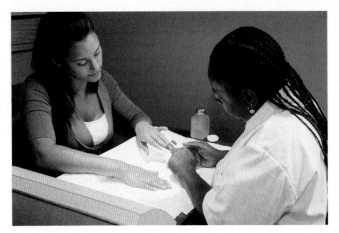

1 Proper home maintenance will ensure that the client's nails look beautiful until your client returns for another service (polish should last 7 to 10 days).

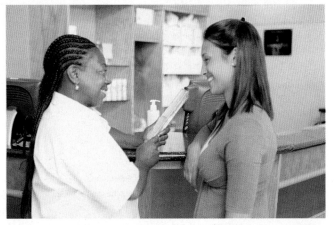

2 Depending on the service provided and the condition of your client's hands, there may be a number of retail products that you should recommend for the client to take home. This is the time to do so. Explain why they are important and how to use them.

B. SCHEDULE THE NEXT APPOINTMENT AND THANK THE CLIENT

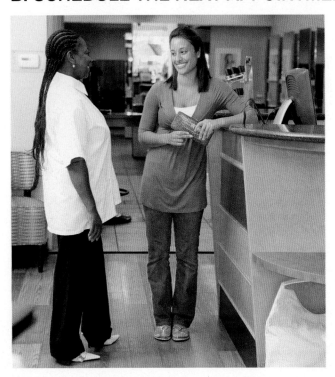

3 Escort the client to the front desk to schedule the next appointment and pay for the service. Set up the date, time, and services. Write the information on your or the shop's appointment card and give it to the client.

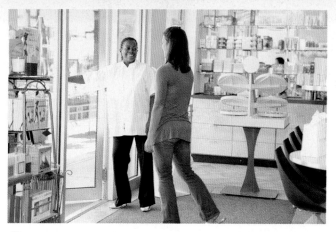

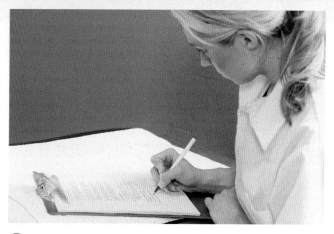

④ Before the client leaves the shop, thank them for their business and mention that you will be looking forward to their next visit.

⑤ Record service information, products used, observations, and retail recommendations on the client service form or computer record.

C. PREPARE THE WORK AREA AND IMPLEMENTS FOR THE NEXT CLIENT

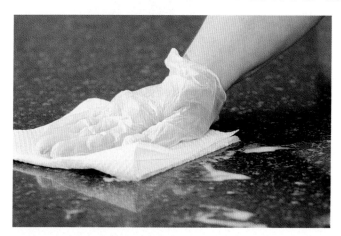

⑥ Remove your products and tools, dispose of all used materials, and then clean and disinfect your work area.

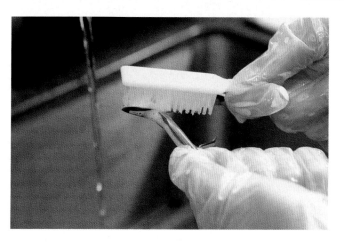

⑦ Follow the steps for disinfecting implements in the Pre-service Procedure.

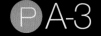

HAND MASSAGE

PROCEDURES

A. HAND MASSAGE TECHNIQUES

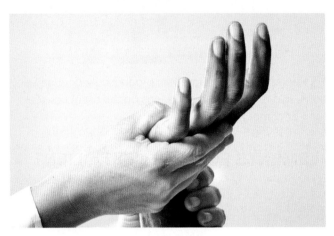

1 *Relaxation movement:* This is a form of massage known as *joint movement*. Apply hand lotion or cream. Place the client's elbow on a cushion. With one hand, brace the client's arm. With the other hand, hold the client's wrist and bend it back and forth slowly 5 to 10 times or until you feel the client has relaxed.

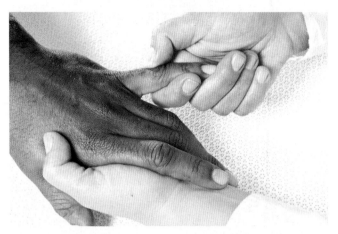

2 *Joint movement on fingers:* Lower the client's arm, bracing the right hand so you can start the massage on the little finger. Hold the finger at the base of the nail and gently rotate to form circles. Work toward the thumb, three to five times on each finger.

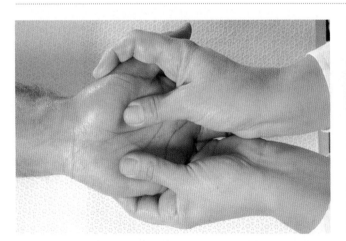

3 *Circular movement in palm:* Use the effleurage manipulation. Place the client's elbow on the cushion and, with your thumbs in the client's palm, rotate in a circular movement in opposite directions.

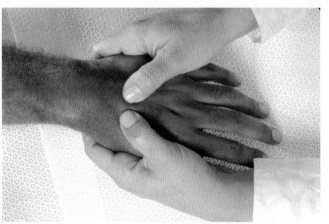

4 *Circular movement on wrist:* Hold the client's hand between your hands, placing your thumbs on top and your fingers below the client's hand. Move the thumbs in a circular motion in opposite directions, from the client's wrist to his knuckles. Move up and down three to five times. At the last rotation, wring the client's wrist by bracing your hands around the wrist and gently twisting in opposite directions.

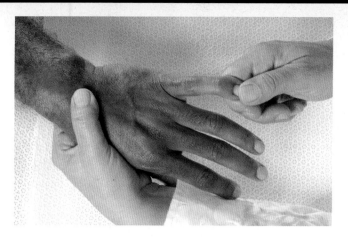

5 *Circular movement on back of the hand and fingers:* Rotate down the back of the client's hand using the thumbs. Rotate down the little finger and the client's thumb, and gently squeeze off at the tips of the client's fingers. Go back and rotate down the ring finger and index finger, gently squeezing off. Now do the middle finger and squeeze off at the tip. This tapering to the fingertips helps blood flow.

B. ARM MASSAGE TECHNIQUES

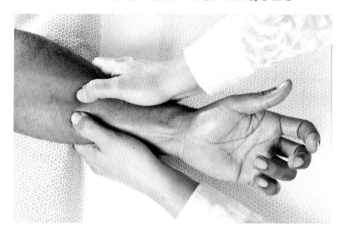

6 Warm cream or lotion in your hands, apply to the client's arm and work it in. Work from the client's wrist toward the elbow, except on the last movement, when work should be from the elbow to the wrist. Finally, squeeze off at the fingertips, as at the end of a hand massage. Apply more cream if necessary.

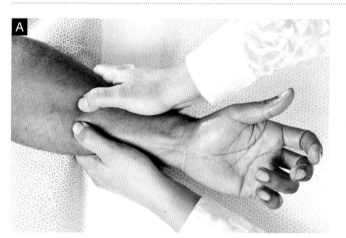

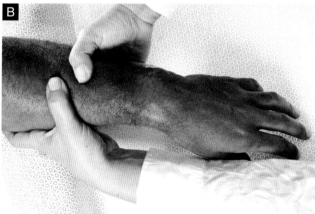

7 *Effleurage on arms:* Put the client's arm on the table, bracing the arm with your hands. Hold the client's hand palm up in your hand. Your fingers should be under the client's hand, your thumbs side by side in the client's palm. Rotate your thumbs in opposite directions, starting at the client's wrist and working toward the elbow. When you reach the elbow, slide your hand down the client's arm to the wrist and rotate back up to the elbow three to five times. Turn the arm over and repeat three to five times on the top side of arm.

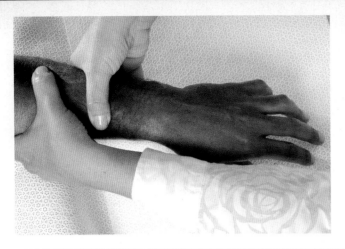

8 *Friction massage movement (wringing movement):* A friction massage involves deep rubbing of the muscles. Bend the client's elbow so the arm is horizontal in front of you, with the back of the hand facing up. Place your hands around the arm with your fingers facing in the same direction as the arm, and gently twist in opposite directions as you would wring out a washcloth, from wrist to elbow. Repeat up and down the forearm three to five times.

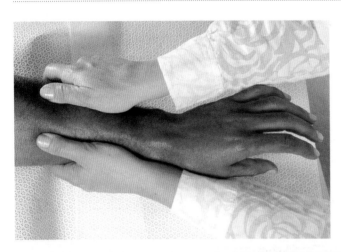

9 *Kneading movement on the arm:* Place your thumbs on the top side of the client's arm so they are horizontal. Move them in opposite directions, from wrist to elbow and back down to wrist. This squeezing motion moves the flesh over the bone and stimulates the arm tissue. Do this three to five times.

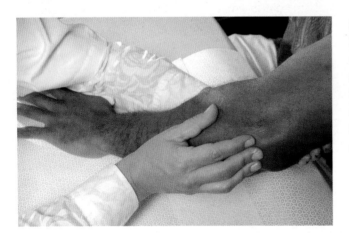

10 *Rotation of the elbow, friction massage movement:* Brace the client's arm with your left hand and apply cream to the elbow. Cup the elbow with your right hand and rotate your hand over the client's elbow. Repeat three to five times. To finish the elbow massage, move your left arm to the top of the client's forearm. Gently slide both hands down the forearm from the elbow to the fingertips as if climbing down a rope. Repeat three to five times.

MEN'S MANICURE

Manicure procedures are basically the same for men and women. Table setup is the same, except that colored polish is not typically used on men. Some men like a clear liquid polish, while others prefer a dry or buffed finish. Using hand cream or lotion is optional and depends on the client's preference. The following is one method of performing a men's manicure.

MATERIALS, IMPLEMENTS, AND EQUIPMENT

☐ Buffing cream

☐ Clear polish

☐ Cotton or pledgets

☐ Disinfection container with disinfectant solution

☐ Disposable implements (abrasive file, wooden pusher, buffers)

☐ Finger bowl and brush

☐ Gloves (if required by regulations)

☐ Hand soap or sanitizer

☐ Linen or paper towels

☐ Manicure table and chairs

☐ Massage cream or lotion

☐ Metal implements (fingernail clippers, nippers, file, metal pusher)

☐ Metal trash receptacle or plastic bags and tape

PREPARATION

1 Perform pre-service and table setup procedures.

2 Greet the client.

3 Wash your hands. Have the client wash his hands or apply a hand sanitizer. Thoroughly dry hands and nails with a sanitized towel. Apply gloves if required.

4 Perform consultation and discuss service options with the client.

5 Begin working with client's left hand so you can work from right to left.

PROCEDURE

1 Remove clear polish if applicable. Begin with the little finger of the left hand, using cotton saturated with polish remover. Repeat on the right hand.

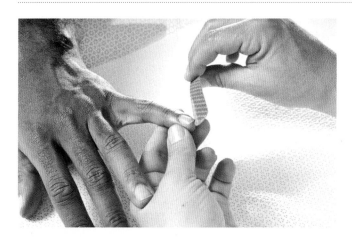

2 Shape the nails. Most men keep their nails fairly short; if the nails are long, shorten them with fingernail clippers before filing. File from the corners to center in one direction; do not saw back and forth.

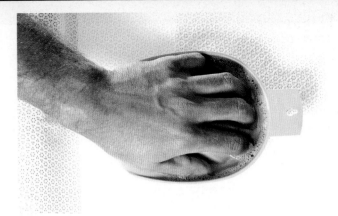

③ Soften the cuticles. After filing the nails of the left hand, soak them in a soap bath while filing the second hand.

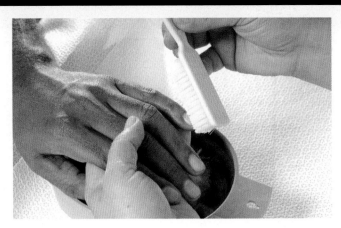

④ Clean the nails. Use a nail brush to clean fingertips and nails and to remove surface debris from nails. Remove the left hand from the soap bath while placing the right hand into the bath, and brush the fingers with downward strokes, starting at the first knuckle and brushing in one direction toward the free edge.

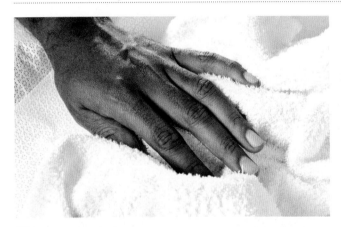

⑤ Dry the hand. Use the end of a clean towel, making sure to dry between the fingers. As you dry, gently push back the eponychium with the towel.

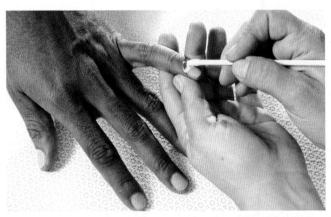

⑥ Apply cuticle remover. Use a cotton-tipped wooden pusher to apply cuticle remover to each nail on the left hand. Put client's left hand back into the bath while repeating cleansing steps on the right hand. Apply cuticle remover to right hand, remove left hand from bath, and replace with right hand.

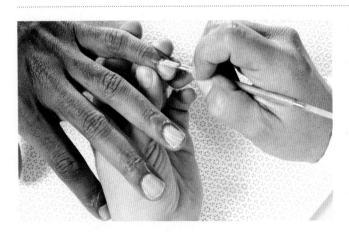

⑦ Loosen the cuticles. Use the spoon end of the pusher or a wooden pusher to gently push back and lift the cuticle off the nails of the left hand. Repeat on right hand.

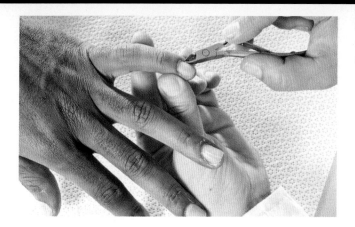

8 Use nippers, if allowed in your state, to remove any loosely hanging tags of dead skin only; do not cut living skin.

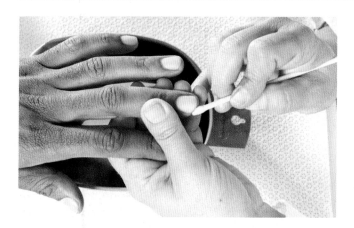

9 Clean under the free edge with a cotton-tipped wooden pusher while holding the left hand over the soap bath, and brush a last time to remove bits of cuticle and nail debris that remain on the nail. Rest the left hand on a clean towel and repeat this procedure on the right hand.

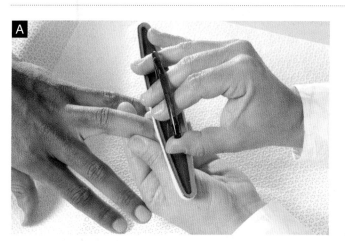

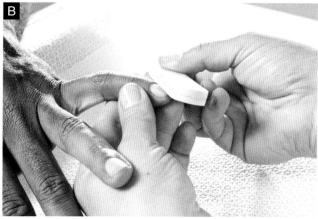

10 Apply buffing powder or cream and buff.

11 Apply cuticle oil. Use a cotton-tipped wooden pusher, a cotton swab, or an eyedropper to apply and massage oil into the nail plate and surrounding skin using a circular motion.

12 Bevel nails if necessary.

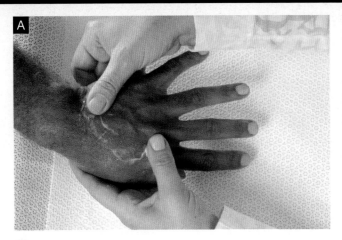

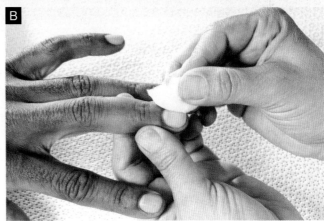

13 Apply hand lotion and massage the hands and wrists; wipe excess lotion off nails.

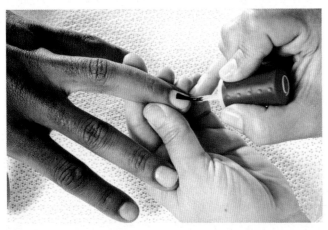

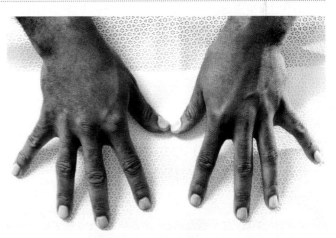

14 Polish the nails with a clear matte polish if desired or re-buff gently.

15 Complete post-service procedure.

POST-SERVICE PROCEDURE

1 Schedule another appointment with the client to maintain the manicure or to perform another service; complete client's record card.

2 Clean up work area. Disinfect table, tools, and implements. Take the time to restore the basic table setup.

3 Place all used materials in the plastic bag at the end of the table and discard into a closed trash can.

4 Wash your hands.

REVIEW QUESTIONS

1 Briefly describe each of the following parts of the nail: nail plate, nail bed, matrix, cuticle, eponychium, perionychium, hyponychium, specialized ligaments, and nail folds.

2 What is the average growth rate of a nail?

3 Name two common nail disorders that may be serviced by a manicurist or nail technician?

4 List the supplies needed to perform a *men's* manicure.

5 What are the five basic nail shapes?

6 Identify nail shapes that look appropriate on a man's hand.

7 Name five hand massage techniques and four arm massage techniques.

8 Briefly list the steps of a basic men's manicure procedure.

9 Explain the manner in which a chair-side manicure is performed.

CHAPTER GLOSSARY

bed epithelium (BED ep-ih-THEE-lee-um)	p. 782	thin layer of tissue between the nail plate and the nail bed
cuticle (KYOO-tih-kul)	p. 783	dead, colorless tissue attached to the nail plate around the base of the nail
discolored (dis-KUL-urd)	p. 784	a condition in which the nails turn a variety of colors such as yellow, blue, blue-gray, green, red, or purple; can be caused by poor blood circulation, a heart condition, topical or oral medications, or a systemic disorder
eponychium (ep-oh-NIK-ee-um)	p. 783	living skin at the base of the nail plate and covering the matrix area
free edge (FREE EJ)	p. 782	part of the nail plate that extends over the tip of the finger
hangnails (HANG-NAYLZ)	p. 784	condition in which the cuticle splits around the nail
hyponychium (hy-poh-NIK-ee-um)	p. 783	slightly thickened layer of skin between the fingertip and free edge of the nail plate
lunula (LOO-nuh-luh)	p. 783	half-moon shape at the base of the nail
matrix (MAY-triks)	p. 783	area where the nail is formed; produces cells that create the nail plate
nail (NAYL)	p. 782	an appendage of the skin; horny protective plate at the end of the finger or toe
nail bed (NAYL BED)	p. 782	portion of the skin on which the nail plate rests
nail folds (NAYL FOHLDZ)	p. 783	folds of normal skin around the nail plate
nail grooves (NAYL GROOVZ)	p. 783	slits or furrows on the sides of the nail
nail plate (NAYL PLAYT)	p. 782	horny plate resting on and attached to the nail bed
onyx (AHN-iks)	p. 782	technical term for nail
perionychium (payr-ee-uh-NIK-ee-um)	p. 783	the living skin bordering the root and sides of a nail
ridges (RIJ-ez)	p. 782	depressions running vertically down the length of the nail
specialized ligaments	p. 783	bands of fibrous tissue that attach the nail bed and matrix to the underlying bone that are located at the base of the matrix and around the edges of the nail bed

E